ROUTLEDGE LIBRARY EDITIONS:
EDUCATION AND GENDER

Volume 5

MIXED OR SINGLE-SEX SCHOOL?

MIXED OR SINGLE-SEX SCHOOL?

Volume II
Some social aspects

R. R. DALE

Routledge
Taylor & Francis Group
LONDON AND NEW YORK

First published in 1971 by Routledge & Kegan Paul Ltd

This edition first published in 2017
by Routledge
2 Park Square, Milton Park, Abingdon, Oxon OX14 4RN

and by Routledge
711 Third Avenue, New York, NY 10017

Routledge is an imprint of the Taylor & Francis Group, an informa business

British Library Cataloguing in Publication Data
A catalogue record for this book is available from the British Library

ISBN: 978-1-138-73736-5 (Set)
ISBN: 978-1-315-18103-5 (Set) (ebk)
ISBN: 978-1-138-04251-3 (Volume 5) (hbk)
ISBN: 978-1-138-04253-7 (Volume 5) (pbk)
ISBN: 978-1-315-17361-0 (Volume 5) (ebk)

Publisher's Note
The publisher has gone to great lengths to ensure the quality of this reprint but points out that some imperfections in the original copies may be apparent.

Disclaimer
The publisher has made every effort to trace copyright holders and would welcome correspondence from those they have been unable to trace.

Mixed or single-sex school?

Volume II

Some social aspects

R. R. Dale

Reader in Education, University of Wales, Swansea

London Routledge & Kegan Paul
New York Humanities Press

First published in 1971
by Routledge & Kegan Paul Ltd
Broadway House,
68–74 Carter Lane,
London EC4V 5EL
Printed in Great Britain by
Butler & Tanner Ltd,
Frome and London

ISBN 0 7100 7024 1

Contents

Tables

Appendix Tables

Figures

Introduction

This volume concludes the presentation of those research results which compare co-educational and single-sex secondary schools in their influence on the social and emotional development of pupils and which examine various attitudes of pupils to these schools. Necessarily teachers play their part and are reflected in the results, but the focus is on the pupils and ex-pupils. It was expected that the present material would make two moderately-sized volumes, but it has proved possible to publish it in a single large one. A third, last volume is projected on the influence of the two types of schooling on academic attainment, and a concluding section of this will present a miscellany of papers relating to co-education containing material which is outside the scope of the previous books.

During the twenty-four years since the first of these researches was commenced there has been in the world a gradually increasing momentum in the trend towards co-education in secondary schools.[1] In the early years of the work a high-ranking delegation of Russian educationists visited the University College of Swansea, enquiring among other things about co-education. The writer's guarded reply that up to then the results of his research were in favour of co-education though it was too early for a definitive pronouncement, may or may not have influenced their decision, but soon after the delegation's return to Moscow it was announced that the Russian educational system was reverting to co-education! Step by step, as a result of several enquiries among their teachers and pupils, more and more of the Swedish secondary schools have, since the 1920s, become co-educational. Soon after the Second World War Japan changed over to this system and in France the experimental 'classes nouvelles' set up in the 1950s tended to be concentrated in co-educational *lycées*. The interest shown in the subject in Italy has prompted an Italian publishing firm to ask permission to translate the first volume of this work into Italian, and even the

[1] This short sketch is not intended to be a history of co-education. Readers who are interested in this aspect should consult W. A. C. Stewart, *The Educational Innovators* (2 vols, London, 1967–8), or B. A. Howard, *The Mixed School*, (1928) (to 1926 only).

Roman Catholic Church, for long a bastion of the single-sex school, now takes a distinctly less rigid attitude.

The State schools of the United States have from the first been for boys and girls together, and, much nearer home, the Scottish schools are traditionally co-educational. In Wales under the Intermediate Act of 1889 many schools had to be built for the two sexes together because of the sparseness of the population, and the same policy was applied in the rural parts of England after the Balfour Act of 1902. Because of the prestige of the best independent boarding and the direct grant schools (lumped together incongruously and somewhat illogically as the 'public schools'—but all then single-sex), some of these co-educational municipal grammar schools were split into two single-sex ones where the increase in population and demand for education made an additional school necessary. This tendency—it could hardly be called a policy—was mainly to be found between about 1925 and 1950, and was even given a little official support in the Hadow Report (1926) and the short-lived Pamphlet No. 1 'The Nation's Schools', issued by the Ministry of Education in 1945. During the last decade, however, the proportion of co-educational secondary (including grammar) schools has been increasing rapidly and in 1968 there were 3,345 mixed compared with 2,231 single-sex schools (Statistics of Education 1968). The grammar schools cannot be separated from the others because of the existence of comprehensive schools, but the trend is to be seen at its strongest in the latter, of which 576 are mixed and 169 single-sex. Recently this tide of change has even reached a few parts of the central stronghold of the single-sex tradition—the public schools.

Though this research has for many years produced results which were favourable to co-education it would be wrong to dismiss the work of the single-sex grammar schools as bad; on the contrary, there was much that was admirable and they established a fine tradition. The findings contained in the two volumes point towards co-education as a means of improving this service to the community. Co-education, however, is not an automatic indication of perfection, and its success will depend, like that of the single-sex schools, on the quality of the men and women serving in such schools.

As with the single-sex type, co-educational schools have their own special problems. Several of these are mentioned in the text, including the need for a reasonable balance between the number of men and women on the staff. A similar problem is occurring with the pupils of some areas in that there is a heavy preponderance of girls in the junior and middle school, arising from a policy of merging boys and girls in a common list in the 11-plus examination or perhaps in some other equivalent instrument of selection. If the examination or its equivalent is weighted too heavily on the verbal side (and if the arithmetic is dominated by the 'mechanical' kind to the virtual exclusion of problem arithmetic), then the girls may gain regularly each year appreciably more than their 50 per cent of places and thus outnumber the boys in the local co-educational school. This is bad for the school and unfair to the boys in so far as the better performance of the girls is probably due partly to their more advanced maturity—a lead which will gradually disappear in the grammar school—and partly to the nature of the examination. Moreover, as the pupils grow older in grammar school and university so the performance of the boys improves in relation to the girls'. In fact in mathematics and the physical sciences boys are soon well in the lead early in their grammar-school life. It might be said that this point should have been reserved for the next volume, in which attainment is to be the main theme, but it is presented here to avoid the delay that would ensue, and also because such an imbalance, if large and continuous, could have an adverse effect on the social life of the school and perhaps (in a more subtle way) on the emotional adjustment of the pupils.

A much more speculative thought is the possible effect of co-educational schooling in reducing the over-aggressive attitudes of the male in the international field. Under Stalin, a few years before the Second World War, the Russians changed from a largely co-educational system of schooling to one which was, where possible, single-sex, because they believed it easier to inculcate a militaristic spirit into their boys in this way. The Nazis also stressed single-sex education for similar reasons. In a world which may depend for its existence on the damping down of aggression this is a topic which is well worth research, however unlikely the theory may seem to some.

The preparation of this book and of the previous volume has been materially assisted at various times by the financial aid of the Department of Education and Science, and by a generous grant from the Leverhulme Trust which enabled the writer to have leave of absence from university teaching and administration for some eight months—including the 'long vacation'. Sincere thanks are extended to both these bodies. Similarly thanks are tendered to those local education authorities, heads, staffs and pupils of schools, principals, staffs and students of Colleges of Education who co-operated so whole-heartedly in the research in spite of their other heavy commitments, and to the members of the advisory committee who gave valuable advice at the start of the Schools project. There is a great debt to be acknowledged to three colleagues, Mr H. Rothera, Mr D. Sharp and Dr P. Miller, who put aside important work of their own in order to give the writer the benefit of their advice on the manuscript.

Finally, thanks are due to my successive research assistants Miss J. MacDonald and Mr G. Lyons for their hard work in the preparation and administration of tests and classification of data; to Dr Patrick Miller for his able assistance with statistics and to Mrs M. Viner for her willing and skilled help in computer programming. Special thanks are due to my secretary, Mrs R. M. Lewis, for her considerable contribution to the preparation of both volumes; her very efficient secretarial work and the insight and accuracy with which she carried out innumerable statistical tests kept the research moving steadily along even when the writer's other duties would otherwise have brought it to a halt.

Earlier versions of Chapters 2, 3, 4, 17 and 18 have appeared in the *British Journal of Educational Psychology* and parts of Chapter 16 in *Occupational Psychology*.

I

The investigations

The research on which this volume is based is derived from those enquiries which were described fully in Chapter 1 of the first volume of the series.[1] The present chapter repeats in a shortened version the account of the procedures and samples in order to make this book independent of the earlier volume, but some changes are made to bring the chapter more into relevance with the new material. However, those readers who do not wish to bother with these details are urged to turn at once to Chapter 2, where the account of the results begins.

This book examines the attitudes of pupils and ex-pupils towards their lives in co-educational or single-sex secondary schools, including their attitudes towards their fellow-pupils. The most important part of the research is probably that which assesses the reactions to school life of those pupils who had experience in both single-sex and co-educational schools. There is an exploration over a wide field of attitudes, rather than a study of one attitude in depth, a choice deliberately made because it seemed appropriate to a survey of unknown territory. The size of the field dictated the technique of research. Attitude scales, in which a large number of questions are asked on a single attitude, were considered inappropriate because of the number of attitudes investigated. This seemed to call for a questionnaire approach, but some of the virtues of the attitude scale were added by making each question in itself a miniature scale. For example, ex-pupils were asked, 'Was your life in school Very happy/Happy/Jogging along/Rather unhappy/Very unhappy?' and they could choose their answer from any one of these points of a linear scale. Throughout the book these judgments are called estimates. An important addition was that the principal questions were usually followed by a few blank lines on which respondents were invited to state reasons for their answer. These are termed the comments or free responses. They proved to be a rich source of additional information, though time-consuming

[1] Dale, R. R., *Mixed or single-sex school?* Vol. I, Routledge & Kegan Paul, 1969.

in analysis. They deepened the understanding of the estimates made, gave an excellent idea of the reliability and seriousness of the answers and also enabled the respondents to protest against any ambiguity or looseness in the question and to qualify their estimates. The evidence derived from these comments, and also from the estimates, in spite of its limitations, has implications for education which reach far beyond the comparison of co-educational and single-sex schools.

The request for these comments or free responses was a technique common to most of the surveys, and the method by which quotations were selected from them is described now to avoid repetition. For those items regarded as the most important the number of replies selected from each category of comment was kept in proportion to the total for that category, except where this would have produced such a small number of comments that they would have been inadequate to illustrate the argument. The co-educational and single-sex samples were always treated alike unless this procedure gave inadequate illustration to the arguments for single-sex schools. Sometimes, however, selection of comments in proportion to the total was considered unnecessary, the classified Tables themselves having set out the proportions of responses in the various sections and whether they were favourable to co-education or not. The responses were then chosen because of their interest, their humour or their contribution towards an insight into the minds of the pupils. Whatever the procedure is, this is clearly stated to avoid giving a wrong impression. A method considered and rejected was selection of the responses randomly; this would have been more scientific but it would have produced a much less interesting book and almost certainly a less useful one.

Not all the survey procedures are described fully in the following section; those which are of a minor character are given as they arise in the text, and one which affects only one chapter is given in that place. The others are outlined here to avoid the repetition that might have been necessary where the findings of an enquiry are scattered through many chapters. The investigations are divided into those concerning ex-pupils and those concerning pupils, but when they examine the same topic, which is quite frequently, the results are assessed together in the same chapter.

The ex-pupils

The three surveys which come under this heading used as subjects students who were training to be teachers. Before describing each of them in detail it is convenient to mention some important aspects of the samples which are common to all three enquiries.[1]

The use of student-teachers has both advantages and disadvantages. The subjects are adult, interested in education, responsible and have a wider experience of schools than have other ex-pupils of similar age. The use of the same type of persons as representatives of both co-educational and single-sex schools also helps to put the two kinds of school on an equal footing. A further safeguard is that one of the surveys consisted only of ex-pupils who had attended both a co-educational and a single-sex grammar (or technical) school. On the other hand certain disadvantages are present. The student-teachers cannot be said with certainty to represent all types of grammar school ex-pupils, though the differences in attitudes between the co-educated and single-sex educated ex-pupils of the research samples are so marked as to make it seem unlikely that these would disappear or even be reversed if the attitudes of the remainder of the ex-pupils were ascertained. If the student-teacher ex-pupils consider prefects in single-sex schools to be much more officious than those in co-educational schools, it seems highly improbable that the other ex-pupils would find no such difference. Some of these results also receive support from a small-scale investigation among sixth-formers, who are at least a wider cross-section of the ex-pupils than are the student-teachers.

In the previous volume it was shown that the high proportion of co-educational colleges in the Second College survey had no undue influence on the estimates, nor did the college courses in general (including teaching practice) *reverse* the preference of more than a negligible number of students for co-educational or single-sex schools. Though the theoretical preference of an appreciable number of ex-pupils for co-education was *strengthened* by their college experience, this influence is likely to have been much less when the ex-pupils were asked specific questions about their experience in the schools they attended; for example, 'Do you think the school's concern with the out-of-school conduct of the pupils was excessive?' This opinion receives some support from the estimates of those ex-pupils (rather more than half the men and slightly less than half the women) who said their college course had made 'no change' in their attitude. Yet one will await with some interest results obtained from entirely different samples.

We now turn to the description of the surveys. The questionnaires themselves, however, are given in *Appendix 1*.

[1] A more detailed discussion of the samples will be found in *Mixed or single-sex School.*' Vol. I, Chapter I.

(*i*) *The First College survey*

This was a first, exploratory survey, made to see whether there appeared to be a prima facie case for investigation. As it concerns only Chapter 11 it is described there.

(*ii*) *The Second College survey*

The Second College survey used a more detailed questionnaire than that of the First College survey, covering a number of the points at issue between the opposing schools of thought. It was sent to those colleges of education and university departments of education that were willing to co-operate, with the request that it should be administered to students in large groups. Sixteen colleges and five departments agreed, and although one college and one department failed to observe the group administration the return of forms was almost 100 per cent. The students were limited to those who had attended secondary grammar or technical or comprehensive schools ; if they had attended such schools for less than one year they were removed from the sample. Almost all had been day pupils and no separate analysis was made for boarders. In order to encourage students to write frankly and to minimize possible external pressure or undue influence, replies were made private and anonymous and directions about this were issued to the questionnaire administrators. Provision was made for those who had attended more than one school of either type. Questions were designed to make a first exploration into such aspects as happiness in school, the state of pupil–teacher relationships, type of school preferred, effect of school life on relations with the opposite sex, attitude to the opposite sex in general, marriage and parenthood, and, for minor reasons, attitude to games and (for women) domestic subjects. As exactly the same questions were asked about the co-educational and the single-sex school the possibility of bias in the questions was reduced. Students were asked to make judgments by means of a five-point scale, e.g. Very happy/Happy/Jogging along/Unhappy/Very unhappy. Requests were also made for free comments in relation to six of the more important questions. The percentage of ex-pupils who selected each value was calculated, and the distributions for co-educated and single-sex educated were compared by the Chi-square test.

For a representative part of the sample, data were secured on parental occupation. Almost 2,000 students participated, scattered throughout England and Wales, so the replies must express opinions about many hundreds of secondary schools (excluding secondary modern). Nine of the colleges were mixed, three were for men and three for women, the proportion of students from mixed colleges being twice those from single-sex colleges. There was no Roman Catholic college and such students are therefore under-represented. The percentage of College of Education students in the sample at 81.7 is only slightly smaller than the 85 per cent in the whole student-teacher population, taking as a basis the number of trainees entering each year.

The written replies again showed that the students had a highly responsible attitude to the investigation. The previous discussion about college samples applies to this inquiry, notably that the college course and experience would not be expected to create any appreciable bias which would influence the comparison between co-educational and single-sex schools, as most of the questions were on the life of the school the students had attended.

(*iii*) *The Third College* (*'Both schools'*) *survey* (*1965–6*)

The Second College survey suffered from the disadvantage that the great majority of respondents had attended only one type of grammar school. At the time this survey was made the number of students who had been pupils at both a co-educational and a single-sex grammar or technical school would probably have been too small to have formed a satisfactory sample, but the recent reorganization of secondary education has been increasing these numbers appreciably.[1]

As its name implies, this third ('Both schools') survey therefore consisted of an inquiry among ex-pupils who had attended both a mixed and a single-sex secondary school, excluding those from secondary modern schools because in that case other unwanted variables would have been brought into action, such as comparative prestige, equipment, building and staffing. The respondents were students in Colleges of Education, and are not therefore a representative sample of *all* ex-pupils of these schools. We wrote to 169 colleges and received offers of co-operation and completed forms from 71, distributed in random fashion all over England and Wales; of these, 5 were men's colleges (out of 10), 29 were women's colleges (out of 72) and 37 were mixed (out of 88). These figures show no heavy imbalance and for reasons already stated it was not considered necessary to persist until a similar proportion of each type of college was reached. There was, however, through no fault of our own, an under-representation of Catholic colleges (one men's and two women's out of two men's, eight

[1] Bilateral and comprehensive schools are included in the sample.

women's and one mixed), and the number of students from each of these colleges was also low (20 in all). This last fact may be due to Catholic families tending to be of lower social class and therefore obtaining a low percentage of grammar school places; another reason may be that Catholic families do not move about the country from one school to another as much as Protestant families. To put the matter into proper perspective, the addition of merely one R.C. women's college—and possibly the mixed for good measure—would correct the slight imbalance. Even if the missing R.C. students were to be appreciably different in their judgments compared with Protestant students (and the differences shown by the 20 in the sample are in fact heavily in favour of mixed schools), the impact of their small numbers on the average 'scores' of the 795 respondents (620 women and 175 men) would indeed be negligible. A corrective factor is that many Catholic students attend non-Catholic colleges.

Colleges were asked to administer the questionnaire (see *Appendix 1*) to the students in large groups under examination conditions, with emphasis on anonymity, privacy and the great importance of the work. To minimize undue influences in any direction the student was asked to place his completed form in an envelope and seal it before handing it in. Most of the colleges observed the request for group administration and returned all the forms completed. A few distributed the forms to individual students and found it administratively too difficult to ensure that each student obtained one and then to collect it when completed. With the many calls on the time of the staff this is understandable and thanks are certainly due for the high degree of co-operation obtained. The number of 'abstentions' is, however, not definitely known, but it would be so small as to have no material effect on the comparison of the two types of school, even if the nature of the replies had been different, and no reason can be given why they should differ. Any 'abstention' would be an abstention from both the mixed and the single-sex school statistics, because the student attended at least one of each.

It will be seen that the first part of the questionnaire (in *Appendix 1*) asks for judgments relating to the co-educational school attended, and the second makes, in most instances, identical requests about the single-sex school attended, the exceptions being questions and statements which were applicable only to a mixed school. If a student had attended two schools of the same type (as well as one of the other) his or her estimates for the two former schools were included, on the principle that the research was assessing schools rather than individuals and the more schools that were assessed the more reliable the results would be. Eighty-four of the 620 women and 27 of the 175 men had attended three schools. Of this sub-sample 45 women had attended two single-sex schools and 39 two co-educational schools, while the corresponding figures for the men were 15 and 12. There is no bias apparent in these figures but there exists the possibility that ex-pupils who had attended three schools might tend to have more severe personality difficulties and, e.g. have a greater incidence of delinquency, than those in the main sample, and that this might have a distorting effect on the results. Though such distortion was considered unlikely in view of (a) the relatively small numbers in the sub-sample, (b) the almost equal proportions who had attended either two single-sex or two co-educational schools, and (c) the usually large differences in opinion which were found in the main sample about the two types of school, the possibility was checked by analysing in detail the replies of the women's sub-sample to six of the principal questions. The analysis compared their replies about single-sex schools with those about co-educational schools, and then compared the results from this sub-sample with those from the main body. The chief feature which emerged from the exercise was the closeness of the verdict of the 'three schools' sub-sample and that of the 'two-schools' (i.e. main) sample, and the continuance in the former of the preference for co-educational schools which is such a feature of the parent sample.[1] If we take this statement as a background, we find in the 'three-schools' sample a *slightly* higher vote on the favourable side, e.g. atmosphere 'very pleasant', for both single-sex and co-educational schools, though the exclusion of the 'three-schools' ex-pupils would have resulted in no change in the findings. The same is true of another slight difference between the two samples—that the 'three schools' group produced more than its proper share of the 'unfavourable' votes, e.g. 'very difficult to make friends' (girls' schools), 'a little difficult to make friends' (co-educational schools), 'atmosphere rather unpleasant' (co-educational schools), 'rather unpleasant' and 'very unpleasant' (girls' schools); the same tendency continued for both girls' and co-educational schools in the replies about happiness—the sub-sample having a slightly greater proportion who were 'rather unhappy' or 'very unhappy'. The numbers involved at this unfavourable end of the scale are, however, so small and the effect is so similar for the two types of schools that the net result on the survey findings is negligible. A reasonable explanation of this trend at the unfavourable end might be as suggested at the outset—that the 'three schools' sample would be likely to contain a

[1] The results of the main and sub-samples were almost identical for the item on type of school preferred.

small proportion of pupils who had been compelled to change schools because of their own temperamental difficulties—a larger proportion than in the 'two schools' sample; but the relatively high vote of the 'three schools' sample at the positive end of the scale shows that these pupils with personality difficulties can be only few in number.

We now return to the description of the survey procedure. Examples of the items used are, 'Do you think that the school atmosphere was Very pleasant/Pleasant/Neutral/Rather unpleasant/Very unpleasant?'; 'The prefects were officious'; 'The presence of the opposite sex of pupil had a good influence'; and 'Which did you prefer, the mixed or single-sex school?' A number of the items were deliberately repeated from the Second College survey.

The students were requested, as with the previous questionnaires, to give judgments or estimates on a five- (sometimes seven-) point scale, such as Agree strongly/Agree/Doubtful/Disagree/Disagree strongly, and were frequently asked to comment. They usually gave reasons for their preferences and where necessary stated any reservations. This process brought to notice three faults that had escaped the pilot run, namely that three of the fifty-five questions contained ambiguities; these questions have been discarded. The nature of the free replies again showed a high degree of responsibility among the students.

The variables for which data were obtained were: Type and sex of secondary schools attended (even if more than two), length of attendance, order of schools attended, boarder or day pupil, occupation of parent, sex, age, length of stay at College of Education, and what type of college, and information on the situation of the school playing field. Schools were coded as either 'first' or 'last', those in the middle being classified as 'first' unless the pupil had a year in the sixth form.

The pupils

(*i*) *The Schools project* (*1964 and 1966*)

This research differed from those already described, by using pupils at school as subjects and by the administration of paper and pencil tests of personality as well as a questionnaire. Up to this point the surveys had dealt only with teachers and ex-pupils—apart from several minor inquiries—hence the project sought to assess the experience of the children in the schools. The ex-pupils had the advantage of being more mature and perhaps better able to make judgments and were removed from the immediate pressure of school loyalties, but for the pupils there was no time gap to affect the memory, or further experience (such as in Colleges of Education) to influence the judgment. On the other hand the ex-pupils of the 'Both schools' survey were better able to make their judgments as they had attended both a co-educational and a single-sex school.

The study was longitudinal, testing the same pupils twice, with two years in between the testings. Two regions—the West Riding and South Wales—were chosen by representatives of the department of Education and Science, subject to the local authorities' approval. The Welsh branch of the department and the West Riding Education Authority then selected the grammar schools, endeavouring to match each co-educational school with a boys' and a girls' school for social background. This produced 42 schools, in which objectively selected samples of pupils aged 11 plus and 15 plus were tested during September and October 1964, and again during 1966, in May in Wales, and in September in Yorkshire. The samples consisted of 20 boys and 20 girls of each age (i.e. 80 in all) from every co-educational school, 20 boys of each age from every boys' school and 20 girls of each age from every girls' school, making an initial total of 2,240. (Pupils were selected alphabetically.)

The tests included a questionnaire (see *Appendix 1*) rather similar in type to those used in the previous surveys, but repeating only the key items and endeavouring to obtain assessments in new areas such as pupil–pupil relationships, exploring whether the presence of the opposite sex had any influence on attitudes to school subjects and to schoolwork, comparative attitudes to the opposite sex, comparative prevalence of bullying, and comparative ease of social relations with the opposite sex, etc. Like the ex-pupils, the pupils were asked to make judgments based on a five-point scale, and were given the opportunity to make free responses, but this facility was much extended in the 1966 version of the questionnaire and important questions were added. Only those items which are relevant to the topics of this book are given in *Appendix 1*. Parts of the results of several paper and pencil tests of personality are also omitted from consideration as either irrelevant to the present theme or as not being of sufficient importance.

In the assessment of aspects of school life, about which pupils might either be sensitive or easily affected by open or subtle pressures and therefore fearful of going against accepted loyalties, good administration of tests is essential. To do their best to ensure this the researcher and his assistant travelled to each school in 1964 and 1966 to administer the tests in person, the researcher taking the boys and his assistant the girls. This was designed to ensure standardization of the testing of each sex, but unfortunately the woman assistant had to leave after a year and was succeeded by a man, thus breaking the standardization for the girls. Though this affected both co-educated and single-sex educated girls it could possibly have made it somewhat harder for the latter to admit to their troubles etc., when a man was present, though the presence of men on the staffs of all but one of the girls' schools might have diminished this effect. In the event the atmosphere during the testing was almost invariably excellent, as is shown by the seriousness of the written replies and the quite remarkable regularity of the patterns produced by the results.

One set of 1964 results includes all 42 schools, but the longitudinal survey of the same pupils over the two years, to which reference may occasionally be made, discards not only the leavers and absentees (from both 1964 and 1966 results), but also two sets of the 'tripled' schools. One set was in Yorkshire where the two single-sex schools of the triple became co-educational, causing the exclusion of the corresponding co-educational school; the other was in South Wales where a wrong administrative decision caused a comprehensive co-educational school to be substituted at very short notice because the school originally selected had an inadequate number of pupils of the right age. During the testing at this school several pupils had to be withdrawn from the sample because they could not read sufficiently well and others were obviously doubtful cases. A later examination of the I.Q. scores showed them to be much below the average of any other school, and as it was the only comprehensive school of the 42 it was omitted from the results, with the two single-sex schools tripled with it for social background. This exclusion was equitable on the objective criterion established at the outset—equality of social background, as the proportion of working-class pupils in the co-educational school was definitely greater than that in the relevant single-sex schools.

The study was originally designed as a pilot study, preparatory to the taking of a national sample of schools, and had consequent limitations imposed on it by restrictions of time and money—the sample of 14 schools of each type, ultimately reduced to 12, though useful, is none the less small. The tripling of them for social background helps to allay fears that the three samples might not be on reasonable terms of equality, but recourse must be had to the general pattern of the results from all of the surveys for confirmation or otherwise. It would be foolish not to recognize that there are many different reasons why schools can be good or bad, and the chance inclusion of two or three very bad—or abnormally good—schools in one of the samples could seriously affect the results. The danger, however, was foreseen and can be taken into account in the final weighing up of evidence. What was not foreseen was that several heads, perhaps for administrative convenience, did not adhere sufficiently strictly to the administrative procedure for the selection of the sample, nor ensure that all selected pupils who were present in the school at the time of the more important second testing took the test. Though these faults would be unlikely to have a large effect, especially in a longitudinal research, they gave rise to some uneasiness. Lest this should be misunderstood the writer pays tribute to all the heads for their warm welcome and their forbearance about the upset to school routine.

As the occupational class distribution of the parents of the pupils has a bearing on the results presented in a number of chapters, it is given here. The schools were matched in triples for social background, but this did not quite result in equality of the samples; as shown in Table 1.1 the single-sex schools had a slightly higher occupational class entry in the full 1964 sample. The co-educated girls of the full schools project sample had also a slightly lower intelligence score than the girls from girls' schools (Table 1.2); the average scores of the opposing boys' groups were equal at age 15; the boys from boys' schools had a slight superiority at age 11. In the longitudinal samples the girls in girls' schools retained their lead, but the average scores of the boys from boys' schools and those from co-educational schools were virtually the same.

TABLE 1.1 *Occupational class composition of the schools sample (1964)*[1]

	Occupational class of pupils' parents											
	1		2		3		4		5		Totals*	
	N	%	N	%	N	%	N	%	N	%	N	%
Girls												
Co-ed. schools	81	14·5	152	27·1	230	41·1	74	13·2	19	3·4	560	100
Girls' schools	90	16·1	143	25·5	241	43·0	56	10·0	25	4·5	560	100
Boys												
Co-ed. schools	70	12·5	130	23·2	274	49·0	55	9·8	27	4·8	560	100
Boys' schools	74	13·2	164	29·3	249	44·5	47	8·4	20	3·6	560	100

* Includes a few unclassifiable. The analysis is based on occupations and follows the classification used in the Early Leaving Report, viz: class 1 Professional, managerial, executive; class 2 Clerical occupations; class 3 Skilled occupations; class 4 Partly skilled; class 5 Unskilled.

[1] The occupational class distribution of the longitudinal sample is in Table A.1. (i.e. Table 1 in *Appendix 2*).

TABLE 1.2 *Average intelligence scores of the schools sample (1964)**
(H.S.P.Q. 'B' factor, maximum 10)

	Co-educational schools	Single-sex schools
Boys—11+	7·09	7·18
15+	7·91	7·90
Girls—11+	6·98	7·29
15+	7·87	8·12

* There are 280 in each of the eight groups. The difference between the co-educated girls and those from girls' schools is statistically significant both at 11 plus and 15 plus.

The scores of the longitudinal samples are in Table A.2. There the differences between the girls' groups are in the same direction but only that at age 13 plus is statistically significant.

(ii) The 'Check' questionnaire (1966)

As some of the early results showed smaller differences between the two girls' groups than those expected from previous work a supplementary investigation was carried out amongst all girls of one relevant age group (i.e. those who were 13 plus in 1966) who had not been included in the original samples. This was partly to test the validity of the project samples from each school. A fifteen-minute questionnaire containing the more important questions and a few additional ones was administered to large groups in each girls' school by a research assistant and in the co-educational schools by the writer. This is given with the other questionnaires in *Appendix 1*. In all there were 1,122 girls from 24 schools, and they provide an additional large sample against which to compare the results from the original inquiry. The occupational class composition of the 'Check' sample was as follows:

TABLE 1.3 *Occupational class composition of the 'Check' sample*

	Occupational class of pupils' parents										
	1		2		3		4		5		
	N	%	N	%	N	%	N	%	N	%	Totals*
Girls in co-ed. schools	88	19·6	95	21·2	184	41·0	51	11·4	22	4·9	449(100)
Girls in girls' schools	149	22·1	152	22·6	289	42·9	54	8·0	23	3·4	673(100)

* Includes 15 unclassifiable.
NOTE: One of the girls' schools of the project had become co-educational and had to be excluded, together with its 'matched' co-educational school.

The data in Table 1.3 show again that in spite of the tripling of schools for social background there remains a small but definite occupational class advantage to the girls' schools. Though this is too small to have more than a slight effect on the results, various analyses of the data according to the occupational class of the fathers of the respondents show that the direction of this effect will be, if anything, in favour of the single-sex schools.

Various other smaller inquiries provided useful supporting evidence but are not sufficiently important for their procedure to be given here. We now move on to the results, which commence with those appertaining to the happiness or unhappiness of pupils and the pleasantness or otherwise of the school atmosphere. The statistical test used to assess the statistical reliability of the differences found in this and succeeding chapters is always Chi-square unless otherwise stated.

2

Happiness in school: (a) the estimates

We have all heard of 'The whining schoolboy, . . . creeping like snail Unwillingly to school', but we like to think that such creatures are scarcer now than they were in those far-off days when the lines were written. Our memories of schooldays are strong; most of us would agree with Byron:

> 'The schoolboy spot
> We ne'er forget, though there we are forgot,'

and we would dearly wish our children's schooldays to be happy. What forces, then, act upon a child to make him happy, or unhappy, at school? We have little precise knowledge about this, but we can make a number of shrewd guesses—and perhaps a few doubtful ones. This chapter doesn't attempt to unravel the complexity of the situation, but merely presents the estimates of several large samples of pupils and ex-pupils about the degree of their happiness in co-educational and single-sex grammar schools. Chapter 3 will enlarge the picture by examining the reasons given in the free responses for these estimates of pupil happiness. First in chronological order, comes the Second College survey.

The Second College survey

In the Second College survey some 2,000 student-teachers in Colleges of Education and University Departments of Education answered the question, 'Was your life in school, viewed as a whole, Very happy/Happy/Jogging along/Rather unhappy/Very unhappy?' They were asked to underline the answer which was true for them. The results are in Figure 2.1.

The most noticeable feature is that few of these ex-pupils (who would have been at least fairly successful in school work) were rather unhappy or worse. On inspection there is no practical or statistically significant difference between the proportion of these 'unhappy' individuals in mixed schools and that in single-sex

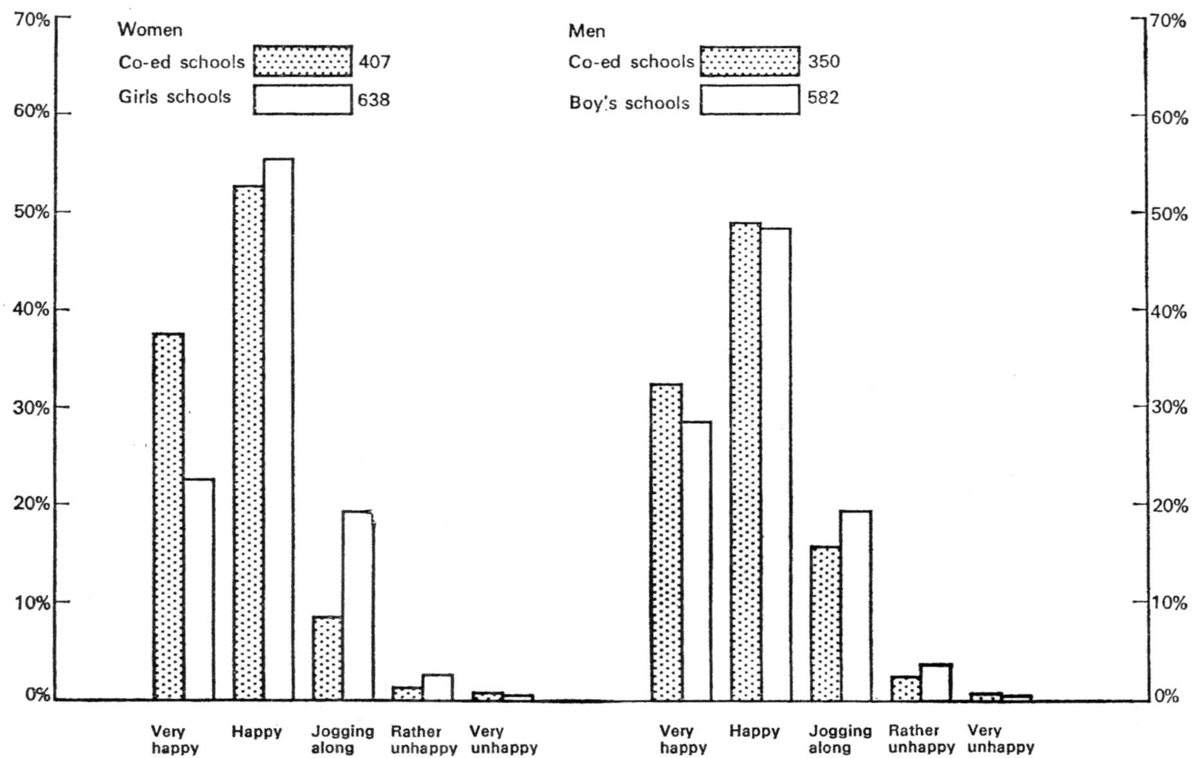

FIGURE 2.1 *Happiness in school: Second College survey*

schools. On the opposite side, however, there is a decided difference between the co-educated and single-sex educated women, the former being more positively happy when at school than the latter. This greater happiness is to be seen in the 15 per cent superiority in the 'very happy' section and in the 11 per cent fewer who admitted to have been only 'jogging along'.[1] The 3 per cent superiority of ex-pupils of girls' schools in the 'Happy' category redresses the balance only slightly. Though the trend for the men is

TABLE 2.1 *Happiness in school (female ex-pupils)—type of college*
Second College survey

Happiness estimate	Ex-pupils of co-educational schools				Ex-pupils of girls' schools			
	Mixed colleges		Women's colleges		Mixed colleges		Women's colleges	
	N	%	N	%	N	%	N	%
Very happy	89	37·4	49	38·9	93	20·5	30	25·4
Happy	128	53·8	64	50·8	250	55·2	69	58·5
Jogging along	16	6·7	13	10·3	95	21·0	18	15·2
Rather unhappy	4	1·7	0	0	15	3·3	1	0·9
Very unhappy	1	0·4	0	0	0	0	0	0
Totals	238	100	126	100	453	100	118	100

TABLE 2.2 *Happiness in school (male ex-pupils)—type of college*
Second College survey

Happiness estimate	Ex-pupils of co-educational schools				Ex-pupils of boys' schools			
	Mixed colleges		Men's colleges		Mixed colleges		Men's colleges	
	N	%	N	%	N	%	N	%
Very happy	35	24·6	44	38·9	56	23·7	58	29·4
Happy	74	52·2	54	47·8	120	50·8	97	49·2
Jogging along	29	20·4	12	10·6	49	20·8	34	17·3
Rather unhappy	3	2·1	3	2·7	11	4·7	8	4·1
Very unhappy	1	0·7	0	0	0	0	0	0
Totals	142	100	113	100	236	100	197	100

[1] The difference between the women's overall distributions for mixed and girls' schools is statistically highly significant (>·001).

the same as for the women, the difference between the two men's groups is not statistically significant.

The full discussion of these results is reserved until the end of the chapter, after comparable results from other surveys have been presented, but an important question arises which is best dealt with here. Did the two-to-one preponderance of students from mixed colleges of education help to produce the favourable results for co-education? The answer is given in Tables 2.1 and 2.2.

ANALYSIS BY TYPE OF COLLEGE

In these Tables there is certainly no evidence that the two-to-one ratio of students from mixed compared with single-sex colleges is biasing *this sample* in favour of co-education; curiously enough there is some trend in the opposite direction. The co-educated women who were in women's colleges rated themselves as slightly happier at school than did the co-educated women who were in mixed colleges, and the women educated at girls' schools who were in women's colleges also rated themselves as slightly happier at school than the similarly educated women who were in mixed colleges; as the latter difference is a little greater than the former the net result is a total women's sample which has a negligible built-in bias towards co-education, i.e. a virtual equality. On the other hand the co-educated men in mixed colleges gave estimates of happiness in school which were appreciably lower than the estimates of similar men in men's colleges, and while the men from boys' schools also gave lower estimates when they were in mixed rather than men's colleges, this difference was clearly smaller; the net result here is that the over-representation of mixed colleges resulted in a bias acting *against* co-education in the happiness estimate.

The 'Both Schools' survey

The large-scale survey previously described might be criticized because the students who were giving their estimates about happiness in school had usually experienced only one type of school and therefore could not validly compare the two under consideration. Another survey was therefore made, again with intending teachers because of the great difficulties of getting other representative—and co-operative—samples, but this time the students were those from Colleges of Education only, who had attended both a co-educational and single-sex grammar school; it was called the 'Both schools' survey. There were returns from 71 institutions representative of hundreds of schools (though public schools will probably be under-represented) and in the replies each student was able to compare his or her experience in one or more single-sex and mixed schools. The questions used were often the same as those used in the previous survey but there were many additions. Here we are concerned with the same question on happiness as that asked in the Second College survey.

FEMALE EX-PUPILS

The results for female ex-pupils are presented in Figure 2.2. The order in which the schools were attended was thought to be a variable of importance; the data are therefore divided in accordance with the theory into co-educational first and co-educational last, and the single-sex schools likewise.

The verdict of these students is clear-cut. If for women we combine first and last schools because, surprisingly, there is little difference between them, we find that well over half of the women said they were 'very happy' while co-educated, but only a quarter gave the same estimate for their girls' schools. At both types rather more than a third were 'fairly happy'. Six per cent gave a 'jogging along' estimate for their mixed school, but 20 per cent at their girls' school. Three times as many were unhappy at the girls' than at the mixed school (117 to 38).

MALE EX-PUPILS

The men were equally emphatic, as may be seen in Figure 2.3. If we combine first and last schools more than 9 out of every 10 of the men said they were happy at the mixed school—half of them 'very happy' and half 'fairly happy', but only a quarter of the total said they were 'very happy' in their boys' school and a third estimated 'fairly happy'. In the middle of the scale only 10 out of 186[1] said they were 'jogging along' when co-educated, but nearly 1 in 5 when they were in the boys' schools. At the bottom end, whereas 1 in 27 were unhappy in the mixed schools, this increased to almost a quarter in the boys' schools. A consideration of first and last schools separately shows that this is a variable which needs watching, the last schools receiving higher estimates for the happiness of boys than the first schools (the girls showing little change), but both sexes estimated that they were much happier at the co-educational schools.

[1] The number is greater than 175 because a few students had estimates for more than one school of the same type.

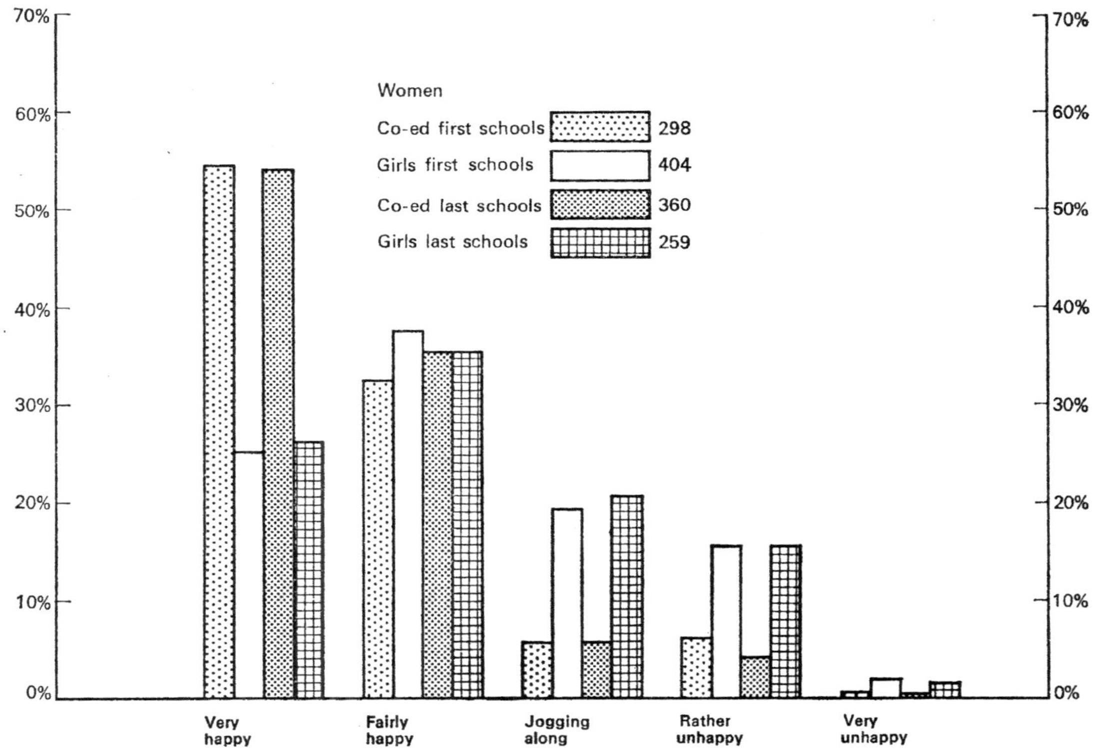

FIGURE 2.2
Happiness in school (women): 'Both schools' survey

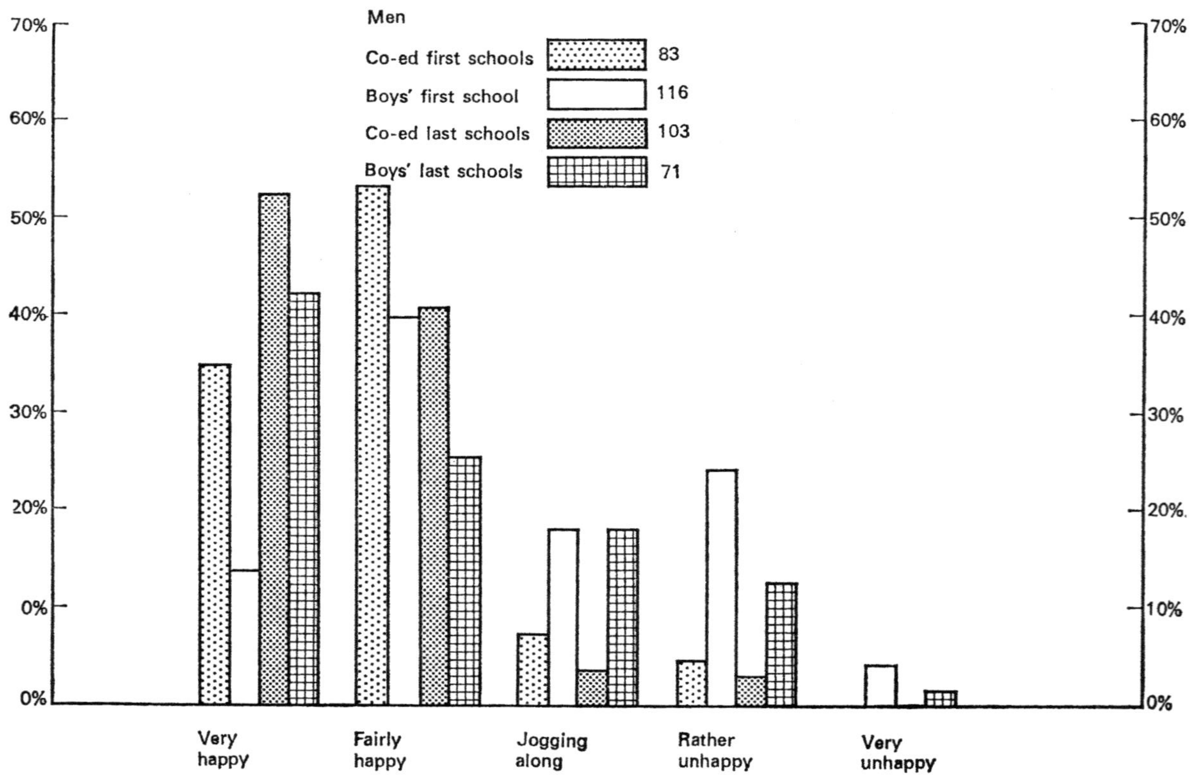

FIGURE 2.3
Happiness in school (men): 'Both schools' survey

Social class

In spite of these apparently decisive results it is possible that they could be produced by variables other than those which have so far been under consideration. One of these variables is the social class of the pupils; if one type of school were predominantly upper and the other type predominantly lower class this could produce a difference in the respective estimates of happiness in school. In order to avoid overweighting the text with Tables the full results have been placed in *Appendix 2*, Tables A.3 to A.4. Here it is merely recorded that *in this sample* there is no clear trend associating degrees of happiness with categories of parental occupational class for the female ex-pupils except some tendency for those from classes 3, 4 and 5 in co-educational schools attended last to be a little less happy than ex-pupils from the other occupational classes, manifested by interchange between 'very happy' and 'happy' rather than by any increase of neutral or negative estimates. Co-educated female pupils have a clear lead over those educated in girls' schools, in every class. No occupational class analysis was made of the male ex-pupils' estimates as the sub-divisions of the sample would have been too small.

Things are not always what they seem, and the lack of a clear association between parental occupational class and ex-pupil estimates of happiness at school might be due either to the tendency for these ex-pupils to be moving towards the same class, i.e. the teaching profession, or to the more highly selected nature of the working-class group.

Pleasant situation of school

Another variable which might affect the happiness estimates is the degree of pleasantness of the situation of the school. The respondents were asked, 'Do you agree or disagree with the following statement about your [co-educational/single-sex] school: "Pleasant situation of the school"?' Respondents could choose between, 'Agree strongly/Agree/Doubtful/Disagree/Disagree strongly', as in Table 2.3. The analysis is again limited to the women as their greater numbers give a more dependable result.

Table 2.3 shows that the co-educated women class their schools as slightly more pleasantly situated than do the women educated in girls' schools, but this difference is not statistically significant. It is certainly too small to have produced the large difference in happiness estimates between ex-pupils of co-educational and girls' schools, and may even have been caused by the greater happiness of the co-educated ex-pupils at school causing them to classify

TABLE 2.3 *Pleasantness of school position (women)*

'Both schools' survey

Estimates about pleasant situation of school	Replies about co-educational schools				Replies about girls' schools			
	First schools		Last schools		First schools		Last schools	
	N	%	N	%	N	%	N	%
Agree strongly	93	31·0	132	36·7	110	27·2	83	31·9
Agree	134	44·9	168	46·7	165	40·7	124	47·7
Doubtful	43	14·4	39	10·8	66	16·3	26	10·0
Disagree and disagree strongly	29	9·7	21	5·8	64	15·8	27	10·4
Totals	299	100	360	100	405	100	260	100

NOTE: The difference between co-educational and girls' schools is not statistically significant, both for first and last schools: Chi-square, however, is sufficiently high to make further analysis desirable.

the situation of their school buildings in a rather more favourable category. On the other hand there may be a real—though small—overall difference. To test for the possible effect of this the happiness scores were classified within the categories concerning the situation of the school, as in Table A.5 (*Appendix 2*) which also allows for social class, and in Table A.6 which dispenses with the social class breakdown after it had been proved to be unnecessary. A perusal of Tables A.5 and A.6 shows that whatever the category of pleasantness the co-educated pupils were the happier, and that this latter variable was much more powerful than 'pleasantness of situation'.

'Amalgamated' schools

The last variable to be examined is a relatively minor one, the existence of a small sub-sample of 'amalgamated' schools among the main sample of co-educational schools. In the first volume of this work these amalgamated schools were consistently shown to be given rather less favourable estimates than those given to the normal co-educational schools, where the boys and girls had grown up in school together. This finding has practical implications for present policy in comprehensive education, as some authorities are planning (or have already commenced) *single-sex* junior high schools and *co-educational* senior high schools, thus creating the problem of suddenly merging classes of adolescent boys with classes of adolescent girls. Whether this less favourable verdict extends to other aspects of social life will be one of the minor themes of this volume (see Chapter 20), and a beginning is made with the estimates for happiness in Table 2.4.

TABLE 2.4 *Happiness of ex-pupils (female): Amalgamated versus remaining 'co-educational last' schools*

Both schools' survey

Estimates of happiness in school	Replies from ex-pupils of amalgamated schools				Replies from ex-pupils of other 'co-educational last' schools			
	About their amalgamated schools		About their girls' schools		About their co-educational schools		About their girls' schools	
	N	%	N	%	N	%	N	%
Very happy	45	48·4	25	26·9	150	56·2	76	24·4
Fairly happy	38	40·9	45	48·4	89	33·3	108	34·8
Jogging along	7	7·5	12	12·9	14	5·2	66	21·2
Rather unhappy	2	2·1	11	11·8	13	4·9	52	16·7
Very unhappy	1	1·1	0	0	1	0·4	9	2·9
Totals	93	100	93	100	267	100	311	100

The data show that the women from amalgamated schools were rather less happy as pupils than were the rest of those who attended a co-educational school last, though the difference is not statistically significant; amusingly enough they were, perhaps by contrast, significantly happier in their girls' school than the rest of the 'girls' school first' sample.

The small sub-sample of men from amalgamated schools were also slightly less happy at school than those who were in normal co-educational schools, but as might be expected from such small numbers the difference was far from statistically significant.

The Schools project

The question on happiness set to the pupils of 42 grammar schools (original 1964 sample) was changed slightly from that set in previous inquiries, the first category of happiness being changed from 'very happy' to 'happy'. This was probably a mistake in judgment as it seemed to make the scale a less sensitive instrument for the samples on whom it was to be used, and might have been anticipated because a principal difference between the co-educated and single-sex educated groups in the surveys already described was in the appreciably higher proportion of the co-educated who endorsed 'very happy' as opposed to 'fairly happy', and some of this distinction between the two groups may have become blurred with the modification of the 'very happy' category to merely 'happy'.

The tables (A.7 to A.10) giving the results about school happiness in the schools project have been placed in *Appendix 2* as their data are so inconclusive, and there is so much other material to be presented. There are two principal ways of looking at the results, one being to regard all eight comparisons as separate entities, and the other to consider the research as four longitudinal studies through time (with only 'before' and 'after' testing).

The first way compares samples of girls from co-educational schools with samples of girls from girls' schools, at the ages of 11, 13, 15 and 17, and correspondingly for boys. None of the differences is statistically significant; six of them give the co-educated pupils as a little happier, one gives the boys' school as slightly happier and one comparison produces virtual equality. In other words the general direction of the difference is in line with the findings of the other surveys but the amount of it is much smaller. The nearest approaches to statistical significance were in favour of co-educated boys aged 11 plus and 13 plus, co-educated girls aged 17 plus, and slightly below the lowest of these, boys aged 17 plus in boys' schools.

Viewed longitudinally there was no major change in any group. Minor ones were that the slightly greater happiness scores of the co-educated 15-year-olds over the group from girls' schools became greater at the age of 17, but it was still not quite statistically significant; also that the virtual equality of the two boys' groups aged 15 changed by the age of 17 into a slight, not statistically significant, lead for those in boys' schools. Analysed in this way no difference can be seen in the effects of the two types of school, but the method has the limitation that it does not allow for any initially greater happiness which a group maintains though does not increase.

It was mentioned in Chapter 1 that the researchers were uneasy about the representativeness of the samples because some heads had not realized how rigidly the administrative instructions for the selection of pupils should be enforced, and that the researchers therefore checked this representativeness by giving the 'Check' questionnaire to the whole of the 13 plus age group, excluding the project pupils of two years previously. It was found that with this much larger group the co-educated girls estimated they were distinctly happier at school than the girls from girls' schools (the results are given in full in the next section). It seems therefore that the project samples of girls aged 11 and 13 were somewhat biased against the co-educational schools compared with the relevant school population aged 13 plus. For practical and financial reasons it was not possible to use the 'Check' questionnaire with the three other groups; they also might have been affected. This illustrates why it is so much better to take an overall view of a number of surveys rather than rely on one.

Yet another factor is the intelligence levels of the opposing groups. In the previous chapter it has been reported that there were statistically significant differences in the average intelligence scores (on a small scale of only ten items) between the co-educated girls of both 11 plus and 15 plus, and the corresponding groups from girls' schools in favour of the latter, and it is presumed that the happiness of pupils would be aided by the ability to master the academic work and reduced by any inability to do so.

The 'Check' survey

In the 'Check' survey, made in 1966 to test the representative nature of the sample in the schools project, all those girls of the 11 plus agegroup who had not been included in the Schools project sample were asked to complete a short questionnaire which included the question on happiness in school. The results are given in Table 2.5.

TABLE 2.5 *Happiness in school (girls)*

'Check' questionnaire

Estimates of happiness in school	Replies from girls aged 13 plus in			
	Co-ed. schools		Girls' schools	
	N	%	N	%
Happy	234	52·1	291	43·2
Fairly happy	189	42·1	320	47·6
Jogging along	16	3·6	53	7·9
Rather unhappy	8	1·8	9	1·3
Unhappy	2	0·4	0	0
Totals	449	100	673	100

NOTE: The co-educated girls are happier (statistical significance beyond ·01 level).

Readers will see that the difference between the co-educated pupils aged 13 plus and those educated in girls' schools is wider than that for the comparable samples drawn from this age group for the schools project. Whereas the co-educated girls in the Schools project gave happiness estimates that were only marginally better than those of girls in girls' schools, here the difference increases appreciably to become highly significant statistically, bringing it more into line with the findings of the previous surveys. As the 'Check' survey was made with a much larger number of pupils (over 1,100) without the necessity of having pupils selected as a sample of their age group within each school, it is also much more reliable. As it is possible to make only surmises about the reasons for the difference between the two results the matter is pursued no further except to emphasize again a principal theme of the previous volume—that in difficult work of this kind, with so many variables and with the necessity of ensuring that the true results are protected from distortion by the strong emotions sometimes aroused, the only safe procedure is to secure a consensus from a number of surveys, while realizing that an occasional departure from this consensus is not unlikely.

The 'Check' questionnaire was not administered to any other age group of girls, nor was it thought profitable to give it to the boys.

Discussion

As it is the object of these books to present results on many topics and from several surveys, the discussion seeks merely to summarize and to indicate a few major points. It seems that girls in general are happier in co-educational secondary grammar schools than in girls' secondary grammar schools. Bilateral grammar-technical schools would be included, and it is the writer's opinion that the statement would also hold good for secondary modern and secondary comprehensive schools, because of the basic social similarities involved, but this has not been proved. Few girls appear to be 'Rather unhappy' or 'Unhappy' in either type of school, but the major difference appears to be in the higher proportion of girls in co-educational schools who endorse the first category (i.e. 'very happy') in the college surveys.

The two groups of males are closer together, though the 'Both schools' survey, where students had experience of both types of school, shows that they estimated that they were much happier in their co-educational than in their boys' school, even when order of school was held constant.

Certain factors contaminate the sample of normal co-educational grammar schools and reduce their estimates slightly, namely the inclusion of amalgamated and comprehensive schools. The slightly greater pleasantness of situation of the co-educational schools (as estimated by the ex-pupils) may work in the opposite direction.

These factors have, however, been examined and have been shown to be only minor influences.

The reasons the students gave for their opinions will be set out and discussed in the next chapter, but it should be indicated here that although the pupil's happiness is very important, and his possible unhappiness at school perhaps more important than anything, critics could still argue that the price to be paid for happiness could be too great if it were for example at the cost of indiscipline. Others would say that the cost is also too great if the happiness is accompanied by a lower academic standard. The argument about academic attainment has, however, been thrashed out in another place (Dale, 1962a, 1962b and 1964), and the balance of that argument cannot be said to be on the side of the single-sex schools.

3

Happiness in school: (b) the free responses

In the preceding chapter the estimates of the ex-pupils and pupils about their happiness in school were examined; in the present chapter the free responses are added. The estimates give a reasonable accuracy while the free responses, not as reliable quantitatively, produce both greater depth and human colour, reminding us that we are not concerned merely with grey statistical abstractions, but with living boys and girls who are our children and other people's children. We seek the greater happiness and well-being of Jack and Jill and their children after them, though we would agree that there are other criteria to be kept in mind.

The results of the various surveys will be presented in the same order as the estimates of Chapter 2, commencing with the Second College survey.

The Second College survey

The students' estimates showed that co-educated women thought they were happier at school than did those who were educated at girls' schools, but we want to know why they were of this opinion. These reasons were supplied by the free responses which the students were requested to give after their estimate, and both men's and women's are included, though as the difference between the two men's groups was smaller these are less interesting and they are therefore given less space.

Owing to a lack of clerical assistance the analysis of the free responses was limited to the first 1,546 respondents whose forms were returned before a supplementary stage was added to the inquiry. Slightly less than half of these contained a comment, and only with the ex-pupils of boys' schools did the proportion rise slightly above one-half. The answers revealed a difficulty that had not shown itself in the pilot testing, namely that a few ex-pupils had trouble in assessing their happiness throughout their secondary school life because it either fluctuated so much, or was very different in the lower school compared with the upper. Of the 115 'old girls' of mixed schools who made comments, 13 expressed this difficulty. Of the similar 182 ex-pupils of girls' schools there were 8 who found the lower school happier, and 15 who were discontented with their sixth-form life; on the other hand there were 32 who were happier in the upper school or sixth form. Only a small proportion of these said they had difficulty in making an overall evaluation and none of them failed in fact to give a judgment. The full classification is given in Table 3.1.

TABLE 3.1 *Classified comments on happiness in school*

Second College survey

School education	Male students		Female students	
	Co-ed. (148)	Boys' (230)	Co-ed. (115)	Girls' (182)
Pupil/staff relations happy	25	39	35	22
Pupil/staff relations unsatisfactory	8	19	6	8
Atmosphere good	20	15	26	21
Atmosphere unpleasant	1	1		2
Discipline good			1	2
Discipline too strict		3	1	11
Societies and sports enjoyable	17	31	15	10
Societies too few	3	5		2
Friendships	21	27	23	27
Work enjoyable	10	19	16	10
Work difficulties*	13	22	7	14
Happiness varied	1	5	2	3
Lower school happier		2	2	8
Upper school happier	11	30	5	32
Sixth form discontent		4	4	15
Mixed school happy	4		4	
Personal difficulties		6	2	
Others	24	33	15	23
Totals (of comments)	158	261	164	210

* 'Work difficulties' includes finding school work not interesting or difficult, the pressure of examinations and excessive homework.

The 1,546 completed forms yielded nearly 700 comments (about 800 when classified, because some included two aspects). When these were divided among the four main groups and classified into ten categories of comment, the resulting numbers in the subgroups were inevitably small. There is also, in spite of precautions, some subjectivity entering into the classification of closely related categories. The Table is, therefore, published not as something conclusive, but as a tentative qualitative illustration of the quantitative results in the previous chapter.

FEMALE EX-PUPILS

If we compare the two groups of female students we find a few clear trends. Those from mixed schools appear, on the whole, to have experienced rather happier relations between pupils and staff than did those who were in girls' schools—though very few of either group said that those relations were unsatisfactory. There may be some measure of support for this in the later comments on the school atmosphere and in those of the previous volume on school discipline, but there may be two opposing views about such a thorny question as discipline. Perhaps the presence of men on the staffs of mixed schools may have influenced these replies, in which case the situation may now be changing somewhat, as more and more girls' schools are appointing a small proportion of men to their staffs. Whatever the reason, we have to record that, whereas four in ten of the comments from women ex-pupils of mixed schools were favourable,[1] the proportion from girls' schools was little more than two in ten; similarly, whereas less than 7 per cent of the comments from the female ex-pupils of mixed schools were adverse, the percentage was 17 from girls' schools. The mixed schools also do better in the comments on work and in the relative lack of sixth-form discontent. It might seem that the girls' schools have an advantage in that a greater proportion of their ex-pupils say they were 'happier in the upper school', but this is merely in apposition to their less happy experience in the lower school; the ex-pupils of mixed schools appear only rarely to experience this variability, or they find the change so slight that they are not impelled to comment.

Female ex-pupils who attended both types

Among the women was a sub-group who had attended both a co-educational and a single-sex secondary grammar (or technical

[1] Combining 'happy staff–pupil relationships', 'good atmosphere', 'good discipline' and 'mixed school happy'. The adverse comments combine the reverse of the above, together with 'sixth-form discontent'.

When these adverse and favourable comments for mixed and single-sex schools are opposed in a 2 × 2 table, the resulting Chi-square is significant well beyond the ·01 level for girls and beyond the ·025 level for boys.

or comprehensive) school. The comments of this group are important and objectivity of presentation is attained by quoting *all* those which compare the two types of school. First are given those remarks which were in favour of co-education, commencing with several which compared the formality of the girls' school with the informality of the mixed:

'Very happy—mixed; rather unhappy (single-sex). Grammar school tended to be less happy because it was more formal (not due to work).'

'Happy in the single-sex school, but very happy in the co-ed. school where there were no barriers between staff and pupils.'

'Happier in the co-ed. school. The atmosphere was better; not so many petty rules.'

'A very friendly atmosphere in the co-ed. school between all pupils and teachers and pupils.'

'The atmosphere of the school was happier when the school was mixed in my fifth year.'

'In single-sex schools in ... and ... I found the discipline unnecessarily severe and girls class-conscious in the extreme.'

'Happy, mixed; very unhappy, single-sex. Because of lack of organization in school, teaching methods and staff, and stupid attitude towards boys.'

Another woman remarks favourably on the presence of boys—or unfavourably on their absence:

'I preferred the co-ed. school and was far happier than in an all-girl community.'

Of the remainder some merely said they were happier at the mixed school while others gave a variety of reasons:

'Happy on an average. But period spent in co-ed. type was exceptionally happy.'

'Happy in the single-sex, very happy in the co-ed.'

'I liked the work and I liked the companionship of the girls.'(Co-ed. school.)

One woman preferred her girls' school:

'Happier at the single-sex school as [i.e. than] at co-ed. I disliked the headmaster.'

Happiness in school: (b) the free responses

MALE EX-PUPILS

When we compare the comments of the two groups of male ex-pupils (Table 3.1), the most marked difference is in the greater variability of the happiness of boys in boys' schools. One seventh of them were happier in the upper than the lower school; in the mixed schools this proportion was less than one-fourteenth. If the categories of pupil–staff relations, atmosphere, discipline and 'mixed school happy' are combined there is a trend in favour of the mixed school, in line with—but emphasizing—the slight trend shown in the *estimates* of happiness by Figure 2.1. Almost one-third of the boys from mixed schools comment favourably, but only one-fifth of those from boys' schools; again, while about one in eighteen from the mixed schools comment adversely in these sections, the proportion from the boys' schools is one in ten.

Male ex-pupils who attended both types

As with the women, the comments of the sub-group of men, 73 in number, who had experienced both types of school, are especially valuable and *all* those that compare the mixed and single-sex school are given here. The favourable ones concentrate mostly on social relations with the girls and the good 'atmosphere', e.g.:

'The attitude of the whole school (mixed) was different. At the first school (co-ed.—happy) we were still willing to learn. At the second school (single-sex—jogging along) there were not any females.'

'It was only towards the later stages of co-ed. school life that I realized how happy school could be.'

'Although the amount of work done in the co-ed. was not as great as in the single-sex school I think the feeling of looking on the girls as companions in work had a good effect on me and influenced greatly my later dealings and friendships with girls or women.'

'First year at the grammar school (single-sex) was terrible due to the change. Last year at grammar school (single-sex) was tense due to failure at "O" levels. Two years at the comprehensive were great, due perhaps to the ability to assert oneself more fully intellectually.'

'A pleasant atmosphere, especially in the co-ed. school.'

'At the mixed school the tutors seemed personally interested in you as an adult—this was, to some extent, true of my first school (single-sex) but less so.'

[Happy co-ed.; very unhappy single-sex] 'Complete change of atmosphere in single-sex school, unable to re-orientate myself. Lost in the artificial segregation I think.'

There were also a few comments which were either unfavourable or less favourable to the co-educational school:

'First school snobbish co-ed.—poor district. Second school single-sex not snobbish—Borough. Also my father died.'

'I gained greatly from the experience I had in the single-sex school and this stood me in good stead for my 2 years in a co-ed. school.'

'Life at the co-ed. school was made unhappy by a headmaster who should never have had a co-ed. school—he obviously wasn't in agreement with both sides mingling freely together.'

'Very happy applies to single-sex as I was in the sixth and staff–pupil relationship was very good. Happy in co-ed.'

A few critical comments written by men who had attended only one type of grammar school are given in the next section because of their general interest:

Jogging along 'I was only an average scholar and did not really feel connected to the school.' (Co-ed.)

Jogging along 'Seemed an aimless existence because you were merely trophy hunting ("O" levels) with no incentive.' (Co-ed.)

Rather unhappy 'Bullying rife in the school, especially felt in the first three forms, imposed by the 4th, 5th and 6th forms.' (Boys' school)

Jogging along 'The public school is not ideal for the artistic temperament.' (Boys' school)

The comments are informative but the estimates given in the previous chapter are a more reliable guide to the comparative happiness of these men when they were pupils in school. The next results to be considered are those from the 'Both schools' survey, where *all* the pupils who took part had actually attended both a co-educational and a single-sex secondary school (excluding secondary modern).

The 'Both schools' survey

FEMALE EX-PUPILS

Each student in the 'Both schools' survey was requested to make a comment on his or her happiness at the co-educational school and another about the single-sex school attended. The comments of the female ex-pupils are classified in Table 3.2, and the totals show at

TABLE 3.2 *Female ex-pupils' comments on happiness*
'Both schools' survey

Categories of comments, classified according to *estimate*		About co-ed. schools	About girls' schools
FAVOURABLE ESTIMATES ON HAPPINESS*			
Atmosphere:	pleasant, free, good school spirit	242	99
	(but impersonal, tense, insecure)		(25)*
	good because no boys		9
	tradition good	3	9
	(but overawed first school)	(5)	
	good facilities		17
	(but not school conscious)		(4)
Staff:	friendly	144	67
	(but unfriendly)	(6)	(14)
	Head good	6	8
	(but head feared, bad)	(1)	(7)
	discipline good	34	25
	(but discipline lax)	(7)	(4)
	(but discipline too strict)	(4)	(17)
Pupils:	friendly	127	150
	(but unfriendly, catty, cliques)	(12)	(26)
	(but prefects officious)		(3)
	good social life	73	17
	(but poor social life)		(9)
	good societies	32	12
	(but unhealthy attitude to boys)		(5)
	boy–girl mixing	115	—
	friends from junior school	8	
	(but difficulties of settling in)	(25)	(10)

[*continued*]

To secure objectivity the free responses are classified according to whether the students underlined a favourable or unfavourable *estimate*. If the estimate and comment differed in this respect the comment is classified in brackets, e.g. a student might underline 'happy' and then comment 'but the atmosphere was too impersonal'; this comment is placed *in brackets* in the 'favourable' section under 'atmosphere'. Comments made after a 'jogging along' estimate are placed in the 'unfavourable' section. In the *totals* for 'unfavourable' are included those category totals in brackets in the 'favourable' section, and vice versa.

TABLE 3.2 (*continued*) *Female ex-pupils' comments on happiness*

'Both schools' survey

Categories of comments, classified according to *estimate*		About co-ed. schools	About girls' schools
FAVOURABLE ESTIMATES ON HAPPINESS			
Work:	good standard	17	81
	(but poor standard, narrow)	(11)	(2)
	enjoyable, education for life	110	2
	(but unsuccessful, boring)	(4)	(1)
	good boy–girl rivalry, discussion	29	
	(but examinations bad, pressure)	(4)	(9)
First school, therefore enjoyed			30
Pleasant surroundings		19	
Sixth especially happy		24	15
Small school liked		19	16
	(but disliked)	(3)	
Girls' school better—less self-conscious			7
Girls' school compares unfavourably			(13)
Others		41	19
UNFAVOURABLE ESTIMATES ON HAPPINESS			
Atmosphere:	poor school spirit	9	10
	(but good tradition, pleasant)		(2)
	overawed—first school	3	8
	convent school		5
	unpleasant, impersonal, tense, insecure		69
	poor facilities		7

[*continued*]

once that the comments give the same picture as the estimates except that the tendencies are more accentuated.

Whereas the students gave 86 per cent of favourable remarks about their co-educational schools, the percentage dropped to 51 for their girls' schools. It made very little difference whether the co-educational school was attended first or last, and the percentage of favourable comments was only a little lower for the girls' schools attended last, compared with those attended first. Sometimes a favourable *estimate* (and perhaps main comment) would be accompanied by a less important unfavourable qualifying clause, usually prefaced by 'but', e.g: 'I loved the school but the building was in a

TABLE 3.2 (*continued*) *Female ex-pupils' comments on happiness 'Both schools' survey*

Categories of comments, classified according to *estimate*		About co-ed. schools	About girls' schools
UNFAVOURABLE ESTIMATES ON HAPPINESS			
Staff:	unfriendly	10	46
	head feared, poor	3	16
	discipline too strict	1	32
Pupils:	unfriendly, catty, cliques	11	62
	(but friendly)	(3)	(13)
	wanted boys		4
	poor social life		11
	unhealthy attitude to boys		9
Work:	poor standard	6	
	(though good standard)		(5)
	examinations bad effect, pressure	2	21
	narrow, boring	8	24
	unsuccessful	2	2
	(but rivalry good)	(1)	
	(but enjoyed)	(2)	(7)
Large school: disliked			7
Small school: disliked		3	
Difficult change, settling down		11	17
But co-ed. better			29
Others		15	7
FAVOURABLE		1049	610
		86·3%	53·3%
UNFAVOURABLE		166	535
		13·7%	46·7%
Totals		1215	1145

shocking state.' Such qualifying clauses are classified in the 'favourable estimates' section but placed in brackets.

As the overall results for the first and last schools are so close together for women, they will be merged for appraisal except where there is any noteworthy divergence. Much of the co-educational advantage is to be found under the heading 'atmosphere', which attracts (on the favourable side) one-fifth of their total comments, and almost no unfavourable ones, while the girls' schools receive far fewer favourable comments under the same heading, and about as many unfavourable as favourable. Other appreciable advantages to the co-educational schools are to be found under the headings 'friendly' and 'unfriendly' staff, and also under 'good social life' and 'good societies'. Under the last two headings the co-educational schools received 105 favourable comments compared with 29 for the girls' schools. Naturally the girls' schools had no counterpart to the 115 comments favouring the mixing of the sexes as in co-educational schools, the nearest being 7 comments favouring girls' schools because the absence of boys makes the girls feel less self-conscious. Perhaps the most dramatic differences are in the 'work' section, where 81 said the girls' schools reached a good standard and only 17 the co-educational schools; on the other hand while only 2 ex-pupils said their girls' schools had enjoyable lessons and educated for life, the co-educational schools received praise in 110 comments for the same topics. As, however, the borderline between these categories is sometimes ill-defined, and the classification subjective, a broad impression is better than these apparently precise numbers. A sound interpretation would be that the ex-pupils of girls' schools tended to stress the good standard of work rather than enjoyment in work, while when reporting on their co-educational schools they stressed the enjoyable nature of the lessons rather than their good standard, but these two qualities will often go hand in hand; it is partly a question of which quality is dominant in the memory of the ex-pupils. In the 'unfavourable' section girls' schools received 21 complaints of overpressure, as against 2 about mixed schools, and 22 complaints about 'narrowness' as against 8 for the mixed.

Though both the co-educational and girls' schools received many comments praising the friendliness of the pupils (127 and 150), the latter had also 62 about unfriendly pupils, compared with 11 from the mixed schools. On the specific point about which kind of school was preferred, including such phrases as 'wanted boys' or 'good because no boys', the co-educational school received an overall total of 46 direct preferences (without including the 115 comments which found boy–girl mixing beneficial), against 18 for the girls' schools. A not insignificant number of ex-pupils found the sixth forms of both types of school to be especially happy.

The usual reminder is given to readers that though an earnest attempt was made to make this classification as objective as possible it must be inferior in this respect to the *estimates* of happiness given by the ex-pupils. As implied at the beginning of the chapter, this is a price which is worth paying for the additional depth, interpretation and colour which the comments give. They also have a watch-dog role as detectors of ambiguities and hidden difficulties in the questions. In these results, however, estimates and comments tell a similar story, except that the latter give an increased emphasis to the unfavourable aspects of girls' schools.

This next section gives a selection of the comments; in each section the favourable ones are given first. *Under each sub-category the proportion of quoted comments to the total for that sub-category is the same for co-educational and single-sex schools, but the proportion quoted is smaller for the larger categories* to avoid overburdening the chapter with quotations. Many of the small sub-categories must necessarily be omitted.

School atmosphere

First let us take that elusive quality said by pupils, staff and even visitors to be the 'atmosphere' of a school, remembering that all the students quoted had attended both co-educational and girls' schools.[1] They speak of their co-educational schools in such terms as the following:

Very happy 'There was an atmosphere in the school of unity. All activities were mixed . . . everyone got on well with each other.'

Very happy 'There were plenty of activities to join in, a friendly atmosphere throughout the school, behaviour on the whole was very good. I just enjoyed going to school.'

Very happy 'Because the social life of the school created a warm atmosphere and made the school a main part of my life, which made the work too more interesting.'

Very happy 'A generally happy atmosphere, an attempt on the part of pupil and teacher alike to make one feel "at home" when new. Also strong element of cheerful competition between sexes.'

Very happy 'The atmosphere was open and friendly with lively discussions in lessons and I used to look forward to going to school every day.'

Very happy 'Happy atmosphere—good teachers and headmaster —friendly children.'

Very happy 'Good young friendly teachers. Enjoyable curriculum. Pleasant surroundings and atmosphere. Active social life connected with school. Variety of school societies and activities.'

[1] Atmosphere is here amalgamated with 'good school spirit'.

Very happy 'The school had happy atmosphere, the staff were co-operative and friendly. The sixth formers were treated well. Many activities.'

The comments on the atmosphere of the girls' schools are much fewer; examples are:

Very happy 'The form was small and so we were all very good friends, we were the top form and on friendly terms with the staff.'

Very happy 'I had a great deal of friends and I boarded so I was with them all the time just like a family.'

Very happy 'It was a small, warm, happy friendly school.'

As there were only a negligible number of criticisms of the atmosphere of the co-educational schools, and these consisted partly of non-typical comments such as being overawed by one's first secondary school, no single comment is as representative as one would like, but the following is quoted:

Rather unhappy 'The atmosphere of the school was hostile.' (In a second co-educational school she was much happier.)

More characteristic of their kind are the quotations from those who criticized the girls' schools:

Rather unhappy 'I hated the petty narrow-mindedness of the women teachers. Most were frustrated old spinsters who wanted us to become the same.'

Rather unhappy 'I found the influence of a rather dictatorial spinster headmistress fermented the atmosphere of the whole school making the staff and pupils tense all the time.'

Rather unhappy 'I found that everyone was narrow-minded and that although I had my own circle of friends I was glad to leave.'

Rather unhappy 'There was a strained feeling among the pupils and the staff. Each trying to out-do the other over trivial things.'

Jogging along 'Rather morbid atmosphere. I had little interest in work.'

Rather unhappy 'The discipline was very strict. Even as a third-year sixth I was marched everywhere and due to the fact that the headmistress was very strict she terrified everyone and the atmosphere was very tense and awful.'

Rather unhappy 'I found the majority of girls giggly over boys and the staff were quarrelsome and catty often in front of the girls. The atmosphere was very wrong.'

Jogging along 'Exam. pressure from school, competitiveness of school. Happy home life, spiteful atmosphere at school—everybody for herself.'

Readers need to be aware that the above strictures present only the pupils' side of the story, and the staffs of girls' schools might argue that a certain amount of discipline is healthy for growing adolescents, even though they sometimes resent it. On the other hand the pupils whose estimates fall into this category seem to have had an experience which goes beyond this and certainly most of them classed themselves as rather unhappy at school—a state of affairs which is without question undesirable. The protagonists of mixed schools would point out that far fewer of the same ex-pupils said they were unhappy at their mixed schools, and though their opponents might reply that the pupils might well be happier because discipline was too lax, the balance of the argument in this sector, after reading the comments and considering the findings of the whole research, would seem to lie with the co-educational schools.

Staff and discipline

The next major category is 'staff', including 'discipline'. Here the co-educational school had 184 favourable references and the girls' schools 100. A twentieth of each total yields a sufficiently representative sample of comments about each type of school, commencing with the co-educational. Readers will notice that the word 'atmosphere' still occurs frequently, and in general this is a marked feature of the comments on the co-educational schools.

Very happy 'There was a happy atmosphere surrounding the school and good pupil–staff and pupil–pupil relationship on the whole.'

Very happy 'A generally happy atmosphere, an attempt on the part of pupil and teacher alike to make one feel "at home" when new.'

Very happy 'The school had a happy atmosphere, the staff more co-operative and friendly.'

Fairly happy 'Happy atmosphere in this fairly new school between staff and pupils, and vice versa. Treated like an equal rather than a pupil.' (Co-ed. school first)

Fairly happy 'General feeling of belonging—sense of team work —meeting people more on a social level.'(Am.)[1]

[1] The comments of pupils from 'amalgamated' schools are distinguished by (Am.).

Very happy 'There was a very pleasant atmosphere and the teachers treated you as adults not as children.'

Very happy 'Free and easy atmosphere. Pleasant staff. Able to have varied conversations with both the girls and the boys.'

Fairly happy 'Good-looking maths, physics and P.E. teachers (male, of course). Young history teacher near my age when in sixth form—good parties.'

Very happy 'Communal atmosphere. Very big school—awe inspiring, many out-of-school activities.' (Here we have a not so usual positive attitude to the very large school)

Though some of the comments on the girls' schools are almost identical there are also differences of which a glimpse is given here:

Very happy 'We were good friends and on good terms with the staff. The attitude of staff to pupils was more personal and our school had a character of its own.' (Am. later)

Very happy 'The staff were all very friendly and everyone knew everyone.' (Am. later)

Very happy 'Good headmistress who was respected.'

Fairly happy 'Nice atmosphere. Well disciplined. There could have been more freedom.' (Am. later)

Very happy 'Girls were catered for and not put second to the interests of the boys. There was lots to do and a greater feeling of a community.'

Three of the comments are about schools which were later amalgamated with boys' schools; one notes also the references to 'well-disciplined' and the complaint that sometimes the interests of the girls are subordinated to those of the boys in a co-educational school. These points were brought to the readers' attention in the first volume of this work.

On the unfavourable side the students made 33 adverse comments about the staff or discipline of their co-educational schools and 135 about their girls' schools. The former are a mixed but amusing collection, of which three are quoted:

Very unhappy 'My father sacked the husband of the mistress who took two subjects and made my life pure hell.'

Rather unhappy 'Disrespect of women teachers by the boys.'

Jogging along 'Because I was in a single-sex school for 6 years and my year in upper sixth when two single-sex schools joined under new headship. Most problems were hardly dealt with, never reviewed, no unity amongst staff—two staffs joined together, each favouring former positions. As school captain I found only three members of staff helpful.' (Am.)

The same proportion of comments is quoted about the girls' schools:

Jogging along 'Most of the staff were old unmarried women and weren't in touch with our generation.'

Jogging along 'I did not like the stiff formal relationship between the staff and pupils.'

Rather unhappy 'At first I tried to like the school and got on quite well, but as time progressed the pettiness of the rules and aloofness of the staff got me more and more irritated.'

Rather unhappy 'Unpleasant headmistress.'

Rather unhappy 'I disliked the atmosphere created by staff of middle-aged spinsters.'

Jogging along 'I didn't like boarding, didn't like so many females, didn't like the snobbery and rigid discipline of the place.'

Jogging along 'At the time it wasn't bad, but when I look back now I don't know how I could have stood it for five years.'

Very unhappy 'It was run by narrow-minded nuns.'

Rather unhappy 'I arrived in time to be thrown into a gigantic pre-G.C.E.-pushing campaign in a vast anonymous building with a vast anonymous staff and collection of girls.'

Rather unhappy 'Far too strict and impersonal.'

Fairly happy 'The dominance of the headmistress tended to make life a little unpleasant.'

Rather unhappy 'The atmosphere was extremely authoritarian.'

Very unhappy '. . . didn't get on with teachers who made life unpleasant, also discipline far too strict.'

Pupil relationships

In the consideration of the section on pupil relationship there is a logical amalgamation of the sub-categories 'friendly pupils', 'good social life' and 'good societies', producing 235 comments favourable to the co-educational schools and 192 for the girls' schools, after omitting from present consideration the '115 plus' comments welcoming the presence of boys. Examples of those praising the co-educational schools are:

Fairly happy 'The first year was very difficult—I found the boys most uncouth and they thought me peculiar. The second year we understood each other and I was extremely happy.'

Very happy 'Got on well with fellow students, more social life, few school rules and restrictions.'

Very happy 'I found a happier and a more easy-going relationship between the pupils themselves and the teacher–pupil relationship.'

Very happy 'There were plenty of activities to join in, a friendly atmosphere throughout the school, behaviour on the whole was very good. I just enjoyed going to school.'

Very happy 'Because there was a good friendly atmosphere between pupils and I did pretty well academically.'

Very happy 'Very pleasant relationship existed between staff and pupils in almost every case.'

In this category the girls' schools are not at such a disadvantage (apart from the postponed sub-category of boy–girl mixing), and typical favourable remarks were:

Fairly happy 'I found it easy to make friends and became less timid because I could talk freely to the girls.'

Very happy 'I had a lot of friends at this school and my work improved beyond recognition. I gained places of responsibility.'

Fairly happy 'There was a happy spirit among members of classes.'

Very happy 'Most people were very friendly to each other and there was no unpleasantness.'

Fairly happy 'The girls were very friendly when I first went there and welcomed me in the school and this impression has always remained.'

By no means all the students had happy experiences at school, and although those who complained were a minority, their remarks can sharpen our insight into conditions that create difficulties.

Criticisms of the co-educational schools were:

Jogging along 'I felt an outsider a lot of the time as many of the pupils had known each other from their infant school days. Also I felt bored.'

Rather unhappy 'I was made unhappy by other girls being jealous of me going out with a popular boy. Except for that I was very happy.' (Am.)

Jogging along 'Suddenly confronted with half a class of boys—took time to fit in properly.'

The following are typical of the unfavourable comments about pupil relationships in the girls' schools. The first complaint is common to both girls' and co-educational schools:

Rather unhappy 'Entered at 17 in 6th form with girls who had been in the school for 10 years, was never really accepted.'

Rather unhappy 'Girls tended to be jealous and catty—I was smaller than the rest and got the butt of everything.'

Jogging along 'I felt rather insignificant and never seemed to excel in any field. Also the social side of school life left much to be desired, one never felt an integral part of the school.'

Very unhappy 'I had to leave because I was unhappy. This was partly because I was too timid, weak and sensitive. They called me a snob but it was really their inverted snobbery and I took it to heart. I was surprised that they were so affectionate when I left.'

Rather unhappy 'I found the girls tended to be rather catty and unfriendly. They all split up into small groups very soon and it just happened that I was the one who was left out.'

Rather unhappy 'Something awful happened to girls when they were altogether—spiteful, etc.'

Very unhappy 'I didn't like the all-female staff of teachers, nor did I like the all-female pupils.'

A few quotations are added from the 115 remarks about the benefits of boy–girl mixing:

Very happy 'I then felt more comfortable with members of the opposite sex and gained more confidence in their presence in out-of-school hours.'

Very happy 'Appreciated the view of the opposite sex and the stimulus it gave in work and socially.'

Very happy 'Being small it was a close community. Boys and girls were at ease together and this diminished adolescent shyness of the opposite sex.'

Very happy 'I prefer to be in mixed, rather than one-sexed, company. This situation seems right to me, it is more like real life.'

Very happy 'I found the early years of secondary education spent in a co-ed. were interesting and exciting. I enjoyed the many different activities in which both sexes took part.'

Work

The last major group of comments to be examined is that devoted to academic work. Here the co-educated have an advantage only because of the large number of ex-pupils of these schools who said they *enjoyed* their school work, and regarded it as an education for life. As mentioned previously, it is interesting that the comments on the girls' schools emphasize the good standard of work, with very little about enjoyment of it, while those on the co-educational schools have a smaller number on the good standard and a much larger number on the enjoyment. Though this general analysis holds good it should not be exaggerated because the enjoyment comments quite often imply a good standard, and the comments which emphasize the good standard sometimes imply enjoyment:

Very happy 'Friendly atmosphere. School completely united. Gentle rivalry between girls and boys stimulated work.'

Very happy 'Strong element of cheerful competition between the sexes.'

Very happy 'I felt secure in a natural surrounding and worked happily, feeling that I was benefiting from the full life this gave me.'

Very happy 'Good, young, friendly teachers. Enjoyable curriculum . . .'

Very happy 'Modern buildings. Rural area quite close to the sea. Was able to acquire good educational standard.'

Very happy 'I enjoyed school life. The mixing of boys and girls made it more enjoyable. Our outlook on life became broader. The staff were good teachers.' (Am.)

Fairly happy 'Most teachers good. Standard improved especially in subjects I liked. Probably liked it better because achieved better results.'

The following comments were about the girls' schools:

Fairly happy 'Worked hard; no distractions from opposite sex.'

Very happy 'There was not the embarrassment resulting from mistakes in lessons etc. which would have been present with boys attending.'

Fairly happy 'I made friends fairly easily and work never troubled me unduly, I enjoyed it as a contrast to strict home.'

Fairly happy 'Able to concentrate on work without boys fighting or making a row.'

Fairly happy 'I enjoyed school work and out-of-school activities.'

Now we examine the *unfavourable* comments on work, taking first as usual those about the co-educational schools. There were 37 of these in all, compared with 59 about the girls' schools, giving a ratio of roughly 3 to 5. Here we see the other side of the coin:

Fairly happy 'Although I enjoyed life in general more at the co-educational school, there was not the same working atmosphere there and I realized that my work was suffering.'

Rather unhappy 'I was studying science and I had the impression that it was wrong for a girl to do science subjects for "A" level G.C.E.' (Co-ed. last two years)

Fairly happy 'The atmosphere in the classroom was sometimes disturbed by the boys fooling about. Didn't seem to get on with the lessons as in a single-sex school.' (Co-ed. first year only)

The unfavourable comments on the work in the girls' schools are more often about strain, examinations and narrowness of outlook, e.g.:

Jogging along 'Finicky school rules, anxiety about exams.'

Fairly happy 'Pressure of work brought tension.' (Girls' school first five years)

Rather unhappy 'I spent two years in (1) and these were rather unpleasant; the work was hard and had little relief.'

Fairly happy 'Many of the lessons were uninteresting.'

Jogging along 'I had a limited circle of friends. There was little stimulus to work (I was in a third stream). Few after-school activities—bar games as in lunch hours.'

Direct comparisons

Perhaps the most interesting section is the one which follows, where ex-pupils have, without being requested to do so, compared the two types of school they attended. As the total yield of such quotations would have overburdened the chapter and to have given a selection would not have been sufficiently objective, recourse was had to publishing *all* those direct comparison quotations which appeared in the first twenty colleges, as coded, the others being unseen. First are given the comments based on the students' co-educational schools:

ABOUT CO-EDUCATIONAL SCHOOLS

Atmosphere

Very happy (Co-ed. first) 'The atmosphere was much easier, the pupil teacher relationship was friendlier. You didn't feel awkward when you met boys of your own age.'

Fairly happy (Co-ed. last) 'But atmosphere tended to be far freer than in single-sex school.'

Very happy (Co-ed. last) 'The whole atmosphere of the school was completely different from that in the single-sex school, probably because the headmaster's study was accessible if we had a problem—it was not a Mount Olympus as in the single-sex school.'

Fairly happy 'Enjoyed the work. Atmosphere more liberal in co-ed. school. Wider curriculum.' (Am.)

Staff–pupil relationships

Very happy (Co-ed. last) 'More life in general than single-sex school. More easy-going.'

Fairly happy (Co-ed. last) 'The atmosphere seemed a lot easier between members of staff, and staff and pupils. The discipline was not so strict and petty.'

Very happy (Co-ed. last) 'People much more friendly both pupils and teachers—atmosphere much more relaxed.'

Very happy (Co-ed. last) 'There was a much happier atmosphere among the children and also the staff. The staff seemed more helpful.'

Very happy (Co-ed. last) 'More freedom than in single-sex school. Better relations with the staff who taught me.' (Am.)

Very happy (Co-ed. last) 'Good atmosphere, the pupils and staff more friendly. It was *so* different to my previous school.' (Which was girls' boarding)

Happiness in school: (b) the free responses

Very happy (Co-ed. last) 'Because although being teased by male section after having been at girls' school the acceptance of you as a person was genuine, also easy relations with all staff. Enjoyed male company.'

Very happy (Co-ed. last) 'The whole atmosphere was happier. There was more friendly contact between staff and pupils. The rules were less rigid.'

Fairly happy (Co-ed. last) 'I found it difficult to become used to the different atmosphere around and people were not so friendly.'

Very unhappy (Co-ed. last) 'Very unhappy to begin with because of change from strict high school. Things improved in sixth form.'

Pupil relationships

Very happy (Co-ed. last) 'I felt it easier to talk to men and boys after my school became co-ed. than before. As a single-sex school I got used to mixing with girls only and felt shy when I had to speak to boys out of school.' (Am.)

Very happy (Co-ed. last) 'I felt that I fitted in better.'

Very happy (Co-ed. first) 'The classroom atmosphere was more relaxed, not so dictatorial. The inter-pupil relationship was more easy-going, not clique forming.'

Very happy (Co-ed. last) 'Healthier, more social atmosphere.' (Am.)

Fairly happy (Co-ed. first) 'The fact that it was a co-ed. school I think made the staff more broad-minded and our social life was more varied.'

Very happy (Co-ed. last) 'Boys and girls mixed easily. Previously the only conversation was about boys.' (Co-ed. boarder)

Fairly happy (Co-ed. last) 'We amalgamated at the beginning of the 5th year—the boys were a rather bad addition—we were much happier without them.' (Am.)

Fairly happy (Co-ed. last) 'Opportunities for viewpoints from opposite sex. A more natural relationship with opposite sex. Advantage of mixed staff.' (Co-ed. boarder)

Fairly happy (Co-ed. first) 'I found that the boys in my co-ed. school tended to be immature and foolish and that as a result the girls had a difficult time.'

ABOUT GIRLS' SCHOOLS

Next are given the direct-comparison comments which are based on the girls' schools:

Atmosphere

Jogging along (Single-sex last) 'I went into the girls' school from the free atmosphere of a co-ed. and found it difficult to adjust. Also, most of the girls had by that time made their friends.'

Very happy (Single-sex last) 'Happy friendly atmosphere. Girls more passive. School quieter than co-ed.'

Rather unhappy (Single-sex last) 'It was a big change to go to a single-sex school after a co-ed. I found it easy to adapt to this, but the whole atmosphere was entirely different.'

Rather unhappy 'I always wanted to return to my co-ed. school.'

Staff–pupil relationship

Fairly happy (Single-sex first) 'The school was all right, although I found the rules much stricter, and the headmistress was one to be feared, not a friend.'

Rather unhappy (Single-sex last) 'After the co-ed. I felt somewhat inhibited and frustrated in a single-sex school.'

Very happy (Single-sex last) 'More individual attention, nicer company, better discipline.'

Rather unhappy (Single-sex last) 'It seemed old-fashioned and narrow after my co-ed. school.'

Fairly happy (Single-sex first) 'Security amongst own sex. Staff very understanding with girls.'

Pupil relationships

Jogging along (Single-sex last) 'Very good friendships but school itself not as happy.'

Fairly happy (Single-sex last) 'In comparison with the previous school (co-ed.) greater tendency to group together—not such a free or pleasant atmosphere: influence of more male staff would have perhaps eased a certain amount of ill-feeling between girls.'

Very happy (Single-sex first) 'Lessons uncomplicated though perhaps not as light-hearted. Much wastage of time when boys present except when offering a different side in discussion.'

Very happy (Single-sex first) 'I was popular in my form, always near the top of the class (brains not being looked down upon in this school). The school was interested in developing whatever talents one had and did not concentrate solely on sport.'

MALE EX-PUPILS

The comments made by the male ex-pupils are presented in Table 3.3, divided into 'favourable' and 'unfavourable' sections according to the *estimates* students gave in answer to this item.

As with the estimates by far the greater number of free responses or comments were favourable with reference to the co-educational schools, but those about boys' schools were approximately equally divided between favourable and unfavourable. Judging by the totals in the different categories, the happiness of the pupils depended much more on personal relationships than on academic work or any other factor, though one presumes that if the standard of work had been clearly unsatisfactory there would have been more pronouncements under this heading. In most major categories the co-educational schools got roughly twice as many favourable mentions as the boys' schools, e.g. 'pleasant atmosphere', 'friendly staff', 'enjoyable socially', and, not so marked a difference, 'friendly pupils'. There is one favourable category on the co-educational side—the mixing of the sexes, with 39 direct mentions, to which the boys' school has no reply. Only in the section labelled 'work' is there a major sub-heading ('good standard') where the boys' schools, at first glance, come off best, though even this is dubious if we look more closely, as under two similar sub-headings, 'enjoyable work' and 'successful in work' the co-educational schools receive 30 mentions without anything to balance it on the boys' school side.

The unfavourable comments are scattered in small numbers throughout the range of categories, with those about the boys' schools being more than three times as numerous as those about the co-educational schools. The largest categories are the 24 mentions of 'poor atmosphere' in boys' schools, 12 of unfriendly staff, 12 of too strict discipline, 10 of unfriendly pupils, and 9 of bullying. Worthy of mention in the light of present trends are the 11 complaints that over-long travel prevented the writers from being happy at school.

Some direct comparisons are given but they are curtailed more rigorously than for the women, where the need for illustration was stronger. To preserve impartiality these comments are selected in proportion to the 'favourable' and 'unfavourable' totals for the two types of school in Table 3.3, using a factor of 30. They are too few for classification.

TABLE 3.3 *Male ex-pupils' comments on happiness*

'Both schools' survey

Categories of comments, classified according to *estimate*		About co-ed. schools	About boys' schools
FAVOURABLE ESTIMATES*			
Atmosphere:	pleasant	55	25
	(though poor, unpleasant)		(4)
	good school spirit	18	3
	(but disliked being first school)		(3)
	(but disliked mixed sexes)	(2)	—
Facilities:	good	2	12
	(but poorer)		(1)
Staff:	friendly	48	22
	(except women)	(3)	
	(but some not)	(2)	(1)
	head good	5	
	(but head poor)	(2)	
	discipline good	15	4
	(but too lax)	(4)	(1)
	(but too strict)	(1)	(1)
Pupils:	friendly	58	36
	(but unfriendly or bullying)	(3)	(4)
	enjoyable socially	19	10
	good societies	5	
	mixing both sexes	39	
	(but shy because girls)	(1)	
Work:	good standard	12	16
	(but narrow or poor)	(4)	(1)
	enjoyable	18	
	(though travel nuisance)		(2)
	successful in	12	
	(unsuccessful, boring)	(1)	(1)
Pleasant surroundings		6	
Though first year strange		6	
Mixed school happier		3	(1)
Boys' school happier			4
Sixth especially happy		7	8
First secondary—enjoyed			6
Others		20	11

[*continued*]

TABLE 3.3 (*continued*) *Male ex-pupils' comments on happiness*

Categories of comments, classified according to *estimate*		About co-ed. schools	About boys' schools
UNFAVOURABLE ESTIMATES*			
Atmosphere:	poor	1	24
	not school conscious	0	1
	(but facilities good)		(2)
Staff:	unfriendly	2	12
	(but friendly)		(2)
	discipline too strict	1	12
	discipline too lax	2	2
Pupils:	unfriendly	2	10
	(but friendly)	(1)	(5)
	bullying	1	9
	snobbish		2
	disliked mixed sexes	1	
	wanted mixed sexes		3
	poor socially		2
Work:	poor standard, boring	3	11
	(but good)		(1)
	narrow	1	6
Sports, etc. over-worshipped			2
Travel:	too far	4	5
Disliked school			3
Mixed school happier			11
Others		6	10
FAVOURABLE		349	167
		88·1%	53·5%
UNFAVOURABLE		47	145
		11·9%	46·5%
Totals		396	312

* Unfavourable includes all comments accompanied by a 'jogging along' estimate or worse, and all comments in brackets in the 'favourable' section. Vice versa for favourable comments.

About co-educational schools

Very happy 'The presence of the opposite sex aided one's social maturity as well as adding colour to the school surroundings.'

Very happy 'The staff–pupil relationship was excellent. They did not set themselves on a pedestal they were easily approachable.'

Very happy 'It was such a change from the single-sex school that I began to enjoy school. Before I had been in a bit of a rut.'

Very happy 'Having been at a very severe and old-fashioned boys' boarding school, the opportunity of working in relative freedom, and mixing with girls, and at the same time being a day-boy, made life much happier.'

Fairly happy 'Previous to single-sex grammar school I had been at a co-ed. secondary modern school. I was glad to return to the freer atmosphere of the co-ed. school system.'

Very happy 'Very friendly atmosphere—a body of people rather than a factory—good staff–pupil relationship.'

Very happy 'We were treated as grown-up in a combined community preparing for later life which would be shared between the sexes.'

Fairly happy 'Lessons seemed to become less stern and more beneficial.'

Fairly happy 'I had friends, the atmosphere of the school was free, and staff was interested in one as people. First years were not treated as an unfortunate necessity.'

Fairly happy 'Seemed to get on well with the other pupils; had a bit more security as older brother also there. There always seemed something to look forward to.'

Very happy 'Excellent preparation in social life, informal atmosphere, high standard of teaching, many great friends in both sexes, wide choice of subjects, excellent headmaster.'

Very happy 'A very happy atmosphere pervaded the school, social life was full and varied and in general there was a good relationship with staff.'

Comments unfavourable to the co-educational schools are few when kept to the same proportion.

Rather unhappy 'Masters not liking the change, new head, lack of school discipline.' (Am.)

Rather unhappy 'Distance involved in travelling, too many female teachers, dislike of mixing with girls.'

About boys' schools

Fairly happy 'Close unit of friends. Also lack of girls was not missed as it had not been experienced.'

Very happy 'The relationship between boys and boys, and boys and staff was excellent.'

Very happy 'School life ran freely and making lasting friends was very easy.'

Very happy 'You always have much more fun with people of the same sex and age groups.'

Fairly happy 'There was a tremendous atmosphere in the school and harmony.'

Very happy 'The school had a friendly, pleasant, personal atmosphere.'

The other side of the coin is to be seen in the following:

Very unhappy 'An unfriendly and unco-operative staff who ran the school in an almost military fashion, led by the headmaster.'

Rather unhappy 'General attitude of fear towards authority (military type staff) and rebellion.'

Rather unhappy 'Didn't like the single sex idea. Games, housemaster, C.C.F. Boarders were highly *privileged*! One of the masters was a homosexual. Proved.' (Boarding) [This is only what the young man wrote, and the writer cannot vouch for its truth]

Rather unhappy 'Hated the change from co-ed. to single-sex—apathetic attitude of pupils—homosexuality in sixth form rife—indifferent teachers.' [Comment as previously]

Rather unhappy 'A lot of bullying, prefects tended to be little Hitlers enjoying power, corporal punishment.'

It is difficult to ensure that such a collection of quotations, even when selected in the correct general proportions, are sufficiently characteristic. Undoubtedly co-educational pupils tend towards praise because of the pleasant 'atmosphere', friendly staff–student relationships, and the presence of the opposite sex, while boys from boys' schools like the friendship and the boy–master relationship when at its best. Whenever co-educational schools are criticized there is a tendency for this to be centred on lack of firm enough discipline, with an occasional comment expressing a preference for the company of the male sex alone. Criticism of boys' schools centres on severity of discipline and the abuses that go with it; the mention of homosexuality is usually in connection with boarding schools and is only occasional.

The Schools project

Though the free responses of the pupils about their happiness at school have been obtained and classified their inclusion would add little that is new to what has already been written. The 'Check' questionnaire did not invite free responses as the time available was inadequate.

4

School atmosphere

The atmosphere of a school is something difficult to define but powerfully felt. Perhaps the word which comes nearest is 'tone'; this, however, seems to have slight overtones of orderliness maintained by the staff, though not with much difficulty. A 'pleasant atmosphere' or 'good atmosphere' seems to go a step further and imply that staff and pupils are a happy co-operative community working and playing together. No such community is without its blemishes—the disliked member of staff, the difficult pupils, the awkward situations that arise from day to day—but the pleasantness of the atmosphere makes them small in significance and quickly forgotten, with no sense of harshness or injustice lingering afterwards. Such a state is obtained only by a finely balanced poise between the discipline that is too consciously imposed and if increased degenerates too easily into authoritarian harshness, and the undue permissiveness or lack of leadership which fails to secure willing pupil co-operation and causes the school to decline quickly into a state of indiscipline.

A good atmosphere is the hallmark of a good school. A poor one may be the result of staff severity or of lack of leadership and control, though occasionally the nature of the neighbourhood may make the task one for strong angels rather than mere mortals. What then do our ex-pupils and pupils say about the atmosphere in their co-educational and single-sex grammar schools? The results of the surveys will be presented in the same order as in the two previous chapters.

The Second College survey

Almost 2,000 students who were training to be teachers were asked, 'Do you think the school atmosphere was Very pleasant/Pleasant/ Neutral/Rather unpleasant/Very unpleasant?' There was no provision for comment, because the questionnaire was already long. The results are given in Table 4.1.

Few pupils in either kind of school found the atmosphere to be 'rather unpleasant' or worse. Both men and women from co-

TABLE 4.1 *School atmosphere*

Second College survey

Estimates of school atmosphere	Replies from male ex-pupils of				Replies from female ex-pupils of			
	Co-educational schools		Boys' schools		Co-educational schools		Girls' schools	
	N	%	N	%	N	%	N	%
Very pleasant	95	27·2	114	19·5	135	33·2	94	14·7
Pleasant	175	50·1	324	55·2	224	55·1	365	57·0
Neutral	67	19·2	114	19·5	42	10·3	140	21·9
Rather unpleasant	10	2·9	33	5·6	5	1·2	37	5·8
Very unpleasant	2	0·6	1	0·2	1	0·2	4	0·6
Totals	349	100	586	100	407	100	640	100

NOTE: The differences between the men's estimates for co-educational schools and boys' schools are statistically significant at ·025 level.

The differences between the women's estimates for co-educational schools and girls' schools are statistically significant well beyond the ·001 level.

educational schools considered it to be more pleasant than did those from single-sex schools, the difference between the two women's groups being much greater than that between the men's groups. Just over one in a hundred of the co-educated women judged the school atmosphere to be 'rather unpleasant', whereas the proportion for women from girls' schools was one in seventeen. It is, however, on the positive side that the chief difference lies; whereas one-third of the girls from mixed schools assessed the school atmosphere as 'very pleasant' only one-seventh of those from girls' schools were as enthusiastic. Whereas a tenth of the co-educated girls evaluated the atmosphere as 'neutral', more than a fifth of the opposite group registered the same assessment. It must be understood that one is here merely reporting results and that these can have various interpretations. Those women who are teaching in girls' schools and are devoted to their profession may understandably feel hurt and misjudged when they read these figures, but unnecessarily so for several reasons. First, because research may reveal other aspects in which girls' schools are superior; second, because we are dealing with averages and there are certainly good girls' schools and poor mixed schools as well as vice versa; third, because the nature of the results may be due mostly to the fact hat a mixed staff and mixed pupils in themselves produce a better atmosphere—and it may be that no woman teaching in a girls' school could prevent this difference arising.

The difference between the co-educated men and those from boys' schools is to be found mostly in the 'very pleasant' and 'pleasant' categories, the former group having nearly 8 per cent more estimating 'very pleasant', though they had 5 per cent fewer estimating 'pleasant'. Rather fewer of those from co-educational schools judged they were rather unhappy or worse than did those from boys' schools.

Let us now look at the estimates of those students in the Second College survey who attended both types of school. Although there were more than 70 women in the group data is available for only 30 owing to lack of clarity in the instructions, but as their special experience is important their results are given in Table 4.2.

TABLE 4.2 *School atmosphere (women): Ex-pupils with experience of both types*

Second College survey

Estimates of ex-pupils who had attended both types	Replies from female ex-pupils about their:	
	Co-educational schools	Girls' schools
	N	N
Very pleasant	15	6
Pleasant	11	7
Neutral	3	11
Rather unpleasant	0	2
Very unpleasant	1	2
Totals	30*	28

NOTE: The difference between the two groups is statistically significant by the Wilcoxon Sign-Rank test for matched pairs.

* Two students each gave estimates for two co-educational schools.

This small group of women thought the atmosphere of their co-educational schools pleasanter than that of their girls' schools, a difference which is statistically significant. It should be noticed that the difference is considerable and, although the numbers are small it is in the same direction as that seen in the large parent sample. The men's sample was too small to be quoted.

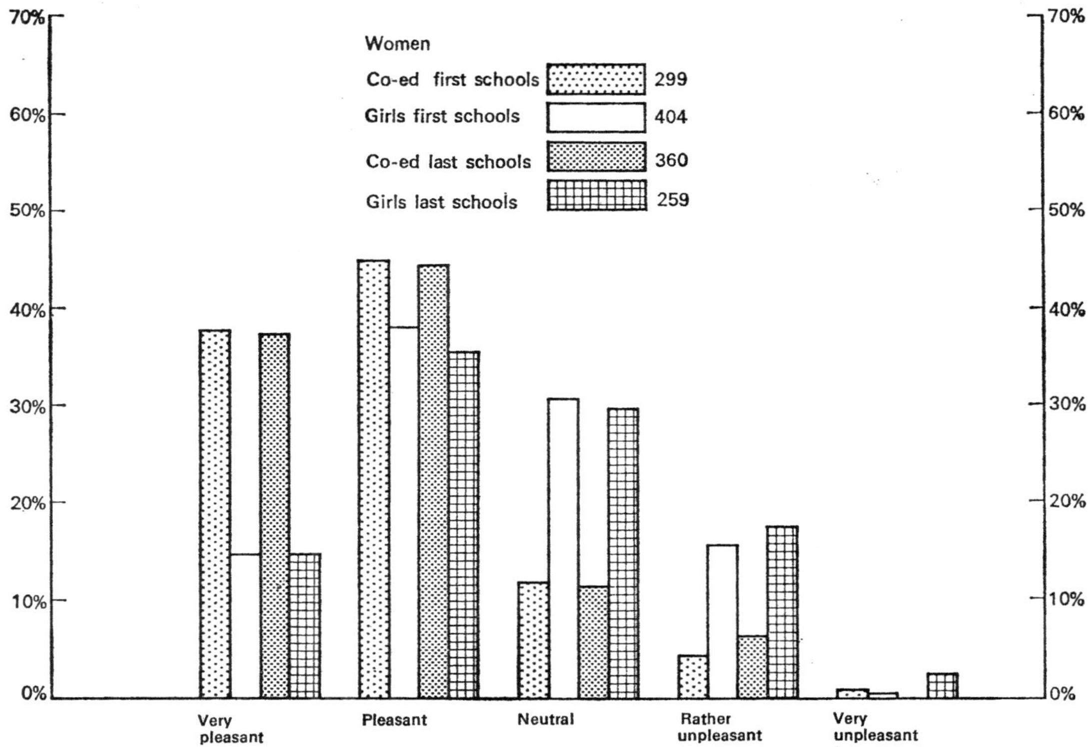

FIGURE 4.1
School atmosphere (women): 'Both schools' survey

The 'Both schools' survey

The next survey to be examined is the 'Both schools' survey (Figure 4.1). Readers will recollect that in order to make sure that the results were not swayed unduly by the order in which the schools were attended (especially as 58 per cent of the women attended a co-educational school last), this influence was removed by classifying the results into ex-pupils who attended a co-educational school first and those who attended a single-sex school first, and similarly for last schools.

Estimates

FEMALE EX-PUPILS

Rather surprisingly the order in which the schools were attended appeared to have little or no influence on the ex-pupils' estimates on the pleasantness of the atmosphere, either in co-educational or girls' schools. Though the estimates for first and last schools of the same type were necessarily given by different sets of people, it is a reasonable presumption that if the influence of the order of the schools attended were strong this would show itself in the results as indeed it does with some items.

The difference in the opinion of the female ex-pupils about the atmosphere in their co-educational compared with their girls' schools is convincingly large; some 37 in every hundred said that the atmosphere in their co-educational school was 'very pleasant' while only 15 in every hundred thought the same about their girls' schools. At the other end of the scale—perhaps the more important end—whereas 1 woman in 18 reported the atmosphere was 'rather unpleasant' or worse at her co-educational school, the corresponding figure for girls' schools was 1 in 6. The analysis increases in significance when it is remembered that it was the same group of women who had attended both types of school.

MALE EX-PUPILS

Through no fault of the researchers the sample of male ex-pupils was much smaller than that of the females, but their results are important because of their experience in both types of school (Figure 4.2).

In Figure 4.2 the influence of the order in which the school were attended is apparent in the estimates for both co-educational and boys' schools. On this occasion the difference between the co-educated men and those from boys' schools is, unexpectedly, greater than that found between the corresponding groups

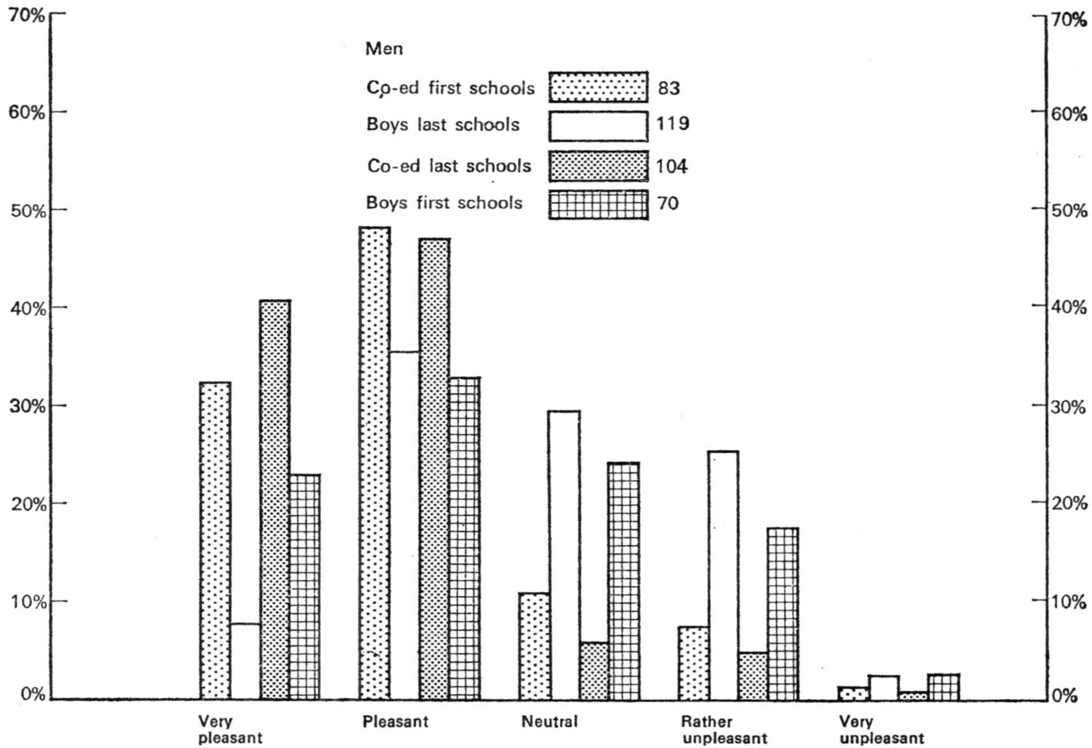

FIGURE 4.2
School atmosphere (men): 'Both schools' survey

of women. Whereas 1 in 3 of the men estimated that the atmosphere of their co-educational schools was 'very pleasant', the figure for the boys' schools was 1 in 8, and while 1 in 14 of them recorded a verdict of 'rather unpleasant' or worse for the co-educational schools, this was the estimate of 1 in 4 of them for their boys' schools. This is a greater difference than that obtained in the other surveys, and its size may be due to the nature of the sample; as all the students had experience of both types of school they were able to compare them, and any change in the atmosphere from one school to the other would be brought sharply to their attention.

Free responses

Though full analyses have been made of the free responses to this question they are not treated in detail because they resemble the answers to the question on happiness; instead, a concise account will be given using the adjectives that constantly recur in the free responses, but illustrating sometimes with direct quotation.

FEMALE EX-PUPILS

Co-educational schools

When writing about the atmosphere of their co-educational schools the women repeatedly brought up three themes. The first clings to the word atmosphere, describing it as 'friendly, happy, relaxed, informal, like a family', or uses the word 'community'. The second is good teacher–pupil relationships, 'friendly, with a spirit of tolerance, the staff enjoying teaching'. Third is 'normal boy–girl relationships'. Other adjectives often used are 'enjoyable, co-operative, balanced, broadness of view, security, humour' and even occasionally 'exciting' and 'enthusiastic'. A few examples are given:

Very pleasant 'The school ran smoothly and was friendly in atmosphere because of this. The atmosphere of co-operation was pervasive. There was no antagonism between staff and pupils.'

Very pleasant 'Discipline was observed by all but not drilled into you. We were not aware we were under rules and regulations.'

Very pleasant 'Teachers and pupils worked together as a team, not against each other, usually. Everyone very friendly.'

Very pleasant 'Boys and girls were learning side by side, as a family almost. This was considered to be perfectly natural and from this stemmed the very pleasant atmosphere.'

Pleasant 'The pupils were treated as far as possible as adults and were given a great deal of freedom which seemed to give a sense of self-discipline.'

Very pleasant 'An all-female community leads to bad feeling arising. Men seem to introduce a practical, logical element which keeps things in perspective.'

Lesser but still important themes are identified as 'individual attention, good discipline, more freedom, co-operation' and 'work enjoyable and interesting', and 'good, lively, enjoyable social life', and 'head good'.

To conclude this section on comments favourable to co-education two quotations are used, one of which is evidently deeply felt:

Very pleasant 'The atmosphere—marvellous school spirit and unity.'

The other discerningly puts its finger on a key quality in a good school:

Pleasant 'Staff seemed to trust pupils, delegate authority and listen to opinions.'

The comments unfavourable to the co-educational schools were few and scattered. Fifteen ex-pupils commented on a poor headmaster, nine on a too-lax discipline, and nine on the school being too impersonal, compared with 175 who praised the atmosphere and 145 who referred to the good pupil–teacher relationship. Mentioned several times were dislike of a large school and dislike of rough lower social class pupils in a comprehensive school.

Girls' schools

The free responses about the girls' schools were more favourable than unfavourable, but, as would be expected from the estimates, the unfavourable aspect was markedly more prominent than in the case of the co-educational schools.

The three chief favourable themes have a strong resemblance to those about the co-educational schools: the friendly, happy, community atmosphere; good pupil–teacher relationship, and good pupil–pupil relationship, but each of these has quite a strong reverse side: strained, tense atmosphere; poor pupil–teacher relationship, and bad pupil–pupil relations ('catty, bickering, spiteful, bitchy'). Less frequently mentioned favourable themes are good discipline and organization, good headmistress, small school, good tradition (13 mentions) and social and extra-curricular life, but all these except good tradition are accompanied by about the same number of opposite responses. Examples of favourable comments are:

Very pleasant 'The teachers and pupils worked with one another in unison—the teachers were highly respected and yet never officious.'

Very pleasant 'Very helpful approach to children's social development—also old with plenty of tradition.'

Very pleasant 'Whole school (apart from odd one or two) was willing to help in all out-of-school activities and there was an air of happiness all the time.'

Very pleasant 'Cultured atmosphere. Fee paying—uniformed etc. Therefore girls of same social status.'

Very pleasant 'It was a community, each working for the good of the whole body.'

Pleasant 'Long established tradition fostered by excellent headmistress.'

The nature of the criticisms is illustrated by the following:

Rather unpleasant 'The small rules and regulations made it difficult to relax, particularly after the co-ed. school.'

Neutral 'Life just went on. Nobody really "fought" but nobody was really friendly. Nobody bothered—it was just a place we attended.'

Rather unhappy 'Tendency for an all-female community to become extremely spiteful and callous.'

Rather unhappy 'Fear was the key word in all discipline.'

Rather unhappy 'The emphasis was on learning for exams, not on preparation for society. It was run on similar lines to a prison, I imagine.'

Rather unhappy 'An unhealthy attitude towards and preoccupation with the opposite sex. They were sex mad and frequently coarse. When I first went there this revolted me.'

MALE EX-PUPILS

Co-educational schools

The reasons given by the male ex-pupils for their high estimates of the pleasantness of the atmosphere in their co-educational schools do not differ fundamentally from those given by the women. Added to the three main themes of friendly family atmosphere, good pupil–teacher relationship and normal social environment (presence of girls) are a few new descriptive words like 'comradeship' and 'genial', with a little more emphasis on 'co-operation', but the similarity is marked. This can be seen in the illustrations:

Very pleasant 'Everything seemed natural, relaxed, complete. The staff and pupil morale was very high indeed.'

Very pleasant 'Pupils and teachers mixed on the same level and pupils admired the teachers for this.'

Pleasant 'Co-operation between boys, girls and teachers.' (Am.)

Very pleasant 'The different sexes treated each other with respect and there was a pleasing atmosphere of co-operation.'

Pleasant 'General ease and relaxed atmosphere. No continual hounding.'

Again, like the women's, the men's comments adverse to co-education were few and widely scattered, the biggest contributions being four complaints about over-lax discipline and three about harsh or restrictive discipline. Prominent, on this small scale, were complaints about 'amalgamated' schools; for example:

Rather unhappy 'Many of the students thought that with the school being twice as big they could do less work and break more rules and get away with it. They did.' (Am.)

Neutral 'There seemed to be some conflict on ideas of punishment between the old members of the staff of the Boys' Grammar School and the members of the staff of the Girls' High School.' (Am.)

Boys' schools

For the boys' schools the principal favourable themes were reduced to two, namely 'friendly community' and 'good pupil–teacher relations', but the latter was opposed by an equal number of comments which complained about the poor pupil–teacher relations and the harsh, restrictive and autocratic discipline. The remainder of the comments, both favourable and unfavourable, were again very diverse in content, the most numerous class being nine protests about bullying. Typical comments were:

FAVOURABLE

Pleasant 'We were all "mates" or comrades. There was plenty of brotherhood which I haven't experienced since.'

Pleasant 'Perhaps just the communal growing up of all the lads together.'

Pleasant 'Everyone knew their place. Prefects were respected and addressed as "Sir". A great deal of tradition was present in the school. It is obviously very old.'

Pleasant 'The headmaster really had the right idea and brought the tone of the school to a high state from nothing.'

Pleasant 'The staff, even if they were a little strict, always made sure that the pupils knew where they stood.'

UNFAVOURABLE

Very unhappy 'Autocratic discipline allowing no freedom of movement or thought. All pupils were finally of the same type.' (Boarding)

Rather unhappy 'I was scared stiff; glad to get home. Staff seemed hard, demanding and bossy.'

Rather unhappy 'There always appeared to be violence of one sort or another in the school.'

Neutral 'Rather unhealthy attitude towards sex.'

Rather unhappy 'Life was so formal that school resembled the army.'

Very unhappy 'A boy of 10 is likely to be affected by very harsh treatment. I've never forgotten this and it seems to have shown itself in stronger forms than it perhaps ought.' (Boarding)

The next set of results to be presented are those from the Schools project, where an attempt was made to tap the experience of some 2,000 boys and girls in grammar schools.

The Schools project

In the Schools project the question on atmosphere was not included in the 1964 administration, but was given in 1966. The results are in Tables 4.3 and 4.4.

The gap shown in Tables 4.3 and 4.4 between the co-educational school estimates and those of the single-sex schools is much narrower than in the previous surveys. This trend is consistent for all questions common to these enquiries. The differences are, however, all in favour of the co-educational schools, as before, except for the two groups of girls aged 13 plus, where there is virtual equality. (In the following section the girls aged 13 plus in

TABLE 4.3 *Pleasantness of school atmosphere*

Schools project (girls aged 13 plus and 17 plus)

	Replies from girls aged 13 plus in				Replies from girls aged 17 plus in			
	Co-educational schools		Girls' schools		Co-educational schools		Girls' schools	
	N	%	N	%	N	%	N	%
Very pleasant	34	15·8	40	18·8	20	17·4	11	9·2
Pleasant	131	60·9	119	55·9	76	66·1	71	59·2
Neutral	43	20·0	44	20·6	17	14·8	28	23·3
Rather unpleasant	6	2·8	9	4·2	2	1·7	10	8·3
Very unpleasant	1	0·5	1	0·5	0	0	0	0
Totals	215	100	213	100	115	100	120	100

NOTE: At the age of 13 there is virtually no difference between the groups. The co-educated girls aged 17 find the atmosphere more pleasant (statistically significant at the ·025 level).

TABLE 4.4 *Pleasantness of school atmosphere*

Schools project (boys aged 13 plus and 17 plus)

	Replies from boys aged 13 plus in				Replies from boys aged 17 plus in			
	Co-educational schools		Boys' schools		Co-educational schools		Boys' schools	
	N	%	N	%	N	%	N	%
Very pleasant	29	12·9	16	7·4	17	12·8	15	10·9
Pleasant	117	52·0	117	54·4	95	71·4	92	67·2
Neutral	65	28·9	60	27·9	18	13·5	21	15·3
Rather unpleasant	13	5·8	19	8·8	3	2·3	9	6·6
Very unpleasant	1	0·4	3	1·4	0	0	0	0
Totals	225	100	215	100	133	100	137	100

NOTE: The difference at age 13 is almost statistically significant.

the much larger 'Check' sample, attending the same schools as those of the Schools project, yielded a statistically significant difference in favour of co-education, though even this difference was smaller than previously.) The advantage of the co-educational schools in the group of boys aged 13 plus, while fairly substantial, was not quite statistically significant. Only in one case did the differences reach this level, that in favour of the co-educated girls aged 17 plus, where it was significant beyond the ·025 probability.

The 'Check' sample

Over 1,100 girls aged 13 in grammar schools answered the 'Check' questionnaire, including the question on atmosphere. The results are in Table 4.5.

TABLE 4.5 *Pleasantness of school atmosphere*

'Check' sample

Estimates of school atmosphere	Replies from girls aged 13 plus in			
	Co-educational schools		Girls' schools	
	N	%	N	%
Very pleasant	91	20·3	92	13·7
Pleasant	255	56·8	373	55·5
Neutral	94	20·9	186	27·6
Rather unpleasant	7	1·6	21	3·1
Very unpleasant	2	0·4	1	0·1
Totals	449	100	673	100

NOTE: The difference between the samples from co-educational and girls' schools is significant beyond the ·01 level.

In this sample the girls from the co-educational schools gave more favourable estimates for their school atmosphere than did those from girls' schools. The difference is not as large as that found in the ex-pupil surveys, particularly in those where the ex-pupils had attended both types of school. The reason for the narrowing of the gap may be the difference in age or the schoolgirls' lack of experience of the other type of school. There was no time in this instance for pupils to write free responses.

Conclusion

In all groups to which this question was put, the co-educational schools were found to have a pleasanter atmosphere, except in one case where there was equality. This does not mean that in all co-educational schools the atmosphere is better than that in all single-sex schools, because other powerful forces affect the situation, such as the quality of the head and staff, the nature of the school recruitment area, and to a lesser extent the type of buildings. Hence there are co-educational schools with a good atmosphere and others with a bad one, and similarly for single-sex schools. We can say, however, that a school being co-educational increases the likelihood that pupils and ex-pupils will find the atmosphere pleasant. As we saw at the beginning of this chapter, this is not the only criterion which should be used for judging the success of a school, but it is an important one.

5

Inter-pupil relationship

One of the powerful forces determining whether pupils are happy at school and whether the school atmosphere is pleasant is the relationship between the pupils themselves, which this chapter begins to explore. As the Second College survey contained nothing directly on this topic the first research to be examined is in the 'Both schools' survey. The central question was 'Within your co-educational/single-sex school did you find it easy or difficult to make friends?' Provision was made also for a free response.

The making of friends

'BOTH SCHOOLS' SURVEY

Female ex-pupils

The results of the girls are treated first (Table 5.1).

TABLE 5.1 *The making of friends*

Both schools' survey (women)

	Replies about first school attended				Replies about last school attended			
	Co-educational		Girls'		Co-educational		Girls'	
	N	%	N	%	N	%	N	%
Very easy	126	42·0	111	27·4	163	45·3	85	32·7
Fairly easy	95	31·8	155	38·3	119	33·1	89	34·2
Neither easy nor difficult	51	17·1	74	18·3	43	11·9	41	15·1
A little difficult	22	7·4	56	13·8	28	7·8	37	14·8
Very difficult	5	1·7	9	2·2	7	1·9	8	3·2
Totals	299	100	405	100	360	100	260	100

NOTE: The difference between the first co-educational and first girls' schools is significant beyond the ·001 level and for last schools beyond the ·01 level.

The results in Table 5.1 show that these 620 women were strongly of the opinion that it was easier to make friends in the co-educational than in the girls' school. If the 'first schools' had not been separated from the 'last schools' it might have been thought that this hidden variable could have caused the difference, but the same result is obtained when co-educational schools which were attended first are opposed to girls' schools attended first, and similarly for 'last schools'. Moreover, the 'order of school' effect seems to be less strong than expected, at least for this topic.

The comments are not as interesting in their distinction between the two types of school as they have often been with other topics; their treatment is therefore curtailed, and 'first' and 'last' schools are taken together.

Easily the most numerous statements about the co-educational schools were those which came rather loosely under the heading 'school atmosphere conducive to easy natural relationship' (67). A long way behind came 'organization of school helped to foster friendship' (25), 'easy natural relationship between boys and girls' (19), 'process aided by common interests, such as sports' (16), 'all friends together from primary school' (14), 'the pleasantness of heterosexual groups in the upper school' (12) and 'compared favourably with girls' schools' (11). Rather apart from the rest were the responses 'always found it easy to make friends' (21).

By far the most serious difficulty encountered in making friends was 'entering school late' (33), with the somewhat related 'pupils in cliques and difficult to join' (14), while some girls, coming from a girls' school, had to overcome a shyness with boys (18). There remained a group which admitted that personally they had difficulty in making friends (18). A few illustrations give a little more light:

Fairly easy 'At first I found it difficult but once I had overcome my shyness about boys I seemed to flourish.'

Fairly easy 'It was difficult where the groups were tightly knit—a new person was considered queer.'

Very easy 'To share a form room and have mixed lessons inevitably ensures easier conversation with the opposite sex.'

Very easy 'Not as petty as single-sex schools.'

Fairly easy 'Easier with boys than girls.'

Very easy 'Pupils in a co-educational school are more friendly towards each other than in a single-sex school where groups tend to form who dislike each other.'

Fairly easy 'I think because boys and girls were together getting in with the girls was better—they tended to be less "catty" than those in the single-sex school.'

Very easy 'At first one gets romantic ideas towards the boys but this soon evaporates as the newness of the idea of a co-educational school wears off and you are soon all good friends.'

Very easy 'The girls were very friendly when I first went there and through them I got to know the boys and lost the shyness of them I had acquired at single-sex schools.'

Very easy 'After having been to about 14 schools I found when I first went to the co-ed. at the age of 13 I made friends far easier than in any other school.'

The suspicion which people (even children) have at first of those who are somewhat different is shown by:

A little difficult 'I spoke with a different accent coming from 8 years in Hertfordshire and the children (Lancs.) would laugh at first. After a while I made friends with some children.'

A little difficult 'I was an English girl in a Scottish school.'

Fairly easy 'I did not [make friends] at first because I went from England to Wales and the pupils seemed to resent my nationality. Later I found it easier.'

Pupils who move from one part of the country, therefore, may have to contend with difficulties arising from accent and nationality, as well as those arising from being a latecomer trying to join rings of already established friends, and girls could be made very unhappy in this way.

The same types of comments were made about the girls' schools, but as would be expected from the estimates the proportion of those favourable was reduced. The most numerous group came, as before, under the general heading 'school atmosphere conducive to easy natural relationship' (29), and 15 under the heading 'tie over from primary school', while 12 said friendship was easy 'because they were all new together'. As with the co-educational schools, for some ex-pupils friendships grew out of common interests (10), and there were 10 students who always found making friends easy.

The principal comments about the difficulties in their girls' schools, as in their co-educational schools, were that it was difficult to make friends if one entered the school late (24) and that it was hard to break into the established cliques of girls (35), but the latter is here more prominent. Eleven women confessed to having personal difficulties in making friends. Minor factors mentioned were social class bias (3) and that the girls discriminated against people who were not identical to themselves (10). The comments ranged from such remarks as:

A little difficult 'There tended to be "cliques" of friends that were difficult to enter. I spent a very bewildering and uneasy few years in this school'

to the ex-pupil who found it 'very easy' and wrote, 'It seemed to be an unwritten rule that it was everyone's duty to make all welcome.' In spite of the estimates and the proportion of comments in favour of the co-educational schools, there were one or two informative and slightly amusing comments showing an influence in the opposite direction; for example:

Very easy 'Because there were no boys to distract them—firmer and more secure friendships were made with girls.'

Very easy 'Girls together and boys together is the best situation in a school where you are rubbing shoulders for the main part of your life. Hatred arises in a co-ed. school if one girl is favoured by a particularly charming young male.'

Interesting comments are the following, for different reasons:

Very difficult 'Very easy at first, then gradually as the atmosphere got me down and the other people conformed to the desired "image" very very difficult. I eventually had no friends at all. Some days the only people who spoke to me were the teachers.'

A little difficult 'This was partly due to the influence of my father who allowed me no opinions or ideas of my own. At school I found difficulty in communication.'

Male ex-pupils

The 172 male ex-pupils were in this instance of very similar mind to the women. They considered it had been much easier to make friends in their co-educational than in their boys' schools. As the order in which the schools were attended had a powerful influence in the boys' schools and a slight one in the co-educational, it being easier in schools attended last, this variable was held constant, but in both first and last schools the co-educational schools had a highly significant advantage (Table 5.2).

From this Table one can see that, whereas almost half of the men said that it had been very easy to make friends in their co-educational schools, only a quarter said the same for their boys' schools. At the other end of the scale the numbers finding it

TABLE 5.2 *The making of friends*

'Both schools' survey (men)

Estimates of ease or difficulty in making friends at school	Replies about first school attended				Replies about last school attended			
	Co-educational		Boys'		Co-educational		Boys'	
	N	%	N	%	N	%	N	%
Very easy	37	44·6	28	23·5	51	49·0	21	30·0
Fairly easy	30	36·2	31	26·1	35	33·7	26	37·1
Neither easy nor difficult	9	10·8	33	27·7	13	12·5	16	22·9
A little difficult	5	6·0	25	21·0	3	2·9	5	7·1
Very difficult	2	2·4	2	1·7	2	1·9	2	2·9
Totals	83	100	119	100	104	100	70	100

NOTE: The difference between the first co-educational and first boys' schools is significant beyond the ·001 level and for last schools beyond the ·05 level.

'fairly difficult', or worse, to make friends, were three times as numerous for the boys' schools as for the co-educational.

The free responses of the men were inevitably less numerous than those of the women, numbering only 89 about the co-educational schools and 67 about the boys' schools. When classified they split into many small categories, the only sizeable group being that which said the school atmosphere in the co-educational school was conducive to easy natural relationship (18), apart from those in both schools who maintained that they personally always found it easy to make friends. The next most important groups, favourable or unfavourable, were those who found friends through common interests (12 in the boys' schools), and those who found difficulty because of cliques or gangs (8 in the boys' schools and 2 in the co-educational). Five comments said it was easier to make friends in the co-educational school, with none saying the opposite. These low numbers are not of course reliable, but are given because we are more concerned with the total effect of all the research than with any small portion in itself. Nothing new would be added by quoting from the free responses, so they are omitted.

Before passing on to the next attempt to explore (in an admittedly superficial way) the relationship between pupils, it should be said that this question on making friends would have been improved if it had been accompanied by a simple definition of what was meant, i.e. making close friends or just friends in general. The lack of greater precision, however, presumably had the same effect on the two groups and was not serious enough to invalidate the findings, though interpretation of these is a little more difficult. In any case the findings do not depend on the one question, but on a number that are related. The one to be considered next was asked in the Schools project.

The friendliness of pupils

THE SCHOOLS AND 'CHECK' QUESTIONNAIRES

These questionnaires included the question, 'Do you find other pupils, in general, Very friendly/Friendly/Indifferent/Unfriendly/Very unfriendly?' Respondents were asked to comment on the estimate they chose. The results of the girls are taken first.

Girls' estimates

This questionnaire was administered in 1966 only, in 36 grammar schools to girls aged 13 plus and 17 plus. The results are not tabulated because they show a clear equality at 17 plus and only the slenderest of advantages to the girls' schools at 13 plus, far below statistical significance.[1] Of some 335 pupils of both ages, there were merely two in each type of school who found their fellow pupils to be unfriendly or very unfriendly.

In the 'Check' survey (1,122 girls) the superiority of the co-educational schools which has been reported for happiness and atmosphere was not continued, the result of the Schools project for 'friendship' being repeated, and the difference again being far from statistical significance. Nearly 4 in 10 girls of both types thought their fellow-pupils 'very friendly', and more than half thought them 'friendly'; the only difference was that 1.4 per cent more of the pupils in girls' schools estimated 'friendly', leaving none in the 'unfriendly' or 'very unfriendly' categories, in which the co-educational schools had 1.5 per cent. This is one of the few occasions where the gap in favour of the co-educational schools, which always narrows in the Schools and related 'Check' surveys, closes and moves minimally in the opposite direction.

Boys' estimates (Schools project, 1966)

The boys' results were similarly inconclusive. At age 13 plus the boys' schools had a slight advantage which could have been a

[1] Chi-square = 1·284 for 3 degrees of freedom.

chance effect,[1] and at age 17 plus the co-educational schools had a bigger advantage which was nearer to statistical significance.[2] This question was not included in the 1964 testing. Discussion is postponed until the picture can be seen as a whole.

Pupils were given the opportunity to comment in the Schools project question, but as the comments add nothing to our knowledge they are not used.

Spitefulness

'BOTH SCHOOLS' QUESTIONNAIRES

The female ex-pupils of the 'Both schools' survey were asked two other questions which are related to 'the friendliness of pupils'. One of these was, 'Do you think that the girls in your form, judged

FIGURE 5.1 *Spitefulness (girls): 'Both schools' survey*

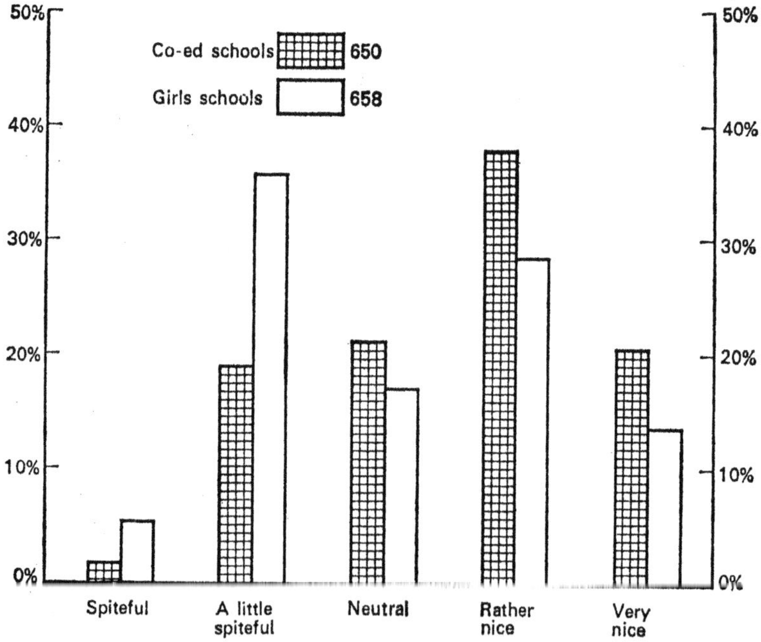

as a whole, were 'Spiteful/A little spiteful/Neutral/Rather nice/ Very nice?' They were also asked to comment on their estimates, which are given in Figure 5.1. As there are no clear social class differences these classes are merged, and similarly for first and

[1] Chi-square = 4·012 for 3 degrees of freedom.
[2] Chi-square = 5·278 for 3 degrees of freedom.

last schools, the difference between last schools (highly significant) being only a little less than that between first schools.

The figures speak for themselves, the respondents estimating twice the amount of 'spitefulness' in their girls' schools as in their co-educational, but most of it not extreme. The free responses are not sufficiently interesting to tabulate, but the principal aspects are summarized. For both the co-educational and girls' schools the proportion of comments complaining of spitefulness was as expected from the estimates. Apparently there are conflicting forces at work. On the one hand the girls tend to refrain from spitefulness in front of boys because boys laugh at them; on the other, girls are sometimes spiteful in a mixed school when they quarrel over a boy-friend, though several free responses mention this in girls' schools also. One of the themes was that a certain amount of spitefulness was to be expected in all-girl groups; some of the individuals confessed to indulging in it themselves! One said that girls are spiteful at heart! A theme which appeared only about the girls' schools (merely three mentions) was 'the malicious teasing of individuals' including 'ganging up on one girl' in a boarding school. Only a few quotations are given:

Co-educational schools

'Some were spiteful but the boys in the class laughed at them, so they were not spiteful in public.'

'Boys were present and would have laughed had the usual spitefulness present among girls been shown.'

'*Very nice* because of the presence of boys. All-girls breeds spitefulness—but a mixture breeds thoughtfulness.'

'When I had a boy-friend before my other girl-friends they were very spiteful towards me but when they had their own boy-friends there was little or no friction.'

A little spiteful 'This was because we had always been together and a spiteful atmosphere had prevailed in the girls' school.' (Am.)

'Any girls getting together in a group are a little spiteful so it cannot be avoided at times when one-sex lessons take place, e.g. gym, or domestic science.'

' "Cat-sessions" between the girls fighting over "best" friends.'

Girls' schools

'Some girls could be very spiteful indeed. I found this only seemed to happen in all-girls schools.'

'Most girls tend to be spiteful if they have to work or live together all the time. It is one of the chief interests.'

'A defect such as wearing national health glasses or being fat—was made fun of often in a very spiteful way. Even I took part in this type of teasing of people.'

'There was a definite split—the big "nobs" and the underdogs.' (Boarding)

'Particularly about other girls' boy-friends.'

'No cattiness because no boys were present.'

We pass on to the second question which was about quarrelling.

Quarrelling

This question was, 'Did the other girls in your form quarrel Very often/Fairly often/Sometimes/Seldom/Never?' The results closely resemble those obtained from the question on spitefulness, as will be seen in Table 5.3.

TABLE 5.3 *Quarrelling (girls)*

'Both schools' survey

Estimates of frequency of quarrelling	Replies about schools attended			
	Co-educational		Girls'	
	N	%	N	%
Very often	10	1·5	37	5·6
Fairly often	61	9·3	148	22·4
Sometimes	324	49·7	333	50·2
Seldom	233	35·7	135	20·4
Never	25	3·8	9	1·4
Totals	653	100	662	100

NOTE: The difference between the co-educational and girls' schools is statistically significant beyond the ·001 level. This is also true if 'first' and 'last' schools are taken separately.

In Table 5.3 well over a quarter of the respondents estimated that quarrels occurred 'often' or 'very often' in their girls' school, and an eighth in their co-educational school. In both cases a large group estimated 'seldom' or 'never', being over 70 per cent about the co-educational schools and 44 per cent about the girls' schools. It could be argued that this difference might be caused by the smallness of the number of girls in co-educational classes, there being, as it were, only half a class to quarrel with, as the girls would rarely quarrel with the boys. If this argument has any force—and the effect is problematic—it would seem to admit that mixed classes result in less quarrelling, thus producing a better atmosphere. This does not, of itself, ensure that mixed classes are better—many other factors would need to be examined before such a pronouncement could be made.

6

Bullying and related aspects

The central theme of this chapter is bullying by boys, and similar behaviour—usually less physical—by girls. Such conduct results in the weaker pupils having a miserable time, particularly in a boarding school, from which the unfortunate boys and girls have no escape, day or night; schools in which this conduct is rife can scarcely be called good schools. It was therefore thought useful to investigate whether the presence of girls in a school toned down such conduct on the part of the boys, and similarly for the influence of boys on girls, in comparison with conduct in single-sex schools. A variable which necessarily has great influence is the age of the pupils, and another might be parental occupational class. Variation between individuals, between heads of schools and between staffs, whether within single-sex or mixed schools, will be countered by the use of a large enough number of pupils and of schools.

The question on bullying was first asked in the 'Both schools' survey, and the nature of the topic makes it perhaps more relevant than usual to remind readers that these ex-pupils were all intending teachers and are not representative of all types of pupil. This, however, should not vitiate the comparison between the two types of school. On this occasion the boys are taken first.

Male ex-pupils

BULLYING

The male ex-pupils were asked, with reference to their co-educational school and later to their boys' school, 'Would you say bullying by boys occurred, Very frequently/Frequently/Not so frequently/Infrequently/Not at all?' For each school they were asked to make a comment. The results are in Figure 6.1

There is no doubt about the result: whereas almost half of these ex-pupils of boys' schools estimated that bullying in them was 'frequent' or 'very frequent', this was reduced to little more than one-fifth when they estimated for their co-educational schools.

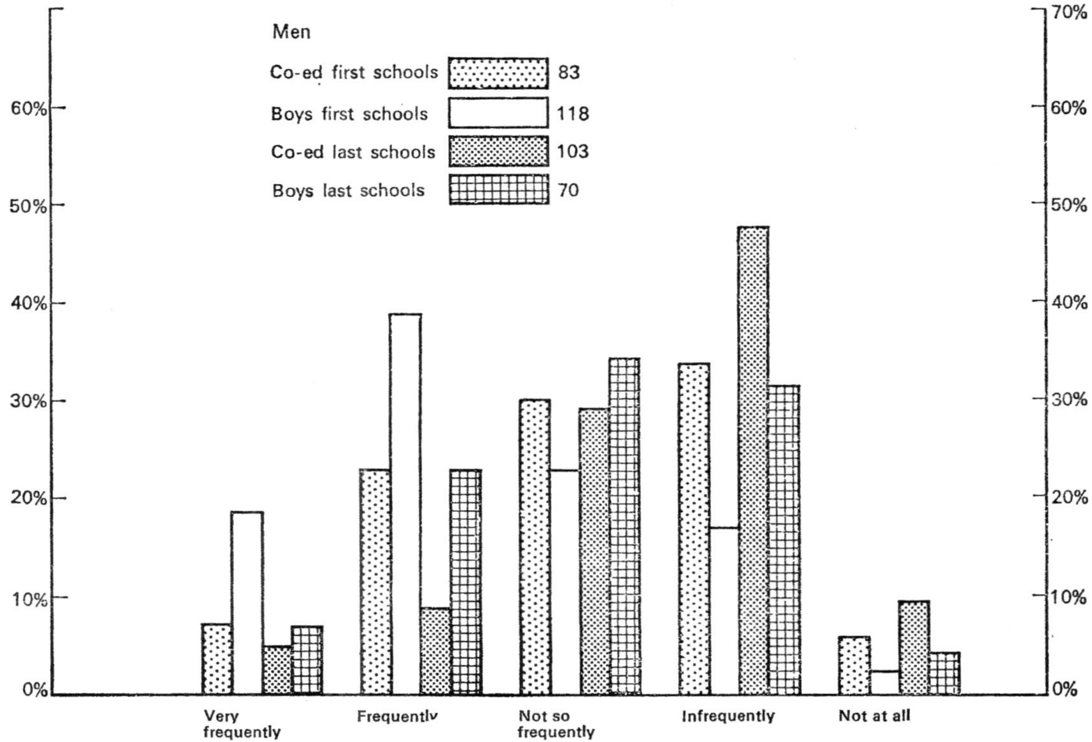

FIGURE 6.1
Incidence of bullying (boys): 'Both schools' survey

Considering first and last schools, the difference between the co-educational and boys' schools is noticeably not as great for last schools as for first, though still of statistical significance, and there is not as much change from co-educational schools attended first to those attended last as there is in the case of the boys' schools; yet in both cases bullying decreases in the senior school. This could, of course, be interpreted to signify that the seniors are big enough to look after themselves and are likely to be the bullies rather than the bullied. This factor would certainly have an influence in spite of the question asking in effect whether the respondents knew about any bullying in general. The free responses in Table 6.1 are especially interesting.

The free responses paint the same picture as the estimates while adding interpretative detail. Additional points of interest are the frequent prevention of bullying, in both types of school, by staff, prefects and pupils themselves, and the stronger support in co-educational schools for the reply that bullying was not a feature of the school because of the friendly atmosphere and the pervading sense of comradeship. In the co-educational school we see opposing forces caused by the presence of girls—bullying to show off in front of them, and restraint because they were there. Rather more space than in recent chapters will be devoted to quotations, as these are illustrative of important differences between boys' and co-educational schools. To preserve objectivity the proportion of favourable to unfavourable quotations given is the same as that in the estimates, considering 'very frequently' and 'frequently' as unfavourable, and 'infrequently' and 'not at all' as favourable.

Co-educational schools

FAVOURABLE 'The school's friendly atmosphere was generally reflected in the attitude of the boys to one another.'

'I found that because of the presence of girls they had much better things to do in their break times.'

'Not at all. This was mainly due to the presence of girls.'

'If at all when girls were not present, which was rare.'

'There was very little of this done due to the strict control of prefects, and if necessary the formation of gangs to sort bullies out either in school or out of school.'

'Mainly any bullying was by a small percentage of prefects. The girls would scorn any boy whom they heard was a bully. This seemed to be a very effective deterrent.'

TABLE 6.1 *Free responses about bullying (boys)*
'Both schools' survey

Estimate	Categories of comments	Co-educational school	Boys' school
Very frequently and Frequently	by individuals (e.g. to assert masculinity)	13	16
	by group	7	5
	to juniors	7	17
	among juniors	5	6
	to own age group	1	
	not restricted by school/staff	2	4
	resisted by group of boys	3	4
	result of environment	1	3
	through traditional rituals		5
	very frequently and frequently		9
	more at single-sex than co-ed.		4
Total		39	73
Not so frequently	by individuals (to assert masculinity)		5
	by individuals—to impress	13	
	by individuals—to impress girls	2	
	by group	1	2
	resisted by boys	3	4
	controlled by staff/prefects	12	5
	restrained by presence of girls	7	
	result of friendly atmosphere	8	
	through traditional fagging		3
	more in single-sex than co-ed.		4
	less in single-sex than co-ed.		1
	more in juniors than seniors		3
	seniors bullying juniors		6
	not so frequently		9
Total		46	42
Infrequently or Not at all	controlled by staff (including through prefects)	23	14
	not a feature of the school	14	3
	seniors asserting position	6	4
	mainly in lower forms		4
	only through traditional rituals	3	
	restrained by presence of girls	13	
	occasionally (impress girls)	7	
	controlled by sense of maturity	6	
	pervading sense of comradeship	4	
	none except out of school	2	
	bullying exceptional trait of particular year	1	
	infrequently		16
Totals		79	41

Bullying and related aspects

UNFAVOURABLE 'I think that boys from rough homes were the bullies and went in gangs. But every day there was a fight or a quarrel.'

'The secondary modern boys would bully weaker first years excessively. Otherwise there was little bullying.'

'An air of bravado often overcame some in the presence of girls and [they] wanted to show off. These, however, were disliked by both sexes.'

Boys' schools

Here the same ratio of quotations (1 in 13) is used as for the co-educational schools.

FAVOURABLE 'Quite a few fights, but a sense of fairness prevailed—an older boy who bullied was disliked by his own age group.'

'The bullying was natural as it always is with boys. But it was not excessive.'

'Boys took it out on themselves during organized games, etc; it was difficult to fight due to prefects.'

UNFAVOURABLE 'You were put in the coal-hole and thumped. The coal-hole was some steps leading to the boiler-house.'

'Frequently. Intimidation was always occurring but seldom was physical force used. The senior boys used the juniors for their own needs—despicable.' (Boarding)

'A kind of outlet for built-up tensions in the classroom—and this was *real* bullying.'

'With no girls around there were no niceties to watch or manners to consider.'

'This was the dominant feature of the school social life.'

The 'direct comparison' technique is now used again, whereby *all* free responses which compare the two types of school are quoted.

Direct Comparisons

FAVOURABLE TO CO-EDUCATION 'There was no fagging of the first years and bullying was punished severely. Far more normal relationship with newcomers was established.'

'There was more bullying than in the co-ed. school.'

'Family atmosphere curbed this. Mixed school had calming effect. Head very strict on this behaviour.'

'From a prefect's point of view I had to stop far less fights here than at my other school.'

'Frequently [in boys' school] that is compared with my other school. Gang warfare at one time was quite a problem and the bullying of individuals quite common.'

'I never recall any large amount of bullying as I experienced it in a single-sex school.'

'Bullying was kept in check by the prefects and it decreased when the school went co-educational.'

'More bullying than at co-ed. school.'

'More bullying than in co-ed. school. There seemed to be a hard core of "teds". Roughness and toughness were admired among boys far more than in co-ed. establishment.'

FAVOURABLE TO BOYS' SCHOOLS 'The older boys when I was younger and the school co-ed., seemed to be more aggressive than we were when I was older and the school single-sex.'

'That bullying which occurred was caused by the notorious dinner queue which older and bigger boys pushed into. Apart from this for practical reasons there was very little superficial bullying as in my mixed school where it was done for fun.'

'This practice seemed to die out after the division of the school. Young boys went readily to see staff so it did not pay to bully.'

'To younger pupils from adolescents. Not as much as co-educational school, less showing off.'

'There was less bullying than in the co-ed. school.'

PREFECTS OFFICIOUS

Pupils were asked to answer another item which sometimes could be related to bullying, namely, 'Do you agree or disagree with the following statement about your co-educational school? "The prefects were officious." Agree strongly/Agree/Doubtful/Disagree/Disagree strongly.' The same question was asked about the girls' schools. It is likely that the wording of the statement suggests agreement, and this tendency would be reinforced by the position of 'Agree strongly' at the start of the continuum, but this matters little as the study is primarily concerned with comparing single-sex and co-educational schools, and the effect would be much the same for each group. The data from the estimates are in Table 6.2; there was no opportunity for free responses.

TABLE 6.2 *Prefects officious (boys)*

'Both schools' survey

Estimates about prefects officious	Replies about first school attended				Replies about last school attended			
	Co-ed.		Boys'		Co-ed.		Boys'	
	N	%	N	%	N	%	N	%
Agree strongly	9	11·0	37	31·6	7	6·9	8	11·3
Agree	29	35·3	38	32·5	18	17·8	26	36·6
Doubtful	14	17·1	31	26·5	22	21·8	12	16·9
Disagree	24	29·3	9	7·7	39	38·6	22	31·0
Disagree strongly	6	7·3	2	1·7	15	14·9	3	4·2
Totals	82	100	117	100	101	100	71	100

NOTE: The difference between the first co-educational schools and the first boys' schools is significant beyond the ·001 level and that between last schools is significant beyond the ·025 level.

Table 6.2 shows in this instance the great effect of the order in which the schools were attended, the seniors of the schools naturally finding the prefects less officious than when they themselves were juniors. Some of the seniors would of course have been prefects themselves and would be eager to decry any charge of officiousness. Because of this big difference between first and last schools the main comparison between co-educational and boys' schools takes first and last separately, and finds the difference to be statistically highly significant for first schools and significant for last schools. (As more of the students finished in co-educational schools the process of combining first and last schools could sometimes produce an invalid result.)

Some 64 per cent of the students agreed that when they were in their boys' schools as juniors their prefects were officious (combining 'agree strongly' with 'agree'); the corresponding percentage for co-educational schools was 46, almost all of the difference being on 'agree strongly'. When the schools compared are those in which students finished last the relevant percentages are 48 and 25. Unfortunately there was not sufficient time at the researchers' disposal to allow them to ask the students for free responses to this question; this lack of data will become evident during the discussion section.

Female ex-pupils

BULLYING ('Both schools' survey)

The women ex-students in the 'Both schools' sample also answered the question on bullying, the wording being: 'In your co-educational school would you say bullying of girls by girls occurred, Not at all/Infrequently/Not so frequently/Frequently/Very frequently?' with the phrase 'single-sex school' substituted for 'co-educational' in the relevant section. The verdict of the students can be seen in Table 6.3.

TABLE 6.3 *Bullying of girls*

'Both schools' survey

Estimates about bullying of girls	Replies about first school attended				Replies about last school attended			
	Co-educational		Girls'		Co-educational		Girls'	
	N	%	N	%	N	%	N	%
Not at all	85	30·9	62	16·5	137	41·5	42	17·5
Infrequently	124	45·1	151	40·3	147	44·6	113	47·1
Not so frequently	51	18·5	83	22·1	28	8·5	43	17·9
Frequently	14	5·1	70	18·7	16	4·8	40	16·7
Very frequently	1	0·4	9	2·4	2	0·6	2	0·8
Totals	275	100	375	100	330	100	240	100

NOTE: The differences between co-educational and girls' schools both for first schools and last schools are statistically significant beyond the ·001 level.

Perhaps the most important feature of Table 6.3 is that in schools attended first, some 1 in 5 of the students thought that bullying was 'frequent' or 'very frequent' in their girls' schools and 1 in 18 in their co-educational schools: in schools attended last the corresponding figures are approximately 1 in 6 and, again, about 1 in 18, both differences being statistically highly significant.

The free responses to this question were not analysed for the women, as they would tend to be duplicates of the replies to the next question on 'made life unpleasant'. Because of its near relationship to bullying this question is here taken before the one on the officiousness of prefects. It was not put to the boys.

'MADE LIFE UNPLEASANT'

The wording of the question was, 'In your co-educational school would you say that a group or groups of the girls "made life unpleasant" for some girls (or girl), Very frequently/Frequently/Not so frequently/Infrequently/Not at all?' The students' estimates are given in Table 6.4.

TABLE 6.4 *Making life unpleasant* (*girls*)

'Both schools' survey

Estimates about making life unpleasant	Replies about first school attended				Replies about last school attended			
	Co-educational		Girls'		Co-educational		Girls'	
	N	%	N	%	N	%	N	%
Very frequently	9	3·1	20	5·0	6	1·7	12	4·7
Frequently	34	11·6	105	26·0	39	11·0	51	19·9
Not so frequently	68	23·3	114	28·3	58	16·3	66	25·8
Infrequently	140	48·0	128	31·8	171	48·2	94	36·7
Not at all	41	14·0	36	8·9	81	22·8	33	12·9
Totals	292	100	403	100	355	100	256	100

NOTE: The differences between co-educational and girls' schools for first and last school are significant well beyond the ·001 level.

In Table 6.4 we see that there was some improvement from 'first' to 'last' school for both the co-educational and the girls' schools. The principal feature, however, is the decidedly lower estimates of the incidence of 'making life unpleasant' for co-educational schools compared with girls' schools, a difference which is highly significant statistically. More insight into these differences is obtained by the study of the free responses (Table 6.5).

In Table 6.5 the comments from ex-pupils who had been seniors in a school (last schools) were amalgamated with those who had been juniors in the same type of school, because there was (surprisingly) insufficient difference between the replies about 'first' and 'last' schools to justify their separate treatment. The data fully confirm the trends in the two previous tables of estimates —that these ex-pupils state that there was less unpleasantness

TABLE 6.5 *Girls 'made life unpleasant' (free responses)*
'Both schools' survey

Estimate	Comment	Co-educational schools	Girls' schools
Not at all and Infrequently	not at all (non-specific)	48	31
	infrequently (non-specific)	134	58
	because of friendly atmosphere, close contact	27	19
	because other girls would stop it	6	5
	only petty things; just quarrels	21	15
	groups kept to themselves	3	5
	occasional sending to Coventry		3
	because no boys present		2
	jealousy over boy	14	3
	presence of boys prevented it	14	
	more than in co-ed. school		2
	jealousy over exam. results	2	
	One girl 'picked on' because different	30	22
	mostly in lower school	13	15
	between groups	8	8
	by 'bossy', by boy-mad girls, by boy haters	1	4
	others	8	11
Totals		329	203
Not so frequently	not so frequently, only normal	32	33
	petty arguments	7	4
	presence of boys and boys as peacemakers	6	
	competition for boys	9	3
	more than in co-ed. school		3
	one girl 'picked on' because different	26	26
	because of boredom		3
	jealousy, changing friends, etc.	3	
	ridicule of dress, hair, etc.		2
	occasional sending to Coventry		6
	occasionally in lower or middle school	8	17
	only in lower streams		2
	between groups	4	15
	one spiteful or dominating girl	2	2
	by boy-mad girls	1	
	by trouble-makers, rebels	7	
	others	2	8
Totals		107	124

[*continued*]

TABLE 6.5 *(continued) Girls 'made life unpleasant' (free responses)*
'Both schools' survey

Estimate	Comment	Co-educational schools	Girls' schools
Frequently and Very frequently	frequently	13	15
	very frequently	3	2
	petty arguments	3	7
	one girl 'picked on' because different	26	60
	jealousy over boys	8	3
	because boys not present		3
	attitude of some groups to boys	1	1
	more than in co-ed. school, all girls		6
	in lower forms, less in higher	6	9
	mostly in higher forms	4	
	by groups, cliques against others	3	20
	between groups		10
	by boy-crazy girls		1
	by rough girls	3	
	by 'catty' girls		6
	others	4	6
Totals		74	149

between girls in their co-educational than in their girls' schools. Table 6.5 endeavours to summarize the responses; apart from the influence of the type of school the salient features were the unhappy lot of the girls who were 'picked on because they were different', and the double role of boys, who caused jealousy in both co-educational and girls' schools and also acted as peacemakers and as a restraining influence in the former. The quotations from these comments are in proportion to the numbers in each category (1 in 20), except that the middle ('not so frequently') category is omitted as adding very little to the illustration, and the number from the combined 'not at all' and 'infrequently' categories is halved to avoid over-loading the chapter. This last category is taken first. All the quotations relate to the 'made life unpleasant' question.

'Not at all' and 'infrequently'

CO-EDUCATIONAL SCHOOLS 'Always tried to be helpful and friendly towards the minority of girls who kept to themselves, and did not interact between the groups. Felt sorry for them.'

'If this happened the boys usually made life so unpleasant for the offensive group that they stopped.'

'They found it might lead to scorn from the boys which they did not wish to incite.'

'After exam results had come out girls could make one girl's life a misery if she had a higher result than them.'

'Often a rise was taken out of some girls because they spoke without accents.'

'They had other people to talk to and about when boys were there and found it a waste of time to quarrel between themselves.'

'The girls tended to be too bothered with making the boys behave!'

'Arguments and disagreements usually settled by discussion—often boys present.'

'Can't remember this happening. Most groups were mixed in sex.'

GIRLS' SCHOOLS 'Quarrels would be of short duration—probably between girls who were friends.'

'A little friction with girls in the 5th year, probably over boys, with whom there was no organized contact.'

'This hardly ever happened, because the school was small and everybody knew everybody else.'

'This happened once or twice, and after we had tasted it, and its after-effects, it never happened again.'

'Nearly all were friendly, not much time for unpleasantness.'

'Tended to be more numerous in the lowest streams.'

'Frequently' and 'Very frequently'

CO-EDUCATIONAL SCHOOLS 'Some sets were worse than others—frequently arose if a girl was dated by a boy who was liked by someone else.'

Often a group would gang up on a girl. Once some girls went to the extent of attacking one girl (sticking pins in her).'

'Mixing of all social classes with a high proportion of working class. Often the working-class girls would pick on the middle-class ones.'

'Some girls were rather mean to one girl because she was less well off than them and rather unattractive.'

GIRLS' SCHOOLS 'A large antagonistic group of sex-obsessed atheists dominated the 6th form.'

'Especially "Rolls Royce" cliques. Anyone slightly different was picked on.'

'There is always a set in a single-sex school, in my opinion, which makes life unpleasant for another.'

'One group of second years terrorized the 1st, 2nd and 3rd years—even fighting!'

'Girls when together are often spiteful and tend to make life unpleasant for a girl who finds it difficult to make friends.'

'Groups of girls made life difficult for girls with rich fathers, good accents, shy girls, clever girls or girls who were "favourites".'

'My own case is a good example. As I was "different" in my speech, etc., I was "ragged" most viciously for the first year. I never believed girls could be so spiteful and unfeeling.'

Direct comparisons

FAVOURABLE TO CO-EDUCATION 'This occurs in a group of children, but not so much in a co-ed. school.'

'This fact was reversed in a single-sex school.' ('Not at all', co-educational school.)

'Can't remember any specific instances. Not nearly as likely as in my single-sex school.'

'A decided lack of spitefulness compared to my single-sex school. I was, however, younger then.'

'It was more obvious in an all-girls school.'

'This often happens among girls and more so in single-sex school than co-educational.'

'Life made unpleasant for single girls by groups—far more than in co-ed.'

'This seemed to occur much more in a single-sex school.'

'There is not the same sense of "fair play" as in school with mixed staff.'

'It happened more than in the co-ed.'

'Much more than in co-educational school.'

'In any girls' society quarrels and backbiting take place but not so frequently in the co-ed. because it was frowned upon by the boys.'

'Just before I left this happened infrequently but just after the change [to co-ed.] and before it was very frequent.' (Am.)

'I have seen one or two cases of this in lower forms. The effects do not seem as great as in a single-sex school.'

'There tended to be more grouping together of girls in individual forms and some girls were left out.'

'More often than previously [i.e. than at the co-educational school].'

'This happened sometimes. I think it is natural in a single-sex community.'

'Seemed to happen more frequently than in the co-educational school.'

'The girls generally seemed to be more aggressive to one another as regards boy-friends.'

'In my opinion it is inadvisable to segregate girls from boys. Both contribute towards growing up. To avoid excessive unpleasantness I recommend mixed school.'

'Sometimes life was made unpleasant for single girls, sometimes little groups from within the class, far more than in the co-educational school.'

'There seemed to be more "ganging up" when the school split up than before it did.'

FAVOURABLE TO GIRLS' SCHOOLS 'Boys were more likely to make life unpleasant for a girl who was quieter and not so friendly.'

'Probably because there was no rivalry for the opposite sex in the single-sex school.' ('Not so frequently')

It is surprising that these direct comparisons are so one-sided, and it is therefore more important than usual that they should be considered against the background of the more dependable estimates, which, though favourable to co-educational schools, are less severe in their criticism of girls' schools. Peculiarly enough, the one comment unfavourable to co-educational schools is quite uncharacteristic of this research, in that the presence of boys is usually welcomed by the girls and judged by them as toning down the 'cattiness' which the quiet girl might find hard to bear.

The section is concluded with a special look at the comments the girls made about the influence of boys. Against the background of welcome in the co-educational school may be discerned both favourable and unfavourable influences. On the onc hand the boys act as the peacemakers and their presence inhibits the catty remarks which the girls admit to occur in their absence. On the other hand there is jealousy about boy-friends, which in turn is a cause of 'cattiness'. The balance evidently tips over heavily on the 'less cattiness' side. Here the quotations are not selected according to the total number of each type, but merely to illustrate each theme.

In the co-educational schools whatever cattiness occurred appeared usually to be about boys, e.g. one young woman writes that the girls 'made life unpleasant' for another girl 'not so frequently', but it was 'generally due to competition for boys and jealousy'. Another estimated 'infrequently' but 'generally over boy-friend snatching'. Similar is 'infrequently: this only happened when two girls liked the same boy or vice-versa', and 'if some girls hadn't a boy-friend they would make fun'. There was, however, a reverse influence: 'Girls would not do this often because they realized that the boys would think them nasty and stupid to do such a thing.' Again, 'The girls were on the whole friendly. We did not want the boys to consider the remark about girls being "catty" was true.'

In the remarks about their girls' schools the women reach virtually a consensus of opinion—that girls will have a strong tendency to 'cattiness' and similar conduct if boys are not present, e.g. 'Girls when together are often spiteful and tend to make life unpleasant for the girl who finds it difficult to make friends'; 'Girls on their own are much more inclined to be spiteful and clan against other girls.' Another woman puts it more humorously: 'I think this may have happened because of boredom with female company.'

We might think that the girls' schools, with no boys present, would be free from jealousy about them, but the girls provide plenty of evidence that this is not the case. This is shown by the frequency of remarks such as, 'Trouble over boys, feuds in classroom'; 'Girls tended to do this when they had nothing else to occupy their time and when some girls had a boy-friend they all liked.' Of related interest are, 'A hard core of boy-mad individuals made life unpleasant for the others', 'There was a definite element of spiteful girls and these were usually boy-mad girls', and 'One group kept spreading rumours indiscriminately, mostly about boys.'

The last question to be considered in this section on girls is about prefects and their attitude to the other pupils.

PREFECTS OFFICIOUS

The same question was put to the girls as was put to the boys: 'Do you agree or disagree with the following statement about your co-educational school? "The prefects were officious." Agree strongly/Agree/Doubtful,' etc. The phrase 'girls' school' was substituted for 'co-educational school' in the parallel questionnaire. The estimates are in Table 6.6; no free responses were requested because of time limitations.

TABLE 6.6 *Prefects officious (girls)*

'Both schools' survey

Estimates of ex-pupils about prefects' officiousness	Replies about first school attended				Replies about last school attended			
	Co-educational		Girls'		Co-educational		Girls'	
	N	%	N	%	N	%	N	%
Agree strongly	12	4·1	67	16·7	13	3·7	31	12·1
Agree	77	26·1	131	32·6	54	15·4	71	27·7
Doubtful	70	23·7	93	23·1	108	30·9	60	23·4
Disagree	116	39·3	97	24·1	134	38·3	80	31·3
Disagree strongly	20	6·8	14	3·5	41	11·7	14	5·5
Totals	295	100	402	100	350	100	256	100

NOTE: The differences between the co-educational and girls' schools both for 'first' and 'last' schools are statistically significant beyond ·001 level.

As with the previous results presented in this chapter, Table 6.6 gives a more favourable result for co-educational than for girls' schools and this is true whether the school was attended as a junior or as a senior, though the seniors of both types of school (some of whom would have been prefects themselves) are less inclined than the juniors to criticize the prefects as being officious. We see that whereas 30 per cent of the women agree about the officiousness of the prefects in their co-educational school when they were juniors, this rises to almost half for those who were juniors at girls' schools. The corresponding figures for seniors are 19 and 30 per cent. This is not reported as a criticism of the working or organization of girls' schools, but merely as something that is recorded by responsible ex-pupils and which might arise simply through the one-sex nature of the schools. It could be argued that the prefects would appear to be more officious in single-sex schools because of the tighter control that these schools seem to entail compared with co-educational schools, and even that the 'consumers' would naturally consider the prefects to be more officious than they really were.

Comment

It cannot be said too often that the co-education/single-sex variable is not the only one which affects pupils' attitudes about such questions as those discussed in this chapter. There is in consequence a wide range of pupil attitude and tone within schools of each kind. The views expressed, though not usually those of the *best* pupils academically, are those of good academic pupils who are obviously endeavouring to give carefully considered judgments and who are able through their experience to compare co-educational and single-sex schools. It is likely that the views of the less academically minded pupils might be more extreme in both types of school.

7

Life in school I

Under the heading 'Life in school' are gathered together a number of inquiries which seek to probe, even if somewhat superficially, various aspects of day-to-day life in co-educational as opposed to single-sex grammar schools. Some questions, such as those on pupil happiness and school atmosphere, are regarded as sufficiently important to merit treatment independently of the others, while the present ones, though not without their own importance, need not be analysed so intensively. It is not pretended that all the important questions have been included, merely that an effort has been made to examine some claims and counter-claims that have been hurled between the contending groups. The first of the inquiries to be reported was concerned with the narrowness of the education.

Narrowness of education

In the 'Both schools' inquiry students were asked whether they agreed or disagreed with the following statement about first their co-educational and then their single-sex school: 'The education I got was extremely narrow. Agree strongly/Agree/Doubtful/Disagree/Disagree strongly.' No provision was made for free responses. The results of the women are taken first.

FEMALE EX-PUPILS

A mere scanning of Figure 7.1 reveals that, as is usual in this survey, the women's replies are decidedly more favourable about their co-educational schools than about their girls' schools.

For both types of school, the women who attended a particular type last thought the education provided in it was rather less narrow than did those for whom this type was their first secondary school. The difference between co-educational and girls' schools, however, is only a little less for 'last schools' than for 'first schools'; in both cases the education provided in the girls' schools was considered to be narrower. Those who disagreed or disagreed strongly

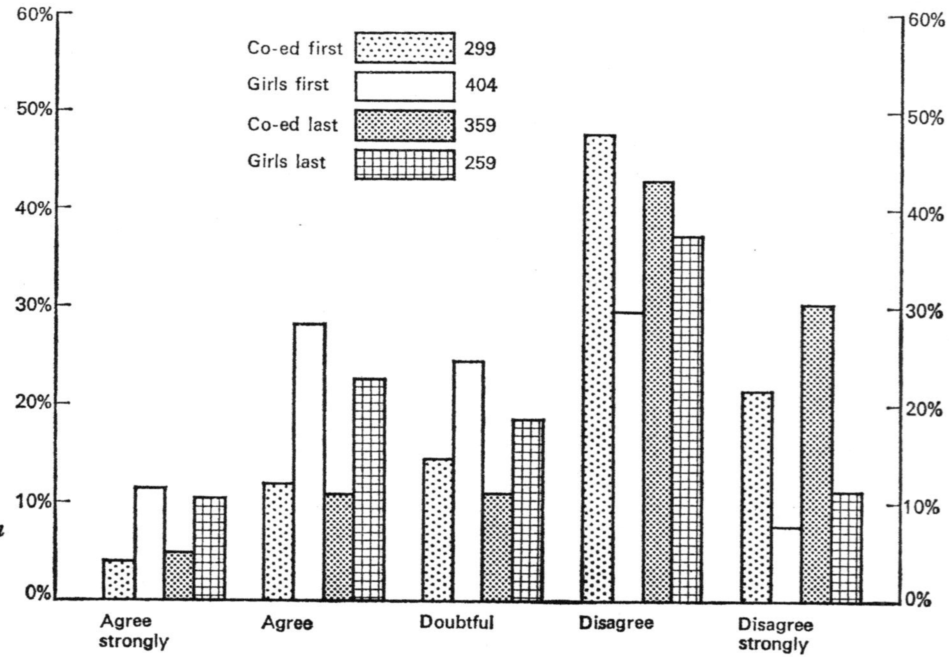

FIGURE 7.1
Narrowness of education (girls): 'Both schools' survey

that the education was narrow in co-educational schools were 70 per cent (first schools) and 73 per cent (last schools), and for girls' schools 35 per cent and 48 per cent. To report these results is one thing, but to interpret them is another. The wording of the statement tended to suggest that it was true; this would increase somewhat the affirmative response, but would presumably have a similar weight for both opposing groups. There is some evidence from the free responses made to other items that the view taken of 'education' was something more than academic instruction. At the same time the students also appear to think that the girls' schools place more emphasis on examination success, at the expense of other matters, than do the co-educational schools.

MALE EX-PUPILS

The results for male ex-pupils are in Table 7.1.

TABLE 7.1 *Narrowness of education (boys)*

'Both schools' survey

Estimates of narrowness of education	Replies about first schools				Replies about last schools			
	Co-educational		Boys'		Co-educational		Boys'	
	N	%	N	%	N	%	N	%
Agree strongly	5	6·0	17	14·3	4	3·8	2	2·8
Agree	14	16·9	38	32·0	16	15·4	17	23·9
Doubtful	12	14·5	18	15·1	18	17·3	12	16·9
Disagree	35	42·1	40	33·6	42	40·4	26	36·7
Disagree strongly	17	20·5	6	5·0	24	23·1	14	19·7
Totals	83	100	119	100	104	100	71	100

NOTE: The difference between co-educational and boys' schools is statistically highly significant for first schools but not significant for last schools, though the difference is in the same direction.

Here again the co-educational schools are considered to provide the less narrow education, but though the difference between the 'first school' groups is statistically highly significant, that between the 'last school' groups is not significant. Approaching half those students who attended boys' schools first agreed or agreed strongly that the education provided in them was narrow, as opposed to almost a quarter of those who attended co-educational schools first. Even for those in the 'last schools' groups the difference was in the same direction, the corresponding percentages being 27 and 19.

This question was not considered to be quite suitable for asking in schools, but the Schools project questionnaire contained a related question on 'preparation for the adult world'; the results from this are, however, placed more appropriately in Chapter 16.

A part of school life which can help to prevent the education from being too narrow is out-of-class activities, such as debating societies, drama groups and various societies catering for hobbies. The next section of the chapter has a somewhat cursory look at this area.

Out-of-school activities

In the 'Both schools' survey the ex-pupils were asked, 'Do you agree or disagree with the following statements about your co-educational school? There were enjoyable out-of-school activities (other than games).' The same question was asked about their single-sex school, and the ex-pupils could choose between the categories of the usual five-point scale, beginning 'agree strongly'. The women's estimates are summarized in Table 7.2.

These female ex-pupils evidently thought their co-educational

TABLE 7.2 *'Were enjoyable out-of-school activities' (female ex-pupils)*

'Both schools' survey

	Replies about first school attended				Replies about last school attended			
	Co-educational		Girls'		Co-educational		Girls'	
	N	%	N	%	N	%	N	%
Agree strongly	82	27·6	23	5·7	123	34·2	34	13·1
Agree	107	36·0	94	23·3	151	41·9	89	34·4
Doubtful	44	14·8	106	26·3	41	11·4	47	18·2
Disagree	48	16·2	114	28·3	36	10·0	49	18·9
Disagree strongly	16	5·4	66	16·4	9	2·5	40	15·4
Totals	297	100	403	100	360	100	259	100

NOTE: The difference between co-educational and girls' schools was statistically highly significant (beyond ·001 level for both first and last schools).

schools were better at providing enjoyable out-of-school activities than were their girls' schools, both in the schools attended as juniors and those attended as seniors. Possible interpretations are that the girls' schools did not provide enough out-of-school activities or that they were not as enjoyable as in the co-educational schools. As there were no free responses we do not know what was in the minds of the students when they gave their estimates. An analysis of the results according to the occupational class of the fathers of the respondents produced no discernible association, but analysis by first and last schools gave a more favourable result for last schools, whether they were co-educational or girls' schools.

The results for male ex-pupils yield the same direction of difference, but the amount is smaller, that between first schools (i.e. those attended as juniors) being statistically significant but that between last schools being far from significant, so that this advantage for co-educational schools attended as seniors is not reliable. As in the case of the females the male ex-pupils gave more favourable estimates of the out-of-school activities when they were seniors in the school—both co-educational and boys' schools—than did ex-pupils who were junior pupils.

Look forward to coming to school

The next item to be considered comes from the Schools project (1966) and was, 'I look forward to coming to school each day. Agree strongly/Agree/Doubtful/Disagree/Disagree strongly.' The estimates of girls aged 13 plus and 17 plus are in Table 7.3.

TABLE 7.3 *'Look forward to coming to school' (girls' estimates)*

Schools project

	Replies of 13-plus girls				Replies of 17-plus girls			
	Co-educational schools		Girls' schools		Co-educational schools		Girls' schools	
	N	%	N	%	N	%	N	%
Agree strongly	14	6·5	16	7·6	6	5·3	2	1·7
Agree	73	34·0	70	33·2	49	43·0	39	32·5
Doubtful	71	33·0	52	24·6	25	21·9	34	28·3
Disagree	41	19·1	50	23·7	30	26·3	35	29·2
Disagree strongly	16	7·4	23	10·9	4	3·5	10	8·3
Totals	215	100	211	100	114	100	120	100

Here the girls from the co-educational schools look forward to coming to school each day rather more than do those from girls' schools, especially the seniors, but neither the difference between the senior groups nor that between the junior groups is statistically significant, though the former approaches it. Support, however, is given to the finding by the direction of the differences being common to both seniors and juniors, and by this direction being the same as that found in most of these inquiries. Incidentally, the differences between the distributions are to be seen more clearly in the two 'disagree' categories than on the positive side.

The pupils' comments about 'looking forward to coming to school' were much more responsible than might have been expected. Though they show only a few differences between co-educational and girls' schools they are given a fairly full treatment

TABLE 7.4 *'Look forward to coming to school' (girls' responses) Schools project, 1966*

Estimate	Comment	Co-educational schools	Girls' schools
Agree and	*School*		
Agree	like school very much	16	3
strongly	fun, interesting, enjoyable, love it	15	15
	friendly atmosphere, happy	10	6
	like usually, on the whole	9	18
	Pupils		
	to meet friends	16	24
	to meet boy-friend	1	
	to meet boy-friend nearby		1
	because mixed	1	
	Teachers and teaching		
	nice, kind, helpful	6	2
	if lessons interesting that day	11	5
	one particular teacher		1
	enjoy lessons	5	3
	lessons useful	1	3
	Activities		
	various, enjoyable, exciting, games	2	6
	Others		
	bored at home, better than home	13	6
	except in rain, getting up early	6	1
	unhappy at home		1
	other single mentions	5	3
Totals		117	98

[*continued*]

TABLE 7.4 (*continued*) *'Look forward to coming to school' (girls' responses)*
Schools project, 1966

Estimate	Comment	Co-educational schools	Girls' schools
Doubtful	doubtful in general	6	5
	depends which teacher, lessons, that day	30	21
	sometimes	10	3
	depends on mood, health, weather	5	6
	depends whether test, homework done	2	3
	dislike getting up early	3	2
	like meeting friends	3	
	all right when get there	5	11
	too much routine, monotonous		3
	others	9	5
Totals		73	59
Disagree and Disagree strongly	*School*		
	hate school	3	3
	dislike school	15	25
	dislike but necessary		2
	but don't hate it	3	5
	but enjoy when get there	3	6
	Teachers and teaching		
	boring	6	6
	depends what day, teacher	9	4
	dislike teacher attitudes	1	5
	pressure too great, too difficult	2	3
	depends homework done		1
	not tests or exams	1	
	Activities		
	prefer leisure activities, home	3	8
	Personal		
	don't like getting up, too early	16	13
	get very tired		4
	depends on mood		2
	Work		
	rather be working	2	1
	Others	3	4
Totals		67	92

because they also have value as a documentation of one aspect of life in school (Table 7.4).

The analysis of the girls' free responses provides good support for the verdict of their estimates. From the 329 girls in co-educational and 331 in girls' schools there came 258 and 249 comments respectively. Of these, 118 favourable comments were from the co-educational and 98 from the girls' schools, and 67 unfavourable comments from the co-educational and 92 from the girls' schools. An analysis which separated the girls aged 13 plus from the 17-year-olds showed that at age 17 plus the co-educated girls looked forward to going to school appreciably more than the 17 plus girls from girls' schools, while at age 13 plus the co-educated girls had decidedly fewer *adverse* comments than did the girls from girls' schools. The difference between the distributions from co-educational and girls' schools is not quite statistically significant at the ·05 level for either the 17-year-old or 13-year-old group. In Table 7·5 these results are presented in numerical form.

TABLE 7.5 *'Look forward to coming to school'. Breakdown of free responses by age of pupil and type of school (girls)*
Schools project

	Favourable				Unfavourable				Doubtful				Totals		
	17+		13+		17+		13+		17+		13+		17+	13+	
	N	%	N	%	N	%	N	%	N	%	N	%	N	N	%
Co-ed. schools	50	51	68	42	31	32	36	23	17	17	56	35	98	160	100
Girls' schools	33	36	65	42	35	38	57	36	24	26	35	22	92	157	100

NOTE: The difference between the co-educational and girls' schools distributions is not significant in either case (13 plus and 17 plus).

If we compare the responses from the two types of school in the detailed Table (7.4), the emphasis is clearly on the similarity of the causes of 'looking forward to coming to school', and the same applies to the negative side; in other words, the underlying basis of human nature asserts itself, whatever the type of school. Some girls do not like getting up early to go to school and this force is not removed or neutralized by either type of school. This therefore 'waters down' any difference caused by the school type. A few of the differences, however, are worthy of mention. In the favourable section ('agree', etc.) there are sixteen mentions under 'like very much' for co-educational schools compared with three for the girls' schools, an imbalance not removed by the results given in the other sub-sections of the 'school' category. On the other hand, in the returns from girls' schools there was greater emphasis on going to school 'to meet friends'. In the unfavourable section the most important difference is between the twenty-seven girls from the girls' schools who disliked going to school as against the fifteen from co-educational schools. One of the most prominent replies, from both types of school, is understandably 'depends on the day, or the teacher', but it is a little surprising to find so many pupils complaining about having to get up early!

The differences in detail reported above are not substantial enough to stand by themselves, but their general trend agrees with the findings in the rest of the research.

A few interesting or amusing quotations are selected to illustrate the text, taking those from co-educational schools first. A few of the co-educated girls look forward to going to school each day because they will meet a boy-friend:

'Because my boy-friend goes to the same school.'

'Because we are in a mixed school!!!' (sic)

Some of the comments are so enthusiastic they are refreshing to read:

'I would stay at school always if I could.'

'School is always happy because of sports, drama etc.'

Then there is a hint that it is not quite done to admit openly that you enjoy school:

'I pretend not to but I enjoy it all the same.'

Occasionally one comes across an unexpected or droll reason:

'I only like a few subjects, but I like the uniform.'

The negative reasons cover a wide range:

'The lessons are dry and I hate getting up.'

'The thought of getting up in the morning is painful.'

'The thought of hard work gets me down.'

'Sometimes I feel queer when I come to school.'

'My mother misses me strongly so I dislike leaving her.'

'Who'd look forward to it?'

The girls from girls' schools give similar reasons, including even the boy-friends:

'To see the boys from the boys' school down the road.'

There is also the same sprinkling of enthusiastic comments:

'School days are really the happiest days of my life.'

'There are usually exciting things to do.'

Again we have the somewhat unexpected reasons, such as the girl who looks forward to coming to school because, 'Sometimes I am very unhappy at home.' Those who dislike school express themselves more forcibly than those from the co-educational schools:

'School stinks.'

'As I have said before, I *hate* school.'

'School's a drag.'

'All I look forward to in school is the dinner and home time.'

'I don't like school and the teachers are like a lot of old maids.'

'I dislike school and the attitude of teachers.'

'I am always tired and the thought of school is awful.'

The general trend of these results was again confirmed in the 'Check' survey, with 1,122 pupils aged 13 plus. The tabulated data may be consulted in Table A.11. Although a rather greater percentage of co-educated girls say they look forward to coming to school each day than do those from girls' schools, and rather fewer disagree with the statement, the difference between the distributions is not quite statistically significant.

The estimates made by the boys in answer to the same question are in Table 7.6.

The estimates of the boys resemble those of the girls in that the co-educated boys look forward to coming to school rather more than do those from boys' schools, but they differ in that the result for the boys aged 13 plus is almost statistically significant, while on the other hand there is a near equality between the two senior groups.

The free responses made by the boys (Table A.12) support the estimates. Although there were 538 of these they produce rather small numbers when divided into the numerous sub-sections, and it is therefore safer and more illuminating to consider the effect of the tabulated results as a whole rather than to consider individual sub-sections. This overview is also made necessary by the subjective element which enters into some parts of the classifying process.

The table indicates that the co-educated boys score rather more heavily in the more important items of the favourable section, such as 'like school much' and 'like school usually', and correspondingly score lower than boys from boys' schools on the unfavourable side, as in 'hate it, depressing, dread it', 'dislike school', and 'too boring'.

The comments from the co-educated boys are perhaps a little more humorous than those of the girls, varying from 'school days

TABLE 7.6 *'Look forward to coming to school' (boys' estimates)*
School project (1966)

	Replies of 13-plus boys				Replies of 17-plus boys			
	Co-educational schools		Boys' schools		Co-educational schools		Boys' schools	
	N	%	N	%	N	%	N	%
Agree strongly	9	4·0	6	2·8	6	4·5	5	3·7
Agree	62	27·8	52	24·1	51	38·8	48	35·9
Doubtful	67	30·0	60	27·8	32	24·2	46	34·3
Disagree	69	31·0	67	31·0	32	24·2	27	20·1
Disagree strongly	16	7·2	31	14·3	11	8·3	8	6·0
Totals	223	100	216	100	132	100	134	100

are the happiest days of your life!' and 'I would be lost without school to go to', to 'I consider every school day as bringing me nearer to a Saturday', and 'would you enjoy going to prison?' One young man wrote, 'some days I do not like coming, so I don't.' Another is doubtful 'because it is like a tape-recorder, it keeps the same each week,' while another looks forward to school 'on Thursday, Friday and Tuesday'. Finally we have a somewhat precocious lad of thirteen saying, 'from a young boy I have always been fascinated by study.'

The comments from boys in boys' schools also have this touch of humour, though it is sometimes unconscious, beginning with the seventeen-year-old who hoped 'in a sense never to leave school, i.e. be a teacher'. Another who agreed that he looked forward to school added, 'but I don't jump for joy at the thought.' One boy turned the question round and asked the inquisitor, 'Do you like doing work—or forced labour?' Similar in opinion—though not in tone—is, 'I find the thought of school each day depresses me.' A boy more thoughtful in outlook wrote, 'Residual working-class distrust of education. Anyway I want to earn money.' Finally there are three comments which succinctly sum up the attitude of the discontented:

'To look forward to school is not normal.'

'Most of the teachers dislike me.'

'I hate masters and I hate school.'

Comment

The major part of the discussion is reserved for the concluding chapter, but here a few comments are necessary. For the themes of this chapter the comparison of co-educational and single-sex schools is advantageous to the former. In the Schools project and its ancillary research, the 'Check' questionnaire, this advantage is slight and occasionally disappears and a state of equality is reached, but in the 'Both schools' project, where the ex-students had experienced both types of school, the co-educational lead became considerable. The difference between these results occurs throughout the book and will be discussed later.

8

Life in school II

The subject of the previous chapter is continued in this, but the merging of the two chapters would have created one of unwieldy length. In addition this chapter describes research which used a slightly different technique. It was thought that some of the pupils and students might have been 'on their guard' and might have answered the more formal questions defensively, trying not to give a bad impression of themselves or betray their loyalty to their school. For example, if asked, 'Do you consider the atmosphere of the school is Very pleasant/Pleasant/Neutral/Rather unpleasant/ Very unpleasant?' pupils might not have cared to admit the worst, or even have been afraid to admit it for fear of the answer being seen by school authorities. By giving them, however, a forced choice between adjectives of opposite meaning (with an intermediate neutral option) which could describe the school, this defensive barrier or the fear of discovery might be surmounted. In addition the words chosen might also get to the heart of any difference in the spirit of the school life in the two types of school community.

To this end respondents were asked, 'Which of the following words *best* fits your school life? Try to choose one of the first two alternatives, even if it doesn't fit exactly. Use "neither" only as a last resort.

Q.45. Lively/dull/neither
Q.46. Variety/monotony/neither
Q.47 Enthusiasm/apathy/neither
Q.48. Kindness/unpleasantness/neither
Q.49. Friendly individuals/cliques or gangs/neither'

These questions were asked of pupils aged 13 plus and 17 plus in the Schools project (1966 only) and of different pupils (girls only) aged 13 plus in the 'Check' questionnaire. To have presented all the results in tabular form would have overcrowded the book, hence no tables are given where the replies from co-educational and single-sex schools are approximately equivalent.

The girls' estimates are presented first. For girls aged 13 plus there was either little or no difference between the co-educated girls and those from girls' schools for all five items; there was equality for Lively/Dull, a slight advantage to girls' schools for Enthusiasm/Apathy, a very slight advantage to co-education for Variety/Monotony, and a slight advantage to co-education in the remaining two items. None of these differences even approached statistical significance.

A more positive result came from the 17-year-old girls. Though the Lively/Dull item again yielded equality, and the Friendly individuals/Cliques item was only slightly favourable to co-education, the better results in the other three items came from the co-educated pupils (Table 8.1).

TABLE 8.1 *Life in school (items 46, 47 and 48)*
Schools project (girls aged 17 plus)

		Replies about co-educational schools		Replies about girls' schools	
		N	%	N	%
Item 46	variety	84	73·7	81	67·5
	monotony	30	26·3	34	28·3
	neither	0	0	5	4·2
	Total	114	100	120	100
Item 47	enthusiasm	78	69·0	73	60·8
	apathy	21	18·6	37	30·9
	neither	14	12·4	10	8·3
	Total	113	100	120	100
Item 48	kindness	103	90·4	97	80·8
	unpleasantness	4	3·5	18	15·0
	neither	7	6·1	5	4·2
	Total	114	100	120	100

NOTE: The difference between the groups from co-educational and girls' schools is statistically highly significant for the kindness/unpleasantness item, approaching significance (Chi-square = 5·04 for 2 D.F.) for enthusiasm/apathy, and for variety/monotony yields a Chi-square of 3·264 for 2 D.F. with Yates's correction.

If we look at item 48 in the table we find that more co-educated girls than girls from girls' schools thought kindness was descriptive of their schools (even here 81 per cent applied this adjective to their girls' school). Correspondingly, fewer of the co-educated girls thought the word 'unpleasantness' characterized their schools. In item 47 appreciably fewer of the co-educated girls than of the girls from girls' schools considered that 'apathy' described their schools, and appreciably more selected 'enthusiasm' as the most suitable word. The advantage to the co-educated girls on Variety/Monotony is smaller and no further comment is made.

Four of these same questions were included in the 'Check' questionnaire, the respondents being all girls of the same age as those aged 13 plus in the Schools project, and in the same schools, but who were *not* included in the 1964 testing. The item on Kindness/Unpleasantness gave a very slight advantage to girls' schools and that on Variety/Monotony a very slight advantage in the opposite direction, neither difference being anywhere near to statistical significance. The question on Friendly individuals/Cliques produced a result which was favourable to the co-educational schools, but not quite statistically significant. When asked, however, whether they thought their schools were 'lively' or 'dull' a significantly larger number of the co-educated than of girls from girls' schools answered 'lively' and fewer answered 'dull' (Table 8.2).

It is not often in all this research that the difference between the

TABLE 8.2 (*a*) *Lively/Dull*, (*b*) *Friendly individuals/Cliques*

'Check' project (girls aged 13 plus)

	Replies about co-educational schools		Replies about girls' schools	
	N	%	N	%
lively	384	86·5	526	78·6
dull	32	7·2	83	12·4
neither	28	6·3	60	9·0
Total	444	100	669	100
friendly individuals	279	63·0	389	58·6
cliques or gangs	135	30·5	242	36·4
neither	29	6·5	33	5·0
Total	443	100	664	100

NOTE: The Chi-square for lively/dull was 11·39 for 2 D.F., and for friendly/cliques 4·812 for 2 D.F.

two boys' groups is greater than that between the two girls' groups, but this is true of the result from their five items considered as a whole (Tables 8.3 and 8.4). We shall see, however, that one of these items does not conform to the general trend.

TABLE 8.3 *Life in school: (a) Lively, (b) Enthusiasm (boys)*

Schools project

	Replies from 13-plus boys				Replies from 17-plus boys			
	Co-educational schools		Boys' schools		Co-educational schools		Boys' schools	
	N	%	N	%	N	%	N	%
Lively	184	82·9	161	75·2	104	79·4	103	75·7
Dull	18	8·1	40	18·7	24	18·3	19	14·0
Neither	20	9·0	13	6·1	3	2·3	14	10·3
Totals	222	100	214	100	131	100	136	100
Enthusiasm	160	73·7	136	65·0	90	69·8	81	60·0
Apathy	31	14·3	39	18·7	35	27·1	34	25·2
Neither	26	12·0	34	16·3	4	3·1	20	14·8
Totals	217	100	209	100	129	100	135	100

NOTE: The 13-year-old and 17-year-old co-educated boys rated their schools as more lively (at ·01 and ·025 significance levels) than did those from boys' schools, and the 17-year-old co-educated boys also rated their schools as showing more enthusiasm. The same trend in the 13-year-olds falls short of statistical significance (Chi-square = 3·778 for 2 D.F.), but gains support from the other results.

The data in Tables 8.3 and 8.4 indicate that the 13-year-old co-educated boys believed their schools to be more lively and less dull, to have more variety and to be less monotonous, to show more kindness and less unpleasantness, and possibly to show more enthusiasm than the boys from boys' schools believed about their own schools. The 17-year-old co-educated boys similarly believed their schools to be more lively and more enthusiastic. For the Friendly individuals/Cliques item there was virtual equality for the two 17-year-old groups, and a very slight advantage, far from being statistically significant, to the 13-year-olds from boys' schools. The 17-year-old boys from boys' schools also had the slenderest of leads on the Variety/Monotony item, with equality for 'unpleasantness' versus 'unkindness'.

TABLE 8.4 *Life in school: (a) Variety (b) Kindness*

Schools project (boys 13 plus)

		Replies about co-educational schools		Replies about boys' schools	
		N	%	N	%
Item 46	Variety	177	80·8	152	71·0
	Monotony	32	14·6	52	24·3
	Neither	10	4·6	10	4·7
	Totals	219	100	214	100
Item 48	Kindness	158	72·5	124	59·1
	Unpleasantness	31	14·2	40	19·0
	Neither	29	13·3	46	21·9
	Totals	218	100	210	100

NOTE: The differences between the groups from co-educational and boys' schools are statistically significant at the ·05 and ·025 levels.

Comment

The results obtained from the slightly different technique used in this part of the research fit into the general picture which has emerged from the main approach. It would seem self-evident that co-educational schools would have more variety than single-sex schools in their social life and even in their classrooms (though what seems self-evident is not always true), but it is interesting to find evidence that this difference in atmosphere probably includes a greater liveliness, enthusiasm, kindness and friendliness between pupils in co-educational schools. In the twenty-four comparisons made in this section between co-educational and single-sex schools one would not expect, in view of all the forces involved, that every difference would be in favour of the co-educational schools, and we do find some of them becoming an equality, but only exceptionally does the difference swing slightly in the opposite direction. There are also distinct variations in atmosphere between schools of the same type; further research is therefore needed on different samples of schools. It would appear, none the less, that in this comparison the co-educational schools have a 'flying start' which may only be lost by the influence of such factors as a very bad head, unusually indifferent staff, or a very deprived catchment area.

Occupational Class

An interesting by-product of the results is a trend associated with occupational class, well defined in both boys' and girls' schools, less certain among co-educated girls and absent among this sample of co-educated boys (Table 8.5). The following section looks at this trend, departing for the moment from the main comparison between co-educational and single-sex schools.

TABLE 8.5 *Analysis by occupational class of items 45 to 49*
Schools project

	Replies from boys in boys' schools								Replies from girls in girls' schools							
	Boys aged 17 plus Class				Boys aged 13 plus Class				Girls aged 17 plus Class				Girls aged 13 plus Class			
	1 and 2		3, 4, 5		1 and 2		3, 4, 5		1 and 2		3, 4, 5		1 and 2		3, 4, 5	
	N	%	N	%	N	%	N	%	N	%	N	%	N	%	N	%
Lively	54	78·3	49	73·2	81	78·6	80	72·1	50	82·0	44	74·6	83	86·4	98	83·5
Dull	6	8·7	13	19·4	17	16·5	23	20·7	10	16·4	12	20·3	11	11·5	15	12·5
Neither	9	13·0	5	7·4	5	4·9	8	7·2	1	1·6	3	5·1	2	2·1	5	4·0
Total	69	100	67	100	103	100	111	100	61	100	59	100	96	100	118	100
Variety	50	72·5	43	65·2	77	74·0	75	68·2	42	68·8	39	66·1	75	78·2	90	77·7
Monotony	13	18·8	20	30·3	22	21·2	30	27·3	15	24·6	19	32·2	20	20·8	20	17·2
Neither	6	8·7	3	4·5	5	4·8	5	4·5	4	6·6	1	1·7	1	1·0	6	5·1
Total	69	100	66	100	104	100	110	100	61	100	59	100	96	100	116	100
Enthusiasm	43	62·3	38	57·5	71	68·9	65	61·3	38	62·3	35	59·3	75	79·0	82	72·9
Apathy	16	23·2	18	27·3	17	16·5	22	20·8	17	27·9	20	33·9	10	10·5	19	16·6
Neither	10	14·5	10	15·2	15	14·6	19	17·9	6	9·8	4	6·8	10	10·5	12	10·5
Total	69	100	66	100	103	100	106	100	61	100	59	100	95	100	113	100
Kindness	51	73·9	50	75·8	62	60·8	62	57·4	51	83·6	46	78·0	73	76·0	91	77·5
Unpleasantness	6	8·7	8	12·1	20	19·6	20	18·5	7	11·5	11	18·6	12	12·5	14	12·4
Neither	12	17·4	8	12·1	20	19·6	26	24·1	3	4·9	2	3·4	11	11·5	12	10·1
Total	69	100	66	100	102	100	108	100	61	100	59	100	96	100	117	100
Friendly individuals	50	71·4	42	64·6	79	75·9	73	67·6	33	54·1	25	42·4	54	56·3	70	56·2
Cliques or gangs	19	27·1	23	35·4	16	15·4	29	26·9	28	45·9	32	54·2	41	42·7	43	36·6
Neither	1	1·4	0	0	9	8·7	6	5·5	0	0	2	3·4	1	1·0	5	7·2
Total	70	100	65	100	104	100	108	100	61	100	59	100	96	100	118	100

In considering Table 8.5 let us follow the negative or less pleasant qualities, e.g. 'dull', 'monotony', in comparing the responses of those whose fathers were in occupational classes 1 and 2 (combined) with those whose fathers were in occupational classes 3, 4 and 5 (combined). If we look first at boys in boys' schools there are ten comparisons, in nine of which the proportion of occupational classes 3, 4 and 5 endorsing the less pleasant qualities is higher than the proportion for classes 1 and 2, the tenth difference in the opposite direction being the smallest of all. This trend is so steady that it would be surprising if it had occurred by chance, though none of the differences is individually statistically significant. When we turn to the girls in girls' schools we find that all five differences between the two occupational class groupings, at age 17 plus, are in the same direction; those for girls aged 13 plus in girls' schools, however, lack consistency. Intriguingly, the trend is less pronounced with the *co-educated* girls aged 13 plus and 17 plus taken as a whole; with the co-educated boys of the same ages the trend is absent. This possible difference in the atmosphere among boys in co-educational schools compared with those in boys' schools would again seem worthy of further research.

The causes of the trend are not clear and one can only theorize. It may be, for example, that the rather smaller proportion of pupils from occupational classes 3, 4 and 5 in these girls' and boys' grammar schools, compared with co-educational, leads to pupils from the lower occupational classes finding less enjoyment in school life. It may be that the co-educational schools are for some reason less snobbish. Whatever the reason, a somewhat greater proportion of pupils whose fathers are from occupational classes 3, 4 and 5 in the boys' and in the girls' schools (but not, in this sample, for girls aged 13 plus) may find school life, on the average, more dull, more monotonous, less enthusiastic, with more unpleasantness, and with more cliques, than their fellow-pupils from occupational classes 1 and 2 find it. Yet, though these items and the results obtained from them are related, they are not identical; for example, in the sample of boys from boys' schools the difference between the two groups is smallest for Unpleasantness/Kindness and greatest for Friendly individuals/Cliques. It should be emphasized that the analysis lacks statistical confirmation and that the theoretical explanation is merely an interesting speculation.

9

Unhappy pupils[1]

In order to obtain a more detailed insight into the significance of the results from the large-scale Schools project a series of short studies was made of all girls who said they were 'unhappy' or 'rather unhappy' at school and had been tested either at 15 years of age in 1964 or at 13 years of age in 1966. It was thought that such a study might also help to explain why in this particular project there was a reduced advantage to the girls in co-educational schools as against girls in girls' schools. Though full case-studies could not be made there was much useful information available, commencing with a detailed questionnaire on attitude to school, teachers, school subjects, careers, marriage, etc., and ranging through tests such as the High School Personality Questionnaire (Cattell), the Mooney Problem Check List and Maudsley Personality Inventory, to teachers' ratings on the Bristol Adjustment Guide[2] and heads' reports about school and home. Some of the most valuable information came from the free responses of the pupils themselves when they were invited to write down (anonymously and confidentially) the problems which were troubling them most.

Of the original sample of 1,028 girls there were only 44 who said they were 'unhappy' or 'rather unhappy' in school. This is a small number but the analysis is not meant to stand independently of the main studies—merely to illuminate them. As limitations of space prevent the publication of the case-studies in full one has to be content with an overall account, designed to illustrate the differences between the 17 pupils from the co-educational schools and the 27 from girls' schools, though other points arise which are of general interest. The pupils assessed themselves on 'happiness' as in Table 9.1, in answer to the question already given in Chapter 2 but here slightly modified, *viz.*: 'Was your life in school, viewed

[1] This chapter is based on the original full sample of 28 schools tested in 1964; and the 26 schools tested in 1966.
[2] Covering such aspects as, 'Withdrawn', 'Nervousness and Timidity', 'Hostility', 'Anxiety about adults'.

as a whole, Happy/Fairly happy/Jogging along/Rather unhappy/ Unhappy?'

TABLE 9.1 *Girls unhappy at school*
Schools project

	Co-educated girls			Girls in girls' schools		
	13 plus	15 plus	Total	13 plus	15 plus	Total
Rather unhappy	6	10	16	7	9	16
Unhappy	0	1	1	5	6	11
Totals	6	11	17	12	15	27
Total sample	231	280	511	237	280	517

Of the 15-year-olds, three out of the eleven from the co-educated group stayed on at school till 17 plus. Two of the three became 'fairly happy' and the other said she was 'jogging along'. Six of the fifteen girls from girls' schools stayed on, of whom one was still 'unhappy', one 'rather unhappy', one 'jogging along', and one 'happy', while one was absent, and the sixth one could not be tested as the school had become co-educational. It should be borne in mind, of course, that chance variations in personality are a possible explanation of these differences, because of the smallness of the numbers.

In attempting to discover why these girls were unhappy or rather unhappy the first area to be explored was pupil–teacher relations, which produced Table 9.2.

TABLE 9.2 *Girls unhappy* at school, pupil–teacher relations*

Teachers	Co-educated girls			Girls at girls' schools		
	13 plus	15 plus	Total	13 plus	15 plus	Total
Very friendly	0	0	0	1	0	1
Friendly	3	5	8	5	4	9
Neutral	1	6	7	5	6	11
Rather unfriendly	1	0	1	1	5	6
Very unfriendly	1	0	1	0	0	0
Total	6	11	17	12	15	27
Very helpful	0	1	1	1	0	1
Helpful	2	6	8	4	7	11
Neutral	2	4	6	5	7	12
Rather unhelpful	2	0	2	2	1	3
Very unhelpful	0	0	0	0	0	0
Total	6	11	17	12	15	27

* Includes 'rather unhappy'.

Though this handful of 'unhappy' girls assessed the teachers at the co-educational schools to be less unfriendly and more helpful than the teachers at the girls' schools, it would again be rash to draw any conclusions from this alone, especially as the difference falls short of statistical significance. We must also recognize that there may be other forces affecting pupils' attitudes in addition to those stemming from the co-educational and single-sex settings. Some school pupils, for example, can become unhappy because they haven't the ability to make a satisfactory job of the work demanded of them, and they dislike the constant failure as compared with the success of their fellow-pupils. Now it has already been demonstrated in the previous volume (Dale, 1969) that although an attempt had been made to equate the co-educated schools with the girls' schools there was a distinct (statistically significant) difference in intelligence levels for the full sample, the girls' schools having the superior average at both age levels. Some of this unhappiness, particularly in the co-educational grammar schools, might therefore have been due not to pupil–teacher relations, but to a less selective intake and consequent inability of those of relatively low intelligence to do the work. Although the only measure of intelligence available was the ten-item sub-scale in the High School Personality Questionnaire, this was much better than nothing, and it produced the results in Table 9.3 for the girls aged 15 plus.

TABLE 9.3 *Intelligence scores* of girls in unhappy categories*
(*aged 15 plus*)

Scores (maximum = 10)	Co-educated girls	Girls in girls' schools
10	1	1
9	4	5
8	0	4
7	0	4
6	4	1
5	1	0
4	1	0
Average	7·18	8·07

* Derived from the miniature scale in the High School Personality Questionnaire. If not high enough in reliability for individuals it suffices for this comparison of groups.

On this scale 7 would be a rather low score at age 15 plus for grammar school work, 6 is definitely low, 5 very low and 4 abysmal.

The girls' schools therefore have only 1 of their 15 unhappy pupils (aged 15 plus) who is clearly too low in score (i.e. below 7), while half of the unhappy co-educated girls are below the line. The 13-year-old girls had a similar distribution of scores (Table 9.4).

TABLE 9.4 *Intelligence scores of girls in unhappy categories*

(*aged 13-plus*)

Scores (maximum = 10)	Co-educated girls	Girls in girls' schools
10	0	1
9	1	1
8	0	5
7	3	2
6	2	3
5	0	0
4	0	0
Average	7·0	7·58

Reference to Tables 9.3 and 9.4 shows that the average score of the girls in girls' schools is in both cases greater than that of the girls in mixed schools. As was anticipated a greater proportion of these co-educated girls than of those in girls' schools could therefore have been unhappy because of their low ability in relation to the grammar school curriculum (cf. McCandless, 1956a and b; Sarason, 1960; Cowen, 1965). Let us then see what the girls themselves said when invited, by free response, to state their special problems (Tables 9.5 and 9.6, see pp. 129–30).

A notable difference about the free responses from the two samples of senior girls (Tables 9.5 and 9.6) is that whereas none of the co-educated girls say they dislike (or hate) school, three of the girls from girls' schools say they 'hate school', another complains that 'our teachers tend to be like icebergs', and another that 'the school atmosphere is rather unpleasant'. Whereas none of the group from girls' schools complain about the difficulty of the work (only one girl had the low intelligence test score of 6 (maximum 10)), with two worrying about passing examinations, such comments are more prevalent in the co-educational group, with its lower I.Q. level. Another pointer is that in the co-educated group, in spite of this lower intelligence level, there is no complaint about too much homework except from the girl who has to stay in to work for examinations, whereas in the group from girls' schools there are several complaints about too much homework and over-emphasis on examinations. It would be wrong, however, to place any reliance on this by itself; it should be viewed as part of the general picture. As the numbers are small it is of some interest to see whether the data obtained from the two groups of junior girls support a similar interpretation (Tables 9.7 and 9.8, see pp. 132–6).

In these tables there are strongly expressed statements showing dislike of school from seven of the pupils in girls' schools, while there is only one, or possibly two, from the co-educated group. Among the latter group it is—as was hypothesized from their lower intelligence level—the difficulty of the work which dominates their free responses. While this aspect is present among the group from girls' schools it seems less dominant.

As this appraisal is necessarily subjective a scheme was devised to obtain a more objective assessment. The free comments of the pupils both in the questionnaire and the Mooney Problem Check List were combined and assessed independently by another psychologist who did not know which groups were from girls' schools and which were from co-educational schools.[1] He was asked to classify the comments as in Table A.13, allocating a score of −2 for strongly unfavourable comments, −1 for adverse comments more moderate in tone, + 1 for normal favourable comment and + 2 for those enthusiastically favourable. A detailed description of each category is given as a footnote to the Tables. The resulting data confirm the subjective findings given above; by far the more important reasons for unhappiness among the 16 co-educational girls are 'out-of-school' or home difficulties (score − 33)[2] and work difficulties (− 20), with teachers' discipline almost the least important (−2), whereas the 25 girls from girls' schools placed general dislike of the school first (−32), with teachers' discipline second (−26),[3] work difficulties at almost the same level (−23), and out-of-school and home difficulties fourth (−19). In interpreting these figures observe that the two groups are unequal in size; the comparison may therefore be aided by the use of the averages, which are added to the table only to assist the reader.

These unhappy girls, as members of their main group, were

[1] One girl from each group failed to make any comments and had to be excluded from this section.

[2] The amount of unhappiness at home compared with that at school being statistically highly significant. The scores are the overall result after plus scores have been subtracted.

[3] A follow-up test after analyses of variance shows that the difference between the scores of the girls at co-educational schools and those at single-sex schools, for teachers' discipline and dislike of school combined, is statistically significant beyond the ·01 level.

given a number of psychological tests and were also rated for maladjustment by their teachers. Most of these data are presented in Tables A.14 to 18, partly for the benefit of those who would like to make a special study of this aspect, and partly to demonstrate the similarities as well as differences between the opposing groups. In view of the smallness of the numbers in each group, however, only large and consistent differences between the co-educated girls and those from girls' schools are mentioned here in the text. Apart from the slight but consistent advantage to the girls' schools in level of intelligence (which is a reflection of the situation in the main groups), and one other much larger trend, the emphasis in these additional tests is on similarity. This is so in ratings on maladjustment (Bristol, 15 plus), in scores on timidity, insecurity, and neuroticism, all of them being high. The greater anxiety score (in the H.S.P.Q. test) of the unhappy girls aged 15 plus in girls' schools, compared with those in co-educational schools, is not paralleled by the results of the younger (13 plus) unhappy girls in the same schools, who record merely the same high anxiety level as those in mixed schools. Similarly the greater number of *problems* recorded on the Mooney Problem Check List by the unhappy junior girls in girls' schools (than by the co-educated girls) is not present at the senior level, where the scores of both groups are again high.

The much larger—and consistent—trend is one of considerable interest. At both the junior and the senior level the unhappy girls from girls' schools record higher scores on extroversion than do those in co-educational schools. Only the difference between the 15-year-old groups of unhappy girls is statistically significant, but the finding receives some support from their main groups of relatively happy pupils, which show the same trend at both age levels, though here the differences are not statistically significant (yet near to it in the case of the 15-year-olds).[1] Incidentally these results are paralleled by the main groups of boys, where those from boys' schools also have the higher extroversion score, the difference between the 15-year-old groups being statistically significant.

Unless this difference is an artefact of some other variable which the research has failed to detect, the finding provides additional evidence for the argument set out previously that the co-educational and single-sex schools are communities with quite different atmospheres, which for years exert different psychological influences on children, and that the pupils are moulded into adults who

[1] The test for senior girls was the Maudsley Personality Inventory and for the juniors the High School Personality Questionnaire.

are psychologically not what they would have been if they had been educated in the opposite kind of school.

Unfortunately this test of extroversion–introversion was only a small part of a large project and the results have not been followed up. It has to be left to later research to determine first whether the difference in score is confirmed, and then whether it denotes that in this respect one type of school or the other gives a 'better' education. An interrelated question is whether the effect—if it exists—is present over a wide range of the extroversion–introversion scale—and whether the 'good' or 'bad' effects of the schooling vary with the temperament of the individual.

As such a test of personality is particularly sensitive to changes in administration it should be recorded that the same researcher administered the test to all the girls, and that no members of staff were present and no names of pupils appeared on the answer sheets. Pupils regarded the test as important but knew they would not be affected personally by the result. None the less it is not impossible that the difference in score might have been produced because of the contrast between the more friendly and less formal pupil–teacher relations of the co-educational school and the stricter discipline of the girls' school. The girls in the girls' schools might have been less ready to admit to tendencies which the school authorities (if they had read the answers) would perhaps have considered less desirable. On the other hand the unnatural deprivation of the company of the opposite sex might cause girls in girls' schools to become more out-going socially, but the difference between the two groups of girls is not large, and whether the higher extroversion is 'good' or 'bad' will be of little consequence for most of them. For some individuals, on the other hand, it could be important. One of the readers of the typescript—Dr Miller—made the interesting suggestion that there might be a greater tendency for extroverts to feel 'out of place' in a single-sex school than in a co-educational one.

This research was too wide in scope for the writer to be able to spend further efforts on this point. However, much of the above paragraph is theory which must be left to be examined by future research.

Discussion

To be unhappy, or merely 'rather unhappy', at school is, putting it mildly, a very undesirable fate for a child. Fortunately the proportion of such children in the grammar schools examined was very small, whether the schools were co-educational or single-sex, and the free responses of the pupils showed unmistakably that some of this unhappiness—especially in the co-educational schools —had its origin in the home, and was so deeply rooted that there was no escape from it wherever the pupil went. Other unhappiness probably stemmed from the temperament of the pupil herself, as many teacher readers must have been murmuring aloud for some time. Rarely is the teacher the villain of the piece, and even when she is it may often be because it is easier to arrive at a breaking point in friendly human relations in one type of school community than in another. We have seen that teachers and ex-pupils believe that the conduct of each sex of pupil is improved in the presence of the other, this opinion being almost unanimous in the case of the boys. The natural level of discipline in a co-educational school would therefore need to be less strict, with a consequent improvement in teacher–pupil relationships; in this atmosphere it would be less easy for pupil–teacher relationships to deteriorate to a point where lasting unhappiness was produced in a pupil.

In this Schools project, however, the results do not give as great an advantage to the co-educational schools as in the surveys involving ex-pupils and teachers. The reasons for this are examined in detail elsewhere, but this chapter has studied one of them through the case-studies of unhappy pupils. It was recognized at the outset of the research that 'happiness in school' is determined by many forces in addition to staff–pupil relationship, and it has been mentioned above that one of these forces is the home, and that this was the most powerful of the influences producing unhappiness in the co-educational schools examined, but not in the girls' schools, though it could by no means be ignored there. In the latter schools it was factors immediately connected with the schools which were dominant.

Unhappiness at school may also be caused by the attempts of pupils to cope with work which is above their level of intelligence, and this factor is much more prominent in the replies from girls in co-educational schools than in those from girls in girls' schools. In support of this it was shown that the intelligence scores of the co-educated unhappy girls were distributed lower in the scale than those of the unhappy girls in girls' schools. We also saw that the average intelligence score of the entire sample of co-educated girls was lower than that of their opposing group.[1]

The happiness of the pupils might not in itself be a guarantee that a school is good, yet it would be true to say that the *unhappiness* of an appreciable number of pupils, if produced by the school, would be a guarantee that the school was bad! In the

[1] The difference is statistically significant for both the 13-year-old and for the 15-year-old groups.

Schools project neither type of school had a large group of these pupils, and the difference between the schools in this respect was small.

The number of pupils providing the central data for the chapter is not as large as was desirable for reliability, but they are the extreme cases and are therefore important. The writer emphasizes again that the chapter is not meant to stand alone, and wherever possible the data have been linked with the data from the main sample of girls, comprising some thousand pupils.

TABLE 9.5 *Outlines of case-studies of unhappy girls*

Co-educated girls aged 15 plus in 1964

Pupil	Self assessment of happiness at school	Intelligence score	Pupil's free responses
1	Rather unhappy	10	None given.
2	Rather unhappy (1964) Fairly happy (1966)	9	'I am not developed enough for my age.' 'I do not like working indoors but I know that I have to. I would rather be out riding and with horses' (1964). 'I have to stay in every evening to work for exams. I worry if my boy-friend is going out with someone else. We have exams in two weeks and I can't settle down to work' (1966).
3	Rather unhappy	9	'My mother had a nervous breakdown last year and had to give up independent work. Now she misses this and doesn't eat anything. She seems to get terribly irritated with myself, father, etc.'
4	Rather unhappy (1964) Fairly happy (1966)	9	'Often ill at ease with friends, not knowing if they really like me (especially boys). I lack self-confidence. We [family] worry too much about friendship, money, everything' (1964). None given (1966).
5	Unhappy	9	None given.
6	Rather unhappy	6	'My parents expecting too much out of me in the way of schoolwork and therefore I'm afraid to fail because of my parents.'
7	Rather unhappy (1964) Jogging along (1966)	6	'School average marks not encouraging. Not allowed to go out except at weekends. Have to be in fairly early' (1964). 'Exams and not enough pocket money' (1966).
8	Rather unhappy	6	'Trying to find a suitable job in which I shall be happy. Worrying about exam results. Thinking about boys I like.'

[*continued*]

TABLE 9.5 (*continued*) *Outlines of case-studies of unhappy girls*
Co-educated girls aged 15 girls plus in 1964

Pupil	Self assessment of happiness at school	Intelligence score	Pupil's free responses
9	Rather unhappy	6	'I am very shy at doing things or talking in front of the people in class. Would very much like to have more self-confidence, and have a job.'
10	Rather unhappy	5	'Not being able to discuss matters with my parents; in matters of sex I just get embarrassed. Not being able to give up smoking.'
11	Rather unhappy	4	'What I am going to do when I leave. I'm not interested in the usual kind of job and I've no idea what to do if I don't find a job. I won't bring any money into the family and as our family is large we need more money.'

TABLE 9.6 *Outlines of case-studies of unhappy girls*
Girls in girls' schools aged 15 plus in 1964

Pupil	Self assessment of happiness at school	Intelligence score	Pupil's free responses
1	Rather unhappy	10	No special problem is given.
2	Unhappy (1964) Rather unhappy (1966)	9	'Lack of self-confidence' (1964). 'School atmosphere rather unpleasant. Getting into trouble with the teachers for no reason' (1966). 'Wondering if I'll ever get married' (1966).
3	Unhappy	9	'Want to earn money to buy myself the clothes my parents cannot afford. Am always quarrelling with my family. I can do nothing right.'
4	Rather unhappy	9	None given.
5	Rather unhappy	9	'Lack of self-confidence.'

[*continued*]

TABLE 9.6 *(continued) Outlines of case-studies of unhappy girls*
Girls in girls' schools aged 15 plus in 1964

Pupil	Self assessment of happiness at school	Intelligence score	Pupil's free responses
6	Rather unhappy (1964) Happy (1966)	9	'Wondering if I am really in love with a boy' (1964). 'Not liking to study; other things always seem more pleasant and I give in very easily. School simply trains you for exams' (1966).
7	Rather unhappy	8	'Problems at home—father—parents disliking my friends. Thinking too much about the opposite sex.'
8	Rather unhappy (1964) Absent (1966)	8	'Whether I will pass my G.C.E. and get a good job.'
9	Unhappy	8	'I hate school and wish I could earn my own money so as not to spend my parents'.'
10	Unhappy	8	'Passing exams before leaving school and getting a job.'
11	Unhappy (1964) Unhappy (1966)	7	'Not having enough money and not enough clothes' (1964). 'I hate school and have lost complete interest in it and I miss someone very much and I am constantly day-dreaming about her during lessons' (1966).
12	Rather unhappy (1964) Jogging along (1966)	7	'Homework takes so much time sometimes it is difficult to get enough sleep. Difficult to concentrate' (1964). 'Wishes to marry but *his* parents oppose' (1966). 'Too much stress on academic work.' 'Our teachers tend to be like icebergs.'
13	Unhappy	7	'Too much homework.'

[*continued*]

TABLE 9.6 (*continued*) *Outlines of case-studies of unhappy girls*

Girls in girls' schools aged 15 plus in 1964

Pupil	Self assessment of happiness at school	Intelligence score	Pupil's free responses
14	Rather unhappy	7	'I hate school and want to start work. At school you are treated much younger than you really are. I am always having arguments with my parents about boys I go out with.'
15	Rather unhappy	6	'School takes up too much of our time and we should have less homework. I don't seem to enjoy myself as much as others.'

TABLE 9.7 *Outlines of case-studies of unhappy girls*

Co-educated girls aged 13 plus in 1966

Pupil	Self assessment of happiness at school	Intelligence score	Pupil's free responses*
1	Rather unhappy	9	She is rather unhappy because, 'People leave me out of things.' The pressure of work worries her because, 'Homework takes too long. In the summer I want to get out in the sunshine.' Later, 'Everything is exams and I get very worried before exams.' 'I can't do as well in school as my parents expect me to do. People don't like me.' (Last two were special problems.)
2	Rather unhappy	7	'I find school dull and uninteresting especially the teachers.' The pressure of work worries her, 'Because it is too strict.'

[*continued*]

TABLE 9.7 (*continued*) *Outlines of case-studies of unhappy girls*

Co-educated girls aged 13 plus in 1966

Pupil	Self assessment of happiness at school	Intelligence score	Pupil's free responses
3	Rather unhappy	7	'I am not a really good pupil. I sometimes never understand the work we do.' The pressure of work worries her, 'Because we get too much homework.' 'The teachers pick on us for every little thing,' and 'I don't like school and some teachers.' 'If I want to get out somewhere special I do not have enough money. Too much homework, don't always understand it. Cannot stay out late at night.'
4	Rather unhappy	7	She disagrees strongly about looking forward to school each day because, 'I want to be a nice person when I grow up.' 'Not being good at French.'
5	Rather unhappy	6	Special problems: 'My father works hard for a good wage but the money does not seem to stretch as there are five of us and mum and dad never get any new clothes. I once went out with someone and worshipped him and when we parted it nearly killed me.' 'I dislike school because I am not clever and some of my friends look down on me.' Agrees the intense pressure of work worries her, 'Because I am not able to understand.' About looking forward to coming to school: 'My mother misses me strongly so I dislike leaving her.' The atmosphere is rather unpleasant, 'Because we have to be forced to come.'

[*continued*]

TABLE 9.7 (*continued*) *Outlines of case studies of unhappy girls*
Co-educated girls aged 13 plus in 1966

Pupil	Self assessment of happiness at school	Intelligence score	Pupil's free responses 1966
6	Rather unhappy	6	She is not worried by the pressure of work: 'I like working.' Most teachers 'Try to help us a lot.' She looks forward to coming to school each day, but she is rather unhappy, 'Because I am not liked by many girls.' 'You see all your friends at school.'

* The quotation marks indicate responses to separate questions. Responses volunteered as Special Problems in the Mooney Test are included.

TABLE 9.8 *Outlines of case-studies of unhappy girls*
Girls in girls' schools, aged 13 plus

Pupil	Self assessment of happiness at school	Intelligence score	Pupil's free responses 1966
1	Rather unhappy (1966) Rather unhappy (1964)	10	'I can't remember things and just cannot study. I also get mixed up.' 'Teachers expect rather a lot of you and they always ignore the ones who are not good enough.' 'The atmosphere is all right for working.'
2	Rather unhappy	9	'It's the teachers' attitude to work and Latin and doing homework that I hate. It takes so much of the evening up and is boring.' The pressure of work worries her: 'All work I hate and worry about unless I like it and people don't boss me too much.' She doesn't look forward to coming to school: 'The discipline and strictness of school is mainly the trouble.' 'There is often a feud between pupils and teachers.'

[*continued*]

TABLE 9.8 (*continued*) *Outlines of case studies of unhappy girls*
Girls in girls' schools, aged 13 plus

Pupil	Self assessment of happiness at school	Intelligence score	Pupil's free responses 1966
3	Rather unhappy	8	'I was really excited when I heard I was coming to this school. Now I wish I had never heard of it. Not being able to keep up with the rest of the class. Afraid of dying and hoping there is no hell.' 'I don't seem to get along very well with either the teachers or my classmates—they seem to find me uninteresting.' Pressure of work worries her: 'Teachers expect more of you than you can do.' She disagrees strongly that she looks forward to coming to school: 'I *hate* school'.
4	Rather unhappy	8	'I cannot settle down well and I don't do homework well.' The teachers 'Do not express much emotion to either good or bad and keep themselves to their colleagues' (sic). 'No teachers in our school could take a joke.' Special problems: 'Parents separating. Skin rash since I was a child. Wanting to start work. I am fed up of school.'
5	Unhappy	8	'I find it difficult to get along with people at school.' Special problems: 'My future. Sex.'
6	Rather unhappy (1966) Rather unhappy (1964)	8	'I dislike most subjects. We get tests every week and I worry about them.' 'I hate school.' Special problems: 'I hate French and I just can't understand a word of it. Can't understand my new maths teacher.'
7	Unhappy (1966) Rather unhappy (1964)	8	'I feel I am disliked by many girls because I am poor.' 'Some teachers are too stern.' 'I just can't face school and friends.' Special problems: 'I am frightened about my mother and father having a

[*continued*]

TABLE 9.8 (*continued*) *Outlines of case studies of unhappy girls*
Girls in girls' schools, aged 13 plus

Pupil	Self assessment of happiness at school	Intelligence score	Pupil's free responses 1966
			divorce. I have a terrible feeling that boys hate me and I'll never get married. I don't mean to swear but it just comes out and when people talk about dirty stories it makes me think.'
8	Unhappy	7	'I am not clever and you are at school for too long.' (But she is not worried by the pressure of work.)
9	Unhappy	7	'I think our school is unhappy because we are shut in too much. We aren't allowed out of school till we go home at night.' 'The teachers pile the work on us and they think it isn't much.' 'Our teachers are usually friendly, they like a joke as much as we do.' 'Our teachers are humorous but I still don't like school.' Special problems: 'Taking things too seriously. Sometimes lying without meaning to.'
10	Rather unhappy	6	'Teachers get annoyed, but sometimes can be pleasant.' (No special problems recorded.)
11	Rather unhappy	6	'There are too many rules to be obeyed.' 'Certain teachers can be very friendly but others are much too bad-tempered.' 'I hate school.' The atmosphere 'Is too serious and precise.' (No special problems.)
12	Unhappy	6	'I hate school and will be glad when I leave.' 'Teachers expect you to know too much, if you don't know they get mad.' 'A lot of teachers at our school are grumpy.' Special problems: 'Before German lessons I always get butterflies in my stomach.'

10

Out-of-school conduct

Most schools take an interest in the out-of-school conduct of their pupils, and many pupils agree that the intention is a good one. The debate is about where the line is to be drawn between parental rights and school demands, between the freedom of the pupil to do as he pleases after school hours, away from the school buildings, and the desire of the school to ensure that its pupils, in their contact with the world, should develop into good citizens and preserve untarnished the school image. The line is inevitably imprecise and is drawn in very different places by individual schools. It is naturally the extremes which attract attention, either undue interference or undue laxity. Though the main purpose of this chapter is to compare co-educational and single-sex schools, there is much that is of general interest, and more than a touch of humour.

This topic was examined in only the 'Both schools' enquiry, which included the question, 'Do you consider that the school's concern with the out-of-school conduct of pupils was, Excessive/Rather strict/Just right/Rather insufficient/Much too lax?' All the ex-pupils had attended at least one co-educational and one single-sex grammar school, and were therefore able to compare the two types. The estimates of the women are given in Table 10.1.

The salient features of Table 10.1 are, first, that whereas over half the estimates for the co-educational schools, both senior and junior, come into the 'just right' category, those for the girls' schools are only one third; second, that the remaining estimates for the co-educational schools are divided evenly above and below the 'just right' line, but those for the girls' schools are concentrated more in the 'rather strict' and 'excessive' categories which comprise over half the estimates. This concentration resulted in a reduction at the opposite end of the scale so that the proportion of those who thought the out-of-school control of the co-educational schools was rather insufficient was greater than in the case of the girls' schools. This finding (like that about the boys in the next section) is again in agreement with those found previously that discipline in single-sex schools is more severe; it also agrees with the theory

TABLE 10.1 *Out-of-school conduct of girls*

'Both schools' survey

Estimates of school's concern with out-of-school conduct of pupils	Replies about first school attended				Replies about last school attended			
	Co-educational		Girls'		Co-educational		Girls'	
	N	%	N	%	N	%	N	%
Excessive	7	2·4	66	16·5	10	2·9	40	15·7
Rather strict	62	21·2	142	35·6	73	21·0	103	40·4
Just right	155	53·1	145	36·3	179	51·2	82	32·1
Rather insufficient	56	19·2	37	9·3	76	21·8	26	10·2
Much too lax	12	4·1	9	2·3	11	3·1	4	1·6
Totals	292	100	399	100	349	100	255	100

NOTE: The differences between co-educational and girls' schools for both first and last schools are statistically significant beyond the ·001 level.

based on this, which ascribes the difference to the contrast between the psychological forces at work within the two school communities. It has been suggested that part of the difference between girls' and co-educational schools might be due to male teachers not noticing minor breaches of the code of conduct (as distinct from not wanting to notice); this, however, does not explain the stricter enforcement of this code in boys' schools.

The free responses under this heading have been classified. (Table A.9) and placed in *Appendix 2*. Their distribution in categories was as expected from the estimates. The examples quoted have been selected in equal proportions in the respective categories, from both girls' and co-educational schools, but the 'excessive interest' and 'much too lax' categories have been given double weighting to secure their adequate representation. As the distributions of the estimates for first and last schools were reasonably similar they were merged. The quotations about the co-educational schools the ex-pupils attended are as follows:

EXCESSIVE 'We were brought up before the senior master if we were known to be courting one of the boys out of school—even if we never saw them during the day—and given a lecture on "how to behave" so we wouldn't disgrace the name of the school.'

'It was thought wrong to mix with pupils from the Sec. Mod. school.'

RATHER STRICT 'The headmaster would frequently stop his car in the middle of a main street and reprimand his pupils for trivial misdemeanours.'

'The headmaster would not give his consent to any member of his school who wished to take art or pottery at night school.'

'The senior mistress fussed about uniform and eating lollipops in the street.'

JUST RIGHT 'Limited to caps and hats and common decency, especially on public transport.'

'Girls and boys were not allowed to associate with each other much straight out of school—when it was known they dated each other.'

'The only time the school went to extremes was when they tried to prevent the school members using a coffee bar—it had no effect.'

'They did not interfere so long as it did not affect school life.'

'Wished pupils to bring credit to the school.'

'Most noticeable on social occasions, polite, well mannered yet enjoyable to be with.'

RATHER INSUFFICIENT 'The women members of staff were more concerned than the men.'

'Behaviour on buses was dreadful at times but nothing was done about this.'

'The staff were concerned with some pupils' out-of-school conduct but I think they had given up hope with some and just ignored them.'

MUCH TOO LAX 'There appeared to be no concern for what happened to anyone out of school.'

'They never appeared to know what we did even though the 6th form as a whole went to the "pub".'

The comments about their girls' schools were:

EXCESSIVE 'They fussed to a ridiculous extent over outdated and silly attitudes, eating a sweet on the bus, etc.'

'If caught without a hat on for any reason you were forced to wear it in school for a day. No eating sweets on buses—no walking in groups, etc.'

'Half-terms, etc. were altered from the same time as the "boys' school" "to prevent unhealthy contacts" as our headmistress told us.'

'We weren't allowed to walk to school with a boy, brother or not.'

'Even told what kind of clothing to wear. In uniform we were not to speak to workers (in overalls) and such.'

'We were not even allowed to walk down certain streets or go shopping after school.'

RATHER STRICT 'Some of the staff carried this noseyness to extremes (older women).'

'One is bound to get some restriction with out-of-school conduct, but perhaps this is rather more so than the co-ed. school.'

'Had to wear hat all year round, no frilly petticoats. Other trivia.'

'You had to act "like ladies" at all times.'

JUST RIGHT 'The school was well known in the area. We ourselves wanted to help its public image.' (Boarding school)

'They were trying to educate us as people, not just encyclopaedias.' (Boarding school)

RATHER INSUFFICIENT 'The school had a bad name in the area owing to lack of interest from senior girls and staff.'

MUCH TOO LAX 'People went mad once they were let out.'

In both types of school the same problems appear, from boy–girl friendships and the use of coffee bars to wearing school hats and not eating sweets on buses! But there is a more rigorous control in the girls' schools—the school doing its best to produce well mannered young ladies and to protect them until they are old enough to protect themselves, and at the same time here and there overstepping the mark, or, as one girl puts it, insisting on out-of-date customs. The pupils express their annoyance at this, and occasionally add that the home itself resented interference. Which reminds one again of that wise French saying, 'Happy is the man who has not the faults of his virtues.' The quotation is so apt in this connection that no apology is made for using it twice. A laudable aim spelled out in too great detail and insisted on with vigilant supervision can rapidly become a cause of deteriorating pupil–teacher relationships, especially when many other equally laudable aims are added and just as zealously pursued, together with the inevitable age gap in customs and attitudes added to the brew. How long ago is it that girls' schools used to insist on girls wearing gloves when travelling to and from school, and how long did the schools persist with the uphill struggle?

Some women teachers in the co-educational schools evidently had the same virtues and the same faults, and there are at times complaints from them and even from some senior girls that the men teachers did not co-operate sufficiently in this control of out-of-school conduct. Perhaps men do not have the same sharp and vigilant eye of the female for the missing hat or the sucked sweet, or perhaps they just don't want to see. A third explanation that is sometimes put forward by women teachers—that the men are too lazy—is in the writer's *opinion* untenable, but being male he himself might be thought prejudiced. Be this as it may, the presence of men on the staff appears in this respect, as well as in others, to exert a moderating influence on the women. Whether this is good or bad is an additional question; there are women teachers in girls' schools who would claim that this influence is either wholly bad or at least that it goes too far. They would add that few young people like to be disciplined, but this is an inevitable part of the training of the younger generation by the older, and the writer is presenting only the views of the pupils and ignoring those of the teachers. In this there is much truth, but two points are made in reply. First, although these views are indeed those of ex-pupils, they are in fact adults and even intending teachers themselves, and looking back on their treatment they can view it more dispassionately; in their replies they show that they now realize more clearly that some of the discipline they then thought was unnecessary was, on mature reflection, justified. This makes their protests of course more reasonable, more balanced and more important. Second, if the result of a certain policy is that an appreciable proportion of the pupils become resentful and express these sentiments long afterwards, it seems as if it might be time to moderate this policy. The little lost on the swings might be gained on the roundabouts in the form of happier and closer teacher–pupil relationships.

Let it be emphasized that there will be many girls' schools where they have been gaining on the roundabouts for a very long time. The writer knows one such school well where a really great headmistress, now passed away, showed qualities of leadership, humanity and tolerance which made her loved and venerated by her pupils. The same qualities will be present in many other women teachers in girls' schools. This book, however, is concerned with average tendencies. The point that the writer is concerned to repeat is that whereas it has often been thought of relatively little moment whether a school is a co-educational or a girls' school, these are in fact very different institutions psychologically. This being so the decision whether to educate boys and girls apart or together is one of the most fundamental that can be asked in education. We have been a long time arriving at this truth, and having arrived there it now seems rather obvious.

The manner in which the estimates and comments about the ex-pupils' co-educational schools cluster closely around the mid-point suggests that there is on the whole satisfaction with most schools in the manner of their control of out-of-school conduct. Yet with the centre of gravity for the estimates situated in the 'just-right' category, it is easier for control in these schools to become 'rather insufficient' than it is the girls' schools, where the comparable centre of gravity is in the 'rather strict' category. The matter is put in proper perspective, however, by a comparison of the proportion of comments in the 'much too lax' category in the two types of school. For girls in girls' schools this was 4.4 per cent and for those in co-educational schools almost 6 per cent.

We now arrive at the male ex-pupils' comments about the control of both of their schools over the out-of-school conduct of pupils. First is presented the most reliable of the two measures—the estimates.

TABLE 10.2 *Out-of-school conduct of boys*

'Both schools' survey

Estimates of schools' concern with out-of-school conduct of pupils	Replies about first school attended				Replies about last school attended			
	Co-educational		Boys'		Co-educational		Boys'	
	N	%	N	%	N	%	N	%
Excessive	4	4·9	10	8·6	8	7·8	5	7·0
Rather strict	20	24·4	35	30·2	27	26·2	24	33·8
Just right	41	50·0	53	45·7	52	50·4	33	46·6
Rather insufficient	12	14·6	11	9·5	12	11·7	4	5·6
Much too lax	5	6·1	7	6·0	4	3·9	5	7·0
Totals	82	100	116	100	103	100	71	100

NOTE: The differences between the distributions for boys' schools and co-educational are not statistically significant, either for first or last schools.

In Table 10.2 there is little difference between the estimates about the schools attended as juniors and those about schools attended as seniors. Though in both junior and senior groups slightly more pupils thought the co-educational school's attitude was just right as compared with that of their boys' school, the difference is only some 4 per cent, with rather small numbers. Similarly, in both junior and senior groups slightly more boys thought their co-educational school had a 'rather insufficient' concern than their boys' school had, while a rather higher proportion of both age groups said their boys' schools were rather strict or excessively so, as opposed to their co-educational schools. If we combine the 'too strict' categories and compare them with the 'too lax' we find that 9 per cent more of the junior sample estimated their boys' schools to be too strict compared with their co-educational schools, and 7 per cent in the seniors, while 5 per cent more of the juniors and 3 per cent more of the seniors estimated the concern of their co-educational schools to be on the lax side. The differences are not great and are not statistically significant, but they agree with the previous findings on the differences between the two types of school in discipline, and with the theory which interprets this as a natural consequence of basic differences in the two kinds of community. When we are considering where the line *should* be drawn we must not forget, first that it may be right that the line is drawn in a different place for the different communities; second, that we are reviewing the experiences of the sufferers rather than those of the imposers; third, that these particular sufferers are in the process of becoming imposers, so that their views are likely to be a compromise between the two sides. This should be borne in mind when readers are considering the verdict of both boys and girls.

The reasons given by the boys for their estimates are not presented in a classified table partly because the number of responses was rather small for sub-division and partly because there was not much difference between the replies from co-educational and those from boys' schools. Those who thought control was excessive maintained that it infringed personal freedom and rights or complained about the narrow-mindedness of head or staff. Most boys who thought control 'rather strict' complained about interference in smaller matters such as the wearing of school caps, especially in middle and senior school, and resented this, but some accepted the strictness and felt it to be justified. Sometimes school tradition or school image was said to be the cause of the strictness, whether in itself the punishment was justifiable or not. Those who said the concern was just right acknowledged a need for control over such things as smoking, drinking, and bad behaviour. A number of boys, however, thought the oversight was rather insufficient because the pupils were drawn from a large area which it was impracticable to supervise.

Out-of-school conduct

Some of the more interesting comments are quoted, first from boys in co-educational schools. The first two quotations are from boys who thought the concern excessive.

Co-educational schools

EXCESSIVE 'In School two prefects had to sign a document that they wouldn't drink, etc., out of school hours even when we were over 18.'

'Deputy head (female) told a prefect not to walk with a girl on Sundays—it was his cousin. She was exceptionally narrow-minded.'

RATHER STRICT Those who thought the concern 'rather strict' included a minority who thought it was justified, but most felt it was unreasonable:

'No holding hands going down the road, no drinking, or smoking in school uniform.'

'All pupils had to wear hats. This (boys') consisted of the usual cap for 1–5 years, but a special beret was introduced for the 6th forms while I was there. Surely there is no need for hats after (say) the 3rd form.'

'It was rather strict but I think that it was justified as the reputation of the school with all its teachers and pupils was at stake, and its reputation for "job value".'

JUST RIGHT The 'just right' group included two more than usually thoughtful replies:

'Co-education was a new venture in the town's educational policy. Consequently the School had to strike the right balance between old narrow-minded attitudes, and the true spirit of co-education—this it did effectively.'

'The School should have a great concern for the pupils' conduct out of school. Child upbringing and education is a 24-hour business not to be undertaken only between 9.00 a.m. to 4.00 p.m.'

MUCH TOO LAX The few comments about laxness included:

'As soon as we were out of school we ceased to be influenced by it.'

'They were concerned about conduct if pupils were wearing school uniform, and then very much.'

Boys' schools

The comments from boys' schools reflect the rather greater strictness shown in the estimates; those who thought it excessive have a sharper tone:

EXCESSIVE 'If it occurred it was heavily punished irrespective of reason.'

'Teachers were known to actually hit pupils outside school hours!'

'Conduct outside the school was to be irreproachable, otherwise the pupil was punished by the head himself.'

'We were pulled up for the slightest thing, such as having a cap on slightly out of line.'

'We were not encouraged to mix with the girls' school next door, for example.'

RATHER STRICT As with the replies about co-educational schools, those who thought the boys' schools' concern was rather strict had a minority who said it was justified.

'The wearing of caps by 16–18-year-olds was rather ridiculous.'

'The school had an "image" to keep up in the North of England.'

'Rather strict in stupid ways, i.e. uniform, but not in ways of behaviour; many pupils were commuters, and warnings only existed for bad behaviour.'

JUST RIGHT Boys who thought the concern 'just right' consisted mainly of a group who wrote of the need to keep the good school 'image' and a group saying that the area the school drew from was too large for close control.

RATHER INSUFFICIENT There were few comments by boys who judged the control to be rather insufficient. One, rather illogically, wrote:

'No concern was shown at all which I think was a good thing.'

There were no comments from the few boys who thought the control to be 'much too lax'.

Little further analysis is needed on the comparison between boys in boys' and in co-educational schools except to mention that the distribution of comments supports the verdict of the estimates in indicating a much closer similarity between boys in boys' schools and those in co-educational schools than between the comparable groups of girls. The same difference is, however, present—the tendency of the single-sex school towards greater strictness of control, and the slightly greater bunching round the 'just right' category for the co-educational schools. The differences, however, are not regarded as statistically reliable.

Comment

As there has already been comment at the end of the various sections only a short note is added. In the matter of out-of-school conduct schools are in a difficult position because their legal right to interfere would appear to be uncertain; yet when pupils in school uniform behave badly the school itself receives the opprobrium of the public. The schools rightly endeavour to educate their pupils to become well-behaved citizens, but what exactly are their legal powers once the pupil sets his foot outside the school? It seems to the writer that schools may have understandably arrogated to themselves powers over out-of-school conduct which could be disputed, though on the whole these powers are exercised in a way which is useful to the community and good for the right social development of the pupils. In some cases, however, there is evidence of parents resenting the schools' attempt to push the boundaries of their claims into areas which the parents regard as their own. Who should decide the style of a girl's hair-ribbon—parent or teacher? In a time of changing fashions has the school the legal right to demand that a boy's hair be cut short? The parent may sign an agreement (does he always?) that he will provide a school hat or cap for his offspring, but has the school any legal—or even moral—right to compel the child to wear it *on the way to school*, against the wishes of both child and parent? These are delicate questions but it is perhaps time that they were asked, though wise guidance and wise oversight *in things that matter* are obviously of benefit to all concerned.

11

School preference

In the previous volume on the rival merits of co-educational and single-sex secondary schools, two of the chapters presented the views of teachers and the reasons for their preference. A decided majority of teachers in maintained day grammar schools considered that co-educational schools provided a better education and preferred them. Those who had taught in both types of school were strongly in favour of co-education, and teachers in co-educational schools were themselves almost unanimously in their favour. Opposition came mainly from those who had had no practical experience of these schools; in other words it is founded upon ignorance. This does not mean that the opponents are not sincere, but it is the writer's opinion that they often confuse effects caused by social class differences between co-educational and single-sex schools (and to some extent differences in status, type of staffing, and degree of selective entry) with differences caused by co-education.

In the present volume we pass on to consider whether co-educational or single-sex schools are preferred by pupils and ex-pupils, naturally placing most stress on the choice of those pupils who have attended at least one co-educational and one single-sex secondary school (excluding secondary modern). Fortunately we also have their reasons for this choice. Their preference, however, is not regarded as being in itself decisive, though its importance is clear. It is a tenable argument that junior and middle school pupils might prefer one school to another because in it they need not do much work and discipline is perhaps more lax than it should be. Against this the verdict of the teachers could be quoted, and it might also be pointed out that the senior pupils and responsible ex-pupils such as intending teachers would be unlikely to make this mistake in judgment. None the less the findings of this and the previous volume are best viewed as a whole, to see whether they result in a consistent picture in favour of one side or the other.

This chapter weighs up evidence on school preference which has been obtained from the ex-pupils of the First and Second College surveys, the 'Both schools' survey, and from two relatively small-scale inquiries among pupils in grammar schools. The results are first presented with a minimum of comment, then reviewed as a whole at the end of the chapter.

The First College survey

In the early days of this research work, in 1946 and 1947, a simple exploratory survey about attitude to co-education was made among ex-pupils of grammar schools who were training to be teachers. (A parallel survey was made at the same time among grammar school teachers.) As the questionnaire was administered in groups the percentage of completed forms was 100 per cent in most institutions, though in a few cases it was low. Institutions with low returns had results similar to those from institutions with high returns. Replies were obtained from seventeen University Departments of Education and (for comparison) four Colleges of Education, comprising in all 1,167 students. As mentioned in Chapter 1, these are not a representative cross-section of ex-grammar school students, but they represent one important type of pupil from both co-educational and single-sex schools, responsible in attitude, and with a deeper than average interest in educational problems. Students from University Departments of Education and those from Colleges of Education are considered separately, as are men and women. They were asked the question, 'Are you in favour of co-education in secondary schools?' and were given the opportunity of choosing between full co-education (Type A), co-education with mostly single-sex classes (Type B), dual schools (a girls' and a boys' school in one building under separate heads), undecided, and single-sex schools. Dual schools were called 'Co-educational, Type C', but were classed with single-sex in the analysis. Each respondent was requested to comment on the preference given.

The results from students in University Departments of Education are given first (Table 11.1); they reveal a change of opinion which few people suspected at that time.

The men's results show two principal trends: first, that a majority of the students preferred co-education, second, that the students educated in co-educational schools were more strongly in favour of these than were those educated in boys' schools. If we logically combine Types A and B (because Type B is much nearer to co-education than to single-sex schooling) and oppose it to Type C plus single-sex, the percentages as one goes down the table are 87 to 9, 59 to 29, 87 to 13, and 52 to 37, there being a majority in favour of co-education in all groups, but a more decisive one among ex-pupils of co-educational schools. The women's results are similar (Table 11.2).

TABLE 11.1 *Type of school preferred:* Male students*

First College survey

Type of student replying	Type of secondary school preferred											
University Departments of Education	Type A		Type B		Type C		Single-sex		Undecided		Totals	
	N	%	N	%	N	%	N	%	N	%	N	%
Co-educated men	98	74·3	17	12·9	6	4·5	6	4·5	5	3·8	132	100
Men from boys' schools	102	45·7	30	13·5	46	20·6	19	8·5	26	11·7	223	100
College of Education												
Co-educated men	47	74·6	8	12·7	3	4·8	5	7·9	0	0	63	100
Men from boys' schools	64	35·8	29	16·2	40	22·3	27	15·1	19	10·6	179	100

* Type C signifies only co-operation between boys' and girls' schools (in the same or adjoining buildings) for joint social activities, and should be counted as against co-education in the generally accepted meaning of the term. Type A is the normal co-educational school, Type B is a school for boys and girls organized in mostly single-sex classes (except perhaps in the Sixth).

TABLE 11.2 *Type of school preferred: Female students*

First College survey

Type of student replying	Type of secondary school preferred Type A		Type B		Type C		Single-sex		Undecided		Totals	
University Departments of Education	N	%	N	%	N	%	N	%	N	%	N	%
Co-educated women	144	90·6	8	5·0	5	3·1	0		2	1·3	159	100
Women from girls' schools	100	44·7	43	19·2	29	12·9	9	4·0	43	19·2	224	100
College of Education												
Co-educated women	42	100·0	0		0		0		0		42	100
Women from girls' schools	30	66·8	11	24·4	2	4·4	1	2·2	1	2·2	45	100

Here one sees the same preference for co-education in all groups and the same powerful influence of the type of school which the respondents themselves attended. Reading from top to bottom of the table, as for the men, the percentages in favour of co-education are 96 to 3, 64 to 17, 100 to 0, and 91 to 7, the last two groups being rather small. The female student teachers of this inquiry are still more favourably inclined to co-education than the men, a finding which will be supported by the results of other investigations described here.

The above findings might be opposed on the grounds that most of the ex-pupils had had experience only of the one type of school he or she had attended. This has been met by separating out those students who had attended both a co-educational and a single-sex secondary school, excluding secondary modern (Table 11.3). The numbers are small but should be considered in relation to other studies discussed later. As all groups had a big majority for co-education all male students are combined, and similarly for women.

TABLE 11.3 *Type of school preferred: Students who attended both types*

First College survey

	Type of secondary school preferred											
	Type A		Type B		Type C		Single-sex		Undecided		Totals	
	N	%	N	%	N	%	N	%	N	%	N	%
Female students	31	64·6	11	22·9	3	6·2	1	2·1	2	4·2	48	100
Male students	33	63·4	7	13·5	3	5·8	5	9·6	4	7·7	52	100

Male and female students who had attended both a co-educational and a single-sex secondary school were heavily in favour of the co-educational school, the male by 77 to 15 per cent, and the female by 88 to 8 per cent, with a negligible number undecided. The numbers in the sample, however, were only 52 men and 48 women.

In their free responses the students set down reasons why they supported or opposed co-education in secondary schools. They could naturally have suppressed some reasons but there seems to be little cause for such an action, particularly as the questionnaires were anonymous. These free responses are classified in Table 11.4, where those from students who were educated in single-sex, mixed and both types of schools are combined because of their basic similarity. The sexes are given separately. In the classification procedure it was often necessary to place sections of a reply into two or even more categories, so that although there were 1,167 questionnaires returned, of which 59 had no comment, the remainder yielded 1,924 classified remarks. The numbers given are therefore more useful for studying the stress placed upon the various arguments than for comparing the preference for and against co-education, for which a comparison based on Tables 11.1, 11.2 and 11.3 is safer.

TABLE 11.4 *Classified comments on co-education (full sample)*

First College survey

	Men	Women
For co-education		
preparation for adult life, training for social life	223	214
school societies and school social life	44	26
segregation is unnatural, healthier atmosphere	68	55
easy relations with other sex, more understanding, healthy sex attitude, less adolescent 'crushes', sex problems, emotional difficulties; sexes are complementary, co-operation learnt	324	315
competition and academic standards	33	68
broader outlook, different points of view and interests	61	78
better discipline, better behaviour	46	16
others	30	40
Totals	829	812
Against co-education		
different abilities, different interests, different rates of development of boys and girls	74	57
discipline difficulty	28	15
distraction by presence of the opposite sex	31	8
staff and head should be the same sex as pupils	24	3
others	32	11
Totals	189	94

From the data in Table 11.4 readers will see that those students in favour of co-education emphasize the social factors involved, indicated by such headings as 'preparation for adult life', 'training for social life', and 'easy relations with the other sex, more understanding'. Related to this but not identical with it is the idea that co-education is more natural and produces a healthier atmosphere. Though the academic side is a lesser factor it attracts an appreciable number of comments stressing the advantages of the broader outlook and the different points of view of the two sexes, and (for male students) the better behaviour of the boys.

The reasons given for opposing co-education are principally concerned with the different abilities, different interests and rates of development of boys and girls, while to a lesser extent there are some fears about distraction by the opposite sex and a few qualms about discipline. One cannot but feel that a section of the opposition did not put down their real fear—that it would be unhealthy and unwise for the two sexes to be in daily propinquity in a school building—though practical experience has shown these fears to be unfounded. It is a characteristic of all these researches that the arguments given for co-education are primarily social and those against co-education are concerned with instruction. The proof of the pudding, however, is in the eating, and as said before, no one has yet demonstrated that co-educated pupils reach a lower standard *because of* co-education than the single-sex educated pupils reach; the available evidence in fact points in the opposite direction (Dale, 1962a, 1962b and 1964).

In order to put a little flesh and blood on the bare bones of the statistics, some of the free responses are given in full, but the numbers for and against are not taken strictly according to the proportion found in the original voting, as this would not have illustrated the case against co-education sufficiently. This proportion, taking all students *who were not undecided*, is 73 to 27 for the men and 89 to 11 for the women.

Comments favourable to co-education[1] *(men)*

The type of education of each respondent is placed in brackets before his comment.

(Both schools) 'Since boys and girls have to mix with each other on leaving school, it strikes me as being ridiculous to segregate them when young. If they have mixed with the other sex in their school days they will have more experience of each other on going out into the world.

'In schools where only boys or girls are educated, there seems to be the opinion that it is wrong to associate with the other sex before reaching manhood or womanhood. This is nonsense and does a great deal of harm.

'The days spent in the co-educational grammar school were the happiest of my life. The atmosphere in the boys' grammar school which I attended later was far less pleasant and natural.'

(Co-educational school) 'It gives the child an opportunity of meeting and working with members of the opposite sex at an age approaching maturity, so letting them "gently" into normal adult life when it is essential for men and women to work together.

'More "colour" is added to school life for pupils and teachers,

[1] Occasionally favourable or unfavourable comments contain qualifying clauses which have the reverse significance, though the overall *estimate* by the student is as indicated in the text. When one respondent makes several points these are paragraphed.

since life can be a very monotonous thing when spent wholly with your own sex.

'It gives a child an opportunity of unconsciously observing the points in members of the opposite sex which later on will mean so much to him when selecting his mate.'

(Boys' boarding school) '(a) Less homosexuality— particularly in boarding schools. THIS IS A VERY SERIOUS POINT AND, I DO ASSURE YOU, IT IS NOT FRIVOLOUS [sic].
'(b) Much more natural attitude to members of the other sex.'

(Co-educational school) 'One aim of education is to enable children to develop as worthy citizens. This can only be achieved if the society of the school resembles society in general.

'In passing on the best of a heritage (or environment) it is essential to preserve a "model society" in the school. This cannot be done on a one-sex basis.

'A child cannot even begin to integrate its personality if it lives and learns in unnatural seclusion from the disturbing but moulding influences exerted by the other sex.

'Co-education will mean mixed staffs—and that *may* lead to the humanization of staffs and their return to the fold of sensible, broad and open-minded people. Teachers with "bees in their bonnets" and petty adherences to "do's and dont's" thrive on the one-sex staff—especially female!!'

(Boys' school) 'Greater opportunities for unusual class-room activities, e.g.—short historical plays with female characters.

'Equal intellectual opportunities for both sexes would lead to a more reasonable appreciation of woman's place in society and would end the deplorable "Back to the Kitchen" attitude which permeates modern society.

'The element of competition would be keener: neither sex would wish to "let the side down".

'The brute in the boys would be curbed by the refining influence of young ladies.'

(Boys' school) 'It is a more natural life and it approximates to conditions in every-day life.

'It does away with shyness and will take women off their pedestals.

'It is essential for plays, drama, dancing, etc.

'For an only child or two boys (or girls) in the same family it is their only chance to meet the opposite sex.

School preference

'Boys from co-ed. schools seem politer and more tolerant of women and old people than those from the other type.'

Comments favourable to co-education (women)

(Co-educational school) 'I think co-education helps children to develop a much more sensible outlook during adolescence: (I have heard it expressed this way—"Girls from a girls' school giggle if they see a boy get on a bus").

'It is good from the point of view of the work. I find that (in general) girls of 11–14 years are more industrious than boys of the same age and the boys in a mixed class just have to do some work to attain a good class position. Boys have a broader vision of a subject, can pick out salient features and tend to discard detail; average girls are more painstaking but tend to get "lost" in the detail and never view the subject as a whole. Surely each sex has something to learn of the other here? After the age of 15–16 years it is the girl who has to work harder than she might otherwise do to keep pace with the boys of the class (in general).

'The presence of the opposite sex in the class has no unsettling effect. It is taken as a matter of course when children have grown up in the system. I feel sure it is a better preparation for life after school when men and women work together in universities, offices, shops, etc.

'As regards Types B and C. To my mind, these types have little to recommend them which a unisexual school has not. In fact I would not class these types as "co-educational". As an experiment in the school I attended boys and girls were placed in separate classes one year on entering the school, and were mixed only on entering the Sixth form. I can only speak of the effect it had on the girls—they were by far the "silliest" section of the school and exhibited all those characteristics of adolescent girls which most people find so objectionable. (At any rate that was the opinion of we senior girls. I do not know what the staff thought of them.)'

(Co-educational school) 'School is part of life, in life there is no segregation of the sexes to such an extent, therefore there should not be a segregation of sexes in schools.

'In all-girl schools the main topic of conversation as far as one can gather seems to be males, whereas in co-educational schools, as the boys are there, girls seem to occupy their minds with other subjects to a greater extent.'

(Both schools) 'As I have had experience of both types of school I can state with personal knowledge on the subject that co-education is preferable. It gives a familiarity with the opposite sex and avoids any curiosity and emotional upset later in adolescence. It provides great opportunities for competition and rouses interest in subjects which might never be dealt with in schools of Type C. In social activities there is greater scope apart from the obvious advantages in school dramatics, etc.'

(Girls' school) 'Since, in their lives after school leaving age, boys and girls have to work together and spend their recreation periods in mixed company, then it is much better training for these adolescents to have experienced mixed company before they leave school. Furthermore, children from segregated schools who proceed to further education in mixed colleges waste valuable time settling down to working in mixed company, it is such a novelty for them that too much time is spent in the social life of the college, too little on the academic side.'

Comments unfavourable to co-education (*men*)

(Both schools—co-educational one year) 'The staff tend to be more heterogeneous than in a school of single-sex and from observation appear to be somewhat mutually antagonistic which is not in the interests of the pupils.

'Discipline must inevitably be a compromise between that suitable for boys and that for girls. At the adolescent stage a girl has far more respect for a woman teacher than she has for a man. Possibly something of the sort is true for boys also to a lesser extent.'

(Boys' school) 'The advantages—social life and joint activities—are in my opinion outweighed by the disturbances caused to both sets—boys and girls. It is far better that each should remain apart as long as possible—there will be plenty of time after leaving school for mixing. As may be seen I favour the monastic type of schooling. Surely co-education is far more difficult for the teacher!??'

(Boys' school) 'The difference in mode of reasoning, the male with his logic, the female with intuition, would not help the various teachers in forming their approach in teaching method. On the whole the average boy prefers segregated education.'

(Boys' school) 'Children appear to have a natural propensity for wasting time. Such wastage tends to be accentuated when the sexes are mixed.

'Judged by observations of Americans and Canadians, the co-educational system appears to have resulted in an exaggerated respect on the part of men for the so-called rights and privileges of women, while conversely women tend to treat men as "universal providers" to whom scant respect is due.'

(Boys' school) 'My secondary school life was spent in a boys' school. By nature I was shy and reserved. On coming up to university I find that my shyness persisted for some time before I became accustomed to mixed classes, tutorials, social activities, etc. There was a girls' school in close proximity to the boys' school but no mixed activities of any kind were allowed. I feel that this segregation was too rigid and severe. In some respects, apart from physical training and games, the needs and interests of boys and girls run apart and for this reason co-education of Type A is not desirable or advantageous.

'Education is preparation for life, and learning to know and respect each other's point of view should be a gradual process in an experience which can well begin in co-education in a school of Type C, where there is a joint social life and school society activities such as dancing, debates, play-producing, etc., where supervision in the nature of advice and guidance is maintained.'

(Boys' school) 'Boys and girls have widely different interests in many ways and in co-ed. schools there is a tendency for the different activities to clash.

'I have noticed a tendency where I was in classes, on occasions when girls were present, that very little work was actually done. A boy of 14 does not mind making a fool of himself before boys—but dreads the thought of doing so before girls.'

Comments unfavourable to co-education (women)

(Girls' school) 'Females become masculine, boys become effeminate.'

(Girls' school) 'Completely different treatment is required for boys and girls.

'Boys and girls distract each other in class.

'Girls are more physically mature than boys of same age although not necessarily more intelligent.

'Boys and girls have different interests and might require different curricula.'

(Girls' school) 'Having had teaching experience in Types A and C of co-educational schools, I find that in Type A interest flags largely because different approach is often necessary for subjects and children feel that they are not considered as individual boys and girls but rather as 'children'. In both A and C question of discipline is difficult for this must be treated differently and any apparent leniency to one sex is resented by the other.'

The Second College survey

The exploratory First College survey was followed in 1948-9 (supplemented in 1963-5) by the more detailed Second College survey, which included several questions on school preference. Among them was, 'If you attended a single-sex school would you have preferred it to have been a mixed school?' Students could answer Yes/No/or Undecided. Students who had attended a mixed school were asked if they would have preferred it to have been single-sex. No opportunity was given for free response because students confronted with an overlong questionnaire might have refused to complete it. The results (Tables 11.5 and 11.6) are similar to those of the earlier survey.

TABLE 11.5 *'If you attended a single-sex school would you have preferred it to have been a mixed school?'*

Second College survey

	Male ex-pupils		Female ex-pupils	
	N	%	N	%
Yes (preferred mixed school)	236	41·9	329	52·6
No (preferred single-sex school)	221	39·3	158	25·2
Undecided	106	18·8	139	22·2
Totals	563	100	626	100

TABLE 11.6 *'If you attended a mixed school would you have preferred it to have been single-sex?'*

Second College survey

	Male ex-pupils		Female ex-pupils	
	N	%	N	%
Yes (preferred single-sex school)	13	3·8	5	1·3
No (preferred mixed school)	311	90·9	382	95·7
Undecided	18	5·3	12	3·0
Totals	342	100	399	100

School preference

Table 11.5 shows that the men who were educated in boys' grammar schools were uncertain whether they would have preferred a co-educational or single-sex school, whereas a majority (53 per cent) of the ex-pupils of girls' schools (with 22 per cent undecided) would have preferred a mixed school. Table 11.6 gives the verdict of former pupils of co-educational schools and is more dramatic. In great contrast to the indecision of the boys from boys' schools and to some extent the girls from girls' schools, both boys and girls from co-educational schools are very decided in their preference for a co-educational school. As many as 91 per cent of the boys and almost 96 per cent of the girls would not have preferred their school to have been single-sex; only 13 boys in 342 and 5 girls in 399 wished that their school had been single-sex. Human nature and human temperaments being so varied one could scarcely expect to get a smaller number in the minority no matter what the question asked!

As with the First College survey the objection could be raised that most of the students of the Second College survey had attended only one type of school and could not therefore validly compare it with another type. This objection was again answered by taking the opinion of a separate sample of students who completed the questionnaire as part of the main sample, but whose results were kept apart; they were students who had attended both types of school.

TABLE 11.7 *School preference: Ex-pupils with experience of both co-educational and single-sex schools*

Second College survey

Type of school preferred	Males		Females	
	N	%	N	%
Single-sex very much	7	9·2	3	4·1
Single-sex a little	11	14·5	1	1·4
Neutral	10	13·2	11	15·1
Mixed a little	17	22·4	10	13·7
Mixed very much	31	40·7	48	65·7
Totals	76	100	73	100

NOTE: The preference for co-educational schools is statistically highly significant for both sexes (beyond the ·001 level).

Although the question which was asked was not identical to that used in the previous survey its significance is very close, sufficiently so for it to be said that the results are mutually supporting. In Table 11.7 some 63 per cent of the men who had experienced both co-educational and boys' schools preferred the co-educational as against 24 per cent preferring the boys' school. Of the women some 80 per cent preferred the co-educational while 6 per cent preferred the girls' school.

The 'Both schools' survey

The 'both schools' survey is the most important one because its sample is composed of a large number of men and women who had been pupils in at least one co-educational as well as at least one single-sex school, and because it is the most recent, the questionnaire being administered in 1965-6. One hundred and seventy-five male and 620 female students who were in Colleges of Education were asked. 'Which did you prefer, the mixed or the single-sex school?' They could choose from one of the following answers: 'Single-sex school much/Single-sex school a little/No preference/ Mixed school a little/Mixed school much.' Reasons for their choice were requested. The question was deliberately made specific to the schools the ex-pupils had attended, and equally deliberately the single-sex schools were given the advantage of the first two places in the list of options—these sometimes attracting extra votes by virtue of their position.

The results are important and will be given intensive treatment. The preferences of the ex-pupils are given in Figure 11.1, and because the order in which the schools were attended could be an important factor, 'last' co-educational schools are compared with 'last' girls' schools and similarly for men. (In this instance to compare 'first' schools in addition would be merely to duplicate the data, as those ex-pupils who attended a co-educational school first are in most instances those who attended a single-sex school last, and vice versa.)

Two trends are apparent in the Figure, first the dominant preference for the students' co-educational schools, second the important influence of the order in which the two (or more) schools were attended. The preference for the co-educational school is much more marked when this was the last school attended, both with males and females,[1] though even when it was attended first there is a decided preference for the co-educational school among the females[2] and a smaller one among the men.[3]

[1] and [2] All statistically highly significant.
[3] Not statistically significant.

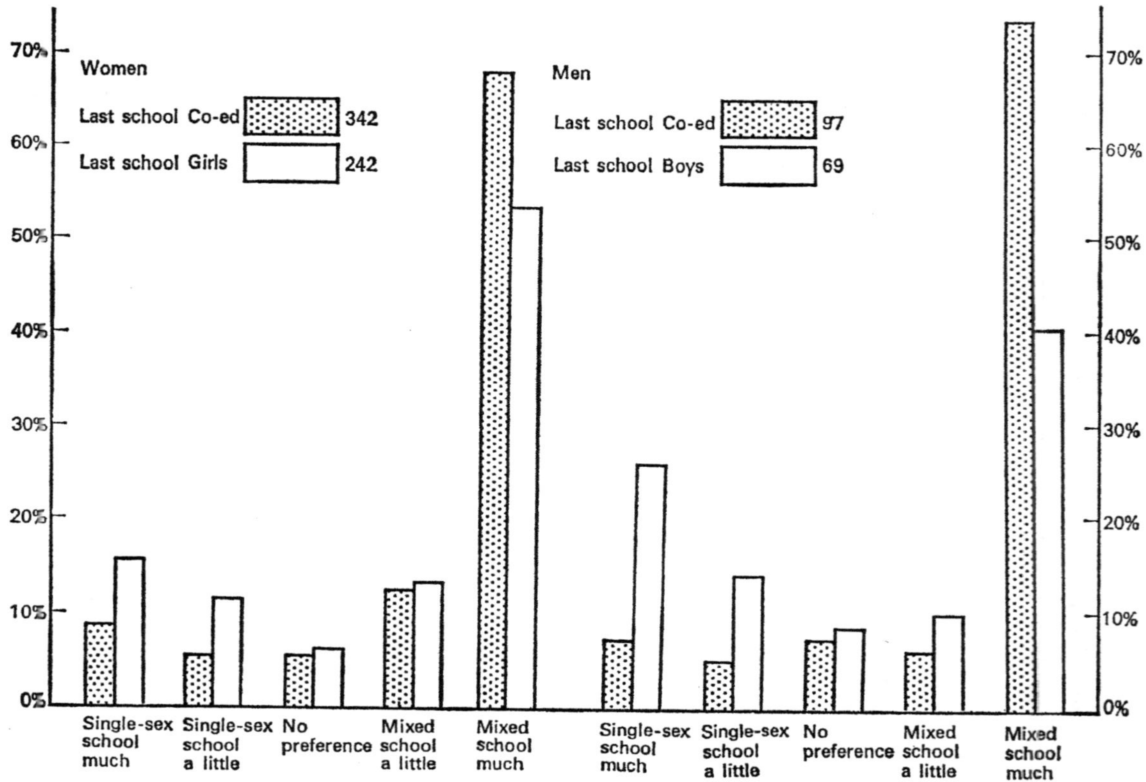

FIGURE 11.1
School preference: 'Both schools' survey

PLEASANTNESS OF POSITION

A hidden factor which might have affected the issue is the pleasant or unpleasant situation of the school, especially since there is a greater percentage of co-educational schools in sparsely populated areas. Accordingly the students were asked, 'Do you agree or disagree with the following statement about your co-educational school? Pleasant situation of school. Agree strongly/Agree/Doubtful/Disagree/Disagree strongly.' The same question was asked about the single-sex school. Though there was a difference in favour of the co-educational schools (which could even have been caused by a halo effect) it was much too small to have produced the large differences in school preference (cf. Table 2.3), and was statistically non-significant. The possibility was double-checked by comparing the school preferences which were based on co-educational schools in very pleasant positions (i.e. where ex-pupils 'agreed strongly' about the pleasantness) with those based on similar single-sex schools, thus neutralizing the influence of the pleasantness factor; the process was continued for other types of school situation and the sum total was taken for all cases where the situation of the two types of school was judged by the students to be similar in 'pleasantness', producing the data in Table 11.8.

TABLE 11.8 *School preference with pleasantness of position held constant*

'Both schools' survey (women)

Preferences of pupils matched on pleasantness of their co-educational and single-sex schools	Co-educational school last		Single-sex school last	
	N	%	N	%
Single-sex school much	10	7·2	8	10·8
Single-sex school a little	6	4·3	7	9·5
No preference	15	10·9	4	5·4
Mixed school a little	21	15·2	13	17·6
Mixed school much	86	62·4	42	56·7
Totals	138	100	74	100

NOTE: The differences between the proportion favouring the single-sex school and that favouring the co-educational is statistically very highly significant both for 'co-educational last' and 'single-sex last' categories.

The evidence shows that the preference for the co-educational school is overwhelmingly strong even when the pleasantness of school position is held constant. The assessment for the men was omitted because of their smaller numbers.

In case there are some readers who consider that the education of the intending teachers in Colleges of Education might have swayed their preference, even when choosing between schools actually attended as pupils, an examination was made of the preferences of the large group of students who said that their training as teachers had made no difference to their opinions about co-educational secondary schools. As an additional safeguard the ex-pupils were also matched as previously on their opinion of the pleasantness of the position of their co-educational school as compared with their single-sex school. Table 11.9 shows that the large co-educational advantage remains, both where the co-educational school was the last attended and where the single-sex school was the last; the influence of the order of schools can also be seen. Though the number in the sample has fallen drastically the interpretation has been made easier by the removal of three extraneous variables from the table.

TABLE 11.9 *School preference with position and College influence held constant*

'Both schools' survey (women)
'No change' on College influence

Position of school held constant by matching in pairs	School preference											
	Single-sex school much		Single-sex school a little		No preference		Mixed school a little		Mixed school much		Totals	
	N	%	N	%	N	%	N	%	N	%	N	%
Co-ed. last	7	10·3	3	4·4	10	14·7	13	19·1	35	51·5	68	100
Single-sex last	4	11·4	5	14·3	1	2·8	5	14·3	20	57·1	35	100

NOTE: The difference between the proportion favouring the single-sex school and that favouring the co-educational is statistically very highly significant both for 'co-educational last' and 'single-sex last' categories.

AMALGAMATED SCHOOLS

A factor which this research has shown to affect the comparison between co-educational and single-sex schools is whether the former is a school which has been created by the merging of two single-sex schools in the previous one or two years, termed here an 'amalgamated' school. An examination was therefore made of the influence of this factor on school preference, and it was found that both the men and the women[1] from amalgamated schools were less in favour of co-education than the rest of the sample who attended a co-educational school last (Table A.20). No change to this finding resulted when the 'pleasantness' of school position was kept constant for the amalgamated schools. (There was the possibility that most of this sub-sample had recently moved into pleasantly situated new buildings.) A broader analysis of the effects of 'amalgamation' is given in Chapter 20; here we move on to consider the free responses of the complete sample of the 'Both schools' survey.

FREE RESPONSES

The comments made by these responsible and interested adults about their preference for one or another of the two types of school they attended, are one of the most valuable pieces of evidence presented in this and the preceding volume, and they are given a full treatment. For those who do not wish to read the quotations a study of Tables 11.10 and 11.11 should suffice, but they will miss the human touch, the insight and the humour.

In the table the dominance of comments favourable to co-education was decided by the original school preference of the students. Except for its special importance, due to the double experience of the respondents, the table is similar to some given earlier. Co-education is favoured because of the natural relationship between the sexes, the educative effect of the presence of the opposite sex, the pleasant friendly relaxed atmosphere, the social life and school activities, the friendliness of staff–pupil relationships, the broad, balanced outlook on life, and the preparation for life in general. Also stressed, however, is that work is more enjoyable, lessons more interesting and more lively, with more discussions and more variety. There is greater freedom, less importance is attached to detail and there are fewer unnecessary rules.

It is difficult, from the table, to find something to say on the opposite side as the comments are so few and scattered, but the clearest feature is that the largest vote is in the 'work' category, where it approximately equals the co-educational vote. Apart from this the surprising feature is the amount of the difference between the two sides, especially as there is an appreciable variation among co-educational and among single-sex schools in academic standards, pleasantness of atmosphere, etc. That this sometimes leads to preference for the single-sex school is shown by the twenty-four students who found this atmosphere pleasant and friendly. Table 11.11 now presents the men's responses.

[1] Statistically significant for the women though not for the men.

TABLE 11.10 *School preference: free responses (women)*

'Both schools' survey — *Preference*

	Mixed much and a little	Single-sex much and a little
Pleasanter atmosphere and community spirit; happy atmosphere; friendly; natural; less tension; more relaxed; natural atmosphere; friendships	175	39
Natural relationship between the sexes; presence of boys educative	179	−1*
Prefers own sex; better attitude in single-sex		6
Staff—friendly, helpful; better staff–pupil relations	65	14
Staff—prefers men teachers in some subjects; more pleasant male staff attitude; mixed staff	21	4
Broader outlook on life; not so narrow; more balanced; healthier; more progressive	55	2
Preparation for life	43	−1
Better social atmosphere and social life, out-of-school activities, more co-operation	60	1 −3
Better for work; lessons more interesting, more lively; work more enjoyable; competition between the sexes	54 −4	43
Variety of interests, etc.; richer topics of conversation, discussion; more colourful; more lively; more opportunities for dramatics	59	
Smaller school		6
Discipline good; efficient		4
Greater freedom and less importance attached to detail; freer atmosphere; less pettiness; fewer unnecessary rules	34	7
Better facilities and opportunities	7	2
Girls less catty; less bitchiness, spitefulness and pettiness	13	
Healthier attitude to sex, less preoccupied with other sex	6	−1
Boys too rough, manners, discipline	−2	6
Others	9	21

* A minus sign indicates that the student's comment qualified his preference.

TABLE 11.11 *School preference: free responses (men)*

'Both schools' survey	Preference	
	Mixed much and a little	Single-sex much and a little
Atmosphere—pleasant, happy, friendly, more relaxed, family, freer	50	3
Relationship between sexes natural; presence of girls, educative	42	
Prefers own sex; restricted by what girls might think		2
Pupil–pupil relations friendly, trust	7	
Prefer boys only		6
Staff—friendly, helpful, better pupil–teacher relations	17	4
Staff—prefer have some women	1	
Staff—prefer no women		2
Preparation for life—helps social behaviour; more adult	12	1
Broader outlook on life, more balanced; healthier	9	
Social—better social life, more varied activities; out-of-school activities	12	
Sports		5
Interests—variety of, more colourful, wider, enjoyable, discussion. More fun.	6	1
Work, better for—higher standard. No distractions	17 −2*	15
Discipline: better	6	6
Better facilities	4	
Better status of school		2
Sex—attitude to, better	3	
Others	7	6

* A minus sign indicates that the student's comment qualified his preference, i.e. modified it.

The free responses of the men portray a story similar to that of the women, except that the dominance of the co-educational side, though strong, is not quite as marked. Because of the similarity comment is curtailed. Again the largest section in favour of the single-sex school is that on 'work' where it equals that for the co-educational. Within this section on the co-educational side is the emphasis on a natural and friendly competition between the sexes, the more enjoyable lessons, mixed staff, etc., and on the other side the lack of distractions and good standard of teaching. The comments under 'better facilities', 'better status' and 'small school' (women) remind us of the presence of other variables contaminating the main comparison.

The proportion of comments favourable to the co-educational school as against those favourable to single-sex schools is so large that to select quotations in this proportion would either produce far too many co-educational ones for the chapter or far too few for the single-sex school arguments to be properly illustrated; the quotations on the single-sex side are therefore increased.

Women: favourable to co-education

SOCIAL 'A natural relationship grew up between boys and girls. The first thing that struck me on going to a single-sex school was the competition there was to try and "get" a boy-friend.'

'The presence of the opposite sex was so very helpful in obtaining a more balanced attitude to many things which I felt somewhat lacking in the girls especially as I had no brother at home.'

'Girls are far too spiteful when together for too long. Boys add competition as well as enjoyable company.'

'Very happy at co-ed. and first single-sex school but cattiness and sex obsession at the second single-sex school left me uncertain as to its merits. (Boarded at first girls' school)

'The relief from the boredom of seeing only females day in and day out.' (Girls' boarding at first)

'More friendly—I lost timidity—I always dread to think what would have happened if the school hadn't amalgamated.' (Am.)

'This allowed boys and girls to develop naturally side by side. The school was far happier when co-ed. It was an artificial situation in the single-sex school.' ('Split' school)

'Because the pleasant atmosphere. The boys were almost always smiling and helped us to "laugh things off" if ever we felt down.'

'Life in a mixed society is decidedly more colourful and helps to bridge the conscious gap between the male and female adolescent.'

'At the single-sex school the girls' only topic of conversation up to the age of 16 was boys.'

'The presence of the opposite sex meant the education in general was easily related to life, which it should be, and a natural attitude to the opposite sex grew out of it.'

PUPIL–TEACHER RELATIONSHIPS 'I felt that there was much more freedom and individuality. Children become independent.' (Co-ed. boarding)

'The narrowness and staid atmosphere of the single-sex school seemed to be crushing my personality.'

'We spent much more time in a state of depression, dejection, feeling unjustly treated, etc. at the single-sex school.'

'In the mixed school everybody was treated as a normal human being instead of being "hushed away" as it were in the single-sex school.'

'I think that the education and atmosphere in a co-educational school is more balanced and a better preparation for life. I only wish I had attended one right from the first form.'

'I felt at ease—the atmosphere was not so strained as in a single-sex school.' (Comp.)

'The attitude of the teachers. In the mixed school they took their work as a pleasure and in the single-sex one as a duty. This altered the atmosphere of the school.'

'Far more pleasant atmosphere between staff and pupils. Men and women together get things in proportion and there is less fuss over minute unimportant details.'

ACADEMIC WORK 'Mainly in the educational field—it is very valuable to know the opinions of the opposite sex in any subjects; this causes the widening of one's own knowledge.'

'There was much more vitality about lessons and debates. Standard of education was higher, people worked harder. Much more fun and team spirit in school activities.'

'In classes the boys were far livelier and amusing at times. The whole atmosphere of the school was more active and alive.' (Co-ed. boarding)

'There was definitely more room for discussion and I am sure that this helped in the maturation of individuals.'

School preference

'Wider choice of subjects and girl/boy rivalry aided work. Education led more to the life you lead after school (self-discipline taught from the start) rather than just academic abilities.' (Comp.)

'The atmosphere both from a work angle and socially is far better. I found that it made people work much harder on the whole.'

'Everything—socially and educationally—was easier and more friendly and people were willing to join in and help towards the group activities and learned to share and became less concerned about "me" and "what I do for me", but "what can I do to help this group?" '

'Social activity and liveliness in the classroom were more apparent in the mixed school. More scope for drama, discussion, work and practical work such as metal work and technical drawing.'

Women—favourable to girls' schools

SOCIAL 'There was more of a feeling of being an individual rather than being one of a huge institution.'

'The general atmosphere was considerably better to other problems of life, though sex was rather prominent.'

'Life was less tense in the upper forms without the other sex—one could concentrate better on work.' (Comp.) (Attended co-ed. boarding school for one year)

'The boys were resented and rather destructive to the building.'

'I preferred the attitude of the single-sex school but if it could have been run on the same lines but as a co-ed. school I feel that it could have been even better.'

'Jealousy plays a big part in the life of a co-ed. school and work does not always come first.'

WORK 'I concentrated far more on my work. On the other hand I think girls who do not meet boys at home *definitely* need a co-ed. school.'

'The attitude of girl to girl was better and of girl to boy was better. The work atmosphere was much much easier.'

'With the happier atmosphere, lacking in the pre-occupation of the other sex [sic] my work reached a much higher standard. It deteriorated on entrance to the mixed school.'

'One was much more able to concentrate on one's work and the work was of a much higher standard in consequence.'

'It was a "better" school, the pupils were "nicer" and the quality of the teaching was on the whole better.' (Girls' boarding)

The men's free responses are particularly frank; as with the women the responses about the single-sex schools are not limited to the proportion allowed to co-educational schools.

Men—favourable to co-education

SOCIAL 'The mannerisms and behaviour of us all towards a mixed society as opposed to a single-sex society was greatly improved. Life was also very enjoyable and interesting discussions arose.' (Am.)

'A healthy atmosphere between boys and girls, good pupil–teacher relationships, excellent school social life, all of which helped develop a healthy pride in school.'

'The whole attitude of both staff and pupils is different—far more pleasant and natural.'

'It meant an opening-out whereby a whole new social horizon was established.' (Am.)

'The presence of girls seemed to make the boys more civilized than they were in my single-sex school.'

'The learning to live together and realizing that the opposite sex is natural and not unnatural and something that you must be shielded from.'

'The mixture seemed thoroughly normal and natural, which the single-sex school never was.'

'It prepared the pupil for the outside world. They could not go on just meeting members of their own sex; eventually they would have to mix; school is the best place for this.' (Am.)

'A much more congenial and relaxed atmosphere designed to produce human beings not computers.'

'The presence of the opposite sex shattered a lot of illusions and helped one make many adjustments to the realities of life—unpleasant as they may be!'

'Gives a chance for the rather timid person to acquaint himself with the opposite sex—*misconceptions in single-sex schools are a fact.*'

'Women and girls' influence calms down excess of lots of things.'

'The single-sex school I went to was frustrating in every way.'

School preference

DISCIPLINE 'It was a school in the most helpful and understanding sense. The single-sex school resembled a concentration camp with frightened guards.'

'The whole atmosphere of school was different—the staff–pupil relationship was much more tenable.'

'More open and friendly relationships, trust, sensible discipline.'

'Much more friendly attitude which is more conducive to work.'

'Less restriction—more of a family unit than the Regimental Barracks.'

SEX 'We were brought up in a community akin to that in which we were to live. Sexual relations are "normal"—boy goes out with girl—and not homosexual as in the single-sex.' (3½ years in boys' school, then 3½ in co-educational)

'I did not like being at a co-ed. school when I was 13. However I think that the absence of girls in my last single-sex school had a bad effect on the pupils and on the teachers with regard to boy–girl relationships and problems of sex which arose in the school.' (Boarding)

'Generally a happier atmosphere. Boys less sex conscious. More natural than segregating sexes. Girls' presence tends to make boys be smarter, less foolish.'

WORK 'The co-ed. school had its atmosphere of healthy regard for other people and for learning. The single-sex did not.'

'Better atmosphere in which to work and play.'

'In the mixed school one felt more relaxed and at times had the feeling that you had to impress the opposite sex, and things and tasks you undertook would be tackled much more efficiently.' (Co-ed. boarding)

'You wanted to work harder often just to impress the girls, but it was a nice atmosphere especially in the Sixth.'

Men—favourable to boys' schools

SOCIAL 'The co-ed. school tended to be rather more impersonal than the single-sex school, also the single-sex school was smaller.'

'Less emotional atmosphere than from women teachers and from girls. Restricted by the thoughts of what the girls might think.' (Am.)

'A delay or rest period before being exposed to the human female.'

'The good atmosphere of boys enjoying life together. Girl-friends were always out of school and much more forgotten during working hours. There is a tendency for shyness to arise, however.'

'No distractions, better feeling between pupils and between pupils and staff. Better sports. More out of school meetings between pupils.'

PUPIL–TEACHER RELATIONSHIPS 'Less interference of staff within societies, etc. Absence of female staff.' (Am.)

'More sport and outdoor activities with teachers taking a greater interest in extra-curricular activities.'

'The fun we had was much better and the attitude of the teachers towards the pupils was a good deal better. The understanding nature of the teachers also made you respect them.' (Small school)

'Better staff–pupil relations. Friendlier atmosphere in class. More progressive work and harder work.'

WORK 'Classroom atmosphere much better—boys have much more fun when no girls are around. Girls are apt to tell teachers if anything is wrong.' (First two years co-ed.)

'In the single-sex atmosphere my academic work was of a far higher standard than at a co-ed. However, the fact that it was a boarding school may have influenced this.'

'There was far more work done, both academically and physically.'

'It enables a better standard of work all the year round rather than just at exams time and there is plenty of time for female company in out-of-school hours.'

PRESTIGE AND TRADITION 'Enjoyed the tradition and pride in belonging to the school.'

'I approve strongly of co-ed. schools. Academically O.K. They don't put this bullying business into everything. I am convinced that girls have something to offer, e.g. in discussion; their points of view often surprisingly different from boys'.' But he strongly preferred the single-sex school he went to and when asked to which type of school he would send his children he replied, 'To my school I hope. Keep up the tradition and all that. (Dad went there).' (Boys' boarding)

PUPILS' PREFERENCE

So far this chapter has described research on the school preference of ex-pupils who were student teachers, and the objection might be raised that these are not a fully representative cross-section of grammar school pupils. Replies to this argument are considered in Chapter 1, but the best answer is evidence from a wider representation of grammar school pupils. Work in this was begun, and although never completed owing to the calls of other research and lack of clerical assistance, it is not without interest.

The first part of this enquiry derives from a questionnaire which was completed by the pupils of a number of sixth forms in grammar schools. In order to make the returns as reliable and as impartial as possible the author visited most of the schools personally and administered the questionnaire himself. Replies were anonymous and pupils were assured that no one at school would be shown the papers. Among a number of other questions pupils were asked, 'Which do you think you would like better, a school of (a) Boys and girls together, (b) Boys or girls only?' The results follow the pattern set by the other enquiries (Table 11.12). This is stressed because the number of schools in the sample is too small for the enquiry to stand as an independent investigation; on the other hand the co-educational schools were almost unanimous. The schools in the table were the only ones approached.

The sixth forms in the co-educational, the boys' and the girls' schools, all proved to be in favour of co-education. In the single-sex schools the majority was sometimes comfortable, sometimes substantial; in the co-educational schools opinion was almost unanimous. Incidentally these were individual opinions, written without consultation with friends or those pupils at the next desks. They were accompanied by free responses, but as these add little to the evidence only a few are quoted.

The comments from the boys' schools were decidedly direct and often forceful; for example, one young man of eighteen who earlier had had experience of co-education wrote, 'A school should be a microcosm. Ours pretends to be but is a false one. We have only one half of the community represented. In the world outside we meet men and women. This should also be the case in schools.' Again, 'A pupil should leave a good educational school with the idea of life as a co-operative adventure, demanding the best efforts of both sexes.' A boy of eighteen writes, somewhat naively, 'So far I have been constantly in the dark as far as girls' general opinions are concerned. I believe emotional association with girls would remove much of the speculation about our opposite sex. As the system exists, end of term parties (with the correspond-

TABLE 11.12 *Pupils' school preference (Sixth forms)*

Type of school sampled	Type of school preferred				
	Co-educational		Single-sex		Percentage for co-education combined sexes
	Boys	Girls	Boys	Girls	
					%
Mixed schools:					
1	13	21	0	0	100
2	5	4	1	0	90
3 (Type B)	7	10	0	0	100
4	10	10	0	0	100
5	12	12	0	0	100*
Girls' schools:					
6		12		1	92
7		24		12	67
8		15		9	63
Boys' schools:					
9	22		4		85
10	14		2		88

* One undecided girl is not included.

ing girls' school) have a stilted atmosphere for those who rarely encounter girls except in cinemas, etc.'

The presence of the opposite sex in the same class may not be merely the distracting influence that some have supposed, as a number of boys thought co-education increased competition in class and raised the standard of work.

Two rather humorous replies against co-education cannot be left out. Brief, but to the point is, 'Because I prefer boys to girls.' The other is more interesting: 'I prefer to keep social life and education separate by dividing the day into two parts, viz. (a) up to 4 p.m. when I do *all* my work and spend all my time in the company of boys; (b) 4 p.m. to 11 p.m. which I spend in the company of my other friends. This variation relieves boredom and makes life very interesting.'

The replies from the girls' schools lacked the unintentional humour of those of the boys. Like the boys' replies, however, they emphasized the value of co-education as a preparation for life. 'If boys and girls were taught together, it usually teaches both to be less self-conscious and does away with any "silliness" they might otherwise show when each would be unexpectedly thrown together. It also teaches the sexes to be more appreciative of the view-points and ideas of the other.' Two comments found frequently were that co-education prepares students for university life and for life in general, and that there is a higher standard of work due to a sense of competition. On the other hand some of the minority thought the presence of the other sex might be a distracting influence. One girl wrote, 'Boys and girls get to know one another without having to roam the streets after dark or sit in the park.'

In the comments from co-educational schools there was almost unanimity on the advantage of co-education, the principal argument being the preparation for social life after school. A boy wrote, 'Association with girls in school often prevents a boy from being narrow-minded later and helps him to achieve self-possession and assurance. His outlook is also broadened.' The girls wrote in a similar strain, e.g., 'By attending mixed schools we come into contact with boys every day and it prepares us for mixing with men in later life. It gives us a chance of understanding men and their outlook on life.'

Among the few comments against co-education from co-educational schools, there was no discernible theme, but a variety of remarks such as, 'Teachers would be all men and I would prefer that,' and, 'There would be easier arrangement of time-tables such as P. T. and Woodwork.'

The second piece of work among pupils in grammar schools was a survey of opinion among the whole age range. This was undertaken because one of the objections to co-education, raised sometimes by men teachers from boys' schools, is that boys want to be with boys and to be taught by men. A variation on this theme is that boys of 12 to 14—and perhaps girls—like to play in groups of their own sex and shun the company of the opposite sex.[1] The writer's intention was to carry out this survey in a number of schools, administering a questionnaire personally, but lack of time has limited the work to one co-educational school. The outcome, however, is not without interest (Figure 11.2).

It is surprising that in spite of the smallness of the sub-group when the 239 pupils are divided according to sex and age, there is a consistency in the results and a trend which fits into the expectations of theory and of previous research. In the first place a decided majority of these boys and girls at all ages between 11 and 18 prefer a school for both sexes, thus refuting the argument that because the sexes prefer to play apart between the ages of 12 and 14, they would prefer separate schools. When they are placed together in a school, and therefore know what they are talking about, they appear to prefer the opposite sex to be there even if the

[1] See also chapter 12, p. 196.

two sexes play apart. As this work was done in only one school, however, confirmation from work in other co-educational schools is needed.

In the second place the graphs show that in spite of the strong preference for co-education there is a dip round about the age of 13. This might be due to boys having a stereotyped impression of

FIGURE 11.2 *Preference for co-education: pupils in co-educational grammar school*

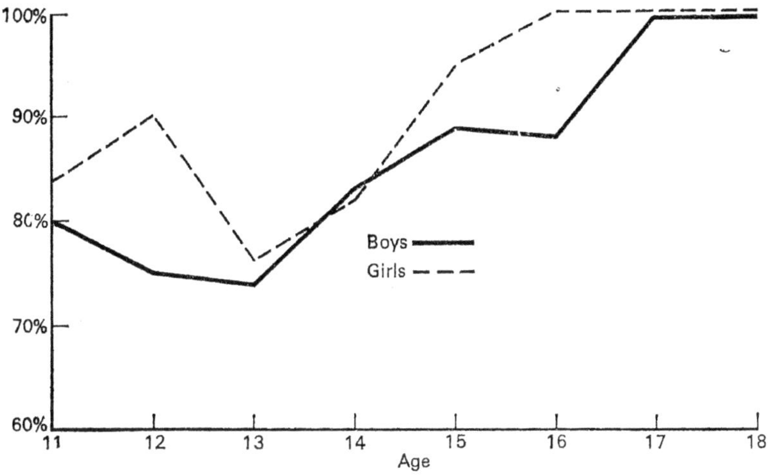

playing with girls as being effeminate, or to boys hesitating to admit at that age that they wanted girls about at all. But what of the girls? Is it similarly 'not done' amongst girls of that age to admit that they like having boys around? Whatever the reason, even at the lowest points of the graph—age 13—three-quarters of the boys and of the girls prefer a school of both sexes, and this preference increases steadily with age. Out of 124 boys in the age range 11 to 18, 103 preferred a mixed school and similarly 101 out of 115 girls. In view of individual differences in temperament, disgruntled individuals, and the instability of young teenagers, this is a very big majority.

Discussion

Though comparisons may sometimes be odious they cannot always be avoided, and there is a danger that established institutions that fare less well in the comparison may become emotionally involved and actively resentful. This would be a pity because reason takes to flight when emotion takes control, and the resentment would be founded on a misconception. For no one should think that this book is in any way a criticism of the dedicated work of the heads and staffs of single-sex schools; it represents rather an assessment of the possibility that the reorganization of these schools as co-educational schools might enable them to serve the children and the community still better. Incidentally it seems that most of the teachers would be happier in such schools (Dale, 1969).

Someone asked why pupils should decide whether secondary schools should be co-educational or single-sex. There is naturally no intention of allowing them to do so, but as consumers—people at the receiving end of education—they have a right to be heard, a right which is made much stronger by their relative maturity and their responsibility. They are mostly ex-pupils and sixth-formers, mostly future entrants to the teaching profession, strongly motivated to want the schools to be as good as possible. These are not 'good time' pupils or disillusioned premature or early leavers, but pupils who are sound academically and should have a better attitude to school than most other pupils. Moreover, the judgment of teachers themselves has also been taken, and there is a most marked similarity between the views of students and of teachers. In both cases the greatest reliance has been placed on the judgment of those who have had practical experience of at least one co-educational and one single-sex school.

In all the inquiries described in this chapter, each with a different sample of respondents, there is a decided preference expressed for co-educational schools. The reasons given seem logically sound—a better preparation for life in a bi-sexual world, a more natural atmosphere between boy and girl, a better attitude to sex, a school life which is more colourful, a staff–pupil relationship which is closer, more friendly, and a staff drawn from both sexes, which is true to life. The three types of school community— co-educational, boys', and girls'— are found to be much more different in 'community spirit' than most educationists considered possible, though we must also remember the wide variations of standard and of atmosphere within the schools of any one of these types.

This range within each could be a principal reason why a small minority of pupils who attended both types of school prefer their single-sex to their co-educational school. Another important reason, given by pupils and ex-pupils themselves, is that the order of schools attended is in itself a force tending to cause a preference for the last school attended, especially for the boys, so that if a student attended a co-educational grammar school for only one year and a single-sex school until he left the sixth, he might well indicate a preference for this last school. As a majority of pupils attended a co-educational school last in the 'Both schools' survey, this factor has been controlled by comparing pupils who attended a co-educational school first with those who attended a single-sex school first, then similarly for last schools.

Other pupils have expressed a preference for the single-sex school because it was small, some because it was an old school with tradition, a number of girls because the pupils were 'more my class' or 'more my type', and a few pupils because of better facilities. Those who are late arrivals at either type of school—especially girls arriving in the fourth form upwards—have difficulty in breaking into established circles and become unhappy; there is therefore a tendency for them to prefer their previous school, though this factor can be outweighed by others.

There remain a number who preferred their single-sex school for reasons which concern the co-educational-versus-single-sex controversy. These include some boys and a tiny minority of girls who said they preferred a school without the opposite sex. There are a number of factors which could cause this attitude. Apart from the handful of individuals who may already have homosexual or lesbian inclinations (and there is evidence that there are a few), there may be others who would prefer the company of their own sex only. They are a very small fraction of the total sample, and it might also be queried whether it is psychologically helpful to them to permit them to withdraw from a bi-sexual world. A related question is whether there might be a connection between high or low scoring on the introversion-extroversion scale and preference for co-educational or single-sex schools. In Chapter 9 on 'unhappy pupils' it seemed likely that unhappy pupils in girls' schools tended to be extroverted more often than unhappy pupils in mixed schools; immediately the opposite case comes to mind—is there a small minority of highly introverted pupils who would prefer to be in a single-sex school? Unfortunately there is no direct evidence available on this point.

The largest group in this minority who preferred their single-sex school is that which based their argument on academic work. Though there is an equal group on the co-educational side, there is a definite overlap here between co-educational and single-sex schools in the standard of teaching and the achievement reached. It would be unfair to the co-educational schools, however, if it were not pointed out that there is a distinct danger of confusion, in so far as a high standard of attainment in a single-sex school may be due either to a good standard of teaching or to a very selective entry, and the latter is a factor which is not an inevitable accompaniment of single-sex education. In large cities direct grant schools, which are almost always for historical reasons single-sex take the cream of the pupils, whereas there are few co-educational schools in this favourable position.

The objection could be made that the preference for the co-educational school might be due to its 'less strict' discipline and even to less stringent demands for academic work. There are three main arguments in reply: first, that research has shown that there is in fact no inferiority in academic standard that can be said to be due to co-education (cf. Dale, 1962a); second, that the students in the samples were academically inclined and would have had no hesitation in protesting if their co-educational schools had not efficiently fulfilled their teaching function; third, that, as shown earlier those teachers who have taught in both types prefer the co-educational and do not criticize the academic standards there.

It has been demonstrated that another factor in the problem—the pleasantness or unpleasantness of the school situation—could not have produced the very large preference for co-educational schools, because the pupils report that the co-educational schools were on average only a little better situated; moreover the large differences in preferences continue when the pleasantness of situation factor is held constant.

The preference for co-educational schools which has been revealed by these enquiries relates to the society in which the pupils and schools are placed. It depends partly upon society's attitude to the relations between the sexes, and to its attitude towards sexual problems, both natural and unnatural. It depends upon the force of tradition and the question of the equality of the sexes. Underneath this, however, is something which is even more fundamental because it is concerned with human nature—the query whether boys and girls naturally benefit more from being educated together or apart. These researches have tried to throw some light on this question, but within the setting of a certain type of civilization.

12

Attitude to the opposite sex

Almost a hundred years ago the Honourable Dudley Campbell, M.A., published a small and ephemeral but prophetic pamphlet entitled *Mixed Education of Boys and Girls in America*.[1] It had little practical result and the pamphlet has been forgotten, but many of its passages show that it was written by a percipient educationist who was, however, before his time. A few passages are here resurrected as a quaint but appropriate introduction to this chapter. Writing of educational influences he argues:

> But there remains to be applied an influence entirely ignored by the principal educators of this country, yet taking rank amongst the most potent agencies for moulding the human mind and character. The moral power of sex upon sex would seem to be regarded as either useless or dangerous. For all the care of the better known institutions, professing to train and completely equip their pupils for the duties of the future, a man might pass his life, from the cradle to the time of taking his degree as a Master of Arts, without ever seeing the face of a woman or hearing the sound of her voice. Yet everyone would admit that such chance opportunities as youths enjoy of associating with ladies are of the utmost value; and that but for the time spent at home before going to school, and, later, for the holidays, they would grow up with very imperfect notions of civilization. Moreover, it is often observed that boys without sisters are less cultivated and refined than their fellows who in this respect have been more fortunate.
>
> Such reflections naturally suggest the inquiry whether an influence so admirable and efficient, in spite of the limited sphere allowed to it, might not be yet more serviceable if permitted to work on a larger scale. Is the society of woman like those Indian spices which, in order to be beneficial, must be sparingly used? or is it like pure air, which men are glad to have in abundance at all seasons of the

[1] London, 1874.

> year? Why should an atmosphere so healthy at home be thought perilous at school? Why should an agency admitted to be good and even necessary in August and September be counted as worthless, if not mischievous, in October and November? If boys and girls, young men and young women, may dance and sing and generally play and amuse themselves together with advantage, is any special danger to be apprehended if they should also study together? Might not the refining influence of the one sex upon the other be expected to continue, so that the boys aiming at a higher standard of conduct would be less prone to selfishness, bullying, and 'rowdyism' of whatever kind, while the girls were less given to frivolity, sentimentalism, and gossip? Might not the fact that each sex demands from the other a loftier standard of action than it is contented with for itself, have an effect in increasing the importance attached by school opinion to study, so that the boys would shrink from showing incompetence or sloth before the girls, or the girls before the boys?

He then mentions the success of mixed schools in Scotland, and even of some in England, a passage which the writer cannot refrain from quoting:

> An excellent instance is afforded by the admirable Home and Colonial School in Gray's Inn Road, near King's Cross, where 1000 pupils of both sexes are trained under the most advanced and enlightened methods of instruction. An example no less striking is afforded by the Birkbeck Literary Institution. The classes there, held every evening, are attended by both men and women. The number belonging to the institution, whether for the sake of the classes or the library, is about two thousand; and it would be difficult to name a body of students, either more respectable in character, or, considering the tax put upon their energies by daily business, more zealous for self-improvement.

Previous chapters have inevitably referred to various aspects of the attitude of the sexes towards each other, but here there is a more direct approach. The results of three surveys are presented.

The equality of the sexes

MEN

In the Second College survey some 900 students in Colleges of Education answered, as part of a questionnaire, the question, 'In your attitude to the opposite sex do you think of them, in general, as being Very superior/Superior/Equal/Inferior/Very inferior?' They were invited to comment if they wished to do so. In Table 12.1 we see that the co-educated men had a slightly stronger belief in the equality of the sexes than did the men who had been in schools apart from the opposite sex, the main interest being in the slightly greater spread of the estimates made by the men who attended boys' schools, rather more of them estimating women as superior and rather more estimating them as inferior to men.[1] That part of the sample for which the information was available was analysed by social class and no significant differences emerged within either type of school. The students in the sample are, however, already moving away from their original social class to a new common one. Another relevant fact is that 38 per cent of these men had spent one or two years in a mixed College of Education.

TABLE 12.1 *Attitude to the opposite sex*

Second College survey

The opposite sex is:	Replies from male students				Replies from female students			
	Co-educational schools		Boys' schools		Co-educational schools		Girls' schools	
	N	%	N	%	N	%	N	%
Very superior	0	0	0	0	1	0·3	2	0·3
Superior	8	2·3	22	4·0	120	30·0	174	28·2
Equal	286	83·4	435	78·5	275	68·7	435	70·7
Inferior	49	14·3	94	17·0	4	1·0	5	0·8
Very inferior	0	0	3	0·5	0	0	0	0
Totals	343	100	554	100	400	100	616	100

NOTE: The differences in the distributions between co-educational and single-sex schools are not statistically significant, but on the men's side they are not without interest.

The free responses showed little difference between the co-educated and single-sex educated men, most of them saying that the sexes are equal but different, are complementary, or that it depends on the individual, but 22 per cent in each group of those who commented regarded women as inferior—a higher proportion

[1] The tendency for the men from boys' schools to be more extreme in attitude is not statistically significant but approaches it.

than in the estimates. A few quotations are given to lighten and in some cases illuminate the text, but here there seemed to be little point in treating them on a proportional basis. From the co-educated men we have:

'Always seemed so hard working, neat and conscientious: gave me a feeling of inferiority! Associated therefore with years just below rather than same.'

(Inferior) 'This is only a general answer. My own girl-friend, e.g. I consider equal, but most females bring their inferiority upon themselves and like it.'

(Inferior) 'Need more care in handling psychologically and emotionally.'

(Equal) 'I feel that male and female are complimentary [sic] to each other. Men have much to offer women and vice versa.'

(Equal) 'At school obvious the girls could hold their own with us. Since then I have found that in our own particular society women can hold their own with us.'

A few comments from the men educated in boys' schools were more extreme:

(Superior) 'Possibly due to the fact that not having had much contact with opposite sex and during adolescence I often feel uncomfortable in their presence.'

(Equal) 'Women are of poor character when in authority—petty.'

(Equal) 'I cannot think that we [men] are on one level and that they [women] are on another level. I only think of humanity on a common level.'

(Inferior) 'God created woman to be in subjection to man as the head of the family unit.'

(Equal) 'After two years in a mixed training college I have grown out of regarding girls as inferiors.'

WOMEN

About a thousand women students answered the same question as the men. Their results are also in Table 12.1 The table shows an almost identical distribution of attitudes for the two groups. It would appear that long exposure to the conduct of boys in a mixed school had done nothing to undermine the feminine assessment of the status of the male, nor had this continual social contact done anything to increase his status. Nor, on the other hand, does the seclusion of the girls in their girls' school seem to have had any effect at all on their estimate of the general status of males. In both groups, however, between a quarter and a third of the women admit to thinking of men as, in general, superior, and only 1 in 100 said they thought them inferior.

The data were then analysed according to social class. No association was found between father's occupation and respondent's view of men as superior, equal or inferior.

Free comments were made by a quarter of each school group, and they were similar in tone. In both groups the commonest statements emphasized the basic equality of the sexes, or implied that they are complementary, or that relationships depend on the individual, or that men are superior to women in some things and inferior in others. Such statements made up 43 per cent of each group's total comments. Thirteen per cent of the comments from the girls' schools group and 14 per cent from the mixed schools expressed a *preference* for men to be superior! About the same proportion actually said man was superior, some 9 per cent on grounds other than physical. A few representative comments are:

'Women will never be men's equals.'

'I tend to get an inferiority complex with most men, but it depends on the man as to whether it affects me.'

'I believe them to be superior in thought, at least the more intelligent ones, because they glean much more from the world around them in politics, government, literature, etc., and have a wider background than most girls but not all.'

'I have much more respect for them than for members of my own sex.'

'I like to be equal in the company of a member of the opposite sex but feel a husband should be superior.'(!)

'More original. Women on the whole mediocre and less interesting.'

'Members of the opposite sex are complimentary.' [sic]

Comment

By the time the ex-pupils have reached the age of eighteen to twenty there is little difference between the view of the co-educated and those educated in single-sex schools on the equality of the sexes. Some students from single-sex schools, however, said that their experience in a mixed College of Education had changed their ideas about the innate superiority of the male.

Attitude pleasant or unpleasant

In the 'Both schools' survey the ex-pupils were asked, 'In your single-sex [or co-educational] school was the general attitude of most of the pupils towards the opposite sex Pleasant/Fairly pleasant/Neutral/A little unpleasant/Unpleasant?' They were also invited to comment.

MEN

The estimates of the men are in Table 12.2. Figures are given separately for schools attended as juniors and those attended as seniors, because of the extent of the difference between them.

TABLE 12.2 *Pleasantness of attitude to the opposite sex (boys)*

'Both schools' survey

	Replies about first school attended				Replies about last school attended			
	Co-educational		Boys'		Co-educational		Boys'	
	N	%	N	%	N	%	N	%
Pleasant	38	45·8	24	20·7	66	63·5	24	35·8
Fairly pleasant	29	34·9	31	26·7	29	27·8	25	37·3
Neutral	12	14·5	35	30·2	9	8·7	4	6·0
A little unpleasant	4	4·8	21	18·1	0	0	13	19·4
Unpleasant	0	0	5	4·3	0	0	1	1·5
Totals	83	100	116	100	104	100	67	100

NOTE: The difference between the distributions for co-educational and boys' schools is statistically very highly significant both for 'first' and for 'last' schools. The difference between 'first' and 'last' schools themselves may well be due mainly to the change in pupils' ages.

Before interpreting the figures a brief comment on the wording of the question is needed. The words 'pleasant attitude' had for a few pupils a slight element of ambiguity; though it is evident from the free responses that most of the boys interpreted the words as meaning 'normally friendly', without any overtones, there were some who interpreted them as 'pleasant because they wanted to date girls'. Fortunately there is no doubt about the incidence of this minority response; the free responses show that it is much more characteristic of the boys' schools than of the co-educational, so that the 'pleasant' estimates are inflated more for the former than for the latter. Additional proof of this is to be seen in the much greater percentage of the ex-pupils who estimated the attitude in their boys' schools towards girls to be 'a little unpleasant' or 'unpleasant' compared with their co-educational schools. The differences in tone between these comments will be seen later in the quotations.

In both the co-educational and boys' schools the ex-pupils who attended as seniors estimated the attitude to girls to be more pleasant among the seniors than among the juniors. The attitude was least pleasant among junior boys in boys' schools, more pleasant among senior boys in the same schools, still more pleasant among junior boys in co-educational schools and most pleasant of all among senior boys in these schools, where some 91 per cent of the students estimated the attitude to be pleasant or fairly pleasant —mostly the former.

Co-educational schools

The seventy-seven free responses from co-educational schools were too few for satisfactory classification, but approaching half of them spoke of a good friendly relationship or that girls were treated as equals or that there was normal interest—often using these phrases. Small groups said that the attitude varied with age and that it depended on the personality of the girl; five said there was a 'romantic relationship'. Because of the central importance of this theme to the co-education debate one in five of these free responses are quoted, except that the relatively uninteresting 'neutral' category is omitted entirely to avoid overloading the text with quotations. The quotations are now proportionate to the total comments in each category for each type of school.

PLEASANT 'In the upper forms the two sexes could talk frankly about each other's problems of growing up which I consider has helped me greatly.'

'The general attitude was that the girls were an asset to the school.'

'As regards members of the opposite sex relations could not have been better.'

'In the Sixth—romances bound to arise. Everyone was broad-minded. Healthy atmosphere.'

'The girls joined in nearly all the "out-of-school" activities which the societies formed and both sexes got on well together.'

Attitude to the opposite sex

'The opposite sex was there and as we grew up in the school that was all there was to it, they were just accepted as being there.'

'There was an acceptance of the fact that it was natural for the two to be together.'

'Never met any woman haters—a few were shy or indifferent at worst—none actually aggressive.'

FAIRLY PLEASANT 'A matter for the individual, depending upon his or her age and social development—on the whole harmonious.'

'There were times when the girls could be a nuisance.'

'A few of the boys were quite open about the fact that they only wanted a girl for the sexual pleasure, rather than the social pleasure that went with it.'

'Some of the girls may have been unpleasant but the majority were enjoyable to work with.'

A LITTLE UNPLEASANT Only three comments came in this category and none of these was in fact 'a little unpleasant', the worst one being:

'The only reason for answering was that it was not neutral but rather disdainful: not really unpleasant at all but neutral would not be right.'

UNPLEASANT As there were no estimates in the unpleasant category, there are no comments either.

Boys' schools

The free responses about the boys' schools, attended by the same pupils who attended the co-educational schools, were of a different nature, the largest single category being accompanied by the estimate 'a little unpleasant'. (The number in the two pleasant categories, however, equalled those in the two unpleasant ones.) There was a wide variety of themes, varying from shyness and ignorance and 'annoying distraction', especially among juniors, through normal interest, friendly relationships and 'romantic', to 'sex mad' and attitude unpleasant sexually. This last type of comment was much more frequent than in the returns about the co-educational school. We must once again remember that this is what the ex-pupils report, and that boasting about sexual adventures which have no basis in reality does sometimes occur among boys in their late 'teens. Yet these are the same ex-pupils reporting on the predominant attitude in the two types of school they attended. Likewise more of the comments in the 'pleasant' category about the boys' schools had 'dating girls' or something similar as a theme whereas the dominant theme about the co-educational schools was 'normal friendly relationship'. Typical free responses are as follows:

PLEASANT 'Most of us met and went everywhere with our girl-friends.'

'It was pleasant in that the opposite sex were completely cut off from us.'

'Dating girls from the High School was common.'

FAIRLY PLEASANT 'The boys tended to look upon girls as a thing to be enjoyed sexually.'

'Sex mad in most boys.'

'We did have a sister school to which we were invited for the Christmas Dance. The atmosphere and attitude of these dances was quite good.'

NEUTRAL 'In my second school I had a much more mature attitude towards girls.' (Attended three schools, the second being co-educational)

A LITTLE UNPLEASANT 'Some were antifeminist, some sexually unhealthy in their attitudes, many immature.'

'Normal attitudes to the opposite sex were sometimes degraded by one or two depraved youngsters.'

'Unbalanced; myself a tendency to fantasies.'

'One or two tried to create the impression of having intimate relations with girls. Probably caused by lack of females in school, therefore ignorance of them.'

'They showed no consideration for girls as people, but rather treated them as animals.'

UNPLEASANT 'With reference to the word "unpleasant" reply is—"Better would be the word 'unhealthy' ".'

'Girls were all right for sex, otherwise they were "sissy".'

Two themes not represented in the above quotations were that the very junior boys were too young to be interested in girls and that some schools or boys were so cut off from girls that they were very ignorant about them. The extent to which an individual may encounter these latter difficulties is illustrated by the following response: 'I don't think I spoke to a single girl for five years.' A direct comparison of some interest is, 'It was completely different from co-ed. and I was frankly shocked by what I considered an unnatural attitude.' Because of the importance of the replies to this question a full tabulation is given in Appendix 2 (Table A.21).

Though surveys in this field should be replicated, it appears highly probable that the Victorians and Edwardians were wrong in their policy of segregating boys and girls in their secondary schools through their fears of encouraging sexual misbehaviour if the two sexes were placed in the same school. In this sample it is in the schools where the boys were deprived of the company of the opposite sex that their attitude is less desirable. It is deprivation of such company that makes them desire it all the more and at the same time tends to create—in their own words—unhealthy attitudes and an outlook towards girls which falls considerably below the 'normal friendship' which is the predominant phrase in the replies about co-educational schools.

The same results were obtained when supplementary questions were asked, such as, 'In your co-educational (or boys') school was the general attitude of most of the pupils (of your own sex) towards the opposite sex, "Rather preoccupied with the opposite sex?" ' and, with a similar preamble, ' "Boy–girl crazy?" ' The ex-pupils thought the senior boys in the boys' schools to be more preoccupied with the opposite sex and more boy–girl crazy than those in the co-educational schools, the differences being statistically very highly significant (cf. Table A.22).[1] When the phrase 'normal interest' was substituted they considered the interest in the opposite sex to be more 'normal' in the co-educational schools than in the boys' schools, the difference being statistically significant for juniors as well as for seniors. Only 8 men out of 177 thought that the attitude in the co-educational schools was not normal or were doubtful (cf. Table A.22).

In the same series of questions were included two which, though related, begin to explore different facets of boy–girl relations. The first was, 'Was the general attitude of most of the pupils (of your own sex) towards the opposite sex "antagonistic"?' Pupils again could choose their answer from True/Partly true/False/Doubtful. The second question substituted the word 'timid' for 'antagonistic'.

[1] Data for 'rather preoccupied', etc., are not given in the table.

The full results may be seen in Table A.23. Here it is sufficient to report that the distributions were closely similar for the two types of school, and though rather more ex-pupils said there was no antagonism in co-educational schools compared with boys' schools, the differences were not statistically significant either for first or last schools. Only 2 per cent of ex-pupils said it was true that there was antagonism, though 20 per cent said it was partly true.

With regard to timidity, segregation in a boys' school produced a greater degree of it according to the ex-pupils' reports, the differences being highly significant statistically for both juniors and seniors (see Table A.23). Some 10 per cent of the students thought this was true of the boys in their boys' school, compared with 1 per cent about the co-educated boys.

WOMEN

When we consider the women's results the question uppermost in our minds is naturally, 'Is the attitude of girls in girls' schools towards the opposite sex subject to the same kind of "deprivation effect" as in the case of the boys?' The answer given by their estimates in Table 12.3 is that at least in this sample it appears to have such an effect.

TABLE 12.3 *Pleasantness of attitude to the opposite sex (girls)*

'Both schools' survey

	Replies about first school attended				Replies about last school attended			
	Co-educational		Girls'		Co-educational		Girls'	
	N	%	N	%	N	%	N	%
Pleasant	136	45·6	117	30·2	206	57·4	107	42·0
Fairly pleasant	112	37·6	125	32·1	117	32·6	84	33·1
Neutral	39	13·1	85	21·9	31	8·6	18	7·1
A little unpleasant	10	3·4	53	13·7	3	0·8	39	15·4
Unpleasant	1	0·3	8	2·1	2	0·6	6	2·4
Totals	298	100	388	100	359	100	254	100

NOTE: The difference between the distribution for co-educational and girls' schools is statistically very highly significant for both first and last schools.

Attitude to the opposite sex

The ex-pupils reported that the attitude of girls in girls' schools towards boys was 'less pleasant' than the attitude of girls in co-educational schools, with regard to both junior and senior pupils. As with the boys an obvious query is, 'What did the ex-pupils mean by "less pleasant" and "unpleasant"?' As one young lady put it when writing of the girls' school she had attended: 'Great interest in boys but depends on your morals as to whether attitude pleasant or not.' Another woman, again commenting on her girls' school, and estimating the attitude to boys to be 'a little unpleasant', wrote, 'Not quite the right word. Bad effect in that many girls were boy-mad.' Fortunately the meaning of the estimates is elucidated by the free responses, a detailed examination of which showed conclusively that whereas in regard to the girls' schools a small minority estimated 'pleasant' and accompanied this with the comment 'boy-crazy' or something similar, this was absent, in regard to their co-educational school, the free responses being dominated by the 'normal friendly relations' category. The difference is epitomized in three 'direct comparisons' which are taken in advance of the main group in order to illustrate this point:

'Pleasant—seemed to be more boy-crazy.' (Girls' school)

'Pleasant—the attitude was "who were you with last night?"—a lot of discussion about boys whereas in a co-ed. they are accepted.'

'Unpleasant—boy-mad. When I returned from co-ed. was shocked at preoccupation for something I took for granted.'

As in the case of the boys this nature of the differences between the girls' and co-educational schools in the 'pleasant' category receives support from the fact that the girls' schools also have the greater percentage of estimates in the two 'unpleasant' categories.

Considering only the estimates in Table 12.3 at present, there is a decided difference between the pleasantness of attitude reported in the co-educational schools and that in the girls' schools, and as we have already seen this extends down into the 'unpleasant' section of the scale. The attitude is both 'pleasanter' at one end of the scale, and less unpleasant at the other, in the co-educational schools. The free responses confirm this in dramatic fashion, those about the co-educational schools being completely dominated by categories of responses such as 'natural friendly relationship', 'took each other for granted' and 'treated them as equals', while the replies about girls' schools were characterized much more by remarks indicating the effects of deprivation, e.g. 'boy-crazy', 'obsessed with sex' and 'unhealthy'. (See Table A.24.) Readers should not infer from this that the attitude affected all girls who went to girls' schools or that the staffs are in some way responsible; the point is merely that because of the form of organization—because of the deprivation of the natural companionship of the opposite sex—there appears to be a sharpening of the desire for them, with boys placed on an artificial pedestal. At the same time there is also evidence that some girls—especially those without brothers—have little opportunity for meeting the opposite sex and are even, in their own words, 'afraid' or 'terrified' of them.

In view of the importance of this question the free responses are quoted extensively, strictly in proportion for each category of estimate and each type of school, but again omitting the 'neutral' category. Those about co-educational schools are taken first.

Co-educational schools

PLEASANT 'In the lower school girls hero-worshipped the boys, but in the Sixth most girls very friendly with the boys although their boy-friends were usually from outside school. Often found schoolboys rather immature. Although we were able to have lively and poignant [sic] discussions about any subject.'

'The boys didn't particularly worry us or affect the way we conducted ourselves—we looked upon them as friends.'

'The boys, for the most part, became an accepted part of a school life, and therefore a pleasant atmosphere surrounded us.'

'Regarded them as companions with whom to work seriously and also share a joke. Sex relationships were the serious problem as most people had ties outside of school life.'

'We were all good friends, but we thought of them as if we were all one sex, and not as an object of the next date as we probably thought of other boys.'

'We all seemed to be on brother and sister terms, very friendly and pleasant towards each other.'

'Many girls got on better with boys than they did with girls.'

'On the whole the girls were less catty when the boys were around. In the 4th year they tended to show off a little, but mainly to impress boys higher up the school. In the Fifth and Sixth forms they treated them more as equals.'

'A lot of the boys in my form I had known from infant schooldays —then we were separated into single-sex schools and then we were mixed again. I find this most satisfying to really get to know a boy for about 13 years. You can in fact watch them developing. Some of these boys I had really disliked during my infant/junior education—yet now I like them all and feel we will always be friends. Perhaps this is not the same for others in my form—but generally I should say relationships were very good.'

'It wasn't often that someone would try to attract a boy or vice versa. We had very platonic friendships.'

'After the initial excitement at first contact, general attitude of acceptance as individuals instead of "boys" and as platonic friends.' (Am.)

'The boys were never looked upon as "from another planet" but only as friends and fellow scholars.'

'Enjoyed their company. Felt the boys really added to the lessons by comments and discussions.'

'One grew to accept the opposite sex, and got to understand their reactions to various situations. Therefore one knew how to behave towards them out of school as well as inside school.'

'It was more pleasant in the senior part of the school. The juniors treated members of the opposite sex in rather a childish manner.'

'One or two boys that some of the girls disliked, but on the whole we thought they were alright. Forgot that they were boys and treated them nearly in the same way that one would treat one's girl-friends.'

FAIRLY PLEASANT 'At an early age the opposite sex were just accepted, then we found an unpleasant argumentative period, but later on during the majority of my time there the attitude was pleasant, friendly.'

'At 14 and 15 tended to be giggly and pester the older boys, but towards their own age group boys and girls always behaved normally.'

'Some went mad the minute we amalgamated, however those mixed lower down the school regard the school as a mixed sexes school—we resented the boys for the most part.' (Am.)

'At first it was a novelty to be co-ed. but after this feeling had worn off the attitude was still pleasant.' (Am.)

'It varied at various ages. In the lower forms it was merely toleration and friendly rivalry but later in the school life closer relationships developed.'

'Pupils learned to accept the opposite sex as friends and not as prospective husbands and wives.'

'The natural interests of teenagers were allowed to exist within a "healthy" background.'

'Regarded them as equals, treated them as such.'

'Generally accepted them. A few of the girls (especially in D stream) were really tarty and either teased or embarrassed the boys.'

A LITTLE UNPLEASANT AND UNPLEASANT 'If you were not friendly with the opposite sex in a boy–girl relationship you were tended to be looked down upon and thought peculiar.'

These comments speak for themselves: the emphasis is decidedly on normality, with boys and girls growing up together in a family-like atmosphere. This is in spite of the existence of the 'amalgamated' schools within the sample of co-educational schools, where adolescent boys and girls were suddenly placed in school together for the first time and the relationship between the sexes might be expected to be troublesome. The tone of the comments about girls' schools is, however, quite different from the 'normality' of those about the co-educational schools:

Girls' schools

PLEASANT 'Absolutely "nuts" about the opposite sex.'

'Pleasant, if you would class obsession as pleasant!!'

'More than pleasant—most adored the opposite sex.'

'Most girls regarded boys as a "must" due to not seeing or being with them all day.'

'The boys seemed more glamorous when we had no contact with them.'

'Social events, etc., with boys' school; not other-sex starved anyway.'

'The boys' school who were invited to our socials and made mixed teams were always welcomed.'

'Man-mad more like it.'

'Most girls had steady boy-friends, whereas in the previous school it was almost unheard of.'

FAIRLY PLEASANT 'General tendency to great excitement the moment almost anyone in trousers appeared!'

'There was a little too much "romantic" glory attached to opposite sex which tainted their attitude to sex.'

'Sixths had grown to regard boys as normal human beings, Fourths still giggled over them.'

'There were extremes; some were boy-crazy, some scared to even speak to a boy, some normally interested.'

'Because we never saw any members of the opposite sex at all, many girls showed interest in builders etc. that they passed.' (Boarding)

'The girls peered through wire netting at the boys peering through from the other side.'

'Everyone boasted about "conquests" but most were painfully shy. All liked boys or would like to know them.'

A LITTLE UNPLEASANT 'Varied from bragging of sexual experience and pseudo-sophistication to indifference because of shyness.'

'Too grasping—too much like a hunt. Boy-friends were status symbols. As I didn't know a single boy that was another black mark for me.'

'If boy walked through the school some girls would immediately turn around, laugh and giggle and generally make a spectacle of themselves.'

'Most of the girls had obsessively morbid interest in boys—as I had grown up with them, could not understand this.'

'Kept away from boys—no attitude could grow healthily.'

'Any male underwent strong scrutiny—they appeared to be starved of male company, didn't know how to behave when with boys.'

UNPLEASANT 'Ridiculous—some were boy-crazy and ignorant; some were priggish, prudish and ignorant. The birth rate was higher than *every* other school in town, secondary modern included.'

In another part of the questionnaire the question dealt with in this section was supplemented by several others. In answer to the question, 'In your co-educational (or girls') school was the general attitude of most of the pupils (of your own sex) towards the opposite sex, Rather preoccupied with the opposite sex?' Respondents chose their answer from True/Partly true/False/Doubtful. Whereas only 9 per cent replied 'true' about their co-educational school, this rose to 38 per cent from the girls' schools. While the proportion estimating 'partly true' was roughly the same for the two types of school, one-third said the statement was false about their co-educational school (compared with one-eighth) and 17 per cent were doubtful (compared with 7 per cent in the case of girls' schools).

Another question, using the same preamble, substituted the words 'girl/boy crazy', with the same choice of replies. Only 5 per cent of the pupils said this was true of the girls in their co-educational school and 29 per cent in their girls' school. The replies for 'partly true' were 26 and 42 per cent respectively, while 52 per cent said the girls in their co-educational school were not boy-crazy compared with 19 per cent about their girls' schools. As might be expected, more of this attitude was reported in the senior schools of both types than in the junior schools. Rather interestingly the social class breakdown showed a slight tendency for this attitude to increase with lower social class girls in the girls' schools but to *decrease* in the co-educational schools.

When the question was phrased in a different way, using the words 'normal interest', 79 per cent said 'true' about their co-educational schools, compared with 42 per cent, and 18 per cent 'partly true' compared with 39 per cent (Table A.25). There was little difference between the reported attitudes of seniors and those of juniors, nor could any social class differences be discerned in either school.

In the same series of items two attacks were made on somewhat different aspects of boy/girl relationship. The first substituted the word 'antagonistic' for the phrase 'normal interest'. There was, however, a remarkable similarity in the distributions of the estimates for the girls in the two types of schools, some 1 per cent of the ex-pupils endorsing 'true' (i.e. 'antagonistic'), and some 17 per cent 'partly true'.

The second new aspect was 'timidity', where the reported difference in attitude was considerable and statistically very highly significant both for juniors and seniors, there being much more timidity amongst girls in girls' schools (59 per cent estimating 'true' or 'partly true') than amongst those in co-educational schools (27 per cent). For both 'antagonism' and 'timidity' the comparison between co-educational and single-sex schools gives a similar result with the girls as with the boys. Fuller results are in Table A.26. To conclude this section of the chapter brief consideration is given to two other questions which relate only to the co-educational schools; though there may appear to be some duplication here, the questions are not identical to those which have gone before, and these linked questions increase the dependability of the results.

Attitude to presence of the opposite sex

It is sometimes said that boys aged about 12 to 14 do not want the company of girls, implying also that they do not want their presence. Though a detailed examination of this could not be attempted[1] a start was made by including for co-educational schools the item, 'The presence of the opposite sex of pupils in my school was Liked very much/Liked/Tolerated/Disliked/Disliked intensely.' The results for both boys and girls are in Table 12.4.

TABLE 12.4 *Liking for presence of opposite sex*

'Both schools' survey

Estimates about co-educational schools	Replies from male ex-pupils				Replies from female ex-pupils			
	First schools (juniors)		Last schools (seniors)		First schools (juniors)		Last schools (seniors)	
	N	%	N	%	N	%	N	%
Liked very much	21	25·3	44	42·7	103	34·4	139	38·8
Liked	47	56·6	50	48·6	163	54·6	196	54·7
Tolerated	14	16·9	7	6·8	30	10·0	20	5·6
Disliked	0	0	2	1·9	2	0·7	2	0·6
Disliked intensely	1	1·2	0	0	1	0·3	1	0·3
Totals	83	100	103	100	299	100	358	100

NOTE: The difference between the distributions for first and last schools does not quite reach the conventional level of statistical significance for males and is insignificant for females.

MEN

In Table 12.4 the male ex-pupils of co-educational schools show a most marked liking for the presence of girls in the school, only one in 186 saying that it was disliked intensely and two saying it was disliked. Some 82 per cent said their presence was liked or liked very much among the juniors, and 91 per cent among the

[1] Some evidence has been put forward in Figure 11.2.

seniors, so that although it is true that their popularity increased with age, they could scarcely be said to be unpopular at the junior stage. The smallness of the numbers precluded a social class analysis.

WOMEN

The women's result is closely akin to that of the men—a similar negligible percentage of dislike (with two out of the three seniors who expressed dislike coming from amalgamated schools) and the same huge preponderance of liking, in both junior and senior schools. As with the men's estimates, however, one can detect among the senior girls a slight increase in the liking for the presence of boys, when compared with the junior girls. Division of the respondents into three social classes according to parental occupation revealed a decided consistency between classes in the 'popularity poll'.

Aspects of attitude to the opposite sex (Schools project)

In order to probe a little more deeply into the effect of separation from the opposite sex compared with companionship, large numbers of present female pupils in some forty grammar schools were given items such as, 'Boys are much too noisy', 'Boys cannot be trusted', 'Boys are unpleasant', 'Boys are nicer than girls', 'Boys are cleverer than girls in school work', 'Boys are better leaders than girls', 'Boys are not as catty as girls', 'Boys are braver than girls', 'Boys are cruel', 'Boys are interested in the wrong things', and 'I would prefer to be a boy'. Other items, some of which were the same, with the word 'girl' substituted for 'boy', were given to the boys. The possible answers were, Agree strongly/Agree/Doubtful/Disagree/Disagree strongly. Unfortunately the test administration time at the researchers' disposal was inadequate for the request of free responses, so that the items lack the elucidation which has so frequently come from this source. The items should therefore be regarded as probes designed to find differences between the groups which might profitably be explored further.

The results were disappointing, in that there were few statistically significant differences between the co-educated and single-sex schools, either for boys or for girls. Possible reasons for this were discussed in the previous volume and are concerned mainly with the intake into the samples of the two types of school. From the four age groups 11 plus, 13 plus, 15 plus and 17 plus were derived forty-four comparisons between girls in co-educational and girls in girls' schools and only five were statistically significant. In spite of this there are two trends which deserve comment. One of these is the tendency for the girls from girls' schools to have a somewhat more romantic view of boys, and those from co-educational schools to have a more down-to-earth outlook, seeing boys' faults as well as their virtues. The second tendency is for the girls in girls' schools to have slightly more extreme opinions. The items which yielded significant differences included that about boys being much too noisy, which produced two out of the five mentioned—in the 13 plus and 15 plus age groups—where the co-educated girls endorsed this more frequently than did those from girls' schools. The third of the five occurred when the co-educated girls aged 15 plus supported more strongly the idea that boys cannot be trusted—though this did not apply among girls from social class 3 or among the other age groups. The fourth was that girls (aged 13 plus) in girls' schools were more inclined to think boys braver than girls, though the other age groups did not agree. Lastly, in the same age group more of the girls in mixed schools agreed that boys are 'interested in the wrong things', though there was very little difference between the co-educated and single-sex educated in the three other age groups.

Four of the boys' items were the same as for the girls except that the word 'girl' replaced 'boy', namely girls are 'nicer', 'cannot be trusted', are 'cleverer', and the boy 'would prefer to be a girl'. Different but in the same vein are, 'Girls are catty and spiteful', are 'kinder', are 'boring', are 'interested in unimportant things', 'giggle and talk too much', and are 'more sensible'. The results strike the same note as those of the girls.

There are only seven statistically significant differences out of forty in the four age groups. One of these comes from the 15 plus boys, where those in boys' schools said that girls are nicer than boys, and the 13 plus and 17 plus boys had the same trend though it was not by convention statistically significant. A second occurred in the boys aged 13 plus where more of those from boys' schools disagreed strongly that girls are boring, supported by a similar non-significant trend in the 15 plus and 17 plus boys. It should be said, however, that a big majority in both types of school did *not* believe that girls are boring.

Two more of the seven differences occurred among boys aged 13 plus and 15 plus in response to the item saying that girls are cleverer than boys in school work, this being endorsed by more boys in the co-educational than in the boys' schools, but this was far from a majority in both types of school. In the same age group the co-educated boys also agreed to a greater extent than their opposites that girls were more sensible than boys; this was, however, still only a relatively small minority opinion. The idea that boys might prefer to be girls had very little support in any age group at either type of school—much less than the 11 to 15 per cent of girls who would have preferred to have been boys.

As with the girls, there was a slight tendency for the boys in boys' schools to be more extreme in their replies, and to present a more romanticized picture of the opposite sex.

Summary

To conclude the chapter let us draw a few threads together. In the Second College survey the ex-pupils from single-sex and those from co-educational schools have closely similar opinions about the basic equality of the sexes, though some men from boys' schools said that their belief in the inherent superiority of the male had been changed by their residence in a mixed college. This question differed from most others in that it asked the ex-pupils about their *present* opinions rather than asking them to make a judgment about their experience in a certain school. The tendency of the ex-pupils of boys' schools to express rather more extreme opinions appears again, even though this difference in spread between the opposite groups did not quite reach statistical significance.

In the question about the pleasantness of the attitude of most of the pupils towards the opposite sex we return to ex-pupils' judgments about the schools which were attended. The male ex-pupils from the 'Both schools' survey considered the attitude towards girls to be more pleasant in their co-educational schools because of a good family relationship there, while the number of judgments describing the atmosphere as a little unpleasant or worse were more numerous about the boys' schools. The same type of 'deprivation effect' is to be seen among the women, there being more 'unpleasant' or 'rather unpleasant' estimates made about the girls' schools than about the co-educational.

The series of supplementary questions about the attitude of pupils towards the opposite sex, which included the one about 'boy/girl crazy', consistently produced the same results—that the attitude was more normal and healthier in the co-educational schools. At the same time this less normal attitude in the single-sex schools appears to be accompanied by a greater timidity about the opposite sex which in a small minority of girls (and a few boys) even becomes fear.

A related problem—whether the younger boys and girls want the presence of the opposite sex in a co-educational school—has been tentatively examined, and although this presence is rather less popular in the junior than in the senior school, a large majority of the junior boys and almost all junior girls welcome it.

Attitude to the opposite sex

For reasons discussed in the previous volume (Dale, 1969), which are mainly concerned with sampling, the Schools project discovered few differences between the attitudes of samples of present pupils of co-educational and single-sex schools towards the opposite sex, though it should also be emphasized that the inquiry was limited to a few aspects. However, a trend was observed for pupils in single-sex schools to use the extremes of the scale slightly more often than those in co-educational schools. Further comment is reserved for the concluding chapter.

13

Social relationships between boys and girls

As might be expected the area of social relationships between boys and girls is considered by both teachers and pupils to produce decided advantages for co-education. A single-sex school clearly cannot give a normal education in these relationships without moving towards co-education. Unless there are serious moral dangers in educating adolescents of both sexes together—and there is not at the moment any research finding to show that this is so—it is necessary for the protagonists of single-sex education to find other powerful arguments to compensate for this considerable deficiency.

This chapter endeavours to supply a little research evidence about the effect of these social relationships, mainly by examining them within the co-educational school itself, using evidence from ex-pupils. A start is made with the influence of the girls on the boys within the co-educational school.

Influence of girls on boys

In the 'Both schools' survey grammar school ex-pupils who were then in Colleges of Education were asked the following question about their schooling: 'Do you consider that the influence of the girls on the boys in this school was, in general, Very good/Good/Fairly good/No effect/Bad/Very bad?' This question might have been better if 'fairly bad' had been included. However, Table 13.1 shows that these mature ex-pupils, looking back on their school-days, judged that the girls had a good influence on the boys. This was the view of both men and women, and was fundamentally the same for junior ('first') and senior ('last') pupils. The men praised the influence of the girls rather more than the women did. Only three women and no men out of 648 replies from women and 181 replies from men estimated that the influence was 'very bad', and the percentage of either sex who considered it 'bad' does not rise above 6.4 per cent. It was shown in the previous volume that this is also the opinion of grammar school teachers and especially of those who had taught in co-educational schools (Dale, 1969, Ch. 4).

TABLE 13.1 *Influence of girls on boys*

'Both schools' survey

Estimates of ex-pupils	Replies from men about co-educational schools				Replies from women about co-educational schools			
	First schools		Last schools		First schools		Last schools	
	N	%	N	%	N	%	N	%
Very good	11	14·1	20	19·4	20	6·8	34	9·6
Good	30	38·5	34	33·0	89	30·4	122	34·4
Fairly good	26	33·3	38	36·9	107	36·5	119	33·5
No effect	6	7·7	8	7·8	59	20·1	70	19·7
Bad	5	6·4	3	2·9	16	5·5	9	2·5
Very bad	0	0	0	0	2	0·7	1	0·3
Totals	78	100	103	100	293	100	355	100

OPINION OF THE MEN ABOUT THE GIRLS' INFLUENCE ON THE BOYS (FREE RESPONSES)

A classification of the free responses made by the ex-pupils as a comment on their estimates is given in Table 13.2. We see that an overwhelming proportion of the men thought the girls had a good influence on the boys. By far the largest group—82 in all—were of the opinion that the behaviour, manners, language or appearance of the boys were improved. In the 'social' section, while 10 made some criticism about 'boys showing off' or girls likewise, no fewer than 8 of these gave favourable estimates about the overall influence of the girls, and there is a strong emphasis on the advantages of learning to mix naturally with the opposite sex, the reduction in shyness and the healthier attitude. On the academic side the dominant opinion is that the conscientiousness of the girls and the friendly rivalry between the sexes improved the standard of work of the boys, while only 5 of the 199 comments mentioned 'distraction from study'. Here we have forces acting in opposite directions, but in the opinion of the men the good influence on academic progress far outweighs the bad, an opinion which is supported by the results of research on the comparative attainment in co-educational and single-sex schools.

TABLE 13.2 *Influence of girls on boys: Men's free responses*
'Both schools' survey

Type of comment	No. of comments
Behaviour	
Improved boys' behaviour, manners, language	65
Appearance	
improved boys' appearance	17
Social	
social life improved	5
social development, easier mixing with opposite sex, less shy, co-operation, mutual understanding	35
healthy attitude to opposite sex, less preoccupation with sex	6
few immoral girls, a few troublesome	2
boys show off before girls	8
girls tried to impress boys	2
Academic	
made boys work harder, girls more conscientious	12
friendly competition	13
distraction from study, lower standard of work	5
girls less ambitious pupils	2
interchange of ideas	2
Depends on age, etc.	7
Others	18
Total	199

A few quotations, again chosen in proportion to the totals in their sections, illustrate the text.

BEHAVIOUR AND APPEARANCE 'Much of the roughness of an all-boys school was removed on the change to a new co-ed. school; different staff came and some of the tradition disappeared.' (Am.)

'Tended to calm the boys down, and also gave incentive to work.'

'A calming influence—*on the whole* improved behaviour.'

'If anything, a modifying effect, on manners, language, bullying, etc.'

'Seemed to keep the boys more in discipline than the school rules.'

'There was a minimum of bad language and an excess of good manners.'

'Increased good manners and decreased bad language.'

'After a certain age (13–15) the boys began to take notice of the girls and respond by (a) trying hard in class, (b) improving their appearance.'

'We all combed our hair after games and wore what we thought the girls would like.'

SOCIAL 'Brought home to me a larger meaning of social behaviour and appearance.'

'Although there was favouritism towards the girls, at last we recognized them as human and not stupid. We saw the upper school mixing much more. We were made to mix in dancing lessons.'

'Gave a good atmosphere.'

'We were in contact with girls all day, therefore we did not find it embarrassing or awkward speaking to members of the opposite sex.'

'To a greater extent there was no effect, but sometimes there was the odd incident where a boy would do something wrong to attract the attention of certain girls.'

'We had an insight into their life. Therefore our outlook became broader. Social events were more natural. Culture varied—more like "life".'

ACADEMIC 'The girls had an extra competitive effect on the boys in both the classroom and in other school activities. I had never felt this before, but I am sure it did nothing but good.'

'Gave a competition in work, which was stimulating to great effort and produced a much freer social life in the school.'

'I think it was bad in so far as it brought the level of the work over the year down which meant that we had to study much more intensely at examination times.'

The tone of the comments is serious and these men obviously think that the girls in their schools had a distinctly good influence. Though there are a few dissenters they form a minute fraction of the whole.

OPINION OF THE WOMEN ABOUT THE GIRLS' INFLUENCE ON THE BOYS

The women ex-pupils answered the same question; their judgments about the influence of the girls on the boys are to be seen in

Table 13.1. Like the men the women thought the girls had a good influence, though some of them are not as certain as the men—the 'no effect' group has risen to 20 per cent of the whole as against the 8 per cent amongst the men. However, those who thought the influence was bad were only 6 per cent for juniors and 3 per cent for seniors—almost identical with the men's figures.

As the free responses from the women are sufficiently large they have been classified in more detail than those of the men in order to give readers a better picture of the reasons underlying the estimates.

The women's judgments in Table 13.3 show that most of them are thinking of the effect of the presence of girls in improving the behaviour, manners, language and appearance of the boys. Secondary in size, but still numerous, are those who write of the healthy academic rivalry of girls with boys and also those who thought the presence of the girls (with the boys) encouraged a natural friendly atmosphere, co-operation between the two sexes and a better understanding of girls by boys. Of lesser importance, but not negligible, are the comments of those women who thought that mixing with girls made the boys less shy and raised their academic standard, but on the negative side there was some showing off and a little distraction. Both these latter groups were again small fractions of the whole.

The large groups of comments are represented by approximately one quotation for every twenty (after consolidation) and the smaller ones by one in ten, in order to give the latter adequate representation.

BEHAVIOUR AND APPEARANCE 'The girls' presence tended to "calm" the boys and teach them to be gentlemen.'

'It made the boys courteous and considerate. Headmaster very firm about this.'

'Girls did help the boys to be more considerate towards them so in fact they acquired a sense of respect.'

'The girls were often able to calm the boys down if riots broke out!'

'Girls make gentlemen out of the boys and also have a "good grooming" influence, e.g. long hair, dyed, etc., would be ridiculed by the girls.'

'They took more care of their appearance and learnt to take care of their manners.'

TABLE 13.3 *Influence of girls on boys: Women's free responses*

'Both schools' survey

Type of comment	No. of comments
Behaviour	
girls steadying influence	30
improved behaviour, manners, language	137
no bullying	2
bad effect	4
Appearance	
improved appearance, dress	55
Social	
not shy	24
natural atmosphere, friendly, respectful, co-operation	56
understood girls better	12
pleasant friendship	2
not preoccupied with opposite sex, not girl-crazy	4
helped boys grow up	12
good co-operation in societies, etc.	6
boys not interested (especially junior)	13
boys interested in girls' sports	3
some showing off	37
no respect for girls	2
thought girls stupid	1
girl-crazy	3
boys dominant	2
Academic	
raised standard, by example	14
healthy rivalry	83
broadened their interests, more balance	9
co-operation	4
no distraction	2
some distraction	10
poor work by boys	1
interests different	1
Moral	
low morals of young girls	1
Depends on age, individuals	5
Don't know	10
No effect	23
Others	56
Total	624

'When school changed to a boys' school I stayed on and noticed that their manners, behaviour and dress became lax.'

'When I look at some of the products of all-boys schools here at College I realize what a good lot ours were on the whole. They were made to be polite and considerate in the beginning and eventually it came naturally. Talking to whose who have left I feel that they appreciate this too, for they are more sure of themselves at all times, especially at social functions.'

'Boys took a little more pride in their dress. Cultivated better manners towards girls, e.g. opening doors, giving up seats, etc. Some did not bother though.'

'Boys tended to be rowdy by themselves. Also disliked being lazy, unintelligent in front of girls.'

'Girls have a sobering influence.'

SOCIAL 'The boys were always aware of the girls' presence and treated them with respect.'

'Because boys and girls mixed together there was no preoccupation with the other sex as sometimes happens in a single-sex school.'

'Boys were aware of the need to respect girls, even though they did not always carry this out in the early years.'

'Boys accepted girls, girls accepted boys. There was no shyness or restraint. We learnt together in an easy atmosphere.'

'It created a more natural atmosphere. They didn't tend to be too shy when talking to girls outside school.'

'I feel it made them understand girls. They worked alongside the girls quite happily. They developed as they grew older a well mannered and naturally friendly attitude to the girls. The boys also learnt not to be embarrassed by girls or company of them. I feel it helped to give them a healthier attitude.'

'I think on the whole influence of the girls was good. Tended to make boys accept the girls naturally. They also learnt some courtesy towards the opposite sex; less rough perhaps than boys from single-sex school.'

ACADEMIC 'Boys appeared to fear being beaten in exams. etc. and were encouraged to work.'

'There was healthy competition between the sexes regarding work—rivalry but also co-operation.'

'Most boys seemed to work harder in order to try and gain superiority.'

'Academically they stretched the boys in discussion, etc. Socially they tended to make them more mature.'

'Attention in class was continually being detracted [sic] from the lesson. General attitudes and behaviour were appalling.'

'They seemed to grow up far more quickly. Childish pranks were in general over by the 4th Form.'

'Boys in my peer group tended to ignore us. If they did pay attention to girls they were usually teasing or "showing off". I suppose politeness (under supervision!) to girls was a temporary "good effect".'

'The girls often encouraged the boys to bad behaviour and showing off.'

The boys showed off and wanted to appear "big" to impress the girls.'

Influence of boys on girls

OPINION OF THE MALE EX-PUPILS

The corresponding question about the boys was: 'Do you consider that the influence of the boys on the girls in this school was,

TABLE 13.4 *Influence of boys on girls*
'Both schools' survey

Estimates of students in Colleges of Education	Replies from men about co-educational schools				Replies from women about co-educational schools			
	First schools co-educational		Last schools		First schools co-educational		Last schools	
	N	%	N	%	N	%	N	%
Very good	8	10·7	14	13·9	16	5·5	33	9·4
Good	18	24·0	24	23·8	103	35·1	130	37·2
Fairly good	33	44·0	37	36·6	104	35·4	112	32·0
No effect	10	13·3	17	16·8	40	13·7	41	11·7
Bad	6	8·0	9	8·9	26	8·9	34	9·7
Very bad	0	0	0	0	4	1·4	0	0
Totals	75	100	101	100	293	100	350	100

Very good/Good/Fairly good/No effect/Bad/Very bad?' The male ex-pupils thought that in their co-educational schools the influence of the boys on the girls was good, only some 8 to 9 per cent thinking it bad, while some 13 per cent (junior) and 17 per cent (senior) thought the boys had no effect. The distribution of estimates of those who were at the schools as juniors and those who were seniors is almost identical (Table 13.4)

TABLE 13.5 *Influence of boys on girls (men's opinions)*

'Both schools' survey

Type of comment	No. of comments
Behaviour	
improved, stabilizing	18
Appearance	
improved	9
Social	
good social development	6
good atmosphere, co-operation	5
girls less preoccupied with opposite sex, understanding, natural mixing	21
less petty-minded, more balanced education	4
less shyness	8
girls rejected 'tearaways'	1
some 'showing off'	4
girls' 'crushes' on older boys	4
jealousy over boy-friends	1
boy/sex crazy	2
Academic	
standard improved, widened interest	5
friendly rivalry	11
bad example of boys	2
moderated girls' preoccupation with work	2
some distraction	2
Sex	
healthy attitude	2
promiscuous impression of some girls	1
some boys corrupted girls	1
good except some boys' sexual offences	1
No effect	12
Others	12
Total	134

The chief reasons for this opinion (Table 13.5) were given as improved behaviour and appearance of the girls, the natural mixing of the sexes with a consequent reduction in shyness, and the friendly rivalry in academic work. The total number of men, however, was only 172, which produced only 134 free responses, so that the numbers in each category were small.

Quotations in the proportion of one in five (approximately) are given from sub-categories containing four or more comments.

BEHAVIOUR AND APPEARANCE 'It made them less petty minded and also made them more mature.'

'Made this *fairly good* rather than good, because girls, even in a single-sex school, *seem* to have a more balanced attitude to opposite sex (so influence of comprehensive is less) but this may only be an appearance, as I also believe the confidence of the comprehensive girl is not just *superficial* but an *inner* confidence arising from working with boys.'

'In general the girls adopted a more sensible attitude to the opposite sex. There was no childish giggling and blushing.'

' "Woke up" some of the quieter ones—thus producing much more balanced community.'

'Girls became more aware of dress sense and far more prepared for out-of-school social life.'

'Kept girls neat and tidy.'

SOCIAL 'Boys are part of everyday life outside of school, to ostracize them in school is to deprive girls socially. Social development is very important especially in later teens.'

'Toughened up the girls' contact with boys, made girls less "romantic".'

'We treated the girls as people and not strange beings.'

'I do think girls build up false impressions about the opposite sex. The presence of the genuine article does I think help in part to break this down.'

'There was a good atmosphere, problems on both sides were discussed freely, seriously and intelligently. The atmosphere was very natural.'

'In quite a few cases the influence was good for it brought some girls out of their shells.'

'In early adolescence the girls tended to become preoccupied with boys—but at least they were always in contact with them—little shyness.'

ACADEMIC 'Raised the standards of the girls.'

'The girls wanted to beat the boys so they worked harder.'

'The boys had an extra competitive effect on the girls in both the classroom and in other school activities.'

Though comments in the adverse categories are too few to be included by the fixed percentage criterion, readers are reminded that there are some, as indicated in Table 13.5.

OPINION OF THE WOMEN EX-PUPILS ABOUT THE INFLUENCE OF THE BOYS ON THE GIRLS

The estimates given by the women ex-pupils about the effect of the boys on the girls (Table 13.4) resemble those given by the men—the same low percentage of ex-pupils thought the influence bad, and a slightly smaller percentage of women than men thought there was no effect. Another slight difference was that rather fewer women considered the influence to be 'very good' as opposed to 'good'; this difference was not considered important enough for testing statistically.

The women's free responses give a definitely favourable opinion about the influence of the boys on the girls in the co-educational schools they attended, though they also indicate some lesser negative aspects. (Table 13.6). Amusingly we find that the improved appearance of girls is an outstanding effect, but combining 'improved behaviour' with 'prevented silliness towards the opposite sex', and 'girls less catty, less giggly and less spiteful' produced an even larger group of comments. The dividing line between 'behaviour' and 'social' is admittedly arbitrary and there is a marked overlap. Classified under 'social' the largest group of comments is concerned with the girls' relationship with boys being normal, girls regarding them as fellow-workers and normal friends, and not being 'boy-crazy', while another sizeable group regards as important the broadening of girls' outlook and ideas. As was indicated at the beginning of the paragraph, these judgments are not unanimous, a few women saying that some girls were boy-crazy, and that some showed off, while other women thought boys set a bad example and encouraged girls to misbehave. In view of the criticism that has in the past—unfairly—been directed against the academic standards of co-educational grammar schools, it is interesting to

TABLE 13.6 *Influence of boys on the girls: (women's opinions)*
'Both schools' survey

Type of comment	No. of comments
Behaviour	
improved behaviour	21
improved appearance	92
too concerned about appearance	3
some tried to attract boys	10
some noisy, rough	5
girls less catty, spiteful, less giggly, silly	46
Social	
prevented silliness towards opposite sex, more natural	65
socially good	4
girls interested in boys' sports	2
boys as normal friends, fellow workers, co-operation	16
understood boys' point of view	13
broadened girls' outlook, ideas; maturity	41
not boy-crazy	15
helped timid girls	5
took notice of boys' opinion	2
bad influence lower forms	3
better in higher forms	3
worse in higher forms	2
some showing off, silliness, rivalry	6
boy-crazy	9
girls encouraged to misbehave	10
boys bad example	5
girls got inferiority complex	3
girls mixed with older boys	1
girls ignored boys and vice-versa (junior)	5
Academic	
good rivalry in classwork	97
helped girls' science	1
encouraged discussion	10
work more interesting	3
boys' humour in lessons, lively	5
lowered standards	1
girls shy about some work	2
distracted girls from work	23
no distraction	2
Others	
(comments inapplicable etc.)	51
difficult to say, generalize	10
too young (juniors)	2
no effect	9
Total	603

see the large body of opinion which praises the friendly academic rivalry of the two sexes, equally in junior and senior school, though the minority view that girls were distracted from their work is not negligible. Little positive pointers that have constantly occurred in this context in answer to related questions, and in other of the writer's researches, are the girls' appreciation of the way class discussions are improved by the presence of boys, and the welcome the girls give to the boys' sense of humour.

The proportion of free responses quoted is one in twenty, but sub-categories with ten or fewer replies have had to be omitted.

BEHAVIOUR 'The girls were inclined to behave in order to make a good impression on boys, especially if rather keen on one particular boy.'

'Nearly 99 per cent of the girls took more care over hair, clothes, etc.'

'Girls' dress improved, although perhaps more for the purpose of attracting the boys, rather than for the good of their souls.'

'The girls tended to act a little more dignified. They didn't shout or run.'

'Girls were less catty and more careful about appearance.'

'Most of the boys were quite rough and as might be expected some of the girls often showed this streak in them.'

'Girls seemed less catty and much less boy-crazy and more mature. Boys' good manners helped femininity.'

'Boys made life less petty and catty. Made girls conscious of having good table manners, etc., because theirs were very poor. Sense of humour from boys infected school.'

SOCIAL 'Boys were accepted as friends, just as we made girl-friends. They helped us to widen our knowledge regarding the opposite sex.'

'I can't think why; boys and girls seemed to provide more natural atmosphere for each other. Sex was not distorted as can happen in single-sex schools. There was more sense of unison, boys and girls working together, both important.'

'Made the timid girls less self-conscious and encouraged them to have more social life.'

'It taught us to get along with the opposite sex, which is important for future life.'

'The girls became interested in the boys' hobbies etc., so had a wider knowledge of life than girls from the nearby girls' school.'

'In general the boys, particularly those with some knowledge of the sciences on a deeper level, had wide knowledge of the Arts too. This broader view showed the girls the limitations of their own knowledge and encouraged them to extend it.'

'They did not seem as "boy-mad" as some girls from girls' schools.'

'The girls were too "boy-crazy" and far more concerned with what they looked like for "Johnny" than what sort of work they presented.'

ACADEMIC 'The girls made a little more effort to look neat and tidy, and worked a bit harder to make sure they kept up with the boys.'

'Having boys in the form made you work harder at the subjects which boys are taken to be better at, e.g. Science, Maths.'

'Girls tried to obtain better results than boys. Element of competition inspired by opposite sexes.'

'In science subjects they were encouraged to "be as good as the boys" who tended towards those subjects.'

'The boys were very good in contributing to class and out-of-school activities, and the girls learned to understand and appreciate their opinions, as the boys did the girls'.'

'In many cases the influence of the boys interfered with the work of the girls and concentration in lessons.'

It has been the practice in previous chapters to publish all those free responses which make a direct comparison between the co-educational and single-sex school. Those relating to this chapter are so numerous and often so repetitive of what has gone before that their presentation as a special section would have overburdened the chapter; some, however, have already been included with the other responses.

Schools project

An attempt was made to compare pupils still at co-educational schools with those still at single-sex schools about their ease of relationship with the opposite sex. They were asked to reply to four items; for the boys these were: 'When I meet girls at a party

I don't know what to say,' 'I feel very awkward when I am with girls', 'I feel perfectly at ease when I am with girls,' and 'I prefer talking to girls rather than to boys.' The possible answers were: 'Very true/Often true/Sometimes true/Seldom true/Not true.'

It was hypothesized that the co-educated pupils would socially be much more at ease with the opposite sex, but the results were quite inconclusive. No differences between the co-educated girls and those from girls' schools were statistically significant, and only two between the boys' groups—more 15-year-old boys from boys' schools preferred talking to girls, and fewer 17-year-old co-educated boys felt awkward when with girls. The reasons for the lack of clear and consistent differences are complex. They appear to include the existence of two opposing forces, first that the separation of the sexes may by perpetuating ignorance, tend to make each sex not at ease with the other, and second that deprivation of the company of the opposite sex may make boys and girls keener to get this company, thereby generating a powerful motivation to overcome shyness. There is in addition a flaw in the multiple choice range of possible answers, because the alternative 'seldom true', for example, could be ambiguous in so far as (a) it was 'seldom true' the pupil felt awkward, because he hardly ever spoke to a girl, and (b) it was 'seldom true' that he felt awkward as a proportion of the many times he spoke to a girl.

Another possible explanation for the lack of reliable differences at the school stage may be that in the co-educational schools the pupils are brought face to face with the problems of social relations with the opposite sex and have a more realistic appraisal of their own position, whereas the girls in girls' schools meet the opposite sex on 'special occasions' rather than on a day-long basis.

Comment

The evidence that the presence of girls improves the appearance, conduct and discipline of the boys is very strong, coming as it does from both male and female ex-pupils and from teachers. Though the evidence that the presence of boys effects a corresponding improvement in the girls is less strong, its existence cannot be denied; the tidiness of the girls and their dress are noticeably better and, according to those women who have attended both a girls' and a co-educational school, they become less catty and vindictive and less inclined to group in cliques. The world, however, is not a simple place, and jealousies over boy-friends are naturally more frequent in co-educational schools. As with so many aspects of the central theme there is an obvious need here for more research.

Social relationships between boys and girls

The lack of supporting evidence from the Schools project on the more specific questions related to the general theme of the chapter may be due to a combination of causes among which the two already mentioned in the previous section—the flaw in the wording of the answer scale and the contrast between the day-long facing of the problems in the co-educational school and the occasional evening venture for girls from girls' schools—may be the most important.

14

Comparative attitude to sex

Whatever reasons may be given openly for opposition to co-education at the secondary stage, there appears to be a deep-seated fear among some people that such schools might lead to an increase in sexual misbehaviour and to an undue interest in sex at too early an age. The introduction to the previous volume included a passage on ways of gathering objective evidence about which kind of school atmosphere encourages or diminishes these tendencies. At an early stage in the inquiry the writer decided that an investigation of that kind would need a research team drawn partly from specialists in social work, and as there were no funds available for the purpose he turned towards a method which was less objective but by no means without value as a preliminary survey of the field. Surprisingly this research has yielded results which are so conclusive in their verdict that they are much more valuable than might otherwise have been the case.

Incorporated in the 'Both schools' questionnaire was the item, 'In which school do you consider the pupils had the healthier attitude towards sex?' The respondents were all intending teachers who had been pupils in both co-educational and single-sex secondary schools (excluding secondary modern), and they were asked to choose one of four alternative replies: Doubtful/Don't know/Single-sex school/Co-educational school. Their replies were obviously sincere and considered, and although there might be quibbles about the exact meaning of 'healthier' there can be little doubt that an unhealthy atmosphere towards sex is undesirable in any school. The estimates themselves, however, do not necessarily indicate that any one of the atmospheres is actually unhealthy—merely that one is healthier than the other. Not until the free responses are examined shall we be in a position to interpret the estimates more precisely.

The attitude of girls

As will be seen from Figure 14.1, a large majority of the women (76 per cent) judged the attitude towards sex to be healthier in their co-educational school than in their girls' school, a mere 7 per cent recording the opposite belief. The only intervening

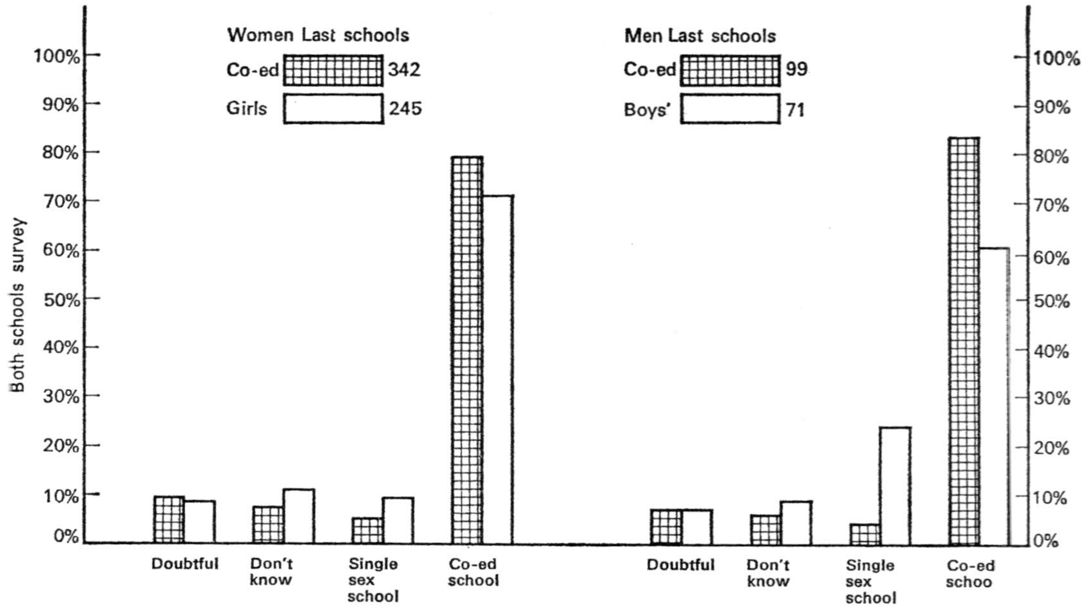

FIGURE 14.1
Healthier attitude to sex: 'Both schools' survey

variable which the writer can think of which might be advantageous to the co-educational schools is that a larger percentage of them have a rural or semi-rural catchment area, but this would in itself be unlikely to produce so great a difference. In these social surveys there are usually so many forces exerting an influence on a problem, and pulling in different directions, that rarely does one find group differences of such magnitude. In spite of the extent of the differences we must remember that for some individuals and maybe for some schools the influence of co-education might be overcome by other forces, among which the individual personality of the pupil and his or her individual experience are obviously important.

There was a greater tendency for women who had been senior pupils in co-educational schools to judge the attitude to sex to be healthier in such schools (than in girls' schools) than for women who had attended girls' schools as seniors, though even among the latter only some 9 per cent thought the attitude was healthier in girls' schools.

TABLE 14.1 *Attitude towards sex (women's opinions)*
'Both schools' survey

Estimate	Type of comment	No. of comments
Co-educational school healthier	co-educational school healthier	20
	natural behaviour, no preoccupation with sex	29
	sex discussed and not kept secret	26
	boys—friends, not obsessed sex, girls equals	25
	outlook broadened; narrow attitude in single-sex	16
	greater knowledge of opposite sex, more realistic	12
	mixed classes in sex education	3
	boys more accessible, not a challenge	2
	not healthy, but more so than single-sex	1
	not healthy, except when junior	1
	girls in girls' school boy-mad, frustrated, segregation unnatural, sex dominated conversation, silly ideas	6
	single-sex—crushes on females, some unhealthy consequences	1
	worse at boarding school	1
	many girls left because pregnant in girls' school	1
	attitude crude, less at co-ed.	2

TABLE 14.1 *Attitude towards sex (women's opinions)*
'Both schools' survey

Estimate	Type of comment	No. of comments
	afraid of men at single-sex school	1
	depends on individual	1
	Other	5
Total		153
Girls' school healthier	sensible, though danger of ignorance	2
	all-female staff, easier to discuss	1
	pleasant and much more tolerable	1
	nicer class of girls	1
	more emphasis on dirtier side in co-ed.	2
	too preoccupied with sex in co-ed., choosing boys	2
	in co-ed. sex considered undesirable	1
	at age when discussed sex sensibly	3
Total		13
Don't know	don't know	6
	more open discussion in co-ed.	4
	co-ed. less embarrassment	1
	depends on upbringing; slightly healthier co-ed.	1
	physical interest single-sex, ethical interest co-ed.	1
	separation in single-sex, therefore went crazy in co-ed.	1
	single-sex perhaps healthier—only wishful thinking	1
	more self-conscious at co-ed. and preoccupied with sex	1
	single-sex some preoccupation with boys, but work better	1
	possible single-sex dirty stories spread more in co-ed.	1
	boys discussed in single-sex because absent	1
	no difference, mixed outside school	1
	depends on home background	2
	not healthy at either	1
	cannot remember co-ed.	2
	varying ages	3
	presence of opposite sex has no effect	1
Total		29

TABLE 14.1 *Attitude towards sex (women's opinions)*
'Both schools' survey

Estimate	Type of comment	No. of comments
Doubtful	doubtful	1
	perhaps co-ed. healthier	1
	indifference at co-ed.	1
	possibly juniors co-ed. healthier	1
	co-ed. little interest sex, reasonable attitude single-sex	1
	lower forms single-sex bad attitude but improved with age	1
	a bit unhealthy in co-ed., single-sex too young	1
	in neither was sex discussed in class	1
	no interest in sex at 13	1
	depends on association out of school	1
Total		10
No estimate	*Other*	
	both the same	2
	difficult question	1
	depends on individual	1
Total		4

The free responses again enable us to interpret more accurately the significance of the estimates. From Table 14.1 we see that the larger groups among those women who judged the attitude to be healthier in their co-educational schools were those who emphasized normal behaviour, the lack of preoccupation with boys, the open discussion, broadened outlook and greater understanding of boys as people. The small minority who found the girls' attitude healthier in their girls' school are too few for their comments to be considered representative of such schools—there were only thirteen.

The classification in Table 14.1 is more detailed than usual, so that there is less need for the quotation of comments, especially quotations in strict proportion to category totals, and only a few of the more discerning or more interesting are given. The first three go to the root cause of the difference between the attitudes prevalent in the two types of school: 'When you see boys every day the novelty wears off,' 'Boys were part of everyday life in the co-ed school, and at times were completely forgotten about,' and 'Mixing with the opposite sex one comes into closer contact than in the single-sex school—it changes one's ideas completely—found I had more respect towards them and a healthier attitude towards sex.' A fourth quotation enlarges this: 'Greater maturity together, therefore far less mystery and intrigue. Accepted each other as personalities and not so much men and women.'

One woman makes the point that the personality of the girl herself can be a strong influence for good or bad: 'Whatever school a girl goes to she makes her own moral values. A girl can be just as "wild" in a girls' school as a co-ed—depends only on the individual,' but she seems to take the argument much too far at the end—as if the environment had no influence.

Two extreme comments are about girls' schools, but they do not rest on any representative basis: 'There was definitely a high proportion of girls leaving school because of pregnancy in the single-sex school, or being married as soon as leaving school, than ever in the co-ed.,' and, 'My single-sex school had unmarried mothers, promiscuous women, a few lesbians, several nuns, one or two mentally unstable young women, and not a few women incapable of friendship with men. I have seen all these come from the form I was in at this school.' One would be sceptical of taking this last comment at its face value if it were not for the transparent honesty of the rest of the woman's replies. A few comments show that sometimes an undesirable atmosphere can also exist in a co-educational school, for example: 'In co-ed. sex was treated as a joke, i.e. "dirty" jokes, etc. were numerous. Obscene remarks from the boys to the girls also evident.' This school, however, was an 'amalgamated' school. In general, remarks of this kind are not characteristic of either type of school, a fairer and more reliable picture being represented by the estimates.

ANALYSIS BY PARENTAL OCCUPATION

When the data are broken down by parental occupation as in Table 14.2 no consistent trend associated with social class appears. The slight drop in the support of the class 2 ex-pupils, i.e. broadly the clerical class, for the healthiness of the attitude in the co-educational schools is intriguing as it occurs among those who were at a co-educational school last as well as among those who attended a girls' school last; but no further examination was made. Any association of the judgments with social class influences would probably be reduced by the tendency for the student teachers themselves to be moving towards the same class. However, the judgment that the attitude towards sex is healthier in the co-educational schools is very decided in each parental occupation grouping.

TABLE 14.2 *Healthier attitude to sex (women's responses): Analysis by parental occupation*

'Both schools' survey

	Replies from women (from 'co-educational last' schools) in Occupational Class						Replies from women (from 'single-sex last' schools) in Occupational Class					
	1		2		3, 4, 5		1		2		3, 4, 5	
	N	%	N	%	N	%	N	%	N	%	N	%
Doubtful	15	8·0	7	10·0	7	8·5	8	6·6	9	18·0	4	5·7
Don't know	13	6·9	6	8·6	7	8·5	13	10·7	6	12·0	8	11·5
Single-sex school	7	3·7	6	8·6	2	2·4	11	9·0	5	10·0	7	10·0
Co-educational school	153	81·4	51	72·8	66	80·6	90	73·7	30	60·0	51	72·8
Totals	188	100	70	100	82	100	122	100	50	100	70	100

The attitude of boys

The estimates of the male ex-pupils were almost as overwhelmingly favourable for the co-educational schools as were those of the females (see Figure 14.1), though the percentage of the men who judged the attitude towards sex in their boys' schools to be

TABLE 14.3 *Attitude towards sex (men's opinions)*

'Both schools' survey

Estimate	Type of comment	No. of comments
Co-educational school healthier	co-educational school most definitely a healthier attitude	11
	perhaps, or slightly more balanced attitude	4
	no secrecy, good healthy relationships	11
	less depravity or homosexual tendencies	8
	mixing made attitudes broader	10
	unhealthy attitude of some of staff of single-sex school	1
Single-sex school healthier	as opposed to co-ed. experience	9
	slightly better attitude	1
Don't know	don't know	3
	varied with individuals	2
Doubtful	doubtful	3
	but slightly in favour of single-sex school	1
Total		64

healthier than in their co-educational schools rose to 24 among those who attended their boys' school as seniors. The number in the sample was too small to permit any meaningful breakdown of the data according to parental occupation.

The free responses were naturally few, but were again informative (see Table 14.3). Most of the replies said that there was a healthier attitude towards sex in the co-educational rather than in the boys' schools, with a more balanced or broader outlook, less secrecy and good friendly relationships. As a sub-section of this majority, eight replies, being one-ninth of the total, said there was less depravity or homosexual tendencies in the co-educational schools. A minority of ten men thought that the attitude was healthier in their boys' school; of these, eight attended the boys' schools as seniors.

Free responses typical of those which said the attitude was healthier in the co-educational schools are quoted below. The proportion of those favourable to boys' schools, given afterwards, has been increased above their due allotment to improve the coverage of the argument. The free responses in favour of co-educational schools are as follows:

'There is less depraved sex-talk amongst the boys—fewer jokes etc. The attitude is far healthier altogether.'

'Close relationships with members of the opposite sex leads to a better understanding of each other's roles in society. A balanced adjustment ensues.'

'They grew up with it, having a respect rather than a desire for one another.'

'Is it healthy to have girls leave school to have babies? I understand there was a homosexual teacher at single-sex school, and I know there were many homosexuals in that school.'

'Some members of staff in the single-sex school had an unbalanced outlook towards sex.'

"The attitude in the single-sex was at least 75 per cent homosexual inside school, and girl-mad outside school.'

'Homosexual tendencies in single-sex schools were obvious and often quite open.'

'Some of the boys in single-sex school seemed more interested in themselves than in girls.'

Four of the ten comments favouring the attitude in the boys' schools were:

'Everyone at the co-ed. school seemed sensitive to the subject. At the boys' school the attitude was one of respect tempered with coarseness.'

'This may be because our attitude grew healthier as we grew older.'

'Promiscuity much more rife in co-ed. school.'

'Even though they were less well acquainted with the opposite sex their attitude to them was far more polite and they were treated with greater respect.'

As with the girls, although a large majority of the men estimate the attitude to be healthier in their co-educational schools there is a small minority whose experience leads them to the opposite view.

A researcher who limited himself to this topic would wish to give additional solidity to the evidence by examining data such as the incidence of unwanted pregnancies, the incidence of juvenile delinquency connected with sex, and even—perhaps as a long shot—investigate whether the incidence of prostitution and of homosexuality was startlingly higher among ex-pupils from one type of school rather than the other, with relevant variables held constant. However, as this evidence is not available we can only say that the data examined in this chapter are strongly in favour of the co-educational school. It should be added that the attitude to sex in co-educational schools does indeed need to be healthy for these schools to be viable institutions.

15

Some sociological questions

The questionnaire used in the 'Both schools' survey contained several items which had an element of sociological significance. One of these—the least sociological—was, 'The school tried to dominate my whole life,' to which respondents could answer one of the following: Agree strongly/Agree/Doubtful/Disagree/Disagree strongly. The results obtained from this are in the first section of the chapter and three sections following will each be devoted to another item.

'The school tried to dominate my whole life'

The demarcation line between the part of a pupil's life which is controlled by the day school and those parts which are controlled by other institutions, such as the family, the Church, the youth club etc. is, as we saw in a previous chapter, exceedingly ill-defined. Have the school authorities any legal right to demand that a pupil should wear a school cap or hat, to and from school, i.e. before he enters the school precincts and comes clearly under the authority of the head of the school? If the family says 'No cap, or hat' and the head insists on the said article, whose legal position is the better? Is a school head within his or her rights in insisting that schoolboys or schoolgirls do not walk through the town eating ice-cream (a) in the dinner-hour, or (b) after school hours? Has a school head any legal right to ban entry to certain rather low-class or noisy cafés during either of these times? If a headmaster sees a boy misbehaving in the streets after school hours, not in such a way that would merit police intervention, has he any *legal* right to stop his car and intervene? More important, if a pupil commits any of these offences, has a head any legal right to punish the offender? Have heads, in a well-intentioned effort to bring up their pupils in the way they should go, arrogated to themselves powers which strictly belong to the family? These questions are not usually asked, probably because the heads of families, the community at large and even most of the pupils recognize that heads are acting for the good of the pupils and for the good of the community. It could happen, however, that an over-zealous head could go too far, and lose this tacit support of families and community. What then?

Another aspect of this item is whether the time demanded by the school *after school hours* is so great that the pupils' good leisure-time activities are seriously curtailed or even prevented. Is this a desirable result of schooling? Some schools frown on pupils attending youth clubs in the evenings because of the effect on homework. Innumerable pupils give up piano lessons when they reach the fourth or fifth because they cannot both practise an instrument and do their homework. Some compromise is probably inevitable but have we sufficiently considered the impact of homework on other legitimate and desirable activities of the pupils? By encroaching on this leisure-time do schools seriously limit those legitimate hobbies and pursuits through which pupils' individualities might normally develop? Do they overstrain their pupils?

There are other ways in which a school could 'dominate the life' of a pupil—by consciously or unconsciously dominating his or her outlook and thoughts. In this respect the writer believes we are much better off than most other countries.

We are concerned, however, with a comparison between co-educational and single-sex schools made by ex-pupils who had attended both. Unfortunately the results are once again limited to

TABLE 15.1 *'The school tried to dominate my whole life'*

'Both schools' survey (women)

Estimates	Replies about 'first' schools attended				Replies about 'last' schools attended			
	Co-educational schools		Girls' schools		Co-educational schools		Girls' schools	
	N	%	N	%	N	%	N	%
Agree strongly	3	1·0	28	6·9	6	1·7	16	6·2
Agree	19	6·4	75	18·5	17	4·7	51	19·6
Doubtful	23	7·7	77	19·0	45	12·5	45	17·3
Disagree	157	52·5	181	44·7	189	52·7	120	46·1
Disagree strongly	97	32·4	44	10·9	102	28·4	28	10·8
Totals	299	100	405	100	359	100	260	100

NOTE: The difference between the estimates about co-educational and girls' schools is statistically significant beyond the ·001 level, both for first and for last schools.

the estimates as there was insufficient time for the ex-pupils to add their free responses to this or the three other items of this chapter. We therefore do not know what type of domination the ex-pupil is referring to if he or she agrees with the statement; yet this overall exploration indicates interesting possibilities for further research. The results for the women are given in Table 15.1.

Table 15.1 shows that the female ex-pupils were strongly of the opinion that their girls' schools 'tried to dominate their whole life' more than their co-educational schools did, whether they were at the schools as junior pupils or as seniors. The possible significance of this has been outlined in the introduction to the chapter and the evidence is inadequate for more precise statements. The finding corresponds with trends found in other parts of the research, e.g. that single-sex school authorities exert more disciplinary power in running their schools.

The results from the male students are given in Table 15.2.

TABLE 15.2 *'The school tried to dominate my whole life'*

'Both schools' survey (men)

Estimates	Replies about 'first' schools attended				Replies about 'last' schools attended			
	Co-educational schools		Boys' schools		Co-educational schools		Boys' schools	
	N	%	N	%	N	%	N	%
Agree strongly	1	1·2	11	9·2	1	1·0	4	5·6
Agree	6	7·2	20	16·8	11	10·6	12	16·9
Doubtful	12	14·5	24	20·2	18	17·3	10	14·1
Disagree	42	50·6	50	42·0	47	45·1	32	45·1
Disagree strongly	22	26·5	14	11·8	27	26·0	13	18·3
Totals	83	100	119	100	104	100	71	100

NOTE: The difference between co-educational and boys' schools is statistically highly significant (beyond ·01) for first schools, but not significant for 'last' schools, though in the same direction.

Here the men give their co-educational schools as less dominating, a result statistically highly significant for 'first' schools but not significant for 'last' schools, though the difference is in the same direction. (This latter difference, however, in the setting of the general findings of the survey and in the light of the differences between the 'first' schools, i.e. junior pupils, is unlikely to have occurred purely by chance.)

The next item was, 'I felt that the school created a gap between myself and my home.' The five possible answers were the same as in the previous section.

Gap between pupils and home

It is sometimes said that the children of manual workers tend to make poorer progress in the grammar school than the children of upper-class parents because they find themselves out of place in the middle-class atmosphere prevalent there. Provided this is not accepted as the only reason or even the most important one, it may be correct. We hear less, however, of the effect of the school on the relationship between the manual worker's child and that child's home. Is it true that the school all unwittingly creates a gap between the child and his home? If it is true, must it be accepted as part of the price to be paid for progress?

Here the analysis is limited to the ex-pupils' opinion about this gap and whether it is felt to be greater in co-educational or single-sex schools (Table 15.3).

TABLE 15.3 *Gap between pupil and home*

'Both schools' (women)

Estimates	Replies about women's 'first' schools attended				Replies about women's 'last' schools attended			
	Co-educational schools		Girls' schools		Co-educational schools		Girls' schools	
	N	%	N	%	N	%	N	%
Agree strongly	7	2·3	21	5·3	4	1·1	9	3·5
Agree	23	7·7	37	9·2	24	6·7	21	8·1
Doubtful	26	8·7	92	23·0	31	8·6	46	17·8
Disagree	142	47·7	188	47·0	173	48·2	132	50·9
Disagree strongly	100	33·6	62	15·5	127	35·4	51	19·7
Totals	298	100	400	100	359	100	259	100

NOTE: The difference between the distributions for co-educational and girls' schools is statistically highly significant both for 'first' and for 'last' schools.

Table 15.3 shows that although a large majority of female ex-pupils from both types of school disagreed that their schools created a gap, they were appreciably more sure that their co-educational school did not have this effect than about their girls' schools. A breakdown of these estimates according to the occupational class of the ex-pupils' fathers revealed only a slightly greater tendency for the girls belonging to social class 3, 4 and 5 in the girls' schools and also those from this class who were seniors in the co-educational schools to agree that a gap was created by the schools.

The men's results resemble those of the women in that although only a small proportion of them agree with the statement as applied to either type of school, they disagree more strongly when it is applied to their co-educational schools. The difference, however, is statistically significant only for 'last' schools (Table 15.4). Breakdown of the data by occupational class of the ex-pupils' fathers could not profitably be undertaken because of the smallness of the sample.

TABLE 15.4 *Gap between pupil and home*

'Both schools' survey (men)

	Replies about men's 'first' schools attended				Replies about men's 'last' schools attended			
	Co-educational schools		Boys' schools		Co-educational schools		Boys' schools	
	N	%	N	%	N	%	N	%
Agree strongly	2	2·4	3	2·5	2	1·9	1	1·4
Agree	7	8·5	17	14·3	6	5·8	6	8·6
Doubtful	10	12·2	25	21·0	5	4·8	11	15·7
Disagree	36	44·0	50	42·0	44	42·3	35	50·0
Disagree strongly	27	32·9	24	20·2	47	45·2	17	24·3
Totals	82	100	119	100	104	100	70	100

NOTE: The difference between co-educational and boys' schools is not statistically significant for 'first' schools but is highly significant for 'last' schools.

Comment

The discovery that these ex-pupils, both men and women, consider that their co-educational schools are less likely to create a gap between pupil and home than are their single-sex schools is not necessarily produced by the type of organization found in those schools—the two are shown to be merely associated. It might be that the rather lower social class composition of the co-educational schools in itself has this effect. Here is yet another field awaiting further research, though the next two items throw a little further light on the problem.

'I felt I didn't belong socially'

In this tug-of-war between school and home there is a danger that the pupil might find himself alienated from both. What proportion of the ex-pupils felt that they 'didn't belong socially' when at school? Was this proportion different in co-educational and single-sex schools? The data gathered in Tables 15.5 and 15.6 indicate that fewer of the ex-pupils, whether they were men or women, felt that they 'didn't belong socially' at their co-educational schools than at their single-sex schools. Again, we cannot say precisely why this is so. As expected there is a tendency for those men who attended as seniors at both co-educational and boys' schools to feel that they belonged socially more than the juniors felt they belonged, while the women's groups showed little difference between junior and senior pupils.

It is a matter of some interest to discover which social class of children felt that they 'didn't belong socially', though again only the sample of women is large enough for this purpose. Accordingly Table 15.7 was prepared.

To simplify the table 'first' and 'last' school estimates are merged, a procedure possible because in this instance the distributions of the estimates for first and last schools were sufficiently similar even when these were broken down according to occupational class. The figures give no support to the hypothesis that there might be a systematic trend associated with occupational class, for example that girls in the lower occupational classes might feel out of place at both mixed and girls' grammar schools. Amusingly enough, in girls' schools rather more pupils of class 1 felt they didn't belong socially (one-quarter of this class) than did pupils of the other social classes, though the difference is not statistically significant. There is, however, a salient difference between the estimates for the co-educational and those for the girls' schools, namely that the ex-pupils are much more emphatic ('disagree strongly') that their co-educational schools did not make them feel they didn't belong socially, than they were about their girls' schools, and this is remarkably consistent for all three occupational class groups.

Social image of the school

A fourth item of a similar nature was: 'I disliked the social image the school tried to capture,' which used the same scale of answers

TABLE 15.5 *'I didn't belong socially'*

'Both schools' survey (women)

Estimates	Replies about women's 'first' schools attended				Replies about women's 'last' schools attended			
	Co-educational schools		Girls' schools		Co-educational schools		Girls' schools	
	N	%	N	%	N	%	N	%
Agree strongly	12	4·0	22	5·4	8	2·2	16	6·2
Agree	28	9·4	71	17·6	27	7·5	27	10·4
Doubtful	30	10·0	57	14·1	28	7·8	47	18·1
Disagree	129	43·2	182	45·1	151	42·3	117	45·2
Disagree strongly	100	33·4	72	17·8	144	40·2	52	20·1
Totals	299	100	404	100	358	100	259	100

NOTE: The differences between the co-educational and girls' schools are statistically highly significant for both 'first' and 'last' schools.

TABLE 15.6 *'I didn't belong socially'*

'Both schools' survey (men)

Estimates	Replies about men's 'first' schools attended				Replies about men's 'last' schools attended			
	Co-educational schools		Boys' schools		Co-educational schools		Boys' schools	
	N	%	N	%	N	%	N	%
Agree strongly	1	1·2	11	9·2	2	1·9	3	4·2
Agree	8	9·8	24	20·2	4	3·8	9	12·7
Doubtful	7	8·6	23	19·3	7	6·7	7	9·9
Disagree	33	40·2	49	41·2	43	41·3	29	40·8
Disagree strongly	33	40·2	12	10·1	48	46·3	23	32·4
Totals	82	100	119	100	104	100	71	100

NOTE: The difference between the distributions for co-educational compared with boys' schools is statistically significant beyond the ·001 level for 'first' schools and is in the same direction for 'last' schools, but here falls just below the conventional significance level.

TABLE 15.7 *'I didn't belong socially' (women): Tabulated by occupational class*

'Both schools' survey

Categories of agreement	Replies from women about co-educational schools (percentages)			Replies from women about girls' schools (percentages)		
	Occupational classes			Occupational classes		
	1	2	3, 4 and 5	1	2	3, 4 and 5
Agree strongly	3·2	1·5	4·1	6·6	5·8	4·1
Agree	8·6	7·4	8·9	18·1	10·9	11·0
Doubtful	6·9	13·2	8·3	12·1	22·5	18·0
Disagree	43·5	40·4	43·2	45·4	41·2	47·1
Disagree strongly	37·8	37·5	35·5	17·8	19·6	19·8
	100%	100%	100%	100%	100%	100%
Number	347	136	169	348	138	172

TABLE 15.8 *Social image of the school*

'Both schools' survey

Estimates concerning dislike of the image	Replies from women about the schools attended				Replies from men about the schools attended			
	Co-educational schools		Girls' schools		Co-educational schools		Boys' schools	
	N	%	N	%	N	%	N	%
Agree strongly	27	4·1	112	16·9	9	4·9	25	13·2
Agree	60	9·2	129	19·6	20	10·8	32	16·8
Doubtful	103	15·9	125	18·9	30	16·2	47	24·7
Disagree	329	50·6	242	36·6	92	49·7	64	33·7
Disagree strongly	131	20·2	53	8·0	34	18·4	22	11·6
Totals	650	100	661	100	185	100	190	100

NOTE: The difference between the distributions for co-educational and girls' schools is statistically highly significant (this is also true when 'schools attended first' or 'last' are taken separately); that between the boys is highly significant for 'first' schools and for combined groups but just fails to reach the conventional ·05 level for 'last' schools.

as the previous items. Table 15.8 indicated that both men and women ex-pupils showed more dislike of the social image projected by their single-sex schools than of that in their co-educational schools, though as many as 45 per cent of both men and women disagreed with the statement as applied to their single-sex school. On the other hand, whereas only 13 per cent of women and 16 per cent of men agreed that they disliked this image in their co-educational schools, these percentages rose to 36 and 30 respectively about their single-sex school. (If we were thinking in terms of 'absolute' standards, we would need to consider the probably favourable nature of the student teacher sample.) In this item those men who attended the co-educational or boys' schools as seniors were more ready to support this 'social image' than were those who attended as juniors, but with the women from both types of school there was a slight tendency in the opposite direction—the 'image' becoming slightly less liked by senior pupils.

An analysis of the women's sample according to the occupational class of the parents of the students was again made. Contrary to expectation, in neither type of school was the social image disliked more by the students from the manual working occupational classes. *Within the present sample* we could find no discernible association with parental occupational class.

Comment

In brief, about a quarter of the women thought their girls' schools 'tried to dominate their whole life' but only some 7 per cent thought this of their co-educational schools; the men produced similar results for 'first' schools, but for 'last' schools a difference in the same direction as that for women was not statistically significant. Likewise more of the women said their girls' schools created a gap between school and home than said the same of their co-educational schools, though they were not so certain of this as about the girls' schools 'trying to dominate their whole life'. With both sexes there was a more emphatic rejection of the idea (i.e. disagree strongly) where the co-educational schools were concerned. The same trend was to be seen in the replies to the item, 'I felt I didn't belong socially,' both for men and women, and this was again repeated for the item, 'I disliked the social image the school tried to capture.' Though a 'halo effect' might conceivably be increasing these differences in favour of the co-educational schools, it is not likely to be creating the gaps themselves, and one has also to ask first the origin of such a halo favourable to co-educational schools and second to consider whether, if such a halo affects the results, it might well be considered part and parcel of the differences between co-educational and single-sex schools. If an ex-pupil considered he or she 'didn't belong socially' in the single-sex school attended, but 'did belong socially' in the co-educational school, this is what really matters to the pupil, whether or not this feeling has been increased by, for example, a generalized liking for the co-educational school. The results reported are what the pupils say about their experience, and as such represent a legitimate comparison of the two types of school.

16

Preparation for the adult world

Research on co-education in this country commenced in the twenties with Tyson's study (1928) of comparative attainment, and continued in a desultory fashion on this theme, only widening its horizons with Moreton's inquiry into the attitudes of teachers to co-education in 1939. No large-scale research on the comparative effects of the two types of schooling on the attitudes and social and emotional development of the pupils appears to have been done anywhere until the work of Moreton (1939), Lotz (1953) in U.S.A., Dale (1948, 1949, 1966 and 1966a) and Atherton (1971). This chapter presents the results of several investigations in one part of this area, all of them examining the extent to which the ex-pupils and pupils considered their school education prepared them for life in the adult world.

The Second College survey

The section of the Second College survey with which we are now concerned related to the attitude of men and women towards the opposite sex, as portrayed by their answers to three questions, viz.:

Did your school life help or hinder you in your relations with the opposite sex? Reply was on a five-point scale from 'very helpful', through 'no effect' to 'great hindrance'.
Do you find it easy to work with the opposite sex? Do you think you would find it easy, in general, to work under the direction of a member of the opposite sex? A seven-point scale was used for these two questions, ranging from 'very easy' to 'very difficult'.

Space for voluntary comment was provided under the last of these questions, partly in order to discover the reasons behind the expressed attitudes, and partly to discover ambiguities or other faults in the questions. The replies of the women are examined first.

THE WOMEN

The results were treated in two ways, first by calculating for each question the percentage of women recording each preference on the scale; second, by weighting (e.g. five for 'very helpful', decreasing to one for 'great hindrance'), and then calculating mean scores for different groups. Though the allocation of the weights is somewhat arbitrary it has compensating advantages for the comparison of large groups, especially combined with the first method.

Results

Table 16.1 shows how women from the two types of school answered the question, *Did your school life help or hinder you in your relations with the opposite sex?*

TABLE 16.1 *Type of schooling and women's relationships with men*

Second College survey

	N*	Percentages						
		Very helpful	Helpful	No effect	Slight hindrance	Great hindrance		
Effect of school life on relationships with men								
women from co-ed. schools	403	31·3	44·7	22·6	1·2	0·2		
women from girls' schools	623	1·6	8·7	50·9	32·4	6·4		
		Very easy	Easy	Fairly easy	Doubtful	A little difficult	Difficult	Very difficult
Ease of working *with* men								
women from co-ed. schools	407	40·0	41·0	17·0	1·0	1·0	0	0
women from girls' schools	610	31·3	32·7	25·4	4·8	4·6	1·0	0·2
Ease of working *under* a man's direction								
women from co-ed. schools	405	44·7	41·6	10·6	2·2	0·7	0·2	0
women from girls' schools	626	40·9	42·1	12·1	3·2	1·1	0·3	0·3

* The totals are not the same for all tables because of differences in the numbers who replied to particular questions.

It requires no great wisdom to forecast which type of school would give the superior estimates, but the extent of the difference is unexpected. Whereas only some 10 per cent of the ex-pupils of girls' schools said their school life was helpful in this respect, the proportion from mixed schools was three-quarters. At the opposite end of the scale almost four in every ten women from girls' schools said their school life was a hindrance, while the proportion from mixed schools was little more than one in every hundred. The difference between the distributions from the two types of school is statistically significant well beyond the ·001 level.

It was known that the social class distribution of the two groups differed, and there might have been a systematic bias. We therefore grouped the women according to the occupational class of their

TABLE 16.2 *Effect of type of schooling on women's relationships with men: Analysis by occupational class**

Second College survey

		Occupational class of father				
		1	2	3	4 & 5	Total
Co-ed. schools N		61	32	91	19	203
Girls' schools N		160	44	148	18	370
	Maximum	Weighted mean scores†				
Effect of school life on relationships with men	5					
Women from co-ed. schools		4·16	4·31	4·27	4·37	4·26
Women from girls' schools		2·65	2·80	2·65	2·50	2·66
Ease of working *with* men	7					
Women from co-ed. schools		6·18	6·44	6·34	6·25	6·29
Women from girls' schools		5·94	5·71	5·85	5·76	5·87
Ease of working *under* a woman's direction	7					
Women from co-ed. schools		6·39	6·47	6·44	6·55	6·44
Women from girls' schools		6·31	6·33	6·24	6·11	6·28

* Data were available for only part of the sample. The categories were: Class 1 professional, administrative, managerial and teachers; class 2 clerical workers; class 3 skilled manual workers; class 4 semi-skilled; and class 5 unskilled.

† Weighted mean scores 7 to 1 on seven-point scale and 5 to 1 on five-point scale, the high scores being the more favourable.

fathers, and calculated the weighted mean scores. These are shown in Table 16.2.

The most striking feature of Table 16.2 is the steadiness of the score from one class to another, within each of the two school groups; further, as one would expect, within each class there is a wide gap between the women from girls' schools and those from mixed schools. It has been mentioned before, however, that the parental occupational class influences are reduced in importance because the respondents all belong to the same (or closely related) future occupational class; also pupils from the lower occupational classes will be a much more restricted sample than those from the higher occupational classes. The figures are therefore reported as true for the present sample and not as representative of the attitudes of the various social classes.

Do you find it easy to work with the opposite sex? The answers to this question are shown in Table 16.1

The hypothesis that women educated in mixed schools would find it easier to work with the opposite sex than women educated in girls' schools finds partial support in these data; the difference between the two distributions is statistically significant beyond the ·001 level.

The possibility of systematic bias from social class factors was again examined. The results, given in Table 16.2, show that, within this sample, occupational class had very little effect on the women's estimate of their ability to work with men. Within each class, however, the women from the mixed schools consistently gave a slightly higher estimate than did women from girls' schools.

It is still traditional and 'normal' in Britain for women to work *under the direction* of a man. There also appears to be a tendency for some—perhaps many—women to dislike working under another woman, but to like working for a man. The questionnaire asked, 'Do you think you would find it easy, in general, to work under the direction of a member of the opposite sex?'

Table 16.1 shows that rather more women from the mixed schools in this sample than from girls' schools thought it would be easy to work under the supervision of a man; but here emphasis should be placed on the similarity between the groups rather than on the small and statistically insignificant difference.

A social class breakdown of the data is given in Table 16.2. There is again a notable consistency in the pattern of the scores.

Respondents were invited to amplify their answers to this question, and about one-quarter of each of the two school groups did so. The comments from these two groups resemble each other closely, apart from one small section of answers. This consisted of some 6 per cent from the girls' schools who expressed difficulties (and even fear in one case) at working under a man; three of these women said it was easier after having attended a mixed college. But the basic similarity is to be seen in the predominant theme of the replies—that men are better in authority, fairer, more patient, gain more respect and are easier to work with. No less than 53 per cent of the replies from the women from co-educational schools come into this category, and almost 49 per cent of those from the girls' schools. A minority of respondents from each group attacked the women instead of praising the men, complaining of cattiness, bossiness, 'bitchiness' and being temperamental and difficult. A few quotations are given:

'I prefer to be dominated by a member of the opposite sex rather than try to dominate him.'

'Men dealt more justly and fairly than women. Women in high positions are usually domineering.'

'Men tend to be more fair in their judgments and certainly not "bitchy".'

'Very difficult to work under a woman.'

'Better than under one of my own sex.'

Other comments of interest were:

'Since being at a mixed college I have found it easier to get on with the other sex. I'm not so shy and self-conscious.'

'I don't get on so easily with the opposite sex as I have a slight fear of them which is not good in a working relationship.'

'Had this been filled in on just leaving school I would have said "very difficult" but four years in mixed Colleges have now overcome the setbacks, but I have taken three years to do so.'

In this last comment there is a hint that the very slight (non-significant) difference between the two groups might have been greater if it had been measured at the time the pupils left school.

The women in this study who attended girls' schools regarded themselves, on the average, as decidedly handicapped in their social life with the opposite sex, and, to a lesser extent, in working with the opposite sex. This is what we might have expected, but it has now for the first time been demonstrated. A factor to be noticed is that almost all the women in the sample, whether from mixed or single-sex schools, were day pupils from grammar schools; the difference in attitudes between the two groups might be greater in the case of boarders. It is still open to the protagonists of girls' schools to argue that the finding might not apply to all types of pupil, though judging by the figures this would seem extremely unlikely. We must also remember that girls' schools may have the advantage in other aspects which have not yet been investigated.

The scores of the women appeared not to vary according to the occupational class of the fathers. We cannot, as we have seen, generalize this finding to the grammar school population as a whole because of the restriction of the sample in respect of occupational class.

Critics might object that the higher estimates of the mixed school group about the ease of their relationships with men could be produced, not by any difference in educational provision, but by girls who felt at ease with the other sex choosing to go to mixed schools rather than to girls' schools. Fortunately we know that in most areas the girls had no choice. In the remaining areas it is likely that, at the age of eleven, the choice would be made for scholastic work and 'atmosphere' or 'tone' rather than because of the girls' attitude to the presence of boys in the school. Where the girls' school is 'Direct Grant', it will tend to take automatically the top thirty or more in the area's 11-plus examination, and few pupils would decline this offer. Further evidence on some of these matters is, however, desirable. We now turn to the men's results for the same questions.

THE MEN

The hypothesis examined was the same as in the case of the women, that educating the two sexes together at the secondary level (as opposed to educating them apart) would affect their social relations and their attitude to each other, and that these effects might to an appreciable extent persist in adult life. Procedure was again by questionnaire, administered in large groups to prevent collusion, with a pledge of anonymity. The sample was drawn from male student teachers in five Departments of Education and sixteen training Colleges, consisting of 569 ex-pupils of boys' schools and 351 from mixed schools. They were asked the same questions as the women and the results were treated in the same way.

Table 16.3 summarizes the answers of the two groups of men. Almost 40 per cent of the men educated at boys' schools thought their school life hindered them in their relationships with women, while nearly three-quarters of those from mixed schools believed that their social life had helped them in this respect. Difference between the two groups is statistically significant ($P < \cdot 001$).

Working *with* women was considered difficult by 9 per cent of the men from boys' schools but only 3 per cent of those from

TABLE 16.3 *Type of schooling and men's relationships with women*

Second College survey

	N*	Percentages						
		Very helpful	Helpful	No effect	Slight hindrance	Great hindrance		
Effect of school life on relationships with women								
men from mixed schools	347	27·4	46·9	20·2	4·6	0·9		
men from boys' schools	569	2·5	10·7	47·4	31·1	8·3		
		Very easy	Easy	Fairly easy	Doubtful	A little difficult	Difficult	Very difficult
Ease of working *with* women								
men from mixed schools	351	30·5	37·6	25·6	3·1	2·6	0·3	0·3
men from boys' schools	542	21·0	34·3	28·2	7·4	7·6	0·9	0·6
Ease of working *under* a woman's direction								
men from mixed schools	345	11·0	26·7	24·7	22·6	7·5	3·2	4·3
men from boys' schools	561	6·6	20·3	26·4	19·4	12·7	8·2	6·4

* The totals are not the same for all tables because of differences in the numbers who replied to particular questions.

mixed schools. The difference between the two groups is statistically significant ($P < \cdot 001$) if those who expressed doubt or difficulty are taken together in contrast with all the others. Working under women also differentiated the two groups; 27 per cent from boys' schools thought this difficult, but only 15 per cent from mixed schools; the difference is significant (P ·001)

Table 16.4 compares these results with the equivalent figures from the parallel study of women's attitudes. Men considered single-sex schooling a greater handicap than did women in their subsequent working relationships *with* the opposite sex.

The data were examined to see whether the expressed attitudes were associated in any systematic way with the occupational class of the men's parents. Table 16.5 shows the number of men in each of the two groups who came from each of four occupational classes; and it also gives the weighted mean score for each of the three questions.

TABLE 16.4 *Type of school and relationships between men and women: Comparison of men and women*

Second College survey

	Men		Women	
	Mixed schools Per cent	Boys' schools	Mixed schools Per cent	Girls' schools
School life a hindrance in relationships with opposite sex	5·5	39·4	1·4	38·8
Difficult to work *with* opposite sex	3·2	9·1	1·0	5·8
Difficult to work *under* opposite sex	15·0	27·3	0·9	1·7

TABLE 16.5 *Effect of type of schooling on men's relationships with women: Analysis by occupational class*

Second College survey

		Occupational class of father				
		1	2	3	4 & 5	Total
Mixed schools	N	32	22	69	17	140
Boys' schools	N	59	20	114	20	213
	Max.	Weighted mean scores				
Effect of school life on relationships with women	5					
Men from mixed schools		4·06	4·05	4·12	4·18	4·10
Men from boys' schools		2·53	2·50	2·49	2·55	2·51
Ease of working *with* women	7					
Men from mixed schools		5·97	5·95	5·89	6·06	5·94
Men from boys' schools		5·84	5·43	5·39	5·40	5·50
Ease of working *under* a woman's direction	7					
Men from mixed schools		4·63	5·09	5·15	5·18	5·02
Men from boys' schools		4·32	4·26	4·41	4·90	4·42

Occupational class appeared not to be associated with any change in these men's estimates of how their school life had affected their relationships with women, but for each class the men from mixed schools gave consistently higher, i.e. more favourable replies than did those from boys' schools. In respect of work *with* women, there was no observed association between class origins and the replies of the men from mixed schools, but among the men from boys' schools those whose fathers were in occupational class 1 had a mean score significantly higher than that of all the others combined ($P < \cdot 05$). Those from mixed schools again scored consistently rather higher than the others. Ease of working *under* a woman's direction also was greater in every occupational group among men from mixed schools; of men from both groups, those in the lower occupational classes tended to score higher, the difference being slightly short of statistical significance.[1]

From the 561 ex-pupils of boys' schools who made estimates there were also 199 free comments on the question of ease of work *under* women. Almost half of these said that sex made no difference or that it depended on the individual's competence or age, but about a quarter replied expressing difficulties, namely that women were inferior, had no natural authority, were petty, domineering and emotional, and not impartial. Of the 345 male ex-pupils of mixed schools, 101 made comments, half of them of the type described above as 'sex made no difference', etc., and like the boys' schools about a quarter mentioned difficulties. A few of the more interesting comments are quoted. From the boys' schools group:

'Women possess an inherent quality of orderliness and method, and love of detail which is unbearable over long periods and eventually terminates in the realm of "hair splitting".' ('Difficult')

'Women were created to be in subjection, not to rule.' ('Very difficult')

'The artificial atmosphere of the single-sex grammar school at first made my present situation intolerable.' ('Very difficult')

'Woman's place is in the home.' ('A little difficult')

'Women cannot govern.' ('Doubtful')

From the mixed schools group:

'Speaking as a senior army officer. My service experience, particularly overseas, has made me very wary of women in positions of authority; there has been less give and take with them and they were unfortunately inclined to be biased in their judgments.' ('Doubtful')

[1] $t = 1 \cdot 81$ opposing classes 4 and 5 with class 1. An examination of the occupational class trend for all men by analysis of variance gave a statistically non-significant result.

Many more of the comments from both groups were of the type, 'Easy, provided she was older and more experienced in the work being done.'

The great majority of the men who completed the questionnaire would be between 18 and 20 years of age. Few would be under 18 and few over 23. Their judgment would be mature, and their memories fresh enough for them to give valid and reliable estimates relating to their life in school. Only one of the questions, however, was based explicitly on school life; the others asked present attitudes. The comments made throughout the questionnaire and the consistent patterns produced by the results indicate that the students were thoroughly interested in their work and showed a high sense of responsibility.

On the other hand the sample, like that of the women, was limited to one type of ex-pupil, and though it can be claimed that this method ensured reasonable equality of sample between mixed and boys' schools it can with equal cogency be argued that one cannot be certain that the findings would be similar for a complete cross-section sample of pupils, even though it appears likely that the findings could be generalized. As with the women, this occupational narrowness of the sample may also have had some influence on the 'reluctance' of the men's estimates to vary with the occupational class of the fathers.

The men from boys' schools in this sample believed that their school life was less helpful to them in their relations with women than did the men who attended mixed schools. Similarly the former considered that it was less easy to work with, and to work under, women than did the latter. In other words, this effect tended to persist after leaving school, though we don't know for how long. In the comments a few individuals said that being students in a mixed college, after having attended a boys' school, had helped them to establish easier social relations with women.

We need to remind ourselves again that attitudes such as those with which this chapter is concerned are powerfully affected, not only by the schools, but by the society around them. The men would have been much less likely in Victorian times, for example, to have been willing to work under the direction of women.

The Schools project

In the Schools project over one thousand pupils aged 13 plus and 17 plus were asked: 'Apart from employment do you think your school prepares you sufficiently for the adult world? Agree strongly/Agree/Doubtful/Disagree/Disagree strongly.' Pupils were also encouraged to add a free response.

For both boys and girls aged 13 plus more of those in the single-sex schools than in the co-educational thought their education did not prepare them for life in the adult world, but neither difference was statistically significant (see Table A.27). For students aged 17 plus the trend was the same, but the difference between the male groups is almost statistically significant and that between the female groups is statistically highly significant (see Figure 16.1). The change between the ages 13 plus and 17 plus might reasonably be thought due to the immaturity of the former group for making a judgment of this kind.

Readers will see that in Figure 16.1 only a negligible percentage of the senior girls in both types of school 'agreed strongly' that their school prepared them sufficiently for life in the adult world, and that whereas 22 per cent of those in girls' schools endorsed 'agreed' this percentage was doubled by the girls in co-educational schools. Correspondingly few of the senior male students in either type of school endorsed 'agree strongly', but whereas only a little more than one third of those in boys' schools estimated 'agree', this figure rose to over one-half for boys in co-educational schools. At the age of 17 plus the sample consists mostly of those who stayed at school until they reached the sixth.

FREE RESPONSES

What were the students' reasons for their estimates? Fortunately their free responses, unmistakably responsible in manner, provide us with a good picture. For both sexes there is a wide variety of reasons for disagreement, ranging from narrowness of curriculum and outlook to lack of the teaching of good manners and sex instruction. The analysis is confined to the older (17 plus) group, as the younger group were rather immature for this question; the girls will be considered first.

Of those girls who agreed that their school prepared them sufficiently for life in the adult world, 16 of those in girls' schools wrote supporting statements, and 31 in co-educational schools. There is little of real interest and information in these individual replies, but the free responses of those who estimated they were doubtful, disagreed or disagreed strongly, are informative, and are given in detail in Table 16.6.

Here the pupils educated in co-educational and those from girls' schools have much in common. In the social area both groups complain that there is no preparation for life's responsibilities and problems, that there is little outside the curriculum, with some lack of guidance on marriage problems, sex, careers and colleges. Girls from girls' schools, however, emphasize more strongly that there is

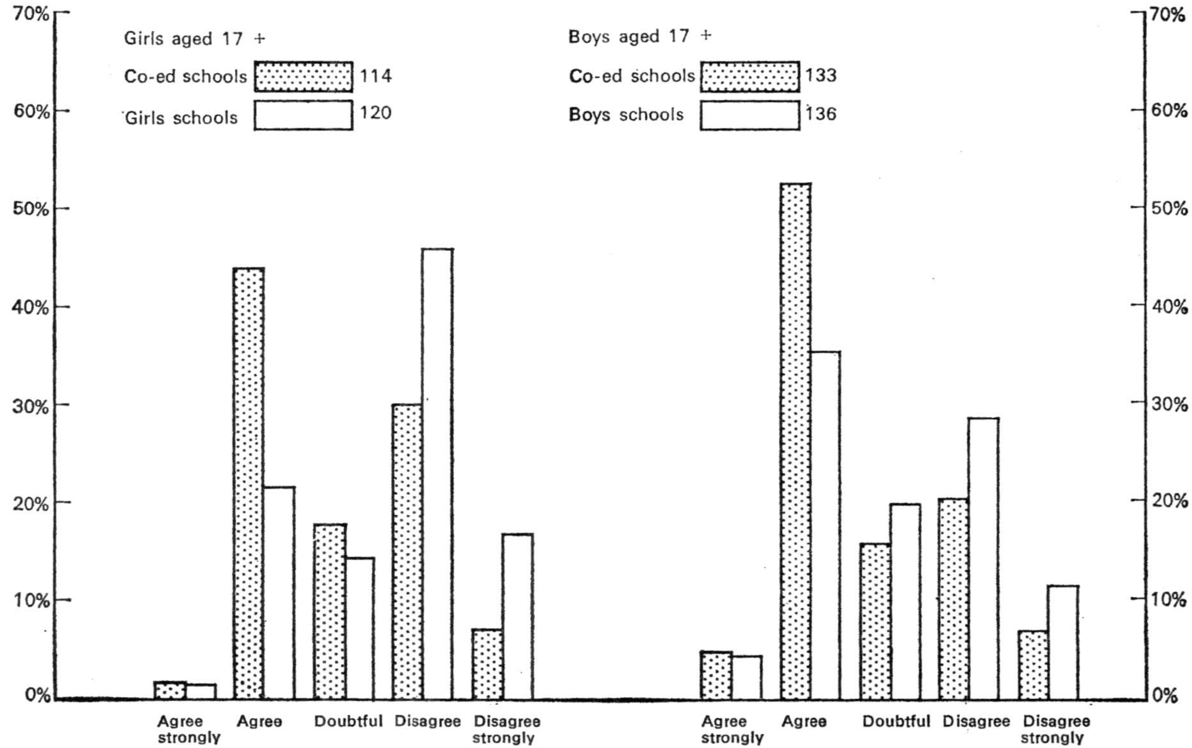

FIGURE 16.1
Sufficient preparation for adult world: Schools project

TABLE 16.6 *Sufficient preparation for world? Girls aged 17 plus: Free responses denoting disagreement*

Schools project, 1966

	Co-ed. schools	Girls' schools
Social		
no experience of life outside school, or preparation for outside responsibilities	10	8
too coddled, sheltered, no freedom, too formal, too organized		7
little outside the curriculum, not enough social activities	9	20
little or nothing on marriage, sex, social behaviour, careers, income tax, college	10	4
no contact with opposite sex		6
Curriculum		
Over-emphasis on curriculum (see under Social)		
more variety of topics needed—too narrow, no relation to life, discussions on life	4	7
need more current affairs, civics	1	2
Discipline		
treated like children—bad preparation for life in adult world	4	3
treated like puppets		1
Others	2	5
do their best but ideas wrong		1
no freedom of thought		1
conduct yes, growing up no		1
have to learn for yourself		2
Totals	40	68

little outside the curriculum, and are alone in protesting about being coddled, sheltered or organized, and in saying they cannot be trained for life in the adult world if they are deprived of social contact with the opposite sex. Both groups believe the curriculum should be less narrow, be more related to life, and should include more current affairs. Again, in the complaints about discipline a few individuals in each group complain that being treated like children is no proper training for life in the world. A few responses are quoted to illustrate the dissatisfaction. (The principle is maintained that the number of quotations should be in proportion to the number of comments made.)

Co-educational schools

'In our school we are treated in a childish manner by the headmaster.'

'Exams are not going to prepare us for the outside world. A lesson on the rights and wrongs of sex life should be held.'

'We are not taught anything about social behaviour.'

'If you fail your exams you are almost totally unprepared.'

Girls' schools

'Little taught on the hardships of life.'

'We are taught nothing of sex.'

'Being in a girls' school—absolutely hopeless!'

'An all-girls school is always a setback.'

'I am taught nothing of etiquette, cooking and current affairs.

'Too much stress laid on academic work.'

'We are confined more or less to our subjects.'

The free responses of the boys (Table 16.7) are strikingly similar to those of the girls. Agreement with the statement was recorded by 38 boys in co-educational schools and by 28 in boys' schools. If those who estimated 'doubtful' are included with the two categories of disagreement there were 35 from co-educational and 66 from boys' schools. The latter made more protests about the lack of preparation for life's responsibilities and problems, but the smallness of the numbers in the sub-categories makes further comment inadvisable.

The quotations are again limited to those expressing concern over deficiencies.

Co-educational schools

'Financial economics should be taught to all.'

'You should be shown different parts of life and other people's ways.'

'One period a week could be put away for sex education.'

'The onus is on intellect and we have no grounding in the techniques for getting on with older people outside school—that we have to do ourselves, which we cannot really do until we are allowed into pubs at 18.'

TABLE 16.7 *Sufficient preparation for world? Boys aged 17 plus: Free responses denoting disagreement*

Schools project, 1966

	Co-ed. schools	Boys' schools
Social		
no experience of life outside school, or preparation for life's responsibilities and problems	2	15
too sheltered, restricted, narrow	4	3
little outside curriculum, social, etc.	5	8
little on morals, sex education, careers, manners	9	3
no contact with opposite sex		5
Curriculum		
over-emphasis on curriculum (see under Social)		
too narrow, no relation to life, theoretical	4	6
need more current affairs, world problems, civics	3	2
insufficient discussion adult world		2
Discipline		
treated like children	2	7
too lax		1
independence not taught		4
Others	3	6
some but not enough	1	
little influence on character		1
depends on teacher		1
up to individual	2	2
Totals	35	66

Boys' schools

'I think we should have more lessons on house buying, banks, insurance, etc.'

'It should be comprehensive and mixed for this.'

'Probably not, because this is a single-sex school.'

'Prepares you for sadism perhaps. No attempt (except by fear) to instil citizenship.'

'Too much emphasis on exams, not enough on world affairs.'

'Some more positive form of sex education should be taught.'

'I think subjects such as cookery should be taught.'

'In the adult world the sexes are not kept apart.'

Comment

As with most of this work there is much to be learnt from the estimates and comments which is quite outside the co-education controversy. A substantial proportion of present pupils and of mature ex-pupils are dissatisfied with their secondary education as a preparation for life in the adult world. Both past and present co-educated pupils, however, show appreciably less dissatisfaction than do their contemporaries from single-sex schools.

17

Marriage

'At first sight of the word marriage at the head of this chapter the reader may understandably have wondered what connection there was between the chapter title and the subject of the book. On reflection, however, he will appreciate that the bringing up together of boys and girls, and indeed young men and young women in the same educational institution might have a permanent effect upon the knowledge that each sex has of the ways, the philosophy and motivations of the other, and that this knowledge might produce a lasting change in the attitude of the sexes towards each other, and consequently influence the keenness of the desire for marriage, and the happiness of marriage. It is of course recognized that the biological urge will be immeasurably more powerful than any effect of schooling.

This chapter, then, differs from most of the preceding ones in being concerned not so much with the immediate attitudes of pupils or of ex-pupils towards their schools but primarily with more lasting effects which may have resulted from their type of schooling. If any difference, say in the degree of marital happiness or in the desire for marriage, exists between the products of single-sex and co-educational schooling, this will be of some interest, though readers will not be unaware that there are many other factors affecting marriage, so that the sample examined would need to be very large in order to randomize out individual differences of temperament, the hazards of misfortune etc., while allowance must be made for factors such as age, social class and length of marriage.

Second College survey

The first attack on the problem was made in the Second College survey, when some 2,000 student teachers who were ex-pupils of secondary schools other than secondary modern were asked, 'Do you wish to marry, provided you can find a suitable partner?' Estimates were requested on a seven-point scale ranging from Very much/Much/A little/Undecided to Very much opposed. The distribution of the estimates of ex-pupils of single-sex grammar schools was compared with that from mixed grammar schools.

For some purposes a comparison of the means of weighted scores was also used. Replies were anonymous and free comments were requested where opposition to marriage was signified. Married students were excluded.

The method of procedure is admittedly not the best, but it was then the only one possible in view of the limitations of finance and time; the section was frankly regarded as exploratory. A more detailed investigation carried out by one of the writer's research students is outlined later in the chapter.

WOMEN'S ESTIMATES

The hypothesis was that social interaction between the sexes at school might slightly increase their desire for marriage, compared with pupils from single-sex schools. For the 972 women the difference was unexpectedly in the opposite direction, though not statistically significant (Chi-square was 5·832 for 6 degrees of freedom); 67·4 per cent of the girls from girls' schools wished 'very much' to marry, and 61·5 per cent from mixed schools, but most of this difference was reversed in the 'much' estimates. In both groups only about 2 per cent gave any of the three 'opposed' estimates. It may be that deprivation—or lack of contact with the opposite sex—slightly increases the desire for marriage and parenthood amongst women, but confirmatory evidence is needed. The effect is interesting but too small to be of practical significance.

As the social class distribution is different in single-sex compared with mixed grammar schools, part of the information was analysed according to this variable. No significant social class differences were found, nor did the variable have any appreciable effect on the main comparison except to reduce the difference slightly. These data were then divided into ex-pupils 'with siblings' and 'without siblings', for the parental skilled artisan class only. Ex-pupils of girls' and mixed schools were combined, as their means and distributions were so similar. The mean score on 'wish for marriage' of those 'with siblings' (163) was 6·42, and 'without siblings' (56) 6·50, i.e. more favourable to marriage, but the difference was far from statistically significant. Almost 6 per cent of those with siblings were undecided or opposed, while none of those without siblings were opposed and only 3·6 per cent were undecided. Unfortunately we do not know how many of the siblings of the women students were male, but there may be here once again a slight hint that lack of social contact with the opposite sex tends to drive people towards such contact more powerfully than the actual experience of it—which may, after all, be tragic or unhappy in some cases.

In all only seventeen comments were given which opposed marriage. The general theme of these is sometimes a frank avowal of selfishness, but more often a mere wish to stay independent or to indulge in an alternative, such as travel. Fear of having children and dislike of the idea of sexual intercourse are both mentioned. Noteworthy are: 'I'm not made for self-sacrifice—natural outcome of marriage for women.' 'Too limited—no scope for independent activity.' 'There are so many things I want to do that to be tied down to one person would not be good for me or him,' and 'I cannot see myself settling down with one person and being happy for the rest of my life.' The smallness of the number of comments severely limited their value.

MEN'S ESTIMATES

In contrast to the women the men's results were in the direction of the hypothesis that co-educational schooling would make them slightly more favourable to marriage. The difference between the two groups was, however, very small and not statistically significant. Of the 304 men from mixed schools, 63·3 per cent wished to marry 'very much', while of the 479 men from boys' schools only 59·5 per cent were in this category. A mere 0·6 per cent of the mixed schools group were opposed to marriage, and 2·3 per cent from the boys' schools. When the two distributions were divided into the favourable and the opposed, the difference between men from mixed and men from boys' schools gave a Chi-square of 3·07 which, for one degree of freedom, is somewhat short of statistical significance.

Analysis by father's occupational class produced a striking similarity between the average scores of the classes within each type of school, but a persistent small difference between the schools within each social class. (As mentioned before, any effect of social class would be reduced because all the students were intending teachers.) These differences between types of school, separately, were not statistically significant, but support each other by their consistent pattern.

Of the 783 men who participated, only thirteen opposed marriage. Two of these thirteen came from mixed schools, and wrote, 'I feel I want to carry on my studies so that I am taxed fully. To have to devote time to a wife and family would hinder me' (A little opposed); and, 'I enjoy my own company and freedom. I don't want the responsibility' (Much opposed). Of the eleven men from boys' schools who opposed marriage (out of 479 who answered), three failed to give their reasons, though requested to do so. The chief reasons advanced are loss of freedom, both personal and financial. There was one objection to 'monogamous marriage', and one man was 'appalled at the thought of such a relationship'. Another was 'very much opposed' because he was too moody and because his parents' marriage had been an unhappy one.

Comment

The slight tendency to greater variability of scores among the group from single-sex schools is interesting and in the case of the men approaches statistical significance. With the latter some opposition to marriage could be caused by a tendency to homosexuality among a small fraction of the pupils in boys' schools. Although there is a very slight indication of this in one comment and in comments about other items in the questionnaire, the evidence is insufficient for any definite conclusion. It was thought that the number of respondents from boys' schools who failed to reply might provide another pointer, when compared with the number of male non-respondents from mixed schools, on the hypothesis that homosexuals would refuse to answer a question on marriage. The difference was in the expected direction, 2·1 per cent from boys' schools, compared with 1·3 per cent of the boys from mixed schools, but it is not statistically reliable,[1] nor in any event could one be at all sure that the difference was due to the homosexual factor. Complaints regarding homosexuality tend to come, however, from boarding rather than day schools, and the former represent only 5 per cent of the present sample from boys' schools. (Of the ten respondents from boys' schools who failed to give any estimate only one was a boarder.) The questionnaire was not, of course, designed to elicit information on this specific point; and even if homosexuality were underlying the cause of opposition it is unlikely that this reason would be stated.

Findings closely similar to those on the marriage question resulted from asking the same sample, 'If you marry—or if you are married—do you wish to have children?' The girls' schools were slightly keener towards parenthood than women from co-educational schools through a slightly greater percentage replying 'very much' as opposed to 'much', there being no difference between the two types of school at the 'opposed' end of the scale, and the overall difference being small and statistically non-significant. For the men there was again a small difference in the opposite direction at the negative end of the scale, some 3.1 per cent of those educated in boys' schools giving one of the 'opposed' estimates, and 0·9 per cent of those from co-educational schools. If the distributions are split into the *realistic* dichotomy of 'against parenthood' versus

[1] Chi-square 0·67 for one degree of freedom.

the rest, the difference falls only a little short of statistical significance. Though the chance element certainly cannot be ruled out there seems here to be a case for more detailed research.

The Atherton survey[1]

The research into this topic was taken a stage further by Atherton, one of the writer's research students at the University College of Swansea. He made an inquiry into the happiness of marriage, comparing co-educated men and women with those from single-sex schools. His sample was over 1,100 men and 1,400 women, selected impartially by a large number of doctors scattered throughout England and Wales, and the procedure was partly by anonymous questionnaire and partly by attitude scale. Results of this work are now available.

The first of two key questions was, 'Do you think that the type of school (mixed or single sex) helped or hindered you in everyday relations with the opposite sex?' Respondents could choose their reply from, 'Helped/Hindered/Neither or Don't know.' For both men and women about 70 per cent of the co-educated group thought their type of school had helped them, 2 per cent thought it had hindered and 25 per cent said 'neither' or 'don't know'. Of the group educated in single-sex schools the percentage of both men and women who said their schooling had helped them fell to 10, while the 'hindered' replies rose to 30 per cent, with the 'neutral' group at over 50 per cent.[2] Some people might say that this result is merely what one would expect—that educating boys and girls together would naturally help them to establish a good social relationship with the opposite sex and that single-sex education would hinder this. The writer would agree, but would add that it is always useful to obtain confirmatory evidence for these beliefs, and that it sometimes happens that such beliefs are shown to be without foundation in fact. A vague belief is also much more open to counter-argument. In the present instance there are certainly supporters of single-sex schools who have argued that co-education made little or no difference because boys and girls these days have plenty of opportunities to meet the opposite sex outside school. This new knowledge, however, makes it more difficult for anyone to sustain this argument. Both the direction of the finding and the decisive difference between the two groups are a replication, with a more representative sample, of the writer's findings as seen especially in the answers to the question. 'Did your school life help or

[1] Cf. the summary in *Where?*, 28 October 1966.

[2] The difference is statistically significant beyond the ·001 level.

hinder you in your relations with the opposite sex?', given in Chapter 12.

With Atherton's second key question it is perhaps not so obvious that the type of schooling might make a difference between the co-educated and those educated in single-sex schools. He asked, 'Do you think the type of school (mixed or single-sex) helped or hindered you in making a happy marriage?' Respondents could reply, 'Helped/Hindered/Don't know'. Many people would think that other factors are so powerful that the influence of the type of school would be negligible. Atherton, however, found that for both men and women roughly 40 per cent of the co-educated judged that their schooling had helped them in making a happy marriage and only 1 per cent thought it had hindered, while among those educated in single-sex schools about 10 per cent thought their schooling had helped, over 5 per cent thought it had hindered and over 75 per cent said 'neither' or 'don't know'. For both men and for women the differences between the distributions of the co-educated and single-sex educated groups were statistically significant beyond the ·001 level. These questions, however, were only supplementary to the main procedure which was the administration of a self-rating questionnaire or 'attitude scale'. This scale for the self-rating of marital happiness also yielded results which gave strong support to these findings. The scale included one question directly on marital happiness and others on such topics as the sharing of interests by husband and wife, agreement on money matters, attitude to in-laws, religion, friends, any regret at having married and either actual separation or divorce or the thought of either. In this way a more objective element was introduced into the survey.

By far the most important difference he found was that between the 'happiness of marriage' scores of the co-educated and those educated in single-sex secondary schools, where schooling went on for five years or more, the co-educated had the better score. (A similar result obtained for those educated in grammar schools only, maybe because they were the principal group with prolonged schooling.) The difference between the two groups who had been at secondary schools for five years or more was statistically highly dependable.[1] The group of women lowest in happiness score were those who had attended convent schools, but even when these were removed (as being non-typical even for the groups educated in single-sex schools) the difference between the women educated at co-educational grammar schools and those educated in single-sex grammar schools remained statistically significant. In spite of the

[1] Beyond the ·01 level for men, ·02 for women and ·001 for men and women together.

consistency of these results an interpreter must tread warily in reaching his conclusions as there are so many other powerful forces acting for or against the happiness of a marriage, such as social class, age and religion, that it is necessary for a number of different researches to come to similar results before a finding can be regarded as established. Atherton's work, though praiseworthy, should be regarded as pioneering a way in a relatively new and difficult area of research.

The Schools project

In the questionnaire administered to groups of girl pupils in some twenty-four grammar schools in South Wales and the West Riding, three items were included which relate to the title of the chapter. They are, 'Marriage is necessary for happiness in later life', 'A woman cannot be married and also successfully carry on with a career', and, 'I feel that marriage and children are more important for a woman than a career'. Girls could choose their answer from a five-point scale ranging from 'agree strongly' to 'disagree strongly'. Their estimates yielded no conclusive results, none of the differences between co-educational and girls' schools being statistically significant for girls aged 17 plus and girls aged 15 plus. A similarly inconclusive result was produced when pupils were divided into social classes, and also when social class 3 (fathers skilled artisans) was split into those with siblings and those without.

Curiously enough, however, when the replies of the 15-year-old girls were analysed by social class, siblings and also geographical area, it was seen that whereas in South Wales there was a trend (remarkably consistent for each social class) for girls in girls' schools to be slightly more favourable to marriage than girls in the sample of co-educational schools from that region, in the West Riding this trend was reversed, again with consistency for social class groups. This reversal may have arisen through the small number of schools of each type in the sample, but whatever the reason it is abundantly clear that no conclusions can be based on such conflicting results (none of the differences was statistically significant).

Comment

An overall view of this evidence suggests that co-educational schooling at the secondary stage produces some improvement in the happiness of marriage, but more research is needed before this finding can be confirmed. More evidence is also needed on the extent of this difference—if indeed it is proved to exist, so that we can judge what weight to give it in the co-educational versus single-sex schools controversy.

The two following chapters may seem to break a certain thread of continuity in the book but they are included in it because like the rest of the material they are concerned with the social and emotional development of children in the two types of school, and are placed at the end because they are both based on a test technique which is not used in the rest of the book.

18

Anxiety about school

The anxious child is a hostage to fortune, liable to physical illness as well as to nervous complaints. No matter how able the child or how high the academic attainment, the future is not bright unless the anxieties can be removed or the anxiety habit modified. Though the home usually has the most important influence on the child, that of the school can be powerful either for good or ill. It is strange that educationists have for so long neglected to see that this good emotional and social development—central to sound education—might be profoundly affected by the alternatives of single-sex or co-educational schooling.

The area of emotional and social adjustment is vast in itself and no pretence is made that the subject is covered in this and the following chapter, nor any claim that the results from this one sample of forty-two schools are conclusive. We need other and larger samples of schools and also, as pointed out elsewhere, more 'objective' measures of emotional adjustment, such as analyses of truancy, juvenile delinquency and school attendance, though in view of other influences that bear on the problem, for example social class and urban versus rural environment, any straight comparison between co-educational and single-sex schools might be misleading.

In this study pupils at the age of 11 plus and 15 plus were given paper and pencil tests of temperament—including anxiety about school—and retested two years later. There are therefore results for the complete group at the first testing, for the remaining pupils two years later, and for a longitudinal sample similar in composition to that secured at the second testing. The tests were a modified Boxall for the juniors, and the Mooney Problem Check List and High School Personality Questionnaire (2nd edition) for both juniors and seniors.

The juniors

THE BOXALL TEST

The results of the Boxall test (for test see Appendix 1) and an analysis of previous research have been reported elsewhere (Dale, 1969), but a summary of the results is given here.

All the tests were administered by the writer and his research assistant, the pupils were told not to give their names, and the importance of the work was stressed. They worked under examination conditions, with no staff present, and their attitude was excellent. On the first occasion twenty pupils were tested in each single-sex school and twenty of each sex in the corresponding co-educational schools, making a full original sample of 1,120 pupils aged 11 plus. Anxiety towards school was measured by the number of situations in which the pupil admitted to feeling anxious, rather than by weighting each item for severity. Each affirmative reply scored one point, making a maximum of 23.

The results of the first testing (when the pupils had been in school for between a few days and two months) are shown in Table 18.1.

TABLE 18.1 *Mean anxiety score by school and occupational class (age 11 plus)*

Schools project

		Fathers' occupational class								
		Class 1		Class 2		Class 3		Classes 4 and 5		All classes
	Pupils*	N		N		N		N		
Girls in girls' schools	275	43	11·63	73	12·20	120	12·86	35	14·40	12·63
Girls in mixed schools	275	42	10·81	70	11·88	116	13·01	45	12·22	12·27
Boys in boys' schools	278	30	11·23	98	10·98	117	12·45	29	12·79	11·83
Boys in mixed schools	275	33	10·45	66	10·74	136	11·87	38	11·26	11·38
All schools	1,103	148	11·05	307	11·43	489	12·52	147	12·60	12·03

* Includes a few unclassifiable pupils.

With each sex the mixed schools have the lower score, this being consistent through all parental occupational classes except for girls of class 3 (skilled manual). Taking the classes separately none of the differences between mixed and single-sex schools is statistically significant for the boys (though the *t* ratio is substantial), and for the girls the only significant difference is the greater anxiety of girls in classes 4/5 in girls' schools compared with those in mixed schools. The consistency of the trend in favour of the mixed schools is so strong, however (seven out of eight differences are in this direction), that it is certainly of interest.[1]

Arithmetic

Questions 2, 3, 8 and 19 were on anxiety about arithmetic. Here the scores of girls in girls' schools and those in mixed schools were unexpectedly almost identical, while for the boys there was a surprisingly highly significant difference in favour of those in mixed schools (see Table 18.2).

TABLE 18.2 *Responses to questions on anxiety about arithmetic (age 11 plus)*

Schools project

	Anxious	Not anxious
Girls in girls' schools	610	500
Girls in mixed schools	603	510
Boys in boys' schools	597	518
Boys in mixed schools	535	579

The pupils of every occupational class contributed to this difference between the boys' groups. In the mixed schools the boys showed a clear increase of anxiety about arithmetic as occupational class became lower, apart from the lowest class (but the difference between extreme classes was statistically significant), with a similar but slighter and more irregular trend in boys' schools.

School (sub-analysis)

Another four questions (4, 5, 20 and 21) had been pre-selected as the more important ones reflecting anxiety about school in general, as compared with those indicating difficulty with work, etc. Here the girls from mixed schools had a significantly lower anxiety score, but the difference between boys, though favouring mixed schools, was not statistically significant (see Table 18.3). These findings are not stressed as the pupils had been at the school only a short time and it cannot be definitely stated that this greater anxiety of the pupils from single-sex schools was not present on entry. In view of the slightly superior entry to the latter (in social class and intelli-

[1] Even though analysis of variance (discarding one-fifth of the group to secure even numbers) yields a non-significant result.

gence) and the whole tenor of this research, the writer's opinion is that the most likely explanation is to be found in a more congenial 'reception' atmosphere, on the average, in the mixed schools.

TABLE 18.3 *Responses to questions on anxiety about school in general (age 11 plus)*

Schools project

	Anxious	Not anxious
Girls in girls' schools	424	676
Girls in mixed schools	379	721
Boys in boys' schools	442	667
Boys in mixed schools	405	691

The longitudinal sample

We pass on to consider the *change* in anxiety about school, i.e. as measured by the whole test, experienced (or recorded) between the two testings. This sample is smaller because of pupils who had left, were absent or, for a variety of reasons, did not arrive at the testing room, and because changes in school organization caused the withdrawal of six schools. The results were at first puzzling. The co-educated boys were at the start rather less anxious about school than those in boys' schools and were also slightly less anxious two years later, but the gap had narrowed; neither the gap nor the slight change was statistically significant. The two girls' groups started with the same average score, but two years later those in girls' schools were slightly less anxious than those in mixed schools, though again the differences between the groups and the change in average scores were quite unreliable. Nor did the results present a regular pattern for each occupational class—both boys and girls of classes 4 and 5 in mixed schools being appreciably less anxious about school than those from single-sex schools, while the closing of the gap in the boys' case was due largely to pupils from the clerical occupational class. The most notable feature was the high consistency in the decline in recorded anxiety between the ages 11 plus and 13 plus for pupils from both groups (see Table A.28).

An exhaustive analysis of the data showed several likely reasons for this departure from the usual trend. One of these held good for most age groups of boys and girls in the research, namely that in spite of the matching of the schools for social background the pupils of the single-sex schools were of rather higher social class than those from the co-educational schools;[1] the girls from girls' schools were also slightly higher in intelligence (see Tables A.1 and A.2 in Appendix 2). Both these factors would be operating to increase the anxiety of the co-educated pupils, thereby handicapping the co-educational schools in a straight comparison with single-sex ones. The study itself shows a persistent tendency for anxiety to school scores to increase from occupational class 1 to occupational classes 4 and 5.[2] On the other hand, a breakdown of the data by occupational class showed that the decrease in recorded anxiety in the two years was slightly greater for boys' and girls' schools in three out of the four occupational class groups when these were separated out, though each of these sub-groups would still contain a slight advantage in intelligence level on the girls' school side.

The likelihood that anxiety would also be increased when I.Q. is lower is substantiated by a number of studies already referred to in Chapter 9 (McCandless, 1956a, b; Sarason, 1960; Cowen, 1965), but in this *longitudinal* sample only the comparison between the girls in co-educational and girls' schools is affected, as the boys' groups have almost the same average I.Q. Additional evidence illustrating this tendency in the case of the girls has already been given in the chapter on unhappy girls.

A third factor played a part when the groups were compared at the first and at the second testing, namely a curious imbalance in the drop-out problem. The drop-outs are those who were reported by the heads as left or absent and those who for any other reason failed to appear in the test room (see Table A.29). The twenty-five girl drop-outs from co-educational schools had an average anxiety score at the first testing which was markedly below that for the whole group, while the average for the twenty-one from girls' schools was well above that of their group. Remarkably, the same held good for the boys, and in neither instance was it due to a few extreme cases, but reflected a general tendency. Whatever the reason for this it disturbs the representativeness of the sample, placing the co-educational schools at a disadvantage.

An examination of the results of individual questions revealed that these were pulling in different ways. Taking the four questions pre-selected for special study in the first testing (full sample) we now find that with the boys in this longitudinal study there is a decided fall in the number in boys' schools who became frightened

[1] Equality for girls aged 15 plus in 1964 in the *longitudinal* sample.

[2] The difference between occupational class 1 and classes 4/5 combined is smaller for co-educational schools and not statistically significant for their girls or boys, but it is almost significant for boys in boys' schools and reaches significance for girls in girls' schools.

when the teacher was cross and this brings them equal with the boys from co-educational schools at the second testing.[1] Similarly with the item on 'often worrying about school' there was less increase for the pupils in boys' schools, bringing them below the opposite group (this of course would include those who worried about work). On the other hand the boys from boys' schools showed a greater increase in pupils who said they hated having to go back to school when they had been away (not quite statistically significant), and less reduction in those who thought that coming back to school after the holidays was frightening. The change for the co-educated boys on this last item was statistically highly significant. This question was the only one of the four in which there was also a decided change in the position of the girls' groups, the girls' schools registering no change in the number of 'frightened' pupils, while the co-educated girls, who started with a score equal to that of their opposite numbers, had a large reduction.[2] The results from this item, from both boys and girls, may have some connection with the finding that discipline is more strict in single-sex schools. Though the *rates of decrease* amongst the two girls' groups to the item 'I hate having to go back to school when I've been away' are similar, rather fewer of the 13-year-old co-educational girls than those from girls' schools endorsed the statement at the second testing.

To summarize, the results of the first testing of the whole sample at 11 plus tended to favour the co-educational schools both in the test as a whole, and in the sections on anxiety towards arithmetic and on anxiety towards teachers, but the longitudinal study's raw scores on the complete test have a slightly opposite tendency though this is statistically unreliable and not consistent for all social classes or all items. It should also be noted that when an analysis was made of each of the four pre-selected questions on anxiety towards teachers, the only statistically significant changes in anxiety were recorded by the co-educated boys who showed a decided reduction in the proportion who said they were frightened at going back to school (a change highly significant); by the boys from boys' schools in the reduced proportion who were frightened when the teacher was cross and by the co-educated girls in the reduction in the proportion of pupils frightened at the idea of going back to school. There was also a nearly significant change statistically among the boys from boys' schools in the increased proportion

[1] Those wishing to study the figures should refer to Table A.30. The drop in the score of the boys from boys' schools is significant at the ·025 level. (This Chi-square used as data the *change* in individuals' scores.)

[2] The reduction for the co-educated girls was statistically significant (by Chi-square allowing for correlation).

of those who hated having to go back to school. The scores at 13 plus for the whole test still showed the co-educated boys slightly less anxious than their opposite numbers, but there is a somewhat greater advantage for girls in girls' schools over those in co-educational schools, neither difference approaching reliability. Evidence has been put forward, however, to show that the girls in girls' schools decreased their scores over questions connected with work, while the scores of the co-educated girls decreased more with items concerning school in general.

We must remember that differences between the groups in average intelligence (girls only), parental occupational class and the type of 'drop-out' pupil all placed the co-educational pupils under a handicap. Further interpretation is given at the end of this juniors' section.

THE MOONEY PROBLEM CHECK LIST

In the Schools project all pupils completed a Mooney Problem Check List.[1] This is a schedule of 210 personal problems, from which the pupils selected any which were troubling them. These are classified into seven problem areas of thirty items each, from 'school' to 'home and family', 'boy–girl problems' and 'people in general'. Examples of the items in the 'school' area are, 'Trouble with mathematics', 'Afraid of failing', 'Too much homework', 'Don't like school', 'Afraid to speak up in class', 'Not getting along with a teacher'. It is with this 'school' section that we are principally concerned, but a brief analysis is made of the test results as a whole and these are also given in tabular form in Appendix 2 (Tables A.31 and A.32). We are here concerned with the longitudinal sample.

The data for the juniors were divided into parental occupational class groups, namely classes 1 and 2 (managerial etc. and white-collar), class 3 (skilled manual) and classes 4 and 5 (semi-skilled and unskilled). As there are seven problem areas this produced 21 mean scores for each type of school for each sex. Of the total of 42 means for boys, 37 rose from age 11 to 13, the number of problems recorded by boys from boys' schools rising rather less than those recorded by the co-educated boys,[2] *except about school*, where the trend was slightly reversed. If we suppose there were 100 boys in each school, 17 of those in boys' schools indicated an increase of one more problem about school compared with the boys

[1] An anglicized version prepared by the writer in conjunction with the N.F.E.R.

[2] The difference between the two boys' groups at age 13, for *all* problems, favoured the boys in boys' schools, but was far from statistically significant.

in co-educational schools, the average number of problems per boy being about four at the first testing and six at the second. Without exception the 21 means of the co-educated boys rose as the occupational class became lower. A result of such a consistent trend is rare and future researchers will need to watch this variable carefully in many kinds of research projects in schools.

For the junior girls in all problem areas for every occupational class, and in both types of school, there is a marked increase of recorded problems between the ages of 11 and 13. The greater intellectual capability (e.g. of speed, of reading and of underlining problem items) of the 13-year-olds might have accounted for some of this, but it is unlikely to be the whole explanation. In five of the seven problem areas the increase of mention between 11 and 13 years of age is slightly less for the sample from girls' schools; in one area (people in general) there is virtual equality of increase, the *school area again being exceptional*, the co-educated girls registering a smaller increase in problems than did the girls from girls' schools. The size of this difference is about the same as that found with the boys.[1] In both co-educational and girls' schools there was a tendency for the girls' means for the two higher occupational classes to be lower than those for classes 4 and 5.

For both boys and girls problems relating to the opposite sex increased slightly more in the co-educational schools than in the single-sex, but this was not consistently maintained within all three occupational class groupings. The problem area showing the largest differences between the two groups in the increase of problems reported was 'home and family', where both girls and boys in the co-educational group had a bigger increase than those educated in single-sex schools. This is in line with the larger proportion of lower-class pupils in the co-educational schools.

As one of the items in the Mooney was similar to one in the questionnaire, it was examined separately for the girls. It was 'School is too strict'; the results are in Table 18.4, the girls in girls' schools being more positive about this than those in mixed schools. This is, of course, the view of the consumers; those making the rules probably have different ideas. Those reporting the school as 'too strict' were, however, only a small proportion of the total (one-fifth in the girls' schools).

A similar examination of the item 'don't like school' for the junior boys groups (longitudinal) at the second testing gave fewer co-educated boys agreeing with the item than boys from boys' schools, but the difference was too small to be reliable.

In a separate section the Mooney 'test' asked pupils, 'What problems are troubling you *most*?' They were instructed to 'write about

[1] Not statistically significant.

TABLE 18.4 *'School is too strict'**

Girls aged 13 plus, longitudinal sample

	Girls in co-educational schools	Girls in girls' schools
Agree	26	42
Disagree	189	173
	215	215

* The difference is statistically significant.

two or three of these if you care to'. Under no circumstances were they pressed to do this, but many pupils gave one or two. (They had been told not to put their names on the tests, which would be read by no-one except the researchers.) We might have expected that the total number of these serious problems would rise sharply between the ages of 11 and 13, but this was true of only the boys. For the juniors, the co-educated boys had slightly fewer serious problems than the boys in boys' schools, including 'boy–girl relationships', but the differences were small except in problems about school, where a negligible initial difference (9 co-educated boys picking out some aspect of school as a special problem compared with 13 in boys' schools) became one of 68 to 84 at age 13.[1] This is the area of greatest change for both sets of boys.

Sub-classification of the problems about school (now allowing more than one problem per pupil in the few cases where these fell into different sub-categories) revealed that the problems were predominantly concerned with work and examinations (about 80 per cent) in both types of school. Poor relationships with teachers or dislike of the school in general were singled out as special problems by only 2.2 per cent of the pupils in the co-educational schools and only 5·5 per cent in boys' schools. In the former these form one-fifteenth of all the special problems recorded in this detailed examination of school problems and in the boys' schools one-eighth, but as numbers recording these personal problems were small the data is not mentioned as being statistically of importance in its own right.[2]

[1] The difference between the groups at the age of 13 is almost statistically significant.

[2] The difference between the two groups of boys in the proportions recording personal relationship problems is, however, not far from statistical significance.

As indicated above, a large majority of the problems, in both types of school, were about work, e.g.:

'Not spending enough time in study.'

'My most troubling problem is not getting high enough marks in exams. I am afraid that I will go to the wrong stream and then I will not be able to do what I like when I grow up.'

'Worried about school etc. and about subjects I don't like such as Maths.'

'Getting low marks when my parents expect me to do better.'

Those about pupil–teacher relations are illustrated by:

'Need more younger teachers. Old-fashioned teachers are no good because they do not understand us.'

'I am worried about being nervous when trying a test. The teachers do not help matters as some of them act as if they are in charge of a concentration camp, they do not look happy, have sad faces and they grumble to themselves.'

'I don't like school very much because it is too strict. Some masters keep whole forms in when only one boy has misbehaved.'

'School is too strict. You should be able to have more freedom.'

One amusing reply came from a co-educated boy: 'The school is too patriotic, i.e. we have to play Rugby when we would rather play football.'

The junior girls did not show the sharp rise in special problems between the two testings which was shown by the boys. The co-educated girls recorded the larger number of *special* problems[1] at both ages, though the opposite was the case when they were concerned with *all problems* (whether 'special' or not). The differences between the two girls' groups came largely from the 'home and family' section. The girls' schools recorded fewer 'boy–girl' special problems at 13 plus, and under 'school' they also had a minimal advantage, far from statistically significant. Both results were again the opposite to the results of the larger Mooney test and must therefore be viewed with some caution, especially as the co-educated girls have distinctly the better result when the number of special 'school' problems for each of the two groups is expressed as a percentage of its total number of special problems. As with the boys the problems are mainly about work and tests etc., those about personal relations at school being rare. We must remember, however, that young pupils, particularly girls, might be reluctant to

[1] See Table A.32a in Appendix 2.

put such problems down on paper as they might be afraid of staff or head seeing these. (For example one headmistress stayed for some time in the test room of the writer's research assistant, although it had been made clear that this might affect the results.)

THE HIGH SCHOOL PERSONALITY QUESTIONNAIRE

All pupils in the Schools project were also given the High School Personality Questionnaire (H.S.P.Q.), and a longitudinal sample consisted of all those who had completed it both in 1964 and 1966. The test yields scores on fourteen personality dimensions, but in this chapter we are dealing only with anxiety, the score for which is a composite of several of these fourteen 'source traits'. The whole test is essentially a self-rating questionnaire, containing items such as 'Do your hands sometimes tremble and your heart beat fast when you get excited about speaking up in class?' There is a choice of three replies: Yes/Perhaps/No. In this case we are not able to derive a score about 'anxiety to school' alone.

The longitudinal samples of junior boys had almost identical scores for the two types of school at the first testing; two years later, at age 13, the boys' schools showed a larger increase in anxiety[1] (see Table A.33). Occupational class 3, however, had a slightly opposite tendency. The junior girls also started off with similar mean scores and like the boys' schools, the girls' schools increased their anxiety score more than the co-educational, but the difference was small and not statistically significant; nor were the results for the separate occupational class groups at all consistent.

Summary (juniors)

The overall analysis is complicated. Clearly no dramatic differences in anxiety between junior pupils of co-educational and single-sex schools have been shown to exist. With regard to the boys the most interesting feature is that in the Mooney Problem Check List the problems recorded by boys in the co-educational schools increase more than those of the boys in boys' schools in every area *except that of the school*, where they increase less. Surprisingly the H.S.P.Q. test shows the boys from boys' schools increasing more in their score on *general* anxiety than those from co-educational schools, but all these differences are small. Readers should note, however, that the Mooney tends to emphasize the statement of problems by the pupil, while the H.S.P.Q. emphasizes

[1] The difference between the changes in scores for the two groups from age 11-plus to age 13-plus is almost statistically significant ($t = 1{\cdot}77$), allowing for correlation within each group.

his anxiety towards them. The powerful influence of occupational class is to be seen throughout the tables, e.g. the differences in score between 11 plus and 13 plus for the co-educational boys in the Mooney test increase consistently with occupational class in all areas in 13 out of the 14 possible comparisons. This is a built-in handicap for the co-educational schools in comparison with the single-sex, though it is not a necessary concomitant of co-education.

The picture is much the same for the girls. In the two tests about general anxiety the differences between the co-educated and pupils from girls' schools are small and are built up from a number of forces which pull in opposite directions. As opposed to the slight advantage of the girls' school in the Boxall test of anxiety to school (longitudinal sample only) we have the fact that in the Mooney Problem Check List it was only in the area of school problems that the co-educated pupils had a smaller increase than the opposing group. It is noteworthy that in the case both of boys and girls it is in the 'home and family' section that the single-sex schools gain their biggest advantage, and one would expect this from their higher social class.

The score on anxiety to school (Boxall test) appears to be built up of several factors which research needs to separate out. It looks especially as if a distinction needs to be made between anxiety about academic progress in school (of several kinds), and anxiety about relationships with people—either staff or pupils. The sub-analysis of items concerned with fear of teachers, being frightened of school, etc., gives a distinct advantage to the co-educational schools, which means they are losing somewhere else, and this is likely to be in the area of academic work, where the lower social class of their pupils, and, with the girls, their lower average I.Q. would of themselves be likely to lead to greater anxiety about school. In the chapter on unhappy girls this factor is shown to be of importance in co-educational schools. In this comparison we should again keep in mind the peculiarly one-sided nature of the drop-out problem.

There are some suggestions—but not proof—in the data that co-education reduces worry about boy–girl problems for boys, but has little effect in this way for girls. This also needs further research, with special regard (once again) to the different occupational class composition of the two types of school.

The seniors

THE MOONEY PROBLEM CHECK LIST

Senior boys

The senior pupils were not given the modified Boxall test. The results from the Mooney Problem Check List had some interesting features (Table A.34). With the boys there was a consistent fall in the average number of problems recorded in each of the seven areas of problems, in each of the two[1] occupational class divisions, for the boys from both types of school—28 averages in all—between 15 and 17 years of age.[2] (Note that these pupils are in a sense specially selected since they chose to stay at school till at least 17.) The average number of problems recorded by the co-educated boys of 15, rather lower than that of the boys in boys' schools[3] (except for small differences in the opposite direction for 'boy–girl relationship' and 'school'), fell slightly more than the scores of the latter, the most favourable change for the co-educated boys being the comparative falls in the two problem areas mentioned.[4] For occupational classes 1 and 2 combined, five of the means (out of 7) fell more in the co-educational sample, with two the reverse, while for occupational classes 3, 4 and 5 combined the two samples differed little in the incidence of change. In every one of the seven problem areas the co-educated boys recorded fewer problems at age 17[5] than did those from the boys' schools, though the averages for *school* problems were not far from equality.

In reply to the question, 'What problems are worrying you *most*?' the same general tendency was continued, the co-educated boys indicating clearly fewer problems in overall total at both 15 and 17 years of age.[6] This was most marked in school problems and continued in 'boy–girl relationships',[7] but there was also an unexpected

[1] Here classes 1 and 2 are combined and 3 with 4 and 5.

[2] Statistically significant, by analysis of variance; (and also for girls).

[3] Substantial but not statistically significant ($t = 1{\cdot}394$).

[4] The analysis of variance for the 'school' problems section showed also a significant sex difference with girls recording fewer problems, but the difference between co-educated boys and those from boys' schools was not statistically significant. The sex difference, however, could conceivably have been affected by a systematic difference in the administration of the tests for the two sexes—there being a different administrator for each. (The research was not assessing sex differences.)

[5] The overall difference approached significance ($t = 1{\cdot}582$).

[6] Almost statistically significant at 15 plus but not at 17 plus.

[7] Not statistically significant for boy–girl relationships at 15 plus or 17 plus.

difference in the same direction for 'Home and Family'. The differences were maintained in each of the occupational class groups.

Senior girls

The same trends are to be seen when we examine the results of the senior girls in the main test (Table A.35). The co-educated girls had very slightly more problems in total at 15 years of age, mostly from the sections 'people in general', 'home and family', and 'work and future', but this was slightly reversed in 'school' problems, with an equality under 'boy–girl'.[1] By the age of 17 plus however, the co-educated girls were appreciably lower in overall total, and lower in all the problem areas except 'people in general' where there was equality. Easily the largest difference between the two types of school in the seven problem sections at the age of 17 *was that of 'school'*[2] and this was also an area in which the change over the two years was the second most favourable to the co-educated girls, the most favourable being 'people in general' (though, as indicated above, the *change* in this last category produced only equality).

A detailed examination of the answers to the four pre-selected items which emphasized 'the school in general' or personal relationships, rather than work, produced fewer co-educated girls who said they were 'not getting along with a teacher'[3] and fewer who thought the school too strict.[4]

Strangely, when these girls were asked to write down those problems which troubled them most, the co-educated girls indicated more in total than did the girls from girls' schools both at 15 and 17 years of age, though the difference had been halved in the two years.[5] It is possible that the co-educated girls were less inhibited about writing the problems down—perhaps less afraid of the consequences if the tests were seen by staff! However, in the 'school' problem section there was equality at age 17, and the co-educated girls had very slightly more problems in the 'boy–girl' area, though this was far from statistically reliable. The principal areas where the girls from girls' schools recorded fewer special problems at 17 years of age were 'people in general' and 'money, work and the future'. In the 'school' problems the co-educated girls recorded more at 15 years[6] and the same as the girls from girls'

[1] None of these differences approached statistical significance.
[2] This verges on statistical significance.
[3] Highly significant at 15 plus and significant at 17 plus.
[4] Not statistically significant at 15 plus but highly significant at 17 plus.
[5] Neither difference reaches statistical significance. See Table A.35a.
[6] Far from statistically significant.

schools at 17 years. In both years these school problems were a slightly lower percentage of the total number of problems for the co-educated group. A detailed analysis of these special school problems, for both co-educated girls and those from girls' schools, yielded a very high proportion of problems directly concerned with school work and examinations, and few about personal relations with teachers. There were no distinct differences between the two types of school in the nature of the special *school* problems.

THE HIGH SCHOOL PERSONALITY QUESTIONNAIRE

In the High School Personality Questionnaire[1] the co-educated senior boys had lower *general anxiety* scores both at 15[2] and at 17 years of age than those at boys' schools; this trend was consistent for both occupational classes, but the *rate of change* favoured the boys' schools, though it was too small to be reliable. Readers are again reminded that this measure of anxiety includes, for example, worry about work as well as about personal relationships, and one of the forces to be considered would be the influence of the lower social class of the co-educated boys in increasing their general anxiety as they approached their important external examinations.

The senior co-educated girls, like the co-educated boys, had lower general anxiety scores both at 15 and at 17[3] years of age, and this was clearly to be seen in each of the occupational class groupings. With the feminine sex, however, the rate of change quite strongly favoured the co-educated girls, the gap between the two types of school being greater at 17 plus than at 15 plus.[4] The co-educational schools had the more favourable rate of change in both occupational classes of this age group.

The finding that the difference in favour of the co-educated girls is greater than that in the case of the co-educated boys (as contrasted with the respective single-sex schools), is in conformity with the trend found at numerous points in these inquiries.

[1] A scientifically constructed American paper and pencil test designed to measure 14 personality factors.

[2] Substantial, but only that for the 15-year-olds reaches the accepted level of significance.

[3] The difference between the co-educated girls and those from girls' schools at age 17 is statistically highly significant.

[4] The difference between the changes in anxiety score for the two types of school (i.e. in the extent of change) is statistically highly significant. ($t = 3{\cdot}002$ allowing for correlation.)

Summary (Seniors)

Among the seniors the co-educated boys showed themselves less anxious both in the main part of the Mooney test and in the section where they were asked about their special problems, but the difference between them and the boys from boys' schools was found to be not statistically significant.[1] The co-educated boys also recorded a rather greater reduction in anxiety between the ages of 15 plus and 17—again not large enough to be statistically reliable, but counter to the trend one would expect from the comparative occupational class distributions of the two samples.

In the H.S.P.Q. test the co-educated boys also had lower scores on general anxiety at 15 and at 17 years of age, but in this case the rate of decrease slightly favoured the boys' schools, though the same qualifying remarks apply as with the Mooney test.

Viewing the results as a whole the co-educated girls were rather less anxious than those from girls' schools especially in the area with which we are most concerned—school, and a more detailed examination of that area showed that the difference was most marked in personal relationships at school. This finding was at first masked by other sources of anxiety such as, in the broad field, anxiety about home and in the narrow area of 'school' by factors such as anxiety about work, which would be accentuated in the co-educational sample by lower social class and lower average intelligence. The finding is in complete agreement with the relevant sections of the other surveys, such as 'happiness in school', 'school atmosphere', and 'friendliness of teachers' and the detailed investigation into 'unhappy pupils'. It should not, however, be exaggerated, as the difference between the two samples in anxiety in general, or even in anxiety towards school in general, is not large.

[1] By analysis of variance.

19

Neuroticism and introversion–extroversion

In addition to the data on anxiety the paper and pencil tests yielded scores on many other personality characteristics, notably on neuroticism and introversion–extroversion. The two latter scores were obtained from the High School Personality Questionnaire and the Maudsley Personality Inventory. The tests were administered by the writer and his research assistant to the sample of pupils in schools (Schools project). Throughout the chapter we shall be concerned with the longitudinal sample, i.e. those pupils who appeared for testing on both the first and the second occasion two years later.

It is undeniable that normally heredity and the home environment will exert the most powerful influence on the personality characteristics of an individual, but the part played by the school may be far from negligible though we know surprisingly little about it from research evidence. Since co-educational and single-sex grammar schools differ substantially as communities—in happiness, atmosphere, discipline, teacher–pupil relationship—it is possible that they may exert different effects on the personality characteristics of the individuals composing them. When comparing the scores of the two types of schools on such characteristics special attention needs to be paid to two other variables which may affect the comparison—the comparative intelligence levels of the groups and the occupational class of the fathers.

Neuroticism

BOYS

The boys' scores on neuroticism, as measured by the High School Personality Questionnaire, are given in Tables 19.1 and 19.2. At age 11 the boys in the co-educational schools had a marginally lower score than those in boys' schools, but by age 13 the difference had increased and become statistically significant (·05 level). This does not signify that the boys from boys' schools were neurotic—

TABLE 19.1 *Neuroticism scores—junior boys*

H.S.P.Q.

		Class 1		Class 2		Class 3		Classes 4 and 5		All*	
Age	Schools	N	Mean	N	Mean	N	Mean	N	Mean	N	Mean
11+	Co-ed.	28	22·19	57	23·72	106	22·61	34	23·16	226	22·93
	Boys'	27	23·64	78	22·62	88	23·64	24	22·23	220	23·13
13+	Co-ed.	28	20·19	57	21·67	106	20·78	34	20·79	226	20·94
	Boys'	27	23·33	78	21·34	88	21·93	24	20·79	220	21·82

NOTE: At age 13 plus the co-educated boys have a statistically significant lower neuroticism score overall, but this is not consistent for all social classes.

TABLE 19.2 *Neuroticism scores—senior boys*

H.S.P.Q.

		Classes 1 and 2		Classes 3, 4 and 5		All*	
Age	Schools	N	Mean	N	Mean	N	Mean
15+	Co-ed.	56	20·71	77	20·85	134	20·83
	Boys'	70	22·47	67	22·11	137	22·29
17+	Co-ed.	56	19·81	77	20·28	134	20·11
	Boys'	70	21·35	67	21·03	137	21·20

* Includes some unclassifiable.

NOTE: At age 15 the co-educated boys had a statistically significant lower neuroticism score, but the gap had closed a little by 17 plus and was then not quite statistically significant.

merely that they had a rather higher score than the co-educated boys on this long scale which runs from 'unduly stable' to 'highly neurotic'.

At age 15 the co-educated boys of the middle school had lower scores for neuroticism than did the boys in boys' schools and the difference was again statistically significant; but the gap between the two samples had narrowed a little by the time they were 17 years of age and now was not quite statistically significant. The overall result of the testing at the four ages shows a clear trend towards rather lower neuroticism scores among the co-educated boys; this seems to differ from the finding of Furneaux (1961) but it should be noted that his was an incidental finding which did not examine other variables which might have had an influence, such as the average intelligence level of the students from the two types of school. In the present longitudinal sample, however, these scores are nearly equal for the boys, though not for the girls.

It should be noticed also that in this partly controlled situation there is no steady trend among the boys for neuroticism scores to increase as the occupational class of the father becomes lower. This is in contrast to the trend in anxiety scores which was commented on in the previous chapter.

As a second measure of neuroticism the Maudsley Personality Inventory was administered to the 15-year-old boys and two years later to the same group again (Table 19.3).

TABLE 19.3 *Boys' neuroticism—mean scores (Maudsley)*

		Classes 1 and 2		Classes 3, 4 and 5		All*	
Age	Schools	N	Mean	N	Mean	N	Mean
15+	Co-ed.	56	26·18	77	25·27	134	25·76
	Boys'	70	26·41	67	29·09	137	27·72
17+	Co-ed.	56	26·16	77	25·84	134	26·05
	Boys'	70	26·06	67	29·16	137	27·58

* Includes some unclassifiable.

As in the H.S.P.Q. test the boys from the boys' schools have the higher neuroticism score at age 15, but the difference between this and the score of the co-educated boys was on this occasion a little short of statistical significance ($t=1{\cdot}754$). Taking classes 3, 4 and 5 alone, however, the co-educated boys had a statistically significant lower neuroticism score. At 17 years of age the co-educated boys still had the lower score, but the difference between the two groups was slightly reduced, being on the verge of statistical significance for students from occupational classes 3, 4 and 5, but negligible for classes 1 and 2.

We also find that in the boys' schools the neuroticism scores of the senior boys on this Maudsley test (at ages 15 and 17) increases as the father's occupational class becomes lower, but there is a smaller trend in the opposite direction in the co-educational schools. It is by no means the first time in these inquiries that there have been hints in the data that pupils of occupational classes 4 and 5 seem to react a little differently in co-educational as compared with single-sex schools. On the other hand the occupational class trend in the Maudsley is not confirmed by the results of the previous test (H.S.P.Q.) though the latter is admittedly a non-specialized test and therefore less reliable.

GIRLS

The girls' neuroticism scores on the High School Personality Questionnaire are given in Tables 19.4 and 19.5.

TABLE 19.4 *Neuroticism—mean scores (H.S.P.Q.)*
Junior girls

		Class 1		Class 2		Class 3		Classes 4 and 5		All*	
Age	Schools	N	Mean	N	Mean	N	Mean	N	Mean	N	Mean
11+	Co-ed.	32	21·82	60	21·89	80	22·87	43	22·65	215	22·40
	Girls'	37	22·21	59	23·00	90	22·93	29	23·25	218	22·87
13+	Co-ed.	32	20·67	60	20·11	80	20·66	43	21·93	215	20·76
	Girls'	37	20·26	59	20·75	90	20·40	29	21·23	218	20·59

TABLE 19.5 *Neuroticism—mean scores (H.S.P.Q.)*
Senior girls

		Classes 1 and 2		Classes 3, 4 and 5		All*	
Age	Schools	N	Mean	N	Mean	N	Mean
15+	Co-ed.	61	21·81	54	20·77	115	21·32
	Girls'	61	21·41	59	20·67	121	21·02
17+	Co-ed.	61	21·66	54	20·79	115	21·25
	Girls'	61	21·96	59	20·46	121	21·25

* Includes some unclassifiable.

Table 19.4 shows that the co-educated girls had rather lower neuroticism scores when aged 11 and that this was maintained in every occupational class,[1] but two years later the average of the girls from girls' schools was very slightly lower[2] than that of the co-educated girls and consistent for three occupational class groups but not for class 2. In Table 19.5 the senior girls' groups reverse this process, those from girls' schools starting at age 15 with slightly lower neuroticism scores than the co-educated (non-significant), and finishing up at 17 years of age with identical

[1] Not statistically significant.
[2] Far from statistically significant.

averages overall and inconsistent differences within the two social class groups.

The results from the more specialized test—the Maudsley—do not change the picture much; they give the co-educated girls a slightly lower average score for neuroticism both at 15 and 17 years of age, but the difference is too small to be reliable and is again inconsistent for the two occupational class groups (Table A.36).

The overall picture, therefore, is that both junior and senior boys in the sample of twelve co-educational schools were lower in neuroticism score than their counterparts in boys' schools, but for the girls the emphasis must be on the near equality of the two groups.

Introversion–extroversion

The same two tests yielded also measures of introversion–extroversion, and the writer was interested in seeing whether the two types of school had any clearly discernible and consistent influence on the pupils in this direction. It could be theorized, for example, that educating the two sexes together would make them less shy of each other and perhaps more extroverted; on the other hand we have seen from this study that *deprivation* of the company of the opposite sex may be a strong driving force impelling pupils to overcome such shyness. Little work has been done on these and related topics, and the writer has been working on such a variety of problems relating to co-education that he does not pretend to have done more here than make a preliminary survey. As the results do not show clear and consistent differences between the co-educational and single-sex schools they are presented concisely and with little comment.

BOYS

The co-educated junior boys were slightly more extroverted as measured by the H.S.P.Q. than the boys from boys' schools, both at 11 and 13 years of age, but the differences were in the opposite direction for children from both occupational classes 2 and 4/5, and were therefore lacking in consistency and reliability (Table A.37). In the case of senior boys the scores of the opposing groups were virtually equal both at 15 and 17 years of age.

When tested by the Maudsley Personality Inventory the extroversion scores of the senior boys from boys' schools at 15 years of age were slightly higher than those of the co-educated boys, though the difference was far from statistically reliable and at 17 years of age had virtually disappeared. The distribution of scores was similar for the two groups, both at 15 and at 17 years of age and they threw up approximately the same number of high scorers (scores over 39).

GIRLS

The junior co-educated girls were slightly more extroverted than those from the girls' schools at 11 years of age as measured by the H.S.P.Q., but by the time they were 13 years old the difference was minimal. There were no consistent occupational class trends (Table A.38). The two senior girls' groups recorded almost the same average score at 15 years of age and two years later the girls from girls' schools were slightly more extroverted. Here there was a slight tendency for the extroversion scores of the girls from occupational classes 1 and 2 to be lower than those of girls from classes 3, 4 and 5 (Table A.39).

The picture obtained from the Maudsley test for the senior girls emphasized this occupational class trend without reaching a difference which was statistically reliable. The 15-year-old girls

TABLE 19.6 *Introversion–extroversion—mean scores (Maudsley)*

Senior girls

		Classes 1 and 2		Classes 3, 4 and 5		All*	
Age	Schools	N	Mean	N	Mean	N	Mean
15+	Co-ed.	61	27·80	54	29·72	115	28·70
	Girls'	61	30·15	59	30·02	121	30·07
17+	Co-ed.	61	27·67	54	30·11	115	28·82
	Girls'	61	29·92	59	31·56	121	30·71

* Includes some unclassifiable.

from girls' schools were rather more extroverted than the co-educated girls and this difference had increased a little two years later (Table 19.6). Once again, however, the variability of score within each group was so high that we cannot rely on the clear difference between the groups being reproduced at another testing. It is true that for this group of senior girls the difference was obtained in both the tests and at ages 15 and 17, and this is strong support for the reliability of the result. On the other hand no such difference between the co-educated and single-sex educated groups of junior girls was found either when 11 or when 13 years old. There was approximately the same number of high scores on both sides at 15 plus, but rather more at girls' schools than at co-educational schools at 17 plus (31 to 21).

Comment

Taking an overall view these tests of introversion–extroversion revealed no decided or consistent difference between the pupils from co-educational schools and those from single-sex schools. This is somewhat fortunate as the interpretation of the significance of such a difference might have been exceptionally difficult. However, the possibly greater extroversion of the senior girls in girls' schools needs further inquiry.

Shyness and leadership

Two of the items on the Maudsley test were pre-selected for a separate analysis of scores because they might have provided an elementary useful lead to research on two of the many problems related to the advantages and disadvantages of co-education, namely shyness in the company of the opposite sex and the possibly reduced opportunities of leadership for girls in co-educational schools.

The first of these questions was, 'Are you inclined to be shy in the presence of the opposite sex?' In none of the four groups of pupils tested—boys aged 15 and aged 17 and two comparable groups of girls—were the differences between co-educated and single-sex educated pupils sufficiently large to be statistically reliable, and most of them were far from being so. Contrary to expectations the 15-year-old boys in boys' schools confessed to being only a little more shy of the opposite sex than did those from co-educational schools, and at 17 years of age there was even a minimal difference in the opposite direction. Rather more co-educated girls than girls from girls' schools said they were shy in the presence of the opposite sex at age 15, but the difference had disappeared two years later. If these small differences in favour of the single-sex schools are confirmed, a tenable theory (as mentioned previously) is that there are conflicting forces at work and depriving each sex of the company of the other acts as a driving force in the overcoming of shyness—a force which may even be stronger than the overcoming of shyness by the natural meeting of the sexes for work at school. However, it should be remembered that the samples of *ex-pupils* are quite sure that mingling with the opposite sex at school helped them with their relationships with members of that sex after they had left school.

The other question was, 'Do you generally prefer to take the lead in group activities?' Again none of the differences between co-educational and single-sex school groups were large enough to be reliable, but the trend was that although at 15 years of age rather more boys from boys' school than from co-educational schools said they preferred to take the lead, this became equality two years later, with co-educational boys from occupational classes 1 and 2 having an advantage. With the girls there was a decided difference between those from different occupational classes, the co-educated girls from classes 1 and 2 being rather more ready to take the lead than their rivals from the girls' schools, but the reverse being the case with girls from occupational classes 3, 4 and 5, this even approaching statistical significance (Table 19.7). Those who do further research into this matter will need to take more account of the nature of the entry into the two types of school. It is, for example, regretted that the merging of the five occupational classes into two may have hidden the real differences of class between co-educational and single-sex schools within these two groups.

The smallness of the numbers within each of the occupational class groupings makes further comment inadvisable except that if additional research confirms that girls of occupational classes 3, 4 and 5 are more reluctant to take the lead in co-educational schools than in girls' schools, then co-educational schools would need to take preventative action as part of their regular policy.

TABLE 19.7 *'Do you generally prefer to take the lead in group activities'*

Maudsley question 28 (senior girls)

	15 plus						17 plus					
	Co-ed. schools			Girls' schools			Co-ed. schools			Girls' schools		
	N*	Yes	No	N*	Yes	No	N*	Yes	No	N*	Yes	No
Social classes 1 and 2	61	19	42	61	15	42	61	25	33	61	19	39
Social classes 3, 4 and 5	54	13	37	59	21	35	54	15	37	59	26	30
Totals	115	32	79	120	36	77	115	40	70	120	45	69

* The totals include a few who marked 'Doubtful'.

20

The amalgamated schools

In the preceding volume it was shown that the students who attended amalgamated schools usually gave rather less favourable estimates relating to these schools than other comparable students gave about the normal co-educational schools they attended. An attempt is made here to summarize the evidence relating to the topic, including that of the first volume *in so far as this involves a comparison with the normal co-educational school.* Throughout the chapter differences between the two types of school are not 'statistically significant' unless this is stated. Some differences which are not statistically significant are mentioned because they form a consistent logical pattern and therefore have an added reliability. As the sample of men from amalgamated schools, however, was only twenty-four their results are not dependable, though they receive some support from the general character of the women's results, where the sample from amalgamated schools numbered ninety-three.

In the earlier research the amalgamated ex-pupils gave a slightly lower estimate for the friendliness of their teachers than did those seniors who were in the other co-educational schools. (Men from amalgamated schools, incidentally, regarded their men teachers as pleasanter than their women teachers to an extent almost statistically significant.)

With regard to discipline there was little difference between the two groups of women, but the men from amalgamated schools provided a much larger proportion of the three 'lax discipline' categories than was warranted by their proportion in the total sample of students from 'co-educational last' schools. The women from amalgamated schools also found their teachers rather less pleasant, including their male teachers, although in reply to another question they considered the presence of male teachers to be as highly favourable as did their parent sample. The corresponding sub-group of men pronounced their men teachers less pleasant than did the other students from normal co-educational schools (though some 83 per cent of the former endorsed the 'fairly pleasant' category or better), but there was very little difference between these groups when they assessed their women teachers. However, in reply to the related item, 'The presence of the opposite sex of teacher has a good influence', the men from amalgamated schools gave less favourable estimates than their opposite numbers.

Readers who would like additional evidence about the effect of amalgamation should consult Chapter 11 of the previous volume (Dale, 1969) where there is a comparison of the estimates of ex-pupils whose single-sex schools became co-educational with those of ex-pupils whose co-educational schools were divided into single-sex ones. This theme would be out of place in this chapter, which is confined to a comparison of the amalgamated with the other co-educational schools.

We have already seen in Chapter 2 that both men and women from amalgamated schools did not give quite as high estimates of their happiness there as the remaining co-educated seniors gave about their schools. In the case of the question on 'school atmosphere the ex-pupils of amalgamated schools considered it to be less pleasant than did the co-educated seniors, the difference being almost statistically significant for men and highly significant for women (Table 20.1).

TABLE 20.1 *School atmosphere: Amalgamated v. other co-educated seniors*

'Both schools' survey

Estimates	Men				Women			
	Normal co-ed. schools		Amalgamated		Normal co-ed. schools		Amalgamated	
	N	%	N	%	N	%	N	%
Very pleasant	35	43·8	8	33·3	109	40·8	24	25·8
Pleasant	39	48·8	10	41·7	117	43·9	44	47·3
Neutral	3	3·7	3	12·5	31	11·6	12	12·9
Rather unpleasant	3	3·7	2	8·3	10	3·7	13	14·0
Very unpleasant	0		1	4·2	0		0	
Totals	80	100	24	100	267	100	93	100

After the survey of pupil–teacher relations followed by the more general 'school atmosphere', we now come to an examination of pupil–pupil relationships, still comparing amalgamated with the normal type of co-educational school. Here the same trends continue. Both male and female ex-pupils from amalgamated schools liked the presence of the opposite sex less than did the ex-pupils from normal co-educational schools, and this difference was statistically significant in both cases.[1] It will avoid misunderstanding if it is pointed out that even in the amalgamated schools some 87 per cent of the women liked the presence of the opposite sex (with only 2 pupils out of 92 disliking it) and 79 per cent of the men similarly (with 2 out of 24 against). However, in answer to the overlapping item, 'The presence of the opposite sex of pupil had a good influence,' the difference between the amalgamated pupils and the rest was not as large, that for the women being slight, though both were still in the same direction.

The question of the influence of the opposite sex was pursued in a little more detail. For example, one of the items asked, 'Do you consider that the influence of the girls on the boys in this school was, in general, Very good/Good/Fairly good/No effect/Bad/ Very bad?' For the two men's groups there was little difference between their judgments (92 per cent of the 'amalgamated' men thought the influence to be 'fairly good', 'good' or 'very good'), but the women from amalgamated schools judged the influence of the girls to be not as good as did the women from the rest of the 'co-education last' group (though 70 per cent said 'good', with 20 per cent undecided).

The opposite question about the influence of the boys on the girls again yielded only a little difference between the judgments of *men* from 'amalgamated' and the other co-educational schools, with a slight advantage to the latter. In the case of the *women* those

TABLE 20.2 *Influence of boys on girls*

Both schools survey (*women*)

Preferences	Normal co-educational schools		Amalgamated schools	
	N	%	N	%
Very good	26	10·1	6	6·6
Good	101	39·2	28	30·7
Fairly good	85	32·9	27	29·7
Neutral	29	11·2	13	14·3
Bad	17	6·6	17	18·7
Very bad	0		0	
Totals	258	100	91	100

NOTE: The difference between the two distributions is statistically significant beyond the ·025 level.

[1] Highly significant for the women and at ·025 level for the men.

from normal co-educational schools were much more sure of the good influence of the boys;[1] but even in the amalgamated schools some 66 per cent of the women ex-pupils placed this influence in the three 'good' categories (see Table 20.2).

To conclude this section the results are presented from two items of the 'Both schools' questionnaire which dig a little deeper into the problem. The first of these was, 'In your co-educational school was the general attitude of most of the pupils (of your own sex) towards the opposite sex "antagonistic"?' The respondents could choose between True/Partly true/False/Doubtful. It will be seen from Table 20.3 that both the women and the men from the amalgamated schools thought the sexes were more antagonistic there than the remaining ex-pupils of other co-educational schools judged to be so in their schools, the differences being statistically significant. The cause would probably be resentment of the 'intruders' and perhaps opposition to drastic change.

TABLE 20.3 *Antagonism between the sexes*

'Both schools' survey

Reply	Men				Women			
	Normal Co-ed. schools		Amalgamated		Normal Co-ed. schools		Amalgamated	
	N	%	N	%	N	%	N	%
True	0	0	0	0	2	0·8	4	4·5
Partly true	5	6·8	10	(41·7)	36	14·3	17	19·3
False	51	69·9	11	(45·8)	163	65·0	48	54·6
Doubtful	17	23·3	3	(12·5)	50	19·9	19	21·6
Totals	73	100	24	100	251	100	88	100

NOTE: The differences between the distributions for the 'normal' and the amalgamated schools are statistically significant for both men and women.

The second item substituted the phrase 'girl/boy-crazy' for 'antagonistic', and in spite of the antagonism (which was true for only one-quarter of the 'amalgamated' women), the women from amalgamated schools were somewhat more boy-crazy at school[2] than were women from normal co-educational schools. There was again little discernible difference between the men's groups. The latter finding is a little surprising but it should be noted that only two of the men (one from each group) gave the extreme answer that it was 'true' the boys were 'girl-crazy', though a quarter of both groups endorsed 'partly true'. (For the boys' schools, the

[1] The difference is statistically significant.
[2] The difference was statistically significant.

answer 'true' was given by nearly 14 per cent of the seniors, while nearly another 50 per cent endorsed 'partly true'.)

From the above items it was an easy transition to the question, 'In which school do you consider the pupils had the healthier attitude towards sex?' The ex-pupils were asked to underline one of the following: Doubtful/Don't know/Single-sex school/Co-educational school. The general results have already been given in another chapter, but here we are interested in the amalgamated schools, who were part of the sample of co-educational schools.

The women from the amalgamated schools produced a distribution of judgments which was almost identical to that of the women who were seniors in other co-educational schools. In both groups some 79 per cent said the pupils in the co-educational schools had the healthier attitude, with only 3 to 5 per cent endorsing girls' schools. The men from amalgamated schools were, however, less certain than those from the other co-educational schools that the pupils in their schools had a healthier attitude than those in their single-sex schools—75 per cent (amalgamated) to 85 per cent (co-educational), the difference between the percentages being made up not by the 'single-sex school' category but under 'doubtful' and 'don't know'.

Finally, was the proportion of pupils who preferred their co-educational school greater among the 'amalgamated' sub-group than among those who attended normal co-educational schools as seniors? This has been reported in Chapter 11 but is summarized here for completeness. The women from the normal co-educational schools were much more certain that they preferred their co-educational school to their girls' school[1] (Table A.20), the preference 'mixed much' being made by 71 per cent of them compared with 60 per cent of those from the amalgamated sample. Again, most of the differences between these percentages did not go to preference for the girls' schools, but were placed in the 'doubtful' or 'don't know' categories.

The men from amalgamated schools had the same trend but the smallness of the numbers made the result statistically not significant (see Table A.20).

Administrators will naturally have realized that the upheaval and resentment occasioned by the sudden combining of two single-sex schools into one co-educational establishment would create problems for some time. The data confirm the existence of these usually temporary problems and suggest perhaps a little more precisely the nature of some of them. The findings indicate that where two junior comprehensive single-sex schools feed a co-educational senior comprehensive school some of these difficulties

[1] The difference being statistically significant.

will be perpetuated, and the school may well be less successful on the social and emotional side than would a school where the boys and girls had grown up together—though other influences would play their part.

For male pupils the numbers are small for reliability, yet it looks as if further research might well show that the girls are more affected by such a reorganization than the boys, and women teachers more than the men.

21

Conclusion

As the present volume and its predecessor *Mixed or Single-sex School?* are separate parts of the same work, this conclusion seeks to integrate the findings of both. The two books analyse and appraise the experience of teachers, ex-pupils and pupils of co-educational and single-sex schools mainly through their own reports. The research has concentrated on respondents' attitudes to their schools and to varying aspects of school life, with a brief look into a few effects of the schooling on their lives afterwards. The most important samples used are those of teachers and of ex-pupils who had each taught or been taught in both kinds of school.

The previous volume was concerned with teachers and pupil–teacher relationship. Teachers in secondary grammar schools were seen to be strongly in favour of co-education, and those teaching in co-educational schools almost unanimously preferred them to single-sex schools. The principal opposition was shown to come from two sources, namely those teachers who had had no direct experience of co-education and were essentially basing their attitudes on ignorance and a stereotyped prejudice, and those women who understandably feared that their opportunities for promotion to headships would disappear if all schools were co-educational. A few teachers thought that the interests of the sexes diverged too much for them to be taught together, and others that academic standards might suffer. Support for co-education was mainly for social reasons, including preparation for life in a bisexual world and the good influence that each sex of pupil and of teacher was believed to have on the conduct of the other. Additional reasons were the fresh life given to school societies, the invigorating effect of increased breadth of interests, the stimulation provided by the greater variety in school life and the beneficial results of a friendly academic rivalry between the sexes.

In order to counter the objection that many of these teachers had taught in only one type of school and therefore knew little about the other, two special samples of teachers, almost 500 in all, who had taught in both types of school were separated out from the others and their returns reclassified. They were strongly in favour of co-education; in one sample the majority was 60 per cent of those teachers who themselves were educated in single-sex schools and 79 per cent of those educated in co-educational schools; in the second sample (analysed differently) those in favour were 93 per cent of men and 97 per cent of women teaching in co-educational schools, 80 per cent of those in boys' schools and 64 per cent in girls' schools, with small percentages undecided. In another inquiry only 9 per cent of staff in University Departments of Education were in favour of single-sex and 'dual' schools.

What is the significance of these results? There are certain limitations of the new evidence which should be mentioned. The teachers are from maintained day grammar schools only, so that the findings cannot be said to be directly applicable to independent schools or to boarding schools, and one can only theorize that if co-education is preferable in grammar schools it would probably also be preferable in secondary modern, technical, bilateral and comprehensive schools.

Some critics may say that teachers prefer co-educational schools not for any purely educational reasons but because they themselves feel happier in such schools. Although almost all the reasons given by the teachers for their preferences were educational in the widest sense, this factor might indeed have affected the preference. However, even if this were true it seems pertinent to ask whether it is not desirable to have a happy staff in a school and whether this happiness might not conceivably be communicated to the pupils, creating thereby an atmosphere which would be conducive to good attainment in the narrow sense of education and better adjusted pupils in its wider sense.

Yet we should recognize that the judgments made by the teachers depend in part upon the established ethos of the society in which they live, and if they had been living in Victorian times, with its fears about the unchaperoned social mixing of the sexes, they might have been swayed in the opposite direction. On the other hand it could be argued that if there had been many more co-educational schools in Victorian times society would not have been so frightened at the idea of educating the two sexes together!

At the present day a noteworthy aspect of the swing towards co-education is that it is occurring in spite of the entrenched prestige of the single-sex 'public' schools, including the direct grant schools, in spite of the single-sex education of most teachers, in spite of there being a majority of teachers teaching in single-sex grammar schools, and in spite of an 'establishment' which is largely the product of single-sex schools. The force of tradition is incredibly strong, yet these teachers have in this one aspect decided for change, and an educational revolution is now taking place in the schools of England by which it seems probable that most of the children will soon be educated in co-educational secondary schools.

The next section summarizes the main findings of the previous volume about the relations between pupils and teachers in co-educational compared with single-sex maintained grammar and technical schools. These results were obtained mainly through questionnaires answered by several large samples of ex-pupils (including a sprinkling who had been taught in comprehensive and bilateral schools). The most important of these samples was that used in the 'Both schools' survey, consisting of some 800 students who had each attended both a co-educational and single-sex secondary school (excluding secondary modern). These students, both men and women, judged the teachers in their co-educational school to be friendlier and more helpful than those in their single-sex schools. The students also thought there was a greater tendency for some teachers in their co-educational schools rather than boys' and girls' schools to have 'a powerful influence for good' (though with equality for senior boys).

The consensus of the findings about the discipline in these schools is that the ex-pupils considered that both boys' and girls' schools tended towards strictness, an appreciable number being judged 'too strict', this becoming over-severity and harshness in a minority of schools, whereas in their co-educational schools the discipline was mostly reported 'satisfactory', but the group judging it 'too lax' was greater than that judging it to be 'too strict'. In the ensuing discussion the theory was put forward that this difference in the conduct of school affairs is probably caused by one type of community having both sexes and the others only one—that boys and girls and also men and women, in such an institution as a school, have an ameliorating effect on each other's conduct and that this makes it possible for authority to use a lighter form of control in a co-educational school than is found practicable in a single-sex school. Hence it is easier for teachers in co-educational schools to appear more friendly and helpful than they do in single-sex schools, where there is more of a barrier between teacher and pupil. Linking up with this theme is the strong liking expressed by girls in co-educational schools for being taught by men.

In reply to some more detailed questions affecting aspects of the pupil–teacher relationship the female ex-pupils of the 'Both schools' survey thought there was much more 'unnecessary fuss about small details' in their girls' schools than in their co-educational, and both males and females in the sample considered that the staffs of their single-sex schools were more 'out of touch with modern adolescents'. The women, whether they attended their girls' school first or last, and those men who had attended their boys' school first, endorsed more frequently for their single-sex schools than for the others that they 'felt grown-up and were treated like children'.

A chapter in the first volume was devoted to a special analysis of the replies of students who had attended an 'amalgamated' school. The results from such schools were not as favourable as were those from the normal co-educational schools in which boys and girls had grown up together from the age of eleven. The estimates from the whole co-educational group were therefore depressed a little in the comparison with single-sex schools. The influence of amalgamated schools persists throughout the results given in the present volume, as demonstrated in a recent chapter. However, another feature which emerged was that the amalgamation affected the girls more than the boys and the women teachers more than the men. Three of the findings were, first, that the pupils from the amalgamated schools were rather less happy than the corresponding group of seniors who had grown up with the opposite sex at school since the age of eleven, though the difference was not sufficiently large to be statistically reliable; second, that the pupils' attitude to sex was reported as being not as healthy in amalgamated schools as in the normal co-educational type (though still healthier than in single-sex schools), and finally that the ex-pupils of the amalgamated were not quite as pronounced in their preference for these (as against their single-sex ones) as were the normally co-educated pupils for their schools.

Returning to the comparison between co-educational and single-sex schools, the chief findings of this volume are outlined in the next few pages. The ex-pupils of the co-educational schools reported themselves as having been happier at school than did those from single-sex schools and they also found the school atmosphere pleasanter. Usually these results are more consistent and stronger for the women than for the men. The reasons both sexes give are that the social life with two sexes is better, it is a more natural preparation for life in the adult world, relations with the staff and between the staff are pleasanter, and the atmosphere is less tense. With regard to academic work they find it more enjoyable in a mixed school and like the friendly rivalry with the opposite sex, though others emphasize the good academic standard of their single-sex school.

In the Schools project the 17-year-old co-educated girls gave higher estimates than those in girls' schools for 'kindness' as opposed to 'unpleasantness' (highly significant), for 'enthusiasm' as opposed to 'apathy' (approaching significance), and for 'variety' as opposed to 'monotony' (substantial but not statistically significant). In the 'Check' questionnaire more of the 13-year-old co-educated girls than of their opposing group estimated their school to be 'lively' as opposed to 'dull'.

In these 'life in school' aspects the co-educated boys, surprisingly, had a bigger advantage than the co-educated girls. The 13-year-old boys believed their schools to be more lively as opposed to more dull, to have more variety as opposed to monotony, and possibly to show more enthusiasm than did the boys from boys' schools. Also the 17-year-old co-educated boys rated their schools as more lively and more enthusiastic.

In this section it appeared likely that pupils from working-class homes found school life in the single-sex schools, on the average, more dull and monotonous, less enthusiastic, more unpleasant and with more cliques than did their fellow-pupils from the higher social classes. This tendency was less certain among co-educated girls and absent among co-educated boys. As this finding is only a by-product of the research a concentrated effort on this aspect might be rewarding.

One of the most startling differences between the men's groups was that whereas almost half of the men in the 'Both schools' survey judged bullying to be frequent or very frequent in their boys' schools, only one-fifth of them made the same estimate for their co-educational schools. The verdict of the women was similar. Following the same general theme, both sexes found the prefects to be 'more officious' in their single-sex than their co-educational schools.

Men and women also judged the education provided in their single-sex schools to be 'narrower' than in their co-educational schools, nor were there as many enjoyable out-of-school activities. In both these cases the difference between the two senior boys' groups was smaller than for junior boys or for girls in general.

In the area of pupil interaction both male and female ex-pupils were strongly of the opinion that it was easier to make friends in their co-educational than in their single-sex schools, and the women thought the girls in the latter were more 'spiteful' and more 'quarrelsome'.

In Chapter 9 the outline case-studies of those girls who had described themselves as 'unhappy' or 'rather unhappy' at school yielded some interesting results. It was demonstrated that the unhappy girls in the co-educational schools were of lower average intelligence than their opposite numbers in the single-sex schools and that their difficulty in coping with their studies was a powerful factor in this unhappiness. By far the more important reasons for unhappiness among the co-educated girls were out-of-school or home difficulties and the above-mentioned lack of ability, with teachers' discipline almost the least important whereas the girls from girls' schools placed dislike of school first, with teachers' discipline second, work difficulties almost equal to this, and out-of-school and home difficulties fourth. A specially intriguing point is that at both junior and senior level the unhappy girls from girls' schools had higher extroversion scores than did those at co-educational schools. Interestingly, hints of this difference are seen between the *boys' main* groups. This finding could not be followed up but it is suggested tentatively either that deprivation of the company of the opposite sex drives these pupils of single-sex schools into slightly increased extroversion, or that those girls in girls' schools who are highly extroverted are more likely to become unhappy at school than similar girls in co-educational schools.

The characteristically stricter discipline of the one-sex school is shown also in the attitude of these schools towards out-of-school conduct. Both male and female ex-pupils judged this interest as 'excessive' or 'rather strict'—mostly the latter (though the difference between the opposing groups of male ex-pupils was not statistically significant), whereas half of the co-educated men and women, for both first and last schools, estimated the interest to be 'just right', with the remaining half spread equally on both sides of this middle line. This was, of course, the judgment of the consumers—though of former consumers who as student teachers were already becoming those who directed the consuming!

A schooling in which boys and girls spend many years at school with the opposite sex, compared with a schooling which segregates boy from girl, would naturally produce a decided difference in attitude in each towards the other. This result was, however, not attained in answer to all the questions in this area. For example, when they were asked if they thought of the opposite sex as being Very superior/Superior . . . Very inferior, the two main groups of women in the Second College survey produced results which were almost identical, though the men from boys' schools did give just a hint of more extreme opinions in both directions. Yet in the replies about the pleasantness or unpleasantness of the attitude of the pupils towards the opposite sex both male and female students of the 'Both schools' survey were sure that the pleasanter attitude was in their co-educational schools. At the same time they reported much more timidity towards the opposite sex among pupils in single-sex schools. Again the latter were more 'preoccupied with the opposite sex' and also more 'boy-girl crazy'.

It is sometimes said that boys do not like the presence of girls in school. The falsity of this argument was demonstrated by the co-educated ex-pupils, as only three males (out of 186) and six females (out of 657) agreed with the statement, in spite of the existence of a number of amalgamated schools in the sample. They also considered that the presence of the opposite sex of teacher had a good influence, but here the male approval (though moderately favourable) was shown to be diminished by the influence of the amalgamated schools.

Ex-pupils of the 'Both schools' survey asserted strongly that the two sexes had a good influence on each other, improving the boys' appearance, manners and turbulent behaviour, and making them work harder, while on the other side improving the atmosphere among girls, widening their interests and making more normal the interest of the girls in boys.

One of the crucial questions which lies hidden in the minds of parents and of some teachers and educationists is whether the presence of boys and girls together in co-educational schools would encourage an excessive interest in sex, and create an unhealthy atmosphere. The ex-pupils who attended both a co-educational and single-sex school have given a very clear reply. Seventy-six per cent of the women believed the attitude towards sex to be healthier in their co-educational school than in their girls' school, only 7 per cent believing the opposite. This is such an important aspect of the problem that three of the reasons given by the women and reported earlier in the text are repeated:

'When you see boys every day the novelty wears off.'

'Boys were part of everyday life in the school and at times were completely forgotten about.'

'Mixing with the opposite sex one comes into closer contact than in the single-sex school—it changes one's ideas completely—found I had more respect towards them and a healthier attitude towards sex.'

The judgment of the men was the same as that of the women. The difference in attitude between the two types of school, for both men and women, was greater than for any other topic explored. A moment's reflection on the problem makes it clear that the propinquity of the sexes in co-educational schools makes it essential for this attitude to be good if the schools are to be viable, whereas the segregation of the sexes in single-sex schools makes a less healthy attitude tolerable as far as the running of the school is concerned, because the consequences in boy–girl relationships are to be seen only away from the school premises if they are known at all. Unfortunately we simply do not know whether the deprivation of the companionship of the opposite sex experienced by pupils in single-sex schools and the consequently less healthy attitude to sex has worse effects outside school than in the case of co-educated pupils.

As was to be expected the topic 'preparation for the adult world' yielded considerable advantage to the co-educational schools. Whereas only some 10 per cent of the ex-pupils of girls' schools, in the Second College survey, said their school life was helpful in their relations with men, the proportion from the co-educated women was three-quarters. Many more of the latter also found it easier to work with men in the adult world. The men's results followed the same pattern except that in addition the men from co-educational schools found it easier to work under the direction of a woman than did the men from boys' schools. In the Schools project the 17-year-old girls from co-educational schools were also more certain than their counterparts that their school 'prepared them sufficiently for the adult world'. The differences between the boys' groups for this question fell a little short of statistical significance, the co-educated boys finding their schooling more helpful.

Marriage would seem a far cry from school—though not as far these days as it used to be. Yet it would seem possible that the two methods of education under consideration—co-education and its opposite—might have very different effects on the social and emotional development of children and even affect the relative happiness of children when later they marry. There have indeed been hints of this possibility in the preceding paragraphs, though it would be folly not to recognize that even if co-education has an influence here it is unlikely that it will be as powerful as a number of other forces.

An amusing beginning in this area was made by the finding that the women of the Second College survey were slightly more keen to marry if they had been educated in a single-sex school, while the reverse was true for the men! Though the differences are not statistically reliable they are not insignificant, and it may be that deprivation of the company of the male sex makes women a little keener on marriage, but men deprived of women (more doubtfully) a little less keen. The same result was obtained from a question on the desire to have children.

Atherton carried this work further by asking a very large sample of married people whether their mixed or single-sex schooling had helped or hindered them in their everyday relations with the opposite sex. His results were overwhelmingly in favour of the co-educational schools. In answer to another question, 'Do you think the type of school (mixed or single-sex) helped or hindered you in making a happy marriage?' his sample again gave a decisive judgment for the co-educational school.

The most important part of his work, however, was that in which he used a self-rating scale of marital happiness, as outlined in Chapter 17, and found that among those who had attended secondary school for five years or more, the co-educated had a better score than those educated in single-sex schools. It is self-evident that in this difficult area of research the finding needs replication before it can be accepted with confidence, but a relevant point is that there appear to be no research findings at present which are in opposition to Atherton's work.

Finally, which schools did the samples prefer? We have seen the views of the teachers and must now consider those of the ex-pupils (the question was omitted from the questionnaire used in the Schools project). In each case there was a decided preference for the co-educational schools, and this was most marked in the two samples, one large and one small where the ex-pupils had attended both a co-educational and a single-sex school and were able to compare their experiences in the two schools. They prefer these schools because—in their own words—there is a natural friendliness between the sexes, and they educate each other; they find the atmosphere pleasant and relaxed, enjoy the social life of the school, the friendliness of the teachers, the broad balanced outlook, and the preparation for the adult world. They also stress that work is more enjoyable, with more interesting and lively lessons and more variety.

A rather small minority preferred the single-sex school, usually for academic reasons, but sometimes because of friendly staff, small school, tradition, etc. Whether they are teachers, pupils or ex-pupils, as soon as they have experienced a co-educational school most of them will have a strong tendency to prefer co-education. Opposition comes mainly from those ignorant of it, and co-education is unthinkingly confused in the minds of some of these teachers and pupils with differences due to the rather lower-social-class intake of some co-educational schools.

Here and there in this work teachers in single-sex schools, particularly women in girls' schools, have been severely criticized by some of their ex-pupils. More than once the writer has shown that this is a minority opinion and that most of these College of Education students give due acknowledgment to the effort and influence of their secondary school teachers. Yet a difference in important aspects of school atmosphere does exist between the two types of school, and this difference could be due entirely to the presence of both sexes in one type of school and the absence of one sex in another type. We must also remember that these researches have been examining average tendencies, and in the endeavour to single out differences between co-educational and single-sex schools other factors in the well-being of a school have rarely been mentioned. Perhaps the most important of these, in the present form of administration used in schools, is the personality and character of the head, but factors such as the calibre of the staff, type and position of buildings, undeniably have a strong influence. On the pupils' side the nature of the school intake, e.g. its ability and its social class, will also be a force of consequence. The result is that there is a wide range of quality within any one type of school and an overlap between types, so that the achievement of a school —in its widest sense—by no means depends only upon whether it is co-educational or single-sex, though these researches have illustrated the importance of this difference in organization.

In the last half of the nineteenth century a few prophetic voices urged the value of co-education, but they were indeed voices crying in the wilderness. The examples of Scotland and the United States were ignored, as were the pleas in the twentieth century of Badley, Pekin and Curry. Victorian and Edwardian society was afraid of the idea, the uncritical worship of the public schools—single-sex by historical evolution—was at its height, and it would have been heresy—as it still is in some circles—to have speculated to what extent the academic achievements and widely acclaimed 'character training for leadership' were due to a combination of special selection of pupils (e.g. in Direct Grant schools) and the pupils' high social class. It was taken for granted—without any scientific examination of the case—first, that the academic achievement was good and second, that it was good because of special merit in the teaching, and these beliefs became connected with a vaguer belief that high achievement and single-sex schooling went hand in hand. It was also assumed—again without any serious examination of the facts—that the acclaimed character training was inclusive of all desirable aspects of personality development, and again, more vaguely, that this was best achieved in a single-sex school. Many teachers in girls' grammar schools tended to think of nearby co-educational schools as 'inferior' and this attitude became linked with the idea that these schools were inferior because they were co-educational, though the weaknesses of which these teachers were critical could have arisen because of the difference in social class intake between the contrasted schools.

Today we now know more facts with which to make a more rational appraisal of the position. The research set out in this volume and in its predecessor has shown that co-educational and single-sex schools are communities with very different atmospheres, with the co-educational school providing the happier, more balanced, more interesting and more complete education. This research does not cover all aspects that need to be covered, nor has the writer been able—for lack of time and resources—to include a sufficient analysis of the more objective evidence which is mentioned elsewhere—the comparative incidence of delinquency, of truancy, homosexuality and schoolgirl pregnancies, etc. Nor has he been able to do more than touch upon the question whether the differences between co-educational and single-sex schools create long-lasting differences in attitudes, personality and social development. It seems likely that the products of co-educational schools have for at least some years after leaving school a more natural and easier relationship with the opposite sex, find it easier to work with the opposite sex and rate themselves as rather more happily married, than do the products of single-sex schools. The writer would be the first to say that we need more evidence on these points, but at the present this is the only evidence that exists.

The Introduction briefly examined how in the last two or three decades the western educational world has slowly moved towards co-education. In Britain more pupils are now in co-educational secondary schools than in single-sex ones. So far so good—the progress appears to be in the right direction. It will not, of course, remove all our troubles—co-education is no panacea for all the ills of the secondary school system, as administrators and teachers in U.S.A. will know. In particular, the success of schools with their pupils depends in part on the attitudes and values inculcated in the children by their parents and by society itself.

Each type of institution, however, is liable to develop its special kind of failing. In this research a few failings of co-educational schools have been mentioned sufficiently frequently by respondents to persuade the writer that they need some consideration. One is the inequality of the status of women on the staff of some of these schools, not indeed in the relationship between male and female assistants, which is usually cordial, but in the fact that not only is the head almost invariably a man (which is accepted by most female critics as necessary in view of the attitude of society, though some relaxation in favour of women is needed), but in some schools *the second in command is also a man*—the senior master. This relegates the senior mistress to third in the hierarchy and this 'image of women' is bad for the girls. Moreover, this accentuates the promotion problem which leads so many headmistresses and some of their staff to oppose co-education; in a world of co-educational schools run in this way they would not only be unable to obtain headships, they would not even be second in command. As mentioned earlier, the best way to deal with this injustice would be to have a headmaster who—in deference to public opinion and because of the scarcity of suitable female applicants—would *usually* be first in command, but also a *headmistress* rather than senior mistress, who would *usually* be second in command rather than first, but would have with the headmaster a right to a seat on the governors' committee. In conjunction with this reform is the necessity to make sure that a reasonable balance of male and female teachers is achieved—a number of schools have now a heavy imbalance of men, and this impairs the true atmosphere of a co-educational school.

A third complaint of women teachers is that the head, being a man, is inclined to sacrifice the interests of the girls to those of the boys, and it is sometimes added that this comes from his lack of experience in co-educational schools before he was appointed. This is something which has not been investigated, but is mentioned as a possible danger—and a possible hint to those organizing training courses for heads that the special needs of co-educational schools ought to be kept in mind.

No mention has been made of parents. This does not mean that the writer is indifferent to them, but they fall outside the limit of this research. In fact the making of a comparison between co-educational and single-sex schools needs either specialized knowledge, which has become available only in the last twenty years and then only in learned journals that are not readily available to parents, or needs actual experience in both kinds of school, and even this is a limited basis for a single individual to make an appraisal. An individual who has no such specialized knowledge or experience may think that he or she is making a judgment about co-education when in reality it is based on the building and its situation, the tradition of the school or its clientele. The net result is that wherever parents' views are ascertained the majority is in favour of the established order, whether it be single-sex or co-educational. It is indeed a tribute to the existing grammar schools of whichever type, that the parents are ready to fight for the local school if there is any proposal to change it from one type to the other. On the other hand, this is a state of affairs which is not of much help to the administrators. It is likely that parental opinion, with that of the teachers (who are, after all, often parents) and student teachers (who will in a few years become parents), is moving slowly towards co-education, but the change will inevitably lag behind the opinion of those people who are themselves working in education.

This brings to an end the reporting of the writer's investigation into those aspects of the comparison between co-educational and single-sex secondary schools which are related to the social and emotional well-being of the pupils. In the next volume it is hoped to present evidence which will help educationists to compare the influence of the two types of schooling on the academic attainment of the pupils.

Finally, although this book has co-education as its main theme, the writer hopes that it will be useful in other contexts. The evidence that has been gathered together about pupil–teacher relationships, about the happiness and unhappiness of pupils, the good and the bad influence of teachers and the anxiety of pupils, bears directly on other central issues of education.

Appendix 1

The questionnaires[1]

[SECOND COLLEGE SURVEY]

Research questionnaire I

For ex-pupils of Secondary Grammar Schools

This questionnaire forms part of a research project on a subject about which there is a great need for reliable information. The compiler asks for the generous co-operation of all those who are invited to assist in the inquiry; it is hoped that they will feel that they are contributing their quota towards the advance of knowledge in this particular field. Great care will be taken to ensure the anonymity of all individuals and of all educational institutions which may take part. You are particularly asked not to put your name on the form.

Sincere thanks to all those who help.

Old Scholars of Secondary Grammar, Comprehensive and Grammar-Technical Schools

All questions relating to school refer to the *secondary school.* Please tick which ever answer is corret. If you attended more than one grammar school, please number your ticks where necessary throughout the questionnaire, using (1) for your first school, (2) for your second, and so on. If your school changed from mixed to single-sex or vice versa, while you were at school, consider this as two separate schools, and instead of numbering your ticks (1) and (2) mark them with M (Mixed) and S (Single-sex).

Please state your sex: Male/Female
Age (unless you prefer not to give it) .... years
Occupation of father ....
Number of brothers ....
Number of sisters ....
Type of Secondary Grammar School attended:
(1) Co-educational/Single-sex[2], for .... years

[1] Only those parts of the questionnaires are given which have relevance to the material in this book.

[2] 'Dual' schools, with girls under a headmistress in one part of the building, and boys under a headmaster in another part of the building, are classed as 'Single-sex', but in such cases please add a D to your tick.

(Answer (2) and (3) if you attended more than one secondary grammar school.)
(2) Co-educational/Single-sex, for .... years
(3) Co-educational/Single-sex, for .... years

Was your life in school, viewed as a whole,
Very happy/Happy/Jogging along/Rather unhappy/Very unhappy?
Comment briefly if you wish, ...
e.g. giving reasons for your opinion ....
....

Do you think the school atmosphere was
Very pleasant/Pleasant/Neutral/Rather unpleasant/Very unpleasant?

If in your secondary grammar school career you attended more than one school, and changed from a mixed to a single-sex school, or vice versa, which did you prefer?
Single-sex school very much/Single-sex school a little/No preference/
Mixed school a little/Mixed school very much

If you attended a single-sex school would you have preferred it to have been a mixed school?
Yes/No/Undecided

If you attended a mixed school would you have preferred it to have been single-sex?
Yes/No/Undecided

Did your school life help or hinder you in your relations with the opposite sex?
Very helpful/Helpful/No effect/Slight hindrance/Great hindrance

Do you find it easy to work with the opposite sex?
Very easy/Easy/Fairly easy/Doubtful/A little difficult/Difficult/Very difficult

Do you think you would find it easy, in general, to work under the direction of a member of the opposite sex?
Very easy/Easy/Fairly easy/Doubtful/A little difficult/Difficult/Very difficult
Comment if you wish ....
....

(When answering the question below, please analyse your attitude very carefully, and give a frank answer)

In your attitude to the opposite sex do you think of them, in general, as being

Very superior/Superior/Equal/Inferior/Very inferior?
Comment if you wish ....
....

(For the unmarried)
Do you wish to marry, provided you can find a suitable partner?
Very much/Much/A little/Undecided/A little opposed/Much opposed/Very much opposed

If you do not wish to marry, please comment ....
....

If you marry—or if you are married—do you wish to have children?
Very much/Much/A little/Undecided/A little opposed/Much opposed/Very much opposed

If you do not wish to have children of your own, it would be helpful if you would give your reasons.
....
....

['BOTH SCHOOLS' SURVEY]

Research questionnaire II

FORM B. *For students who have attended both a co-educational and a single-sex grammar, or comprehensive, or grammar technical school in Britain*

This questionnaire forms part of a research project on a subject about which there is a great need for reliable information. The project is financially supported by the Department of Education and Science. The compiler asks for the generous co-operation of all those who are invited to assist in the inquiry; it is hoped that they will feel that they are contributing their quota towards the advance of knowledge in this particular field. Great care will be taken to ensure the anonymity of all individuals and of all educational institutions which may take part. You are particularly asked not to put your name on the form.

Sincere thanks to all those who help.

Please answer these preliminary questions. (In ink please—not pencil)
Age ...... years Sex ... Male/Female
How long have you been a student in a College of Education (or Training College)? ...... years ...... months
Occupation of Father or Guardian (former occupation if unemployed or deceased). Please give this as fully as you can, e.g. not merely MINER but *Miner-Deputy* or *Cutter*; not ENGINEER but

Maintenance Engineer or *Graduate Engineer*; not MANAGER but *Manager of small shop*; not FARMER but *Tenant Farmer* or *Smallholder*; not just CIVIL SERVANT but *Civil Servant—Clerk* or *Executive*; not just FACTORY WORKER but *Fitter*, or *Works Labourer*, or *Machine Operator*.

OCCUPATION...

All questions refer to your *secondary schools*
If while you were at school your school changed from a mixed to a single-sex school, or vice versa, consider this as two separate schools. If one school you attended was secondary modern exclude this from your answers.

When answering the following questions please underline the answer which is correct for you, e.g. Co-educational

Type of Secondary (or Comprehensive etc.) school attended, in *chronological order*.
(1) Co-educational/Single-sex ... years (approx.)
(2) Co-educational/Single-sex ... years (approx.)
(3) Co-educational/Single sex ... years (approx.)
If you were a boarder write 'B' after the school where you boarded.
If you attended a Comprehensive school write 'C' after this school.

Your co-educational school

If you attended more than one co-educational secondary school (apart from secondary modern) please give answers for each of these schools and distinguish between them by numbering each answer, (1) for the first co-educational school you attended and (2) for the second. Please give these numbers even where the answer is the same for both schools.
Underline the answer which is correct for you.

1. Was your life in your co-educational school, viewed as a whole, 1. Very happy/2. Fairly happy/3. Jogging along/4. Rather unhappy/5. Very unhappy?
Please give your reasons ....
....
....

7. Do you think the school atmosphere in your co-educational school was 1. Very pleasant/2. Pleasant/3. Neutral/4. Rather unpleasant/5. Very unpleasant?
Give the most important reason for your answer ....
....
....

8. Do you agree or disagree with the following statements about your co-educational school? *Underline* your answers.
   (2) Pleasant situation of the school.
   1. Agree strongly/2. Agree/3. Doubtful/4. Disagree/5. Disagree strongly.
   (3) Presence of the opposite sex of teacher had a good influence.
   1. Agree strongly/2. Agree/3. Doubtful/4. Disagree/5. Disagree strongly.
   (4) Presence of the opposite sex of pupil had a good influence.
   1. Agree strongly/2. Agree/3. Doubtful/4. Disagree/5. Disagree strongly.
   (6) There were enjoyable out-of-school activities (other than games).
   1. Agree strongly/2. Agree/3. Doubtful/4. Disagree/5. Disagree strongly.
   (7) There was unnecessary fuss over small details, e.g. hair, uniform, etc.
   1. Agree strongly/2. Agree/3. Doubtful/4. Disagree/5. Disagree strongly.
   (8) The prefects were officious.
   1. Agree strongly/2. Agree/3. Doubtful/4. Disagree/5. Disagree strongly.
   (9) I disliked the social image the school tried to capture.
   1. Agree strongly/2. Agree/3. Doubtful/4. Disagree/5. Disagree strongly.
   (10) I felt I didn't belong socially.
   1. Agree strongly/2. Agree/3. Doubtful/4. Disagree/5. Disagree strongly.
   (11) The staff were out of touch with modern adolescents.
   1. Agree strongly/2. Agree/3. Doubtful/4. Disagree/5. Disagree strongly.
   (13) The education I got was extremely narrow.
   1. Agree strongly/2. Agree/3. Doubtful/4. Disagree/5. Disagree strongly.
   (14) The school tried to dominate my whole life.
   1. Agree strongly/2. Agree/3. Doubtful/4. Disagree/5. Disagree strongly.
   (15) I felt I was grown up and was treated like a child.
   1. Agree strongly/2. Agree/3. Doubtful/4. Disagree/5. Disagree strongly.
   (16) I felt that the school created a gap between myself and my home.
   1. Agree strongly/2. Agree/3. Doubtful/4. Disagree/5. Disagree strongly.

13. Within your co-educational school did you find it easy or difficult to make friends?
1. Very easy/2. Fairly easy/3. Neither easy nor difficult/4. A little difficult/5. Very difficult.
Comment if you wish..
....

14. In your co-educational school was the general attitude of most of the pupils (of your own sex) towards the opposite sex
1. Pleasant/2. Fairly pleasant/3. Neutral/4. A little unpleasant/5. Unpleasant?
Comment if you wish..
....

15. In your co-educational school was the general attitude of most of the pupils (of your own sex) towards the opposite sex

Antagonistic?	1. True/2. Partly true/3. False/4. Doubtful
Indifferent?	1. True/2. Partly true/3. False/4. Doubtful
Normal Interest?	1. True/2. Partly true/3. False/4. Doubtful
Rather preoccupied with opposite sex?	1. True/2. Partly true/3. False/4. Doubtful
Girl/Boy crazy?	1. True/2. Partly true/3. False/4. Doubtful
Timid?	1. True/2. Partly true/3. False/4. Doubtful

16. The presence of the opposite sex of pupils in my school was
1. Liked very much/2. Liked/3. Tolerated/4. Disliked/5. Disliked intensely.

20. Do you consider that the influence of the girls on the boys in this school was, in general,
1. Very good/2. Good/3. Fairly good/4. No effect/5. Bad/6. Very bad
Please comment ....
....
....

21. Do you consider that the influence of the boys on the girls in this school was, in general,
1. Very good/2. Good/3. Fairly good/4. No effect/5. Bad/6. Very bad?
Please comment ....
....

22. Do you think that the school's concern with the out-of-school conduct of the pupils was
1. Excessive/2. Rather strict/3. Just right/4. Rather insufficient/5. Much too lax?

Comment if you wish..
....

23. WOMEN ONLY
Do you think that the girls in your form, considered as a whole, were
1. Spiteful/2. A little spiteful/3. Neutral/4. Rather nice/5. Very nice?

Comment if you wish..
....

24. WOMEN ONLY
Did the other girls in your form quarrel
1. Very often/2. Fairly often/3. Sometimes/4. Seldom/5. Never?

25. WOMEN ONLY
In your co-educational school would you say that a group or groups of girls 'made life unpleasant' for some girls (or girl)
1. Very frequently/2. Frequently/3. Not so frequently/4. Infrequently/5. Not at all?

Please comment ....
....

26. MEN ONLY
In your co-educational school would you say bullying by boys occurred
1. Very frequently/2. Frequently/3. Not so frequently/4. Infrequently/5. Not at all?

Please comment ....
....

WOMEN STUDENTS ONLY

A. In your co-educational school would you say bullying of girls by girls occurred
1. Not at all/2. Infrequently/3. Not so frequently/4. Frequently/5. Very frequently?

Comment if you wish..
....
....

Your single-sex school

If you attended more than one single-sex secondary school (apart from secondary modern) please give answers for each of these schools and distinguish between them by numbering each answer, (1) for the first single-sex school you attended and (2) for the second. Please give these numbers even where the answer is the same for both schools.

[The questions under this heading were exactly the same as for the co-educational school except when not applicable.]

WOMEN AND MEN STUDENTS

48. Which did you prefer, the mixed or single-sex school?
Single-sex school much/Single-sex school a little/No preference/
Mixed school a little/Mixed school much.
State the most important reason for your preference:
....
....
....

49. Has your study and experience in your training for the teaching profession changed your opinion about co-educational secondary schools? *Underline* which statement applies:
Made no change.
Strengthened preference for single-sex secondary schools.
Strengthened preference for co-educational secondary schools.
Changed my preference from co-educational to single-sex secondary schools.
Changed my preference from single-sex to co-educational secondary schools.
Comment if you wish ....
....

50. In which school do you consider the pupils had the healthier attitude towards sex?
Doubtful/Don't know/Single-sex school/Co-educational school
Comment if you wish ....
....
....

[SCHOOLS PROJECT]

Age...   Sex...Boy/Girl (Please tick)

Name of school.. Date...............
Please answer the following questions according to the instruction given. *Do not* write your name on this sheet. Your answers will be kept strictly private, so please be *completely frank and truthful.*

Here is a list of statements about school. Underneath each statement is a list of opinions. Underline the opinion with which you agree.

6. Altogether my life at school is:
   1. Happy/2. Fairly happy/3. Jogging along/4. Rather unhappy/5. Unhappy.
   Please comment ....
   ....

ALL QUESTIONS ON THIS PAGE ARE TO BE ANSWERED BY 'GIRLS ONLY'
Here are some statements about boys of your own age. *Underline* the opinion which in general is true for you.

26. Boys are much too noisy.
    1. Agree strongly/2. Agree/3. Doubtful/4. Disagree/5. Disagree strongly
27. Boys cannot be trusted.
    1. Agree strongly/2. Agree/3. Doubtful/4. Disagree/5. Disagree strongly
28. Boys are unpleasant.
    1. Agree strongly/2. Agree/3. Doubtful/4. Disagree/5. Disagree strongly
29. Boys are nicer than girls.
    1. Agree strongly/2. Agree/3. Doubtful/4. Disagree/5. Disagree strongly
30. Boys are cleverer than girls in school work.
    1. Agree strongly/2. Agree/3. Doubtful/4. Disagree/5. Disagree strongly
31. Boys are better leaders than girls.
    1. Agree strongly/2. Agree/3. Doubtful/4. Disagree/5. Disagree strongly
32. Boys are not as catty as girls.
    1. Agree strongly/2. Agree/3. Doubtful/4. Disagree/5. Disagree strongly
33. Boys are braver than girls.
    1. Agree strongly/2. Agree/3. Doubtful/4. Disagree/5. Disagree strongly

34. Boys are cruel.
1. Agree strongly/2. Agree/3. Doubtful/4. Disagree/5. Disagree strongly

35. Boys are interested in the wrong things.
1. Agree strongly/2. Agree/3. Doubtful/4. Disagree/5. Disagree strongly

36. I would prefer to be a boy.
1. Agree strongly/2. Agree/3. Doubtful/4. Disagree/5. Disagree strongly

38. When I meet boys at a party I don't know what to say.
1. Very true/2. Often true/3. Sometimes true/4. Seldom true/5. Not true

Please comment ....
....

39. I feel very awkward whenever I am with boys.
1. Very true/2. Often true/3. Sometimes true/4. Seldom true/5. Not true

40. I feel perfectly at ease when talking with boys.
1. Very true/2. Often true/3. Sometimes true/4. Seldom true/5. Not true

41. I prefer talking to boys rather than to girls.
1. Very true/2. Often true/3. Sometimes true/4. Seldom true/5. Not true

Please comment ....
....

FOR ALL PUPILS

Which of the following words *best* fits your school life? Try to choose one of the first two alternatives, even if it doesn't fit exactly. Use 'neither' only as a last resort.

45. 1. lively/2. dull/3. neither

46. 1. variety/2. monotony/3. neither

47. 1. enthusiasm/2. apathy/3. neither

48. 1. kindness/2. unpleasantness/3. neither

49. 1. friendly individuals/2. cliques or gangs/3. neither

ALL QUESTIONS ON THIS PAGE ARE TO BE ANSWERED BY 'BOYS ONLY'

Here are some statements about girls of your own age. *Underline* the opinion with which you agree.

61. Girls are nicer than boys.
1. Agree strongly/2. Agree/3. Doubtful/4. Disagree/5. Disagree strongly
62. Girls are catty and spiteful.
1. Agree strongly/2. Agree/3. Doubtful/4. Disagree/5. Disagree strongly
63. Girls cannot be trusted.
1. Agree strongly/2. Agree/3. Doubtful/4. Disagree/5. Disagree strongly
64. Girls are kinder than boys.
1. Agree strongly/2. Agree/3. Doubtful/4. Disagree/5. Disagree strongly
65. Girls are interested in unimportant things.
1. Agree strongly/2. Agree/3. Doubtful/4. Disagree/5. Disagree strongly
66. Girls are boring.
1. Agree strongly/2. Agree/3. Doubtful/4. Disagree/5. Disagree strongly
67. Girls are cleverer than boys in school work.
1. Agree strongly/2. Agree/3. Doubtful/4. Disagree/5. Disagree strongly
68. Girls giggle and talk too much.
1. Agree strongly/2. Agree/3. Doubtful/4. Disagree/5. Disagree strongly
69. Girls are more sensible than boys.
1. Agree strongly/2. Agree/3. Doubtful/4. Disagree/5. Disagree strongly
70. I would prefer to be a girl.
1. Agree strongly/2. Agree/3. Doubtful/4. Disagree/5. Disagree strongly
71. Girls do not bully each other as much as boys do.
1. Agree strongly/2. Agree/3. Doubtful/4. Disagree/5. Disagree strongly.
Please comment ....
....

[Questions 72 to 75 were the same as Questions 38 to 41, but with 'girls' inserted instead of 'boys' and vice versa.]

FOR ALL PUPILS

93. I look forward to coming to school each day.
1. Agree strongly/2. Agree/3. Doubtful/4. Disagree/5. Disagree strongly

94. Apart from employment do you think your school prepares you sufficiently for the adult world?
1. Agree strongly/2. Agree/3. Doubtful/4. Disagree/5. Disagree strongly

96. Do you find the other pupils, in general,
1. Very friendly/2. Friendly/3. Indifferent/4. Unfriendly/5. Very unfriendly?

97. Do you consider that the atmosphere of the school is
1. Very pleasant/2. Pleasant/3. Neutral/4. Rather unpleasant/5. Very unpleasant?

[SCHOOLS PROJECT]

'Check Questionnaire'

Name of school .... Grammar/High School
Occupation of Father or Guardian (former occupation if unemployed or deceased). Please give this as fully as you can, e.g. not merely MINER but *Miner-Deputy* or *Cutter*; not ENGINEER but *Maintenance Engineer* or *Graduate Engineer*; not MANAGER but *Manager of small shop*; not FARMER but *Tenant Farmer* or *Smallholder*; not just CIVIL SERVANT but *Civil Servant-Clerk* or *Executive*; not just FACTORY WORKER but *Fitter*, or *Works Labourer*, or *Machine Operator*
OCCUPATION..
Please answer the following questions according to the instructions given.
Do not write your name on this sheet. Your answers will be kept strictly private, so please be *completely frank and truthful.*
Read the following items and *underline* the answer which is true for you.

3. I look forward to coming to school each day.
1. Agree strongly/2. Agree/3. Doubtful/4. Disagree/5. Disagree strongly

4. Do you find the other pupils, in general,
1. Very friendly/2. Friendly/3. Indifferent/4. Unfriendly/5. Very unfriendly?

5. Do you consider that the atmosphere of the school is
1. Very pleasant/2. Pleasant/3. Neutral/4. Rather unpleasant/5. Very unpleasant?

6. Altogether my life at school is:
1. Happy/2. Fairly happy/3. Jogging along/4. Rather unhappy/5. Unhappy

Which of the following words best fits your school life? Try to choose one of the first two alternatives, even if it doesn't fit exactly. Use 'neither' only as a last resort.

11. 1. lively/2. dull/3. neither
12. 1. variety/2. monotony/3. neither
13. 1. kindness/2. unpleasantness/3. neither
14. 1. friendly individuals/2. cliques or gangs/3. neither

Modified Boxall Anxiety Test[1]

Here is a list of statements. *Underline* either 'YES' or 'NO' for each one according to whether or not it is true for you. Answer *all* the questions.

ALL ABOUT SCHOOL

1. I feel all funny inside if I have to stand up and speak in front of the class. YES/NO
2. I get very worried if I see a new kind of sum on the blackboard and I do not know how to do it. YES/NO
3. It worries me if some of my sums are wrong. YES/NO
4. My teacher makes me frightened when he or she is cross with the class. YES/NO
5. At home I often worry about school. YES/NO
6. I am very worried if I promise to bring to school a book and then forget. YES/NO
7. I dread making a mistake when reading aloud to the class. YES/NO
8. I don't like other children to know if I get a bad mark for arithmetic. YES/NO
9. I do not like having new teachers. YES/NO
10. Shivers go up and down my spine if I hear that a child in school is to be severely punished. YES/NO
11. I feel so awful if I haven't got gym shoes for P.T. lessons. YES/NO
12. I go all hot and cold inside if I think that I am late for school. YES/NO
13. I dread the thought of my parents coming and talking to my teacher. YES/NO

[1] Revised by the writer.

14. I should hate to go into a new class with strange children. YES/NO
15. I am miserable if my teacher grumbles at me. YES/NO
16. I dread the thought of examinations. YES/NO
17. I hate it if my teacher looks over my shoulder while I am writing. YES/NO
18. I dread having to see the school doctor. YES/NO
19. I get all dithery and muddled if my mathematics teacher asks sudden questions. YES/NO
20. I hate having to go back to school when I have been away. YES/NO
21. I think that coming back to school after the holidays is frightening. YES/NO
22. I am sure that I would go white if I got a message that I am to go to see the headmaster/headmistress. YES/NO
23. Sometimes I have horrid dreams about school. YES/NO

Appendix 2

Some additional tables

TABLE A.1 *Occupational Class composition of the longitudinal sample*

Schools project

		Occupational class of pupils' parent											
		1		2		3		4		5		Totals*	
		N	%	N	%	N	%	N	%	N	%	N	%
Girls aged 11+ and 13+	Co-ed. schools	32	14·9	60	27·9	80	37·2	33	15·3	10	4·7	215	100
	Girls' schools	37	17·0	59	27·0	90	41·2	23	10·6	6	2·8	218	100
Girls aged 15+ and 17+	Co-ed. schools	24	20·9	37	32·2	39	33·9	12	10·4	3	2·6	115	100
	Girls' schools	28	23·1	33	27·3	41	34·0	9	7·4	9	7·4	121	100
Boys aged 11+ and 13+	Co-ed. schools	28	12·4	57	25·2	106	47·0	22	9·7	12	5·3	226	100
	Boys' schools	27	12·3	78	35·5	88	39·9	16	7·3	8	3·6	220	100
Boys aged 15+ and 17+	Co-ed. schools	20	14·9	36	26·9	60	44·8	10	7·5	7	5·2	134	100
	Boys' schools	31	22·6	39	28·5	52	37·9	12	8·8	3	2·2	137	100

* Includes a few unclassifiable. The analysis is based on occupations and follows the classification used in the Early Leaving Report, viz.: Class 1 Professional, managerial, executive; Class 2 Clerical occupations; Class 3 Skilled occupations; Class 4 Partly skilled; Class 5 Unskilled.

TABLE A.2 *Average intelligence scores (H.S.P.Q. 'B' Factor)*

Schools project longitudinal sample (maximum 10)

		Co-educational schools		Single-sex schools	
		N	Mean	N	Mean
1964					
Boys aged	11+	226	7·23	220	7·23
	15+	134	8·15	137	8·19
Girls aged	11+	215	7·11	218	7·27
	15+	115	8·24	121	8·27
1966					
Boys aged	13+	226	7·55	220	7·56
	17+	134	8·39	137	8·33
Girls aged	13+	215	7·38	218	7·80
	17+	115	8·44	121	8·56

NOTE: The co-educated girls have a lower score than those from girls' schools at all four ages: one of these differences (at 15 plus) can obviously be dismissed but that at 13 plus is statistically significant.

TABLE A.3 *Happiness of female ex-pupils (first schools): Analysis by parental occupational class*

'Both schools' survey

Estimates of happiness in school	Replies about first co-educational schools						Replies about first girls' schools					
	Occupational classes						Occupational classes					
	1		2		3, 4, 5		1		2		3, 4, 5	
	N	%	N	%	N	%	N	%	N	%	N	%
Very happy	76	49·7	39	63·0	45	56·3	49	21·9	24	29·6	28	28·0
Fairly happy	55	35·9	18	29·0	24	30·0	85	38·0	32	39·5	35	36·1
Jogging along	10	6·5	2	3·2	5	6·2	46	20·5	15	18·5	17	17·5
Rather unhappy	11	7·2	2	3·2	6	7·5	39	17·4	8	9·9	16	16·5
Very unhappy	1	0·7	1	1·6	0	0	5	2·2	2	2·5	1	1·0
Totals	153	100	62	100	80	100	224	100	81	100	97	100

TABLE A.4 *Happiness of female ex-pupils (last schools): Analysis by parental occupational class*

'Both schools' survey

Estimates of happiness in school	Replies about last co-educational schools						Replies about last girls' schools					
	Occupational classes						Occupational classes					
	1		2		3, 4, 5		1		2		3, 4, 5	
	N	%	N	%	N	%	N	%	N	%	N	%
Very happy	118	60·2	37	50·0	40	45·5	34	27·2	13	22·8	20	28·0
Fairly happy	60	30·6	28	37·8	38	43·2	37	29·6	25	43·8	30	40·0
Jogging along	11	5·6	5	6·8	4	4·5	27	21·6	14	24·6	12	16·0
Rather unhappy	6	3·1	4	5·4	5	5·7	24	19·2	5	8·8	11	14·7
Very unhappy	1	0·5	0	0	1	1·1	3	2·4	0	0	1	1·3
Totals	196	100	74	100	88	100	125	100	57	100	74	100

TABLE A.5 *Pupil happiness and school situation (females): Analysis by first and last school and occupational class*

'Both schools' survey

Happiness estimates of those who agree strongly on pleasant situation of school	Replies about first schools												Replies about last schools											
	Co-educational						Girls'						Co-educational						Girls'					
	Occupational classes						Occupational classes						Occupational classes						Occupational classes					
	1 and 2		3, 4, 5		All*		1 and 2		3, 4, 5		All*		1 and 2		3, 4, 5		All*		1 and 2		3, 4, 5		All*	
	N	%	N	%	N	%	N	%	N	%	N	%	N	%	N	%	N	%	N	%	N	%	N	%
Very happy	40	59·7	15	62·6	56	60·9	32	39·0	12	44·5	44	40·0	64	68·0	22	59·5	86	65·2	21	36·8	9	37·5	30	36·6
Fairly happy	24	35·8	5	20·8	29	31·5	29	35·4	11	40·7	40	36·4	28	29·8	10	27·0	38	28·8	21	36·8	10	41·7	31	37·8
Jogging along	0	0	2	8·3	2	2·2	12	14·6	2	7·4	14	12·7	1	1·1	2	5·4	4	3·0	11	19·3	2	8·3	14	17·1
Rather unhappy	3	4·5	2	8·3	5	5·4	9	11·0	1	3·7	10	9·1	1	1·1	3	8·1	4	3·0	3	5·3	3	12·5	6	7·3
Very unhappy	0	0	0	0	0	0	0	0	1	3·7	2	1·8	0	0	0	0	0	0	1	1·8	0	0	1	1·2
Totals*	67	100	24	100	92	100	82	100	27	100	110	100	94	100	37	100	132	100	57	100	24	100	82	100

* Includes a few unclassifiables. Those percentages which are based on small numbers are liable to large fluctuations.

TABLE A.6 *Pupil happiness and school situation (females): Analysis by first and last schools**

'Both schools' survey

Estimates of happiness in school	Replies about first schools												Replies about last schools											
	Co-educational						Girls'						Co-educational						Girls'					
	Pleasant school situation						Pleasant school situation						Pleasant school situation						Pleasant school situation					
	Agree		Doubtful		Disagree†		Agree		Doubtful		Disagree		Agree		Doubtful		Disagree		Agree		Doubtful		Disagree	
	N	%	N	%	N	%	N	%	N	%	N	%	N	%	N	%	N	%	N	%	N	%	N	%
Very happy	74	55·3	20	46·5	13	44·9	34	20·6	18	28·1	5	7·7	81	48·2	21	53·8	7	33·3	30	24·2	3	12·0	5	17·9
Fairly happy	42	31·3	14	32·6	12	41·4	74	44·9	17	26·6	22	33·8	66	39·3	12	30·8	11	52·4	47	38·0	9	36·0	5	17·9
Jogging along	9	6·7	5	11·6	1	3·4	32	19·4	15	23·4	17	26·2	13	7·7	3	7·7	1	4·8	23	18·5	8	32·0	9	32·1
Rather unhappy	9	6·7	3	7·0	2	6·9	23	13·9	14	21·9	16	24·6	6	3·6	3	7·7	2	9·5	23	18·5	5	20·0	7	25·0
Very unhappy	0	0	1	2·3	1	3·4	2	1·2	0	0	5	7·7	2	1·2	0	0	0	0	1	0·8	0	0	2	7·1
Totals	134	100	43	100	29	100	165	100	64	100	65	100	168	100	39	100	21	100	124	100	25	100	28	100

* The social class analysis is not given as the data showed no consistent trend.
† Combines 'Disagree' with 'Disagree strongly'.

TABLE A.7 *Happiness in school (girls)*

Schools project (longitudinal)

Estimates of happiness in school	Replies from 11 plus girls				Replies from 13 plus girls			
	Co-educational schools		Girls' schools		Co-educational schools		Girls' schools	
	N	%	N	%	N	%	N	%
Happy	129	60·0	116	53·9	102	47·7	103	47·9
Fairly happy	69	32·1	74	34·4	82	38·3	77	35·8
Jogging along	14	6·5	18	8·4	24	11·2	23	10·7
Rather unhappy	3	1·4	6	2·8	6	2·8	7	3·3
Unhappy	0	0	1	0·5	0	0	5	2·3
Totals	215	100	215	100	214	100	215	100

TABLE A.8 *Happiness in school (boys)*

Schools project (longitudinal)

Estimates of happiness in school	Replies from 11 plus boys				Replies from 13 plus boys			
	Co-educational schools		Boys' schools		Co-educational schools		Boys' schools	
	N	%	N	%	N	%	N	%
Happy	110	48·9	83	38·2	96	42·6	72	33·3
Fairly happy	88	39·1	98	45·1	90	40·0	98	45·4
Jogging along	24	10·7	29	13·4	35	15·6	38	17·6
Rather unhappy	2	0·9	6	2·8	2	0·9	7	3·2
Unhappy	1	0·4	1	0·5	2	0·9	1	0·5
Totals	225	100	217	100	225	100	216	100

TABLE A.9 *Happiness in school (girls)*

Schools project (longitudinal)

Estimates of happiness in school	Replies from 15 plus girls				Replies from 17 plus girls			
	Co-educational schools		Girls' schools		Co-educational schools		Girls' schools	
	N	%	N	%	N	%	N	%
Happy	63	54·7	63	52·5	61	53·0	48	40·0
Fairly happy	41	35·7	37	30·8	34	29·6	48	40·0
Jogging along	8	7·0	17	14·2	16	13·9	22	18·3
Rather unhappy	3	2·6	2	1·7	4	3·5	2	1·7
Unhappy	0	0	1	0·8	0	0	0	0
Totals	115	100	120	100	115	100	120	100

TABLE A.10 *Happiness in school (boys)*

Schools project (longitudinal)

Estimates of happiness in school	Replies from 15 plus boys				Replies from 17 plus boys			
	Co-educational schools		Boys' schools		Co-educational schools		Boys' schools	
	N	%	N	%	N	%	N	%
Happy	64	48·2	59	43·1	44	33·0	61	44·5
Fairly happy	48	36·1	58	42·3	62	46·7	56	40·9
Jogging along	16	12·0	18	13·1	20	15·0	17	12·4
Rather unhappy	4	3·0	2	1·5	6	4·5	2	1·5
Unhappy	1	0·7	0	0	1	0·8	1	0·7
Totals	133	100	137	100	133	100	137	100

TABLE A.11 *Look forward to coming to school (girls aged 13 plus)*

'Check' questionnaire

	Replies from girls in			
	Co-educational schools		Girls' schools	
	N	%	N	%
Agree strongly	33	7·3	34	5·1
Agree	219	48·9	305	45·3
Doubtful	153	34·1	251	37·3
Disagree	33	7·3	72	10·7
Disagree strongly	11	2·4	11	1·6
Totals	449	100	673	100

TABLE A.12 *Look forward to coming to school (boys' responses)*

Schools project (1966)

Estimate	Comment	Co-educational schools	Boys' schools
Agree	*School*		
and	like school much, enjoy, fun	31	25
Agree	like usually, on the whole	18	13
strongly	useful, essential	1	10
	variety of school life	8	1
	boring at home, school better	7	6
	Pupils		
	for friendships	12	11
	Teachers and teaching		
	friendly teachers, good	5	3
	like school work	7	6
	depends on teachers, lessons	6	5
	Personal		
	but don't like getting up		3
	sometimes get very tired	1	1
	but prefer other pastimes		2
	others		3
Totals		96	89
Doubtful	doubtful in general	6	11
	doubtful sometimes	14	13
	depends which day, teacher	12	9
	only useful	2	3
	all right when I get there	7	4
	monotonous, routine, boring	7	6
	no choice		4
	worry about homework, tests	3	
	prefer earn money, do other things	8	5
	dislike getting up, too early	13	7
	others	2	6
Totals		74	68

TABLE A.12 (*continued*) *Look forward to coming to school* (*boys' responses*)

Estimate	Comment	Co-educational schools	Boys' schools
Disagree and Disagree strongly	*School*		
	hate it, depressing, dread it	2	8
	sometimes hate it	3	
	dislike school	18	21
	dislike but necessary	4	5
	but don't hate, dislike	5	5
	but enjoy when there	2	
	not normal to look forward to it		1
	Teachers and teaching		
	too boring	7	15
	dislike some teachers	7	8
	depends on the day, teachers	10	9
	dislike tests, homework, examinations		4
	depends if homework done, right	1	2
	depends on mood, weather	2	
	disliked by teachers		1
	Activities		
	prefer leisure activities, games, home	10	3
	Personal		
	dislike getting up early	17	19
	sometimes too tired	2	
	Work		
	rather be working		3
	others	6	11
Totals		96	115

TABLE Å.13 'Unhappy' girls—classification of free responses: Schools project

	Number of pupils		Teachers'† discipline	Working pupils too hard	General† dislike of school	Work difficulties	Trouble with classmates	General anxiety	Out-of-school or home difficulties
Girls aged 13 plus									
Co-educated	6	Unfavourable	−4	−1	−5	−13	−4	0	−9
		Favourable	+2	0	0	+1	0	0	0
in girls' schools	12	Unfavourable	−28	−4	−22	−14	−7	−7	−4
		Favourable	+7	0	+1	0	0	0	0
Girls aged 15 plus									
Co-educated	10	Unfavourable	0	0	−3	−8	−2	−3	−24
		Favourable	0	0	0	0	0	0	0
in girls' schools	13	Unfavourable	−5	−1	−11	−9	0	−3	−15
		Favourable	0	0	0	0	0	0	0
Combined co-ed. girls	16	Unfavourable	−4	−1	−8	−21	−6	−3	−33
		Favourable	+2	0	0	+1	0	0	0
		Balance	−2	−1	−8	**−20**	−6	−3	**−33**
Combined girls in girls' schools	25	Unfavourable	−33	−5	−33	−23	−7	−10	−19
		Favourable	+7	0	+1	0	0	0	0
		Balance	**−26**	−5	**−32**	**−23**	−7	**−10**	**−19**

NOTE: The principal reasons given for unhappiness are heavily underlined to facilitate the contrast for the two types of school. The smaller numbers are recorded merely to complete the table. Though the scoring system is arbitrary it should be fair enough for the comparison of the two groups, but it should be noted that the contrasted groups are unequal in numbers.

* Teachers' discipline is scored minus if there is trouble or dislike evident, or if school rules are mentioned as irksome or irritating. Under general dislike are scored boredom with school (−1) and hatred of school or similar phrase (−2). 'Work difficulties' comprises difficulty in studying or understanding, or if, in the Mooney special problem response, dislike of a particular subject is expressed. Those comments showing a general anxiety not traceable to problems at home or school are placed under 'anxiety'. Out-of-school or home difficulties includes trouble about boy-friends. Of the 15-year-old girls two from girls' schools and one from a co-educational school made no comment; they were omitted in calculating the averages. In the table heading, 'unhappy' includes those who said 'rather unhappy'.

† A follow-up test after analysis of variance shows that the difference between the scores of the girls at co-educational schools and those at single-sex schools, for teachers' discipline and dislike of schoo combined, is statistically significant beyond the ·01 level.

TABLE A.14 *Average scores of 'unhappy' and 'rather unhappy' girls*

	Number of pupils	Bristol Social Adjust. Guide	High School Personality Questionnaire				Maudsley		Mooney
			Anxiety*	Factor H† 0–20	Factor O‡ 0–20	Intelligence 0–10	Neurot. 0–48	Extrov. 0–48	Problems (210 possible)
Co-ed. 15 plus	6	10·3	66·8	4·5	14·6	7·2	37·1	23·8	43·3
Single-sex 15 plus	12	9·0	77·7	6·2	15·5	8·1	39·4	36·3	43·5
							H.S.P.Q. 4–40	H.S.P.Q. 7–70	
Co-ed. 13 plus	11	Not given	74·5	4·2	14·3	7·0	21·1	27·5	42·0
Single-sex 13 plus	15	Not given	72·3	5·5	14·4	7·6	22·0	32·8	54·7

* Possible range not given (10 extremely low and 100 extremely high).

† Factor H: Low scoring indicates a person who is withdrawn, retiring in face of opposite sex, aloof, conscientious, considerate and danger-sensitive as opposed to adventurous, likes meeting people, overt interest in opposite sex, genial, frivolous, carefree. It is interesting to note the slight signs of possible differences between 'unhappy' girls in co-educational and girls' schools, but the fewness of the numbers and shortness of the test make statistical analysis unwise. All four groups score below the average for their main groups, the co-educational more so than the others.

‡ Factor O: Low scoring indicates *self-confidence*, cheerfulness, rudely vigorous, no fears, as opposed to worrying, depressed, sensitive, strong sense of duty, *insecure*. Here also the four groups score above the average for their main groups, i.e. in the direction of greater insecurity, etc.

TABLE A.15 *Test scores: unhappy girls in co-educational schools (aged 15 plus in 1964)*

Occupational class	Code No.	Intelligence score	Extroversion–introversion (Maudsley)	Neuroticism (Maudsley)	Mooney Problem Check-list	Anxiety (H.S.P.Q.)	Factors H and O (H.S.P.Q.)	Bristol score (teacher's)
3	1	10	25 Normal	41 High	31 Fairly high	82 High	Withdrawn and insecure	9
1	2	9	31 Normal	26 Normal	31 Fairly high	66	Active, social	21 Maladjusted
2	3	9	38 Fairly high	24 Fairly low	5 Very low	41 Low	Active, social	4
1	4	9	32 Normal	44 High	61 High	80 High	A little shy, insecure	6
3	5	9	11 Introverted (low)	47 High	50 High	84 High	Shy and rather insecure	6
2	6	6	30 Normal	19 Low	18 Normal	49	Active, social	None given
4	7	6	8 Low (introverted)	44 High	40 High	72 High	Shy, withdrawn	0
4	8	6	16 Low (introverted)	42 High	39 Fairly high	59	Rather shy	15 Unsettled
3	9	6	29 Normal	44 High	82 Very high	56	Timid	18 Unsettled
3	10	5	32 Normal	33 Normal	36 Fairly high	73 High	Some bitterness, not shy	13 Unsettled
3	11	4	10 Introverted (low)	44 High	83 Very high	73 High	Extremely shy and insecure	11 Unsettled

TABLE A.16 *Test scores: unhappy girls in girls' schools (aged 15 plus in 1964)*

Occupational class	Code No.	Intelligence score	Extroversion–introversion (Maudsley)	Neuroticism (Maudsley)	Mooney Problem Check-list	Anxiety (H.S.P.Q.)	Factors H and O (H.S.P.Q.)	Bristol score (teacher's)
2	1	10	40 High	36 Normal	49 High	74 High	Rather shy	8
5	2	9	33 Normal	36 Normal	47 High	82 High	Rather shy, insecure, depressed	15 Unsettled
4	3	9	24 Normal	44 High	32 Fairly high	78 High	Shy and timid, insecure	8
2	4	9	46 High	44 High	68 Very high	76 High	Fairly normal	17 Unsettled
3	5	9	36 Normal to High	46 High	81 Very high	80 High	Very timid, shy, insecure	2
1	6	9	46 High	46 High	23 Not high	66	Active, friendly	10 Unsettled
2	7	8	33 Normal	44 High	70 Very high	88 Very high	Not shy or timid, insecure	19 Unsettled
1	8	8	44 High	26 Normal	15 Low	82 High	Shy, rather insecure, depressed	5
2	9	8	39 High	43 High	44 High	84 High	Rather shy	3
1	10	8	34 Normal	45 High	62 High	80 High	Shy, timid	7
3	11	7	44 High	32 Normal	41 High	82 High	Not shy or timid, insecure, depressed	17 Unsettled
2	12	7	33 Normal	46 High	21 Not high	64	Friendly, impulsive, little insecure	6
5	13	7	26 Normal	36 Normal	19 Average	64	Rather confident	5
2	14	7	40 High	32 Normal	50 High	81 High	Not shy or timid, a little insecure	9
3	15	6	27 Normal	35 Normal	30	84 High	Not shy, rather insecure	10 Unsettled

TABLE A.17 *Test scores: unhappy girls in co-educational schools (aged 13 plus in 1966)*

Code No.	Occupational class	Intelligence score	Extroversion (H.S.P.Q.)*	Neuroticism (H.S.P.Q.)*	Anxiety (H.S.P.Q.)	Factors H and O (H.S.P.Q.)	Mooney Problem Check-list	No. of school problems	% school problems to whole	Looks forward to coming to school	Pressure of work worries me
1	2	9	26 Fairly low	20·7	87 Very high	Rather shy and unsettled	37	8	22	Disagree	Agree strongly
2	3	7	21 Low	21·8	78 High	Shy	77	17	22	Doubtful	Agree strongly
3	3	7	37 Normal	18·2	62	A little shy	86	22	26	Disagree strongly	Agree strongly
4	4	7	30 Normal to low	24·4	74 High	A little shy and insecure	26	15	58	Disagree strongly	Agree strongly
5	2	6	25 Fairly low	15·2 Fairly low	62	Shy and insecure	9	3	33	Disagree strongly	Agree strongly
6	2	6	26 Fairly low	26·4	84 High	A little shy	15	5	33	Agree	Disagree strongly

* Note that the tests on extroversion and introversion are different for the two age groups (15 plus and 13 plus).

TABLE A.18 *Test scores: unhappy girls in girls' schools (aged 13 plus in 1966)*

Code No.	Occupational class	Intelligence score	Extroversion (H.S.P.Q.)	Neuroticism (H.S.P.Q.)	Anxiety (H.S.P.Q.)	Factors H and O (H.S.P.Q.)	Mooney Problem Check-list	No. of school problems	% school problems to whole	Looks forward to coming to school	Pressure of work worries me
1	3	10	20 Fairly low	27·7	67 High	Shy	89	15	17	Disagree strongly	Agree strongly
2	2	9	18 Low	27·0	80 High	Withdrawn and rather insecure	92	20	22	Disagree strongly	Agree
3	3	8	26 Fairly low	23·6	86 Very high	Very shy	59	11	19	Disagree strongly	Agree
4	1	8	27 Fairly low	23·6	86 Very high	A little shy and insecure	26	7	27	Doubtful	Agree strongly
5	2	8	22 Low	29·4 Rather high	74 High	Very shy	95	19	20	Doubtful	Agree strongly
6	3	8	42 Normal	21·5	75 High	Average socially, insecure	26	14	54	Disagree	Agree strongly
7	3	8	28 Fairly low	22·9	79 High	Rather insecure	97	11	11	Disagree strongly	Doubtful
8	5	7	53 High	12·5 Low	65	Active, social	21	9	43	Disagree strongly	Disagree
9	4	7	41 Normal	21·8	58	Average socially	34	10	29	Disagree	Agree
10	4	6	31 Normal	22·4	64	Average socially a little insecure	38	9	24	Doubtful	Agree
11	3	6	33 Normal	16 Fairly low	60	Average socially	53	8	15	Disagree strongly	Agree strongly
12	3	6	37 Normal	15·4 Fairly low	74 High	Rather timid and insecure	26	17	65	Disagree strongly	Agree strongly

TABLE A.19 *School's control of out-of-school conduct*

(*Women's responses, 'Both schools' survey*)

Estimate	Comment	Co-educational schools	Girls' schools
Excessive			2
	because boarding	2	6
	school image too important	4	8
	no talking to boys, parties, etc.		8
	no boy/girl friendships	2	5
	too much interference, out of date petty rules, eating in streets, hats, cafés	6	21
	severe punishment		2
	staff, heads too nosey		3
	others		2
Totals		14	57
Rather strict		8	4
	too much stress image	5	8
	concern about public opinion		7
	hats, cafés, weekends, evenings, Saturday jobs, eating in streets, too much interference	10	23
	when in uniform, buses	9	18
	on smoking, drinking, swearing	1	
	head too strict	7	
	boy/girl relationships	2	
	too concerned private life	2	2
	no talking to boys		3
	strict but necessary	16	7
	but ineffective	1	2
	others	7	5
Totals		68	79

TABLE A.19 (*continued*) *School's control of out-of-school conduct*

Estimate	Comment	Co-educational schools	Girls' schools
Just right		16	6
	correct stress reputation of school	14	
	when in uniform, to and from school	20	
	sufficient interest, when necessary	23	7
	good behaviour stressed	17	5
	strict but necessary		3
	not dominated; few restrictions, interference	17	
	respect for school	3	3
	no boy/girl friendships	3	2
	out-of-school conduct good		3
	staff not interested		5
	others	10	2
Totals		123	36
Rather insufficient		8	
	only concerned re school reputation	4	
	few rules	3	
	wrong concern—hats, etc.		1
	staff took no interest	11	11
	staff attempts ineffectual	9	4
	head weak, not strict	3	
	rowdy behaviour buses	8	
	only on buses		1
	school poor reputation	2	
	homes too scattered	7	
	but not needed	1	1
	others	7	5
Totals		63	23
Much too lax	poor behaviour in public	2	
	pupils bad discipline		2
	poor behaviour of boys	1	
	no interest unless complaints	13	7
	homes too dispersed	1	
Totals		17	9

TABLE A.20 *School preference: Amalgamated pupils versus the remainder of the 'co-educated last'*

'Both schools' survey

Preference	Men				Women			
	Normal co-educational		Amalgamated		Normal co-educational		Amalgamated	
	N	%	N	%	N	%	N	%
Single-sex school much	4	5·5	3	(13)	24	9·5	6	6·7
Single-sex school a little	3	4·1	2	(8)	14	5·5	3	3·3
No preference	5	6·8	2	(8)	8	3·2	11	12·2
Mixed school a little	4	5·5	2	(8)	27	10·7	16	17·8
Mixed school much	57	78·1	15	(62)	179	71·1	54	60·0
Totals	73	100	24	100	252	100	90	100

NOTE: The men from amalgamated schools were less in favour of mixed schools than the remainder (non significant): the women were also less in favour than the rest of the 'co-educated last' women (statistically significant).

TABLE A.21 *Attitude to girls pleasant or unpleasant (men's comments)*

'Both schools' survey

Estimate	Comment	Co-educational schools	Boys' schools
Pleasant		3	2
	good friendly relationship	21	
	taken for granted—normal interest	5	
	no experience of girls' company —immature		2
	mixed in class, but not out of it	2	
	opposite sex completely cut off		3
	travelled with and dated girls		5
	romantic relationship	4	
	interesting discussions	2	
	often wistfully pleasant		2
	sex talk but not unpleasant		1
	friendly rivalry with sister school		2
	young—shyness, avoidance	2	
	depends on individual	1	
	better with girls than boys	2	
Totals		42	17
Fairly pleasant			6
	good friendly relationship	7	
	romantic relationship	1	
	most boys sex-mad		3
	at first shy, avoidance	1	
	bawdy but not excessively		2
	little contact in school hours		2
	varied with age, too young	7	1
	depends on individual	2	
	better with girls than boys	1	
	but annoying distraction	1	
	better than single-sex school	1	
	others	1	3
Totals		22	17

TABLE A.21 (*continued*) *Attitude to girls pleasant and unpleasant (men's comments)*

Estimate	Comment	Co-educational schools	Boys' schools
Neutral		1	1
	good friendly relationship	1	
	opposite sex not discussed much		4
	taken for granted	1	
	unknown factor		5
	romantic relationship	1	
	did not bother with girls		4
	more mature as grew older	1	2
	occasionally smutty talk		1
	boys will talk of girls		1
	shy but interested	1	
	depends on individual	2	
	varied with age	2	
Totals		10	18
A little unpleasant			3
	only 11-year-olds—normal	2	1
	improved in VIth		3
	at first thought girls foolish	1	
	pupils 'sex starved'		2
	girls looked on purely from sex angle		8
	no positive attitude towards opposite sex		1
	crude conversation, unhealthy		5
	some boasting of sex experience, some depraved		3
	others	1	
Totals		4	26
Unpleasant	girls all right for sex, otherwise 'sissy'		1
	dirty and unhealthy		2
	scared of girls—immature		4
Totals		0	7

TABLE A.22 (*a*) *Normal interest in girls* and (*b*) *Boy–girl crazy*

'Both schools' survey (males)

Estimates of boys' attitudes to girls	Normal interest				Boy–girl crazy			
	Co-educational schools		Boys' schools		Co-educational schools		Boys' schools	
	N	%	N	%	N	%	N	%
True	138	78·0	74	43·8	7	4·0	25	14·1
Partly true	31	17·4	63	37·3	48	27·3	66	37·3
False	4	2·3	15	8·9	86	48·8	63	35·6
Doubtful	4	2·3	17	10·0	35	19·9	23	13·0
Totals	177	100	169	100	176	100	177	100

NOTE: The difference between the co-educational and boys' schools is statistically highly significant for 'normal interest' for both juniors and seniors, but that for 'girl–boy crazy' is only highly significant for the seniors. The differences between the juniors and seniors were surprisingly not very large but they were reversed in the two types of school, the estimates showing less boy–girl craziness in the senior than in the junior co-educational school. This Table omits the junior/senior breakdown.

TABLE A.23 (*a*) *Antagonistic and* (*b*) *Timid, with girls*

'Both schools' survey (males)

Estimates of boys' attitudes to girls	Replies 'Antagonistic'				Replies 'Timid'			
	Co-educational schools		Boys' schools		Co-educational schools		Boys' schools	
	N	%	N	%	N	%	N	%
True	4	2·3	4	2·3	1	0·6	17	9·8
Partly true	34	19·3	35	20·3	52	30·2	69	39·6
False	107	60·8	96	55·9	90	52·3	56	32·2
Doubtful	31	17·6	37	21·5	29	16·9	32	18·4
Totals	176	100	172	100	172	100	174	100

NOTE: The differences between the estimates for the co-educational and boys' schools are highly significant for juniors and seniors for timidity but not for antagonism.

TABLE A.24 *Attitude to boys pleasant or unpleasant (women's comments)*

'Both schools' survey

Estimate	Type of comment	Co-ed. school	Girls' school
Pleasant	good friendly relationship, normal	89	10
	friendly rivalry	7	
	interesting discussions	8	
	depends on individual boys, age, etc.	15	
	better with boys than girls	2	
	more natural than girls' school	8	
	romantic relationship	8	
	man-mad, boy-crazy	4	23
	boys novelties		12
	some discussed boys all day		5
	some girls showed off	2	
	boys adored by most		7
	more interested in boys than the co-ed.		2
	most had steady boy-friends		5
	boys' school near, mixed frequently		10
	some shy, especially young	3	3
	depended on morals		2
	others, e.g. 'pleasant'	16	8
Totals		162	87
Fairly pleasant	good friendly relationship, normal	29	4
	friendly rivalry	3	
	depended on the boy, age, etc.	21	
	interesting discussions	2	
	tendency to show off	5	
	romantic relationship	5	
	some shy, especially young	2	4
	attitude better in co-ed. school	2	
	boy-crazy groups		14
	boy-crazy individuals	3	
	silly, immature sometimes (because boys taboo)		9
	varied from boy-crazy to naturally interested		3
	good relationship with adjacent boys' school		6
	great excitement if male appeared		3
	mixed groups and boy-friends outside school		5
	too segregated to know		4
	others, e.g. 'fairly pleasant'	23	17
Totals		95	69

TABLE A.24 (*continued*) *Attitude to boys pleasant or unpleasant (women's comments)*

Estimate	Type of comment	Co-ed. school	Girls' school
Neutral	normal interest	12	
	interest increased with age	6	19
	annoying distraction	3	
	depends on individual		5
	enforced neutrality, little contact		13
	mild interest in near-by boys' school		2
	'boy-mad' usual with young girls, silly	3	5
	immature, boy-crazy compared with co-ed.		3
	a little in awe of boys, scared		3
	others	10	6
Totals		34	56
A little unpleasant	good friendly relationship	1	
	many girls boy-mad	1	11
	morbid obsession, unhealthy		5
	sex mad, main conversation		3
	many girls boasted about conquests		6
	boasting sexual experience		1
	exhibitionist, flirting, badly behaved		4
	some hysteria when boys visited school		3
	boys taboo, therefore idolized		2
	more rivalry over boys than co-ed.		1
	out of things if no boy-friends		4
	juniors giggled over boys		4
	frightened of them		4
	more unmarried mothers		2
	foul jokes		1
	others, e.g. a little unpleasant	6	10
Totals		8	61
Unpleasant	man-mad, idol worship	1	2
	sexual desire		2
	much giggling and talk about sex and boys, silly		4
Totals		1	8
No estimate	too young		2
	unnatural and unhealthy		1
	went mad when saw a male		2
	others	1	
Totals		1	5

TABLE A.25 (*a*) *Normal interest in boys and* (*b*) *Girl–boy crazy*

'Both schools' survey (females)

Estimates of girls' attitudes to boys	Normal interest				Girl–boy crazy			
	Co-educational schools		Girls' schools		Co-educational schools		Girls' schools	
	N	%	N	%	N	%	N	%
True	506	79·1	260	41·6	33	5·3	179	29·1
Partly true	112	17·5	246	39·4	163	26·3	260	42·1
False	9	1·4	57	9·1	322	52·1	119	19·2
Doubtful	13	2·0	62	9·9	101	16·3	59	9·6
Totals	640	100	625	100	619	100	617	100

NOTE: The difference between the distributions for co-educational and girls' schools is statistically very highly significant for 'normal interest' and for 'girl–boy crazy'. In neither type of school is there much difference between juniors and seniors.

TABLE A.26 (*a*) *Antagonistic and* (*b*) *Timid, with boys*

'Both schools' survey (females)

Girls' attitudes to boys	'Antagonistic'				'Timid'			
	Co-educational schools		Girls' schools		Co-educational schools		Girls' schools	
	N	%	N	%	N	%	N	%
True	9	1·5	11	1·8	14	2·3	84	14·0
Partly true	110	17·8	104	17·1	152	24·8	270	45·0
False	382	61·6	383	63·0	313	51·2	162	27·0
Doubtful	118	19·1	110	18·1	133	21·7	83	14·0
Totals	619	100	608	100	612	100	599	100

NOTE: The difference between the estimates for co-educational and girls' schools is statistically highly significant for 'timidity' for both juniors and seniors, but not for 'antagonism'.

TABLE A.27 *Sufficient preparation for adult world? (age 13 plus)*

Schools project—1966 estimates

Estimates of sufficiency of preparation for adult world	Replies from boys				Replies from girls			
	Co-ed. schools		Boys' schools		Co-ed. schools		Girls' schools	
	N	%	N	%	N	%	N	%
Agree strongly	24	10·8	15	7·0	19	8·9	21	9·9
Agree	127	57·2	119	55·7	113	52·8	101	47·4
Doubtful	46	20·7	48	22·4	55	25·7	49	23·0
Disagree	20	9·0	27	12·6	22	10·3	32	15·0
Disagree strongly	5	2·3	5	2·3	5	2·3	10	4·7
Totals	222	100	214	100	214	100	213	100

NOTE: The differences between co-educational and single-sex schools for both boys and girls aged 13 plus are not statistically significant.

TABLE A.28 *Anxiety to School: Mean scores (Boxall) by parental occupation*

Schools project: longitudinal sample

Occup. class	Boys in co-ed. schools				Boys in boys' schools			
	N	Age 11+	Age 13+	Change	N	Age 11+	Age 13+	Change
1	28	10·61	10·07	−0·54	26	10·77	10·46	−0·31
2	56	10·82	10·50	−0·32	78	10·71	9·54	−1·18
3	103	11·51	10·31	−1·20	87	12·39	10·60	−1·79
4 + 5	34	11·03	9·79	−1·24	24	12·96	11·42	−1·54
All*	222	11·17	10·27	−0·90	218	11·65	10·35	−1·30

Occup. class	Girls in co-ed. schools				Girls in girls' schools			
	N	Age 11+	Age 13+	Change	N	Age 11+	Age 13+	Change
1	32	11·59	10·56	−1·03	36	11·53	9·75	−1·78
2	60	11·80	11·97	+0·17	59	11·92	11·41	−0·51
3	79	13·35	12·09	−1·23	90	12·77	11·79	−0·98
4 + 5	40	12·33	12·18	−0·15	29	13·76	12·69	−1·07
All*	211	12·45	11·84	−0·61	217	12·43	11·47	−0·96

* Includes a few unclassifiable.

TABLE A.29 *The drop-out problem*

School Anxiety Test 1964

Comparison of mean scores for leavers and the remainder of the sample

	(Age 11 plus—longitudinal sample)					
	1964 sample		Leavers and absentees		Remainder 1964 sample	
Girls						
co-educated	236	12·32	25	11·2	211	12·45
from girls' schools	238	12·61	21	14·3	217	12·43
Boys						
co-educated	235	11·10	13	9·8	222	11·17
from boys' schools	238	11·73	20	12·55	218	11·65

TABLE A.30 *Anxiety about school*

Longitudinal sample

		Co-educated boys Yes	No	Boys in boys' schools Yes	No	Co-educated girls Yes	No	Girls in girls' schools Yes	No
Teacher makes me frightened when cross with class									
Age	11+	57	165	72	146	71	140	79	138
Age	13+	52	170	52	164	72	139	71	145
At home I often worry about school									
Age	11+	85	134	83	133	72	137	81	134
Age	13+	105	114	92	124	91	120	97	118
I hate having to go back to school									
Age	11+	117	99	115	101	103	104	120	93
Age	13+	123	99	131	86	92	119	106	111
Coming back to school after holidays is frightening									
Age	11+	61	159	69	148	52	158	51	165
Age	13+	39	183	57	161	36	175	50	167

The following differences were statistically significant:

1. The drop in score on the frightening effect of the teacher amongst boys in boys' schools between age 11 and 13.
2. The reduction in score of co-educated boys between age 11 and 13 about going back to school being frightening.
3. The reduction for co-educated girls aged 13 compared with those aged 11 on coming back to school being frightening.

Almost significant was the increase in score between age 11 and 13 of boys in boys' schools about hating going back to school.

TABLE A.31 *Mooney Problem Check list: Longitudinal survey 1964–6 (36 schools)*

Girls aged 11 plus and 13 plus—mean scores

Occup. class	N	Age	Health and physical develop-ment	School	Home and family	Money, work and future	Boy–girl	People in general	Self-concern	Overall
Co-educated girls										
1 and 2	92	11+	2·27	2·75	1·26	1·39	1·48	2·47	3·42	15·04
		13+	2·87	5·07	2·54	2·92	4·02	3·46	4·14	25·03
3	80	11+	2·43	3·33	1·65	2·04	2·18	3·51	3·88	19·00
		13+	3·99	6·56	3·90	4·08	5·00	4·35	4·89	32·76
4 and 5	43	11+	2·44	2·72	1·26	1·70	1·93	2·02	3·26	15·33
		13+	3·21	6·05	2·72	3·35	3·88	3·51	5·21	27·93
all	215	11+	2·36	2·96	1·40	1·69	1·83	2·77	3·56	16·57
		13+	3·35	5·82	3·08	3·44	4·36	3·80	4·63	28·49
Girls in girls' schools										
1 and 2	96	11+	2·53	3·07	2·26	2·10	2·43	2·89	4·45	19·73
		13+	3·00	5·64	3·05	3·39	4·08	3·93	4·07	28·05
3	90	11+	2·03	3·22	1·59	1·99	1·87	2·93	4·03	17·67
		13+	3·30	6·24	3·20	3·81	4·62	4·10	4·97	30·24
4 and 5	29	11+	2·55	3·21	1·52	1·59	1·59	3·00	3·72	17·17
		13+	3·72	7·93	3·17	3·41	4·28	4·03	5·62	32·17
all	215	11+	2·33	3·15	1·88	1·99	2·08	2·92	4·18	18·52
		13+	3·22	6·20	3·13	3·57	4·33	4·01	5·06	29·53

All 42 means rise. The greater speed of working of the 13-year-olds may have had something to do with this, but is unlikely to be the whole explanation. In five of the problem areas the increase of mentions between 11 plus and 13 plus is slightly less for the sample from girls' schools, in one area there is virtual equality of increase, and in the remaining area, *the school*, there is a small advantage to the co-educational sample.

TABLE A.32 *Mooney Problem check list: Longitudinal survey 1964–6 (36 schools)*

Boys aged 11 plus and 13 plus—mean scores

Occup. class	N	Age	Health and physical develop-ment	School	Home and family	Money, work and future	Boy–girl	People in general	Self-concern	Overall
Co-educated boys										
1 and 2	85	11+	2·59	4·13	2·55	3·08	2·53	3·32	4·92	23·12
		13+	3·27	6·07	2·72	3·60	4·53	3·49	4·75	28·44
3	106	11+	2·44	3·58	2·28	2·74	2·16	3·21	4·25	20·66
		13+	3·53	6·08	3·52	3·77	3·82	3·97	5·03	29·73
4 and 5	34	11+	2·00	3·41	2·65	2·56	2·32	3·29	3·50	19·74
		13+	3·79	6·24	4·18	3·97	4·59	4·41	4·79	31·97
all	225	11+	2·43	3·76	2·44	2·84	2·32	3·26	4·39	21·45
		13+	3·47	6·10	3·32	3·74	4·20	3·86	4·89	29·58
Boys from boys' schools										
1 and 2	105	11+	2·19	3·18	2·11	2·60	2·40	2·82	3·64	18·94
		13+	3·04	6·17	2·88	3·23	4·07	3·17	4·39	26·94
3	88	11+	2·83	4·20	2·86	3·19	2·60	3·38	4·52	23·59
		13+	3·03	6·30	2·72	3·42	4·26	3·45	4·35	27·53
4 and 5	24	11+	2·96	5·33	3·54	3·00	3·25	4·71	5·21	28·00
		13+	3·63	7·21	3·21	3·50	3·92	4·38	6·17	32·00
all	217	11+	2·53	3·83	2·58	2·88	2·58	3·25	4·17	21·83
		13+	3·10	6·34	2·85	3·34	4·13	3·42	4·57	27·74

Of the 42 means, 37 rise from age 11 to 13, the single-sex educated groups rising less than the co-educated in all sections *except school*, where the trend was slightly reversed. It should be noted that if the co-educated of combined occupational classes 1 and 2 are compared with the single-sex educated of the same classes, the co-educated have rather lower increases than the single-sex educated, and that this trend is reversed in the other two occupational class groups. Without exception the co-ed. means rise with occupational class, but with boys from single-sex schools there is a tendency for them to fall.

TABLE A.32a *Mooney Problem Check list: Special problems. Longitudinal survey 1964–6 (36 schools)—11 plus and 13 plus girls*

Occup. class	N	Age	Health and physical development	School N	School %*	Home and family	Money, work and future	Boy-girl	People in general	Self-concern	Overall
Co-educated girls											
1 and 2	92	11+	19	23	25·0	20	3	5	9	13	92
		13+	16	20	20·8	22	7	19	8	4	96
3	80	11+	14	20	24·4	13	4	8	11	12	82
		13+	10	20	20·4	24	13	15	11	5	98
4 and 5	43	11+	15	11	22·4	5	4	2	3	9	49
		13+	6	9	17·6	10	5	8	6	7	51
all	215	11+	48	54	24·2	38	11	15	23	34	223
		13+	32	49	20·0	56	25	42	25	16	245
Girls from girls' schools											
1 and 2	96	11+	23	14	16·3	13	5	4	9	18	86
		13+	10	16	15·8	20	12	19	15	9	101
3	90	11+	11	26	30·6	10	5	3	11	19	85
		13+	11	21	27·6	12	5	9	9	9	76
4 and 5	29	11+	3	10	33·3	5	5	1	2	4	30
		13+	5	6	21·4	5	1	3	5	3	28
all	215	11+	37	50	33·1	28	15	8	22	41	201
		13+	26	43	26·5	37	18	31	29	21	205

* Number of 'School' problems as a percentage of Overall problems.

NOTE: In any section the pupil who had problems was counted only once but the same pupil has sometimes recorded problems in several sections.

TABLE A.33 *H.S.P.Q. Anxiety mean scores with occupational class*

Longitudinal survey

Occup. class	Boys in co-educational schools: N	Age	Mean	Difference 11+/13+	Boys in boys' schools: N	Age	Mean	Difference 11+/13+	Difference between differences*
1	28	11+	60·82	−2·86	27	11+	56·41	7.63	+10·49
		13+	57·96			13+	64·04		
2	57	11+	57·56	0·40	78	11+	57·06	4·04	+3·64
		13+	57·97			13+	61·10		
3	106	11+	58·43	1·13	88	11+	60·51	0·48	0·65
		13+	59·56			13+	60·99		
4 + 5	34	11+	58·35	4·24	24	11+	59·79	5·17	+0·93
		13+	62·59			13+	64·96		
all†	226	11+	58·56	0·94	220	11+	58·85	3·19	+2·25
		13+	59·50			13+	62·04		

* A + sign before a difference indicates that the single sex-schools had the greater increase in anxiety.

† Includes a few unclassifiable.

TABLE A.34 *Mooney Problem Check list: Longitudinal survey 1964–6 (36 schools)*

Boys aged 15 plus and 17 plus—mean scores

Occup. class	N	Age	Health and physical development	School	Home and family	Money, work and future	Boy–girl	People in general	Self-concern	Overall
Co-educated boys										
1 + 2	56	15+	2·73	5·73	3·13	3·46	4·41	3·52	4·73	27·71
		17+	2·11	3·86	2·14	3·34	2·73	2·48	3·36	20·02
3, 4 & 5	77	15+	2·86	6·14	2·58	4·22	4·04	4·05	4·69	28·58
		17+	2·70	4·68	2·00	4·06	2·96	2·78	3·70	22·88
all	133	15+	2·80	5·97	2·81	3·90	4·20	3·83	4·71	28·22
		17+	2·45	4·33	2·06	3·76	2·86	2·65	3·56	21·68
Boys in boys' schools										
1 + 2	70	15+	3·14	4·83	3·24	4·33	3·57	3·73	5·67	28·51
		17+	2·69	3·73	2·50	3·57	2·94	2·80	3·96	22·19
3, 4 & 5	67	15+	3·52	6·27	3·63	5·18	4·46	4·19	5·88	33·13
		17+	3·07	5·12	3·00	5·06	3·43	3·51	4·36	27·55
all	137	15+	3·33	5·53	3·43	4·74	4·01	3·96	5·77	30·77
		17+	2·88	4·41	2·74	4·30	3·18	3·15	4·15	24·81

Every boys' group mean falls between 15 plus and 17 plus, within each type of school and within each occupational class—28 instances. The co-educational means fall rather more than the single-sex though not in all sections, the most favourable to co-education being the school and boy–girl relationship sections. For occupational classes 1 and 2 five means fall more in the co-educational sample and two the reverse, while for classes 3, 4 and 5 the two samples differ little in their change of problem incidence.

TABLE A.35 *Mooney Problem Check list: Longitudinal survey 1964–6 (36 schools)*

Girls aged 15 plus and 17 plus

Occup. class	N	Age	Mean scores: Health and physical devel.	School	Home and family	Money, work and future	Boy–girl	People in general	Self-concern	Overall
Co-educated girls										
1 + 2	61	15+	2·59	4·66	2·84	3·64	3·49	3·80	4·79	25·80
		17+	2·84	3·61	2·79	3·54	3·03	3·48	4·93	24·21
3, 4 & 5	54	15+	2·28	5·06	2·33	3·37	3·15	4·00	3·93	24·11
		17+	2·48	3·41	1·85	3·37	2·06	2·74	3·85	19·76
all	115	15+	2·44	4·84	2·60	3·51	3·33	3·90	4·38	25·01
		17+	2·67	3·51	2·35	3·46	2·57	3·13	4·43	22·12
Girls in girls' schools										
1 + 2	61	15+	2·16	4·16	1·89	2·97	2·93	2·67	4·02	20·80
		17+	2·62	4·21	2·64	3·87	2·67	3·41	4·23	23·66
3, 4 & 5	59	15+	2·68	5·81	3·08	4·29	3·68	3·51	5·00	28·05
		17+	3·03	4·39	2·90	4·25	2·71	2·80	4·86	24·95
all	120	15+	2·42	4·98	2·48	3·62	3·30	3·08	4·50	24·37
		17+	2·83	4·30	2·77	4·06	2·69	3·11	4·54	24·29

The reduction in problem mentions between 15 plus and 17 plus are greater for the co-educational sample in all sections except self-concern (equality) and health and physical development where the same trend is to be seen in the slightly lower increase for the co-educational. The sections with the largest differences between co-educational and single-sex are 'people in general' and 'school'.

TABLE A.35a *Mooney Problem Check list: Special problems: Longitudinal survey 1964–6 (36 schools)—15 plus and 17 plus girls*

Occup. class	N	Age	Health and physical devel.	School N	School %*	Home and family	Money, work and future	Boy–girl	People in general	Self-concern	Overall
Co-educated girls											
1 and 2	61	15+	6	23	22·1	18	27	13	6	11	104
		17+	4	17	18·9	13	22	16	13	5	90
3, 4 & 5	54	15+	9	20	29·4	12	6	9	4	8	68
		17+	8	15	19·5	13	16	7	6	12	77
all	115	15+	15	43	25·0	30	33	22	10	19	172
		17+	12	32	19·2	26	38	23	19	17	167
Girls from girls' schools											
1 and 2	61	15+	9	18	30·5	7	4	11	4	6	59
		17+	6	16	19·3	13	16	11	7	14	83
3, 4 & 5	59	15+	9	18	25·0	11	9	8	7	10	72
		17+	3	17	28·3	13	14	8	1	4	60
all	120	15+	18	36	27·5	18	13	19	11	16	131
		17+	9	33	23·1	26	30	19	8	18	143

* Number of 'School' problems as a percentage of Overall problems.

NOTE: In any section the pupil who had problems was counted only once but the same pupil has sometimes recorded problems in several sections.

TABLE A.36 *Girls' neuroticism—mean scores (Maudsley)*

Age	Schools	Classes 1 and 2		Classes 3, 4 and 5		All	
		N	Mean	N	Mean	N	Mean
15+	Co-ed.	61	28·87	54	31·56	115	30·13
	Girls'	61	29·33	59	31·48	120	30·36
17+	Co-ed.	61	29·02	54	30·74	115	29·83
	Girls'	61	29·93	59	30·19	120	30·06

TABLE A.37 *Introversion–extroversion mean scores (H.S.P.Q.)*

Junior boys

Age	Schools	Class 1		Class 2		Class 3		Classes 4 and 5		All*	
		N	Mean	N	Mean	N	Mean	N	Mean	N	Mean
11+	Co-ed.	28	36·79	57	35·95	106	37·49	34	36·56	226	36·82
	Boys'	27	36·11	78	36·28	88	34·83	24	39·00	220	36·05
13+	Co-ed.	28	38·32	57	36·26	106	37·76	34	34·82	226	36·96
	Boys'	27	33·59	78	37·71	88	34·59	24	35·63	220	35·73

* Includes some unclassifiable.

TABLE A.38 *Introversion–extroversion mean scores (H.S.P.Q.)*

Junior girls

Age	Schools	Class 1		Class 2		Class 3		Classes 4 and 5		All*	
		N	Mean	N	Mean	N	Mean	N	Mean	N	Mean
11+	Co-ed.	32	38·16	60	38·20	80	36·59	43	38·88	215	37·73
	Girls'	37	35·00	59	39·05	90	36·80	29	35·28	218	36·87
13+	Co-ed.	32	37·81	60	37·58	80	36·56	43	36·49	215	37·02
	Girls'	37	36·57	59	38·27	90	36·21	29	36·28	218	36·87

* Includes some unclassifiable.

TABLE A.39 *Introversion–extroversion mean scores (H.S.P.Q.)*
Senior girls

		Classes 1 and 2		Classes 3, 4 and 5		All*	
Age	Schools	N	Mean	N	Mean	N	Mean
15+	Co-ed.	61	36·30	54	36·72	115	36·50
	Girls'	61	37·49	59	36·66	121	37·04
17+	Co-ed.	61	35·92	54	37·41	115	36·62
	Girls'	61	36·28	59	38·78	121	37·48

* Includes some unclassifiable.

Bibliography

NOTE: A compendious annotated bibliography of books and articles on co-education has been published by Faculté des sciences de l'éducation, Université de Montréal, Montréal, Canada, (1970), entitled *La Coéducation dans les écoles officielles et les écoles Catholiques des 45 pays* by Marcel de Grandpré.

ATHERTON, B. F., (1971), 'The relative merits of co-educational and single-sex schools with particular reference to happiness in marriage of former pupils', M.A. thesis, University College of Swansea.

(1966), 'Co-education and happiness in marriage', *Where?*, 28.

BADLEY, J. H., (1914), *Co-education in Practice*, Cambridge.

(1923), *Bedales: A Pioneer School*, London.

(1929), *Co-education and its part in a complete education*, Cambridge.

BOARD OF EDUCATION, (1926), *The Hadow Report. Report on the education of the adolescent*, H.M.S.O.

BOXALL, JEAN, (1961), 'A study of some of the relationships between anxiety and failure in learning to read', Thesis for the Diploma in the Psychology of Childhood, University of Birmingham.

Bristol Social Adjustment Guide, see STOTT, D. H.

CAMPBELL, DUDLEY, (1874), *Mixed Education of Boys and Girls in America*, London.

CATTELL, R. B. AND BELOFF, H., (1963), 'Jr.–Sr. High School Personality Questionnaire', Form A, (Second Edition), Champaign, Illinois.

COWEN, E. L., et al., (1965), 'The relationship of anxiety in children to school record, achievement and the behavioural measures', *Child Development*, 36, 685–95.

CURRY, W. B., (1947), *Education for Sanity*, London.

DALE, R. R., (1948), 'Co-education: An Enquiry', *Times Educational Supplement*, 28 August 1948.

(1949), 'Co-education and the Modern Age', Association of Assistant Masters, Sept.

(1962a), 'Co-education—I: A critical analysis of research on the effects of co-education on academic attainment in grammar schools', *Educational Research*, 4, 3.

(1962b), 'Co-education—II: An analysis of research on comparative attainment in mathematics in single-sex and co-educational maintained grammar schools', *Educational Research*, 5, 1.

(1964), 'Co-education—III: Research on comparative attainment in English in single-sex and co-educational grammar schools', *Educational Research*, 6, 3.

(1966), 'The happiness of pupils in co-educational and single-sex grammar schools', *British Journal of Educational Psychology*, XXXVI, 1.
(1966a), 'Pupil–teacher relationships in co-educational and single-sex grammar schools', *British Journal of Educational Psychology*, XXXVI, 3.
(1969), 'Anxiety about school among first-year grammar school pupils, and its relation to occupational class and co-education', *British Journal of Educational Psychology*, 39, 1.
(1969), *Mixed or Single-sex School?, Vol. I*, London.
DEPARTMENT OF EDUCATION AND SCIENCE, (1969), *Statistics of Education*, Vol. 1, Year 1968: Schools, H.M.S.O.
EYSENCK, H. J., (1959), 'Maudsley Personality Inventory', London.
FURNEAUX, W. D., (1961), *The Chosen Few*, London.
HIGH SCHOOL PERSONALITY QUESTIONNAIRE, JR.–SR., (H.S.P.Q.), *see* CATTELL.
HOWARD, B. A., (1928), *The Mixed School*, London.
LOTZ, H. B., (1953), 'The relationship between emotional and social adjustment of individuals and their attendance at co-educational and single-sex high schools', Ph.D. thesis, New York University.
MCCANDLESS, B. R., AND CASTANEDA, A., (1956a), 'Anxiety in children, school achievement and intelligence', *Child Dev.*, 27, 379–82.
(1956b), 'The Children's form of the Manifest Anxiety Scale', *Child Dev.*, 27, 317–26.
MAUDSLEY PERSONALITY INVENTORY, (H. J. Eysenck), (1959), London.
MINISTRY OF EDUCATION, (1945), Pamphlet No. 1, *The Nation's Schools: their plan and purpose*, H.M.S.O.
MOONEY, ROSS L., and GORDON, L. V., (1950/64 revision), 'Mooney Problem Check List, Junior High School Form', (anglicized version), N.F.E.R. Slough.
MORETON, F. E., (1939), 'Co-education—a statistical enquiry into the attitude of teachers . . . and a comparative study of the emotional development of children . . .', Ph.D. thesis, University of London. (Summarized in *British Journal of Educational Psychology*, 1946, XVI, 2.)
PEKIN, L.B., (1934), *Progressive schools: their principles and practice*, London.
(1939), *Co-education in its historical and theoretical setting*, London.
SARASON, S. B., et al., (1960), *Anxiety in Elementary School Children*, New York.
STEWART, W. A. C., (1967 and 1968), *The Educational Innovators*, 2 vols. (particularly vol. 2, 'The Progressive Schools 1881–1967'), London.
STOTT, D. H., and SYKES, E. G., (1956), 'Bristol Social-Adjustment Guides', No. 1 and No. 2 *The Child in School.*
TYSON, G., (1928), 'Some apparent effects of co-education suggested by a statistical investigation of examination results', M.Ed. thesis, University of Manchester.

INDEX

For Product Safety Concerns and Information please contact our EU representative GPSR@taylorandfrancis.com Taylor & Francis Verlag GmbH, Kaufingerstraße 24, 80331 München, Germany

Batch number: 10725973

Printed by Printforce, the Netherlands

Making Medicines in Early Colonial Lima, Peru

Atlantic World

EUROPE, AFRICA AND THE AMERICAS, 1500–1830

Edited by

Benjamin Schmidt (*University of Washington*)
Wim Klooster (*Clark University*)

VOLUME 34

The titles published in this series are listed at *brill.com/aw*

Making Medicines in Early Colonial Lima, Peru

Apothecaries, Science and Society

By

Linda A. Newson

BRILL

LEIDEN | BOSTON

over illustration: Drawing of mechoacan in Antonio de Robles Cornejo's "Examen de los simples medici-
ales," 1617. Courtesy Spain. Ministerio de Cultura. Archivo del Real Jardín Botánico, Madrid. División 1, leg
fol. 204.

ibrary of Congress Cataloging-in-Publication Data

James: Newson, Linda A., author.
itle: Making medicines in early colonial Lima, Peru : apothecaries, science
and society / by Linda A. Newson.
Description: Leiden ; Boston : Brill, 2017. | Series: Atlantic world :
Europe, Africa and the Americas, 1500-1830, ISSN 1570-0542 ; VOLUME 34 |
Includes bibliographical references and index.
dentifiers: LCCN 2017029635 (print) | LCCN 2017031403 (ebook) | ISBN
9789004351271 (E-book) | ISBN 9789004350632 (hardback : acid-free paper)
ubjects: LCSH: Pharmacists--Peru--Lima--History. |
Medicine--Peru--Lima--History. | Materia medica--Peru--Lima--History. |
Pharmacy--Social aspects--Peru--Lima--History. | Science--Social
aspects--Peru--Lima--History. | Lima (Peru)--Social conditions. | Lima
(Peru)--Intellectual life. | Lima (Peru)--Relations--Spain. |
Spain--Relations--Peru--Lima. | Peru--History--1548-1820.
lassification: LCC RS67.P42 (ebook) | LCC RS67.P42 L538 2017 (print) | DDC
615.10985/25--dc23
C record available at https://lccn.loc.gov/2017029635

ypeface for the Latin, Greek, and Cyrillic scripts: "Brill". See and download: brill.com/brill-typeface.

SSN 1570-0542
SBN 978-90-04-35063-2 (hardback)
SBN 978-90-04-35127-1 (e-book)

his book is printed on acid-free paper and produced in a sustainable manner.

For Keith

Contents

Appendices

Acknowledgments

This monograph had its genesis is a previous book I published with Susie Minchin entitled, *From Capture to Sale: The Portuguese Slave Trade to Spanish South America in the Early Seventeenth Century* (Leiden: Brill, 2007). In that book we examined the medicines and medical practices that were involved in the treatment of African slaves both during their transhipment from Senegambia to Peru as well as in Lima. Arising from this previous study, I speculated that a conjunction of political, cultural and environmental conditions in Peru favoured early experimentation with native *materia medica*. I started with the propositions that the Counter Reformation encouraged medical practitioners of a more "progressive" persuasion to migrate from Spain to escape scrutiny by the Inquisition and that, while the development of empirical methods was generally encouraged by Spain's encounter with the New World, this was especially so in Peru given its rich botanical and mineral resources. As such, I postulated that medical practice in Peru might have been more "progressive" than in Spain at the time. I chose to focus on apothecaries since more than other professional medical practitioners they were pivotal in supplying Lima with medicines and, unlike physicians, had to hand the raw materials with which to experiment and thus possessed the potential to be pioneers in the development of medicine. As this book reveals, many of these original ideas proved to have limited foundation, at least for the period studied. Nevertheless, the research yielded a number of interesting findings that challenge some existing understandings of the nature of early modern medical practice. At the same time it revealed some underexplored facets of Lima's early colonial social history.

Another stimulus behind this book lay in the very exceptional archival sources for the study of early colonial medicine that exist in Lima, which I had encountered during research for *From Capture to Sale*. Of particular importance is the Archivo de Beneficencia Pública, which contains hospital and *cofradía* records from the mid-sixteenth century. Records of this kind are quite exceptional for Europe, let alone for Spanish America. I felt they deserved more extensive research, and they still do, especially since studies of professional medical practice in early colonial Spanish America have generally been hampered by the lack of archival sources.

I owe scholarly debts to a number of researchers who have generously supported this project by bringing to my attention unfamiliar sources. First, I would like to thank the brilliant and generous young scholar, Samir Boumediene, who I met while we were researching in the Jesuit archive in Rome. It was

Samir who drew my attention to the unpublished manuscript by Antonio de Robles Cornejo in the Archivo del Real Jardín Botánico in Madrid that proved to be a vital source for this study and one which made me think through many of the ideas in this book. Second, I would like to thank Pablo Gómez for bringing to my notice a manuscript recently acquired by the John Carter Brown Library referring to the installation of the pharmacy of Diego de Tineo in Lima in 1555. Finally, I would like to thank Susie Minchin, who worked with me on *From Capture to Sale*. Without the groundwork that we undertook for that project, this book would not have been either conceived or possible.

In the course of this research I have worked in many archives and libraries in Peru, Colombia, Spain, and Italy. In particular I would like to acknowledge the service provided by Yolanda Auqui at the Archivo General de la Nacion and Laura Gutiérrez Arbulú at the Archivo Arzobispal in Lima. Finally, this research would not have been possible without the generous financial support provided by the British Academy, the Wellcome Trust, and the Leverhulme Trust.

List of Illustrations

Figures

Tables

Abbreviations

Archival Sources

AAL	Archivo Arzobispal de Lima
ABPL	Archivo de Beneficencia Pública, Lima
AGI	Archivo General de Indias, Seville
AGNC	Archivo General de la Nación, Bogotá, Colombia
AGNP	Archivo General de la Nación, Lima, Peru
	SO CO Santo Oficio Contencioso
AHIRA	Archivo Histórico Instituto Riva-Agüero, Lima
AHML	Archivo Histórico Municipal de Lima
AHNM	Archivo Histórico Nacional, Madrid
AMS	Archivo Municipal de Sevilla
ARJBM	Archivo del Real Jardín Botánico, Madrid
ARSI	Archivum Romanum Societatis Iesu, Rome
BNM	Biblioteca Nacional, Madrid
JCB	John Carter Brown Library, Providence, Rhode Island
RAHM	Real Academia de Historia, Madrid
UNMSM	Archivo Histórico "Domingo Angulo," Universidad Nacional Mayor de San Marcos

CHAPTER 1

Medicines: Empire, Science and Society

> … the medicines of people around the Atlantic rim were intermingled, affecting not only the history of places Europeans went, but the history of Europe itself. They did so because medicine was not only a set of ideas and practices but was also part of the fabric of the commercial and colonial enterprises of the day.[1]

Harold Cook and Timothy Walker have observed that one of the great ironies of the study of the history of medicine is that very little attention has been paid to medicines.[2] This is not wholly true in the case of Spanish America since a few scholarly studies exist of a limited number of American plants, such as guaiacum, sarsaparilla, mechoacan, cinchona (quinine) and tobacco, which made it into European pharmacopoeias in the early colonial period.[3] The relative shortage of studies of New World medicines reflects Spain's

1 Harold J. Cook and Timothy Walker, "Circulation of Medicine in the Early Modern Atlantic World," *Social History of Medicine* 26 (3) (2013): 348.

2 Ibid., 345.

3 Simon Varey, Rafael Chabrán and Dora B. Weiner, eds., *Searching for the Secrets of Nature: The Life and Works of Dr. Francisco Hernández*, 2 vols.(Stanford: Stanford University Press, 2000); Londa Schiebinger, *Plants and Empire: Colonial Bioprospecting in the Atlantic World* (Cambridge, Mass.: Harvard University Press, 2004); Londa Schiebinger and Claudia Swan, eds., *Colonial Botany: Science, Commerce, and Politics in the Early Modern World* (Philadelphia: University of Pennsylvania Press, 2005); Antonio Barrera-Osorio, *Experiencing Nature: The Spanish American Empire and the Early Scientific Revolution* (Austin: University of Texas Press, 2006); Antonio Barrera-Osorio, "Knowledge and Empiricism in the Sixteenth-century Spanish Atlantic World," in *Science in the Spanish and Portuguese Empires: 1560–1800.*, eds. Daniela Bleichmar, Paula de Vos, Kristin Huffine and Kevin Sheehan (Stanford: Stanford University Press, 2009), 219–32. For cinchona see Fiammetta Rocco, *Miraculous Fever-Tree: Malaria, Medicine and the Cure That Changed the World* (New York: HarperCollins, 2003); Samir Boumediene, *La colonisation du savoir: une histoire des plantes medicinales de "Nuevo Mundo" (1492–1750)* (Vaulx-en-Velin: Éditions des mondes à faire, 2016), 187–292 ; Matthew J. Crawford, *The Andean Wonder Drug: Cinchona Bark and Imperial Science in the Spanish Atlantic, 1630–1800* (Pittsburg, PA: University of Pittsburgh Press, 2016).

 | DOI 10.1163/9789004351271_002

continued reliance in the sixteenth and early seventeenth centuries on Asia as its main source of both drugs and spices, and also that its interest in American medical products was restricted to finding substitutes for those which were in short supply in Europe or were expensive. As such, no large-scale transatlantic trade in American medicinal products developed in the early colonial period.[4] Meanwhile, very little is known about the medicines that were employed by professional medical practitioners in the Americas at that time.

In the New World the Spanish encountered a diversity of environments and cultures, including healing traditions, which should have encouraged intellectual curiosity and experimentation with native botanical and mineral products. However, focussing on Peru, and Lima in particular, this study reveals that contrary to what might be expected, professional medical practitioners in the period prior to 1650 adopted very few New World products and continued to rely largely on *materia medica* of Old World origin, whether they were imported or grown locally. It argues that the development of experimental methods was discouraged by state regulation, the activities of the Church and Inquisition, and by entrenched values and cultural traditions that governed not only medical practice but also colonial society as a whole.

The study focuses on the daily practices of apothecaries since they were primarily responsible for the acquisition of *materia medica* and the preparation of medicines. As recent historians of science and medicine have argued, scientific practices can only be understood within particular historical, cultural, and geographical contexts. Consistent with this judgment, the book considers how apothecaries were trained, ran their business, traded and prepared medicines, and established their place in society, activities that reflected a complex set of cultural values and beliefs that reflected both transatlantic connections and local circumstances. Apothecaries and the medicines they

---

4 Francisco Guerra, "Drugs from the Indies and the Political Economy of the Sixteenth Century," in *Analecta Medico-Historica: Materia Medica in the XVIth Century*, ed. Marcel Florkin (Oxford: Pergamon, 1966), 48–52; J. Worth Estes, "The European Reception of the First Drugs from the New World," *Pharmacy in History* 37(1)(1995): 11–21; Miguel Cordero del Campillo, *Crónicas de Indias: ganadería, medicina y veterinaria* (Salamanca: Junta de Castilla y León, 2001), 125–27. In fact, the interest in Asian plants led to early experiments with the large-scale production of ginger, cloves, and China root (probably ginseng) in Mexico and the Caribbean islands (Paula S. De Vos, "The Science of Spices: Empiricism and Economic Botany in the Early Spanish Empire," *Journal of World History* 17(4)(2006): 409–26; John Slater, "The Green Gold Fallacies: Myth and Reality in the Transatlantic Trade in Medicinal Plants (1493–1663)," in *Geografías médicas: orillas y fronteras culturales de la medicina hispanomericana (siglos XVI y XVII)*, eds. José Pardo-Tomás and Mauricio Sánchez Menchero (Mexico DF: Universidad Autónoma de México, 2014), 99–122.

prepared therefore open a window on colonial society in Lima as a whole in the early colonial period and in particular on the neglected role, organisation, and status of professional groups in general. The book goes beyond being a case study, however, and contributes to understanding of the relationship between medicine and empire, the nature of early modern medicine, and the role of different types of professional medical practitioners in the development of medicine, and indeed science in general. An overview of these wider processes and debates is therefore presented below in order that the significance of the book's empirical findings can be fully understood and their significance appreciated.

Medicine and Empire

Historians have often linked the spread of modern scientific medicine to the expansion of empire, seeing it as facilitating overseas exploration, settlement, and administrative control.[5] Most research in this field has focussed on the nineteenth century by which time most Spanish American regions had achieved political independence. Yet, recent research has demonstrated that the spread of western science was not necessarily dependent on imperial support or control. In Latin America, newly-independent states often adopted modernising agendas that incorporated public health initiatives based on Enlightenment ideas and scientific medicine, which in common with colonial powers served to legitimise state control through their perceived beneficial and civilisational effects.[6] Science in general is usually regarded as being beneficial to society

5 David Arnold, ed., *Imperial Medicine and Indigenous Societies* (Manchester: Manchester University Press, 1988), 11; Roy MacLeod, "Introduction," in *Disease, Medicine and Empire: Perspectives on Western Medicine and the Experience of European Expansion*, eds. Roy MacLeod and Milton Lewis (London: Routledge, 1988), 2–4; Andrew Cunningham and Bridie Andrews, eds., *Western Medicine as Contested Knowledge* (Manchester University Press: Manchester, 1997), 1–12.

6 For a review of recent work in this field see Diego Armus, ed., *Disease in the History of Modern Latin America: From Malaria to Aids* (Duke University Press: Durham, 2003) part translated as "Legados y tendencias en la historiografía sobre la enfermedad en América Latina moderna," in *Higienizar, medicar, gobernar: Historia, medicina y sociedad en Colombia*, eds. Jorge Márquez, Álvaro Casa, and Victoria Estrada (Medellín: Universidad Nacional de Colombia, 2004), 13–39. The Spanish version includes a more extensive bibliography. See also Marcus Cueto and Stephen Palmer, *Medicine and Public Health in Latin America: A History* (New York: Cambridge University Press, 2015), 58–105, and pp. 279–81 for a useful bibliography on the topic.

in bringing rationality and freedom from superstition, though has also been viewed by some as being detrimental in facilitating state control and repression.[7] Arguably the link between medicine and imperialism is more evident in the case of scientific medicine since its objective methods aim to produce the "truth," making state control and intervention in public health both easier to justify and more difficult to challenge. Scientific medicine it is argued was, and is, inherently imperialistic.[8]

In examining the relationship between medicine and empire, David Arnold has suggested that prior to the nineteenth century medicine was not employed to extend and consolidate state control,[9] while others have argued that in as much as there was a relationship, colonial powers were primarily concerned with the health of Europeans and made few formal attempts to transform indigenous medical practices.[10] This conclusion is generally reached by those conducting research on Asia and Africa, where the tropical fevers took a heavy toll of European lives.[11] In early colonial Spanish America circumstances were different. The disease environment was less threatening to the health of colonial servants, such as bureaucrats, soldiers and the clergy;[12] there it was the indigenous population that died in millions.[13] Even if the health of Europeans

---

7 Charles W.J. Withers and David N. Livingstone, "Introduction: On Geography and Enlightenment," in *Geography and Enlightenment*, eds. David N Livingstone and Charles W.J. Withers (Chicago: The University of Chicago Press, 1999), 8 and Charles W.J. Withers, *Placing the Enlightenment: Thinking Geographically about the Age of Reason* (Chicago: the University of Chicago Press, 2007), 4, referring to Max Horkheimer and Theodor Adorno's seminal work, *Dialectic of Enlightenment* (New York: Herder and Herder, 1972).

8 Cunningham and Andrews, *Western Medicine*, 6, 10.

9 Arnold, *Imperial Medicine*, 11–12, 18.

10 MacLeod, "Introduction," 6–9.

11 See for example, Philip D. Curtin, *Death by Migration: Europe's Encounter with the Tropical World in the Nineteenth Century* (Cambridge: Cambridge University Press, 1989).

12 In fact the disease environment became more threatening with the introduction of the tropical fevers, malaria and yellow fever, but their full impact was not felt until after the mid-seventeenth century (J.R. McNeill, *Mosquito Empires: Ecology and War in the Greater Caribbean, 1620–1914* (Cambridge: Cambridge University Press, 2010).

13 There is an extensive literature on this topic. For an introduction see Alfred W. Crosby, "Virgin Soil Epidemics as a Factor in the Aboriginal Depopulation in America," *The William and Mary Quarterly* 33 (2) (1976): 289–299; Noble David Cook, *Born to Die: Disease and New World Conquests, 1492–1650* (Cambridge: Cambridge University Press, 1998) and for Peru *Demographic Collapse: Indian Peru 1520–1620* (Cambridge: Cambridge University Press, 1981).

in the New World was not of prime concern to the Spanish state, two other motives encouraged state intervention in the medical field, which both had the potential to transform the nature of medical practice and the *materia medica* employed.

First, as Antonio Barrera-Osorio and Paula De Vos among others have shown, from earliest years of conquest Spain was interested in native medicinal products from the perspective finding *materia medica* that could be commercialised and generate profits to strengthen its financial position.[14] While early state-sponsored expeditions in search of new products may not have affected medical practice or the types of medicinal products used in the colonies directly, as will be demonstrated in this study, the process of acquiring knowledge about New World products indirectly fostered new empirical approaches to medicine, which had the potential to affect the nature of medical practice and indeed science more generally.

Second, state intervention into medical realm was also driven by the Catholic Spain's desire to discharge its Christian duty to provide charity and care for the sick and, through the vehicle of healing, fulfil its providential mission to "civilise" and convert native peoples to Christianity.[15] In order to achieve its colonial ambitions, the Habsburg state worked closely with the Church, and as will be shown in some circumstances, including in healthcare, even depended

14 Barrera-Osorio, *Experiencing Nature*, 5; De Vos, "The Science of Spices," 399–427; Schiebinger, *Plants and Empire*; Jorge Cañizares-Esguerra, *Nature, Empire, and Nation: Explorations of the History of Science in the Iberian World* (Stanford: Stanford University Press, 2006), 56–60; Daniela Bleichmar, Paula De Vos, Kristin Huffine, and Kevin Sheehan, eds. *Science in the Spanish and Portuguese Empires, 1500–1800* (Stanford University Press, 2009) *passim*; Pratik Chakrabarti, *Medicine and Empire 1600–1960* (Basingstoke: Palgrave Macmillan, 2014), 20–26. For a similar argument see Pamela H. Smith, *The Business of Alchemy: Science and Culture in the Holy Roman Empire* (Princeton: Princeton University Press, 1997), 5, and in the context of the Dutch empire Harold J. Cook, *Matters of Exchange: Commerce, Medicines, and Science in the Dutch Golden Age* (New Haven: Yale University Press, 2007).

15 John H. Elliott, *Empires of the Atlantic World: Britain and Spain in America 1492–1830* (New Haven: Yale University Press, 2006), 184–87; Francisco Guerra. "The Role of Religion in Spanish American Medicine," in *Medicine and Culture*, ed. F.N.L. Poynter (London: Wellcome Institute, 1969), 179–88; Francisco Guerra, *El hospital en hispanoamérica y filipinas 1492–1898* (Madrid: Ministerio de Sandiad y Consumo, 1994); David Sowell, *The Tale of Healer Miguel Perdomo Neira: Medicine, Ideologies, and Power in the Nineteenth-Century Andes* (Wilmington, Delaware: Scholarly Resources Inc., 2001), 14–18; Gabriela Ramos, "Indian Hospitals and Government in the Colonial Andes," *Medical History* 57 (2)(2013): 186–205.

upon it to deliver its colonial mission. It was only with the Bourbon reforms of the eighteenth century that the Crown sought to wrest control of medical practice from the Church and religious orders and promoted the professionalization of medicine.[16] This study shows how the Church's involvement in the medical sphere directly affected the philosophical basis of medical practice and even the particular medicines employed. It will argue that in some respects these influences, while different in kind, were no less interventionist than those later associated with scientific medicine sponsored by the secular state.

In the fifteenth and sixteenth centuries the Spanish state regulated the practice of medicine more than any other European country.[17] It did this through the founding of chairs in universities for the teaching of medicine and through the establishment of medical boards, known as *protomedicatos*, which licensed practitioners and inspected pharmacies and hospitals.[18] Crown regulation was strongest in Castile; in Valencia, Navarra and Aragón it did not exert the same degree of power.[19] It was the bureaucratic and regulatory framework that was being developed in Castile that served as the basic model for Spanish state control of medical practice in the New World. However in crossing the Atlantic, some modifications were made, notably to the jurisdiction and responsibilities of the *protomedicato*. These aimed to take account of American circumstances, particularly the general shortage of trained personnel and the presence of native *curanderos*.[20] It is worth noting that even in Castile state medical institutions were still in the process of formation and much medical practice remained unregulated; as in the rest of Europe, popular healers and priests played a vital role in caring for the sick.[21]

16 Adam Warren, *Medicine and Politics in Colonial Peru: Population Growth and the Bourbon Reforms* (Pittsburgh, PA: University of Pittsburgh Press, 2010), 20, 35–77.

17 Guenter B. Risse, "Medicine in New Spain," in *Medicine in the New World: New Spain, New France, and New England*, ed. Ronald L. Numbers (Knoxville: University of Tennessee Press, 1987), 15; Paula S. De Vos, "The Art of Pharmacy in Seventeenth- and Eighteenth-Century Mexico." PhD diss., University of California, Berkeley, 2001, 6.

18 Michele Clouse, *Medicine, Government and Public Health in Philip II's Spain: Shared Interests, Competing Authorities* (Farnham: Ashgate, 2011). For apothecaries in particular see pp. 111–41.

19 María Luz López Terrada, "Medical Pluralism in the Iberian Kingdoms: The Control of Extra-academic Practitioners in Valencia," *Medical History Supplement* 29 (2009): 9–13.

20 Pilar Gardeta Sabater, "El nuevo modelo del Real Tribunal del Protomedicato en la América española: trasformaciones sufridas ante las Leyes de Indias y el cuerpo legislativo posterior," *Dynamis* 16 (1996): 237–59.

21 Francisco Guerra, "Role of Religion," 179–81; Luis S. Granjel, *La medicina española renacentista* (Salamanca: Ediciones Universidad de Salamanca, 1980), 133–50; Nancy G. Siraisi, *Medieval and Early Renaissance Medicine: An Introduction to Knowledge and Practice* (Chicago: University of Chicago, 1990), 7–9; Enrique Perdiguero, "Protomedicato y

In Spanish America the establishment of this medical infrastructure was never fully achieved. Universities capable of awarding medical degrees were only established in Mexico and Lima in 1631 and 1634 respectively; in many other regions they did not appear until the eighteenth century.[22] The result was a severe shortage of licensed physicians. Although the Salamancan physician Hernando de Sepúlveda was appointed as *protomédico* in Lima in 1537, it was only in 1568 that Antonio Sánchez Renedo was appointed as royal *protomedico* with powers equivalent to *protomédicos* in Spain; similarly it was only in 1570 that the Crown established the *protomedicato* in New Spain with the appointment of the naturalist and court physician, Francisco Hernández.[23] The delay in the establishment of the *protomedicatos* in Spanish America has been attributed not to Philip II's lack of interest in medical care, but rather his overambitious health programme and the lack of funds to carry it through.[24] As will be demonstrated in this book, the medical infrastructure that was established was therefore more partial, fragmented, and hence often less effective than was envisaged in the metropolis, which potentially at least created space for the emergence of alternative forms of medical practice.

Practices of Medicine

The medical infrastructure that was being developed in Spain and its colonies occurred against a backdrop of changes in the nature of medical practice in

---

curanderismo," *Dynamis* 16 (1996): 101–102; Mary Lindemann, *Medicine and Society in Early Modern Europe* (Cambridge: Cambridge University Press, 1999), 123–29; Guenter B. Risse, *Mending Bodies, Saving Souls: A History of Hospitals* (New York: Oxford University Press, 1999), 73–109; David Sowell, *Tale of Healer*, 14–15.

22 John Tate Lanning, *The Royal Protomedicato: The Regulation of the Medical Professions in the Spanish Empire*, ed. John Jay TePaske (Durham: Duke University Press, 1985), 325–31.

23 Hernando de Sepúlveda was appointed as *protomédico* in 1537. He accompanied Pedro de Alvarado's expedition to Peru and he remained there as a supporter of Francisco Pizarro. Although he received the title from the Crown, his appointment was approved by the *cabildo* who exercised its power to license medical practitioners according to Spanish pragmatics (*Libros de cabildos de Lima*, 1: 141–142 27 Apr. 1537; Lanning, *Royal Protomedicato*, 29–30; Luis Deza Bringas, *Testimonios del linaje médico peruano en los libros del cabildo de Lima, siglo XVI* (Lima: Universidad de San Martín de Porres, Facultad de Medicina Humana, 2004), 31–35, 173).

24 Lanning, *Royal Protomedicato*, 11; David C. Goodman, *Power and Penury: Government, Technology and Science in Philip II's Spain* (Cambridge: Cambridge University Press, 1988), 261–64.

Europe and the growing power of the Inquisition. Humoral medicine dominated in late Renaissance times.[25] At that time, sickness was thought to derive from an imbalance in the humours that could be redressed through diet, bleeding, and the application of medicines that acted as purgatives or emetics. Ill health was regarded as a divine punishment for sin and therefore required no further explanation. Humoral medicine was based on a natural philosophy that was elaborated through the study of classical texts. However, new approaches to medical practice, associated with the names of the chemists (Theophrastus Bombastus von Hohenheim) (1493–1541) and Jan Baptist Van Helmont (1580–1644) among others, were emerging. These argued that illness was caused by some external factor that through observation and experiment could be identified and the ailment treated. For them the development of medical knowledge lay in understanding nature rather than in scholasticism.[26] The empirical methods they adopted challenged the existing natural philosophy that was based on Christian interpretations of classical texts, which had largely been undertaken by clerics or by scholars working for institutions allied to the Church. Any opposition to the prevailing natural philosophy might therefore be seen as an attack on Christianity itself.[27] Moreover the empirical methods advocated by Paracelsians often used chemicals and minerals and were regarded as dangerously close to witchcraft. For these reasons, what came to be known as Paracelsianism, was opposed by the Catholic Church particularly during the Counter Reformation when the Inquisition sought to suppress it.[28]

In an effort to maintain orthodox medical practice, in 1559 Philip II banned Spaniards from studying abroad thereby reducing their access to the main European centres of medical education at Bologna, Padua, Paris and Montpellier.[29] Like many European countries at the time, Castile sought to control the

---

25 George M. Foster, *Hippocrates' Latin American Legacy: Humoral Medicine in the New World* (Langhorne, PA: Gordon and Breach:, 1994), 4–7, 12–14; Rebecca Earle, *The Body of the Conquistador: Food, Race and the Colonial Experience in Spanish America, 1492–1700* (Cambridge: Cambridge University Press, 2012), 19–41.

26 Steven Shapin, *The Scientific Revolution* (Chicago: University of Chicago Press, 1996), 69.

27 Ibid., 126, 136; William B. Ashworth, "Catholicism and Early Modern Science," in *God and Nature: Historical Essays on the Encounter between Christianity and Religion*, eds. David C. Lindberg and Ronald L. Numbers (Berkeley: University of California Press, 1986), 148–53; Cueto and Palmer, *Medicine and Public Health*, 23.

28 José Maria López Piñero, "Paracelsus and His Work in Sixteenth and Seventeenth Century Spain," *Clio Medica* 8 (2) (1973): 119–31.

29 Allen G. Debus, "Paracelsus and the Delayed Scientific Revolution in Spain: A Legacy of Philip II," in *Reading the Book of Nature: the Other Side of the Scientific Revolution*, eds. Allen G. Debus and Michael T. Walton (Kirksville-Missouri: Sixteenth Century Journal

inflow of foreign literature. From 1558 the Crown banned foreign book imports and obliged printers to obtain licences to print. At the same time the Inquisition was entrusted with censoring the publication of books deemed to be heretical.[30] Some debate exists about the impact of the Counter Reformation and Inquisition on the development of medicine, and indeed science generally, in Spain.[31] Some scholars see these measures as having a detrimental effect, while others argue that their impact was limited because few Spaniards sought training abroad, the laws were often circumvented or ignored, and works by Paracelsus were not unknown. A tribunal of the Inquisition was established in Lima in 1570 and this book explores the possible impact of the Inquisition in both Spain and Peru on local medical practices. First, it evaluates the success of the Inquisition in restricting the introduction and circulation of what might be called "progressive" medical texts, here defined as those based on empirical and experimental methods that among other things might advocate the use of chemical and mineral *materia medica*. Second, it explores whether the creation of a conservative intellectual environment in Spain that opposed the development of new approaches to medicine might have encouraged certain medical practitioners to migrate to Spanish America in order to practise more freely;[32] they might include medical practitioners of Jewish or Muslim heritage, known as *Conversos*, who although they had converted to Christianity, were particularly vulnerable to scrutiny by the Inquisition and being charged with heresy. Research for this book began with the proposition that for both groups the distant geographical location of Peru would have made it a particularly

Publishers, Inc., 1998), 148. All those studying overseas were ordered home except those enrolled in the theologically more orthodox colleges at Bologna, Rome, Naples, and Coimbra.

30 Henry Kamen, *The Spanish Inquisition: An Historical Revision* (London: Weidenfeld and Nicolson, 1997), 103–34.

31 José Maria López Piñero, *Ciencia y técnica en la sociedad española de los siglos XVI y XVII* (Barcelona: Labor Universitaria 1979), 141–44; David C. Goodman, "Philip II's Patronage of Science and Engineering," *The British Journal for the History of Science* 16(1) (1983): 50–53 and *Power and Penury*, 220–21; Kamen, *Spanish Inquisition*, 104–108. For recent evaluations of the impact of Paracelsus in Spain see: José Rodríguez Guerrero, "Censura y Paracelsismo durante el Reinado de Felipe II," *Azogue* 4 (2001) URL: http://www.revista-azogue.com [Accessed 19 May 2016]; Miguel López Pérez, "Spanish Paracelsus Revisited and Decontaminated," *Azogue* 7 (2013) URL: http://www.revistaazogue.com [Accessed 19 May 2016]; Mar Rey Bueno, "Los paracelsistas españoles: medicina química en la España moderna," in *Más allá de la Leyenda Negra: España y la revolución científica*, ed. Victor Navarro Brotons and William Eamon (Valencia: Instituto de Historia de la Ciencia y Documentación López Piñero, 2007), 41–55.

32 See for example, the Sevillian surgeon Pedro López de León who is discussed in Chapter 5.

attractive destination for those groups, but as will be shown in Chapter 5 it has found little evidence to support it.

While the regulation of medical practice and the control of the literature entering the New World by the Inquisition may have promoted a conservative intellectual environment for the practice of medicine in early colonial Peru, several factors promoted innovation. As in Spain, the medical infrastructure in the New World had its limitations, leaving space for the emergence of alternative methods of healing. Equally important was the rich diversity of plants, minerals, and other natural products found in the Andean region that aroused curiosity and encouraged experimentation. Of particular importance was the abundance of minerals, including mercury, which was a common ingredient in medicines promoted by Paracelsians.

Medicine and Science

Spain's encounter with New World peoples and environments generated new knowledge that challenged existing practices and beliefs. In fact, scholars such as Jorge Cañizares-Esguerra, Antonio Barrera-Osorio, and Mauricio Nieto have demonstrated that Spain's experience in the Americas, particularly during the early years of exploration had a profound effect on intellectual developments in Europe, including the Scientific Revolution.[33] They have argued that Spanish scientific achievements, notably in the fields of cartography, cosmology and natural history, were fundamental to the development of modern science. More specifically, others have suggested that the abundance of minerals found in the New World furthered an interest in the development of chemical methods associated with modern scientific medicine.[34] Despite the putative contributions of Spanish science to the development of modern science, Cañizares-Esguerra argues that they have generally been neglected in

---

33 Jorge Cañizares-Esguerra, "Iberian Science in the Renaissance: Ignored How Much Longer?," *Perspectives on Science* 12(1)(2004): 86–124; "Iberian Colonial Science," *Isis* 96 (2005): 64–70, and *Nature, Empire, and Nation*, 14–45; Mauricio Nieto Olarte, "Scientific Practices in the Sixteenth-Century Iberian Atlantic," in *Theorising the Ibero-American Atlantic*, eds. Harald E Braun and Lisa Vollendorf (Leiden: Brill, 2013), 149; Barrera-Osorio, *Experiencing Nature* and "Knowledge and Empiricism." For the importance of the encounter with foreign lands in contributing to the Enlightenment see Withers and Livingstone, "Introduction," 12.

34 Alix Cooper, *Inventing the Indigenous: Local Knowledge and Natural History in Early Modern Europe* (Cambridge: Cambridge University Press, 2007), 87–92; Chakrabarti, *Medicine and Empire*, 9.

the discourse around the Scientific Revolution and Enlightenment. This he attributes to the focus of historians of science on the contributions of astronomy, physics and mathematics to the exclusion of other scientific fields and to the prejudice of Protestant Northern Europeans against Catholic Spain. As such, the usefulness of the concept of the Scientific Revolution itself has been questioned especially by scholars of Spanish science.[35] It is not the aim of this book to demonstrate the intellectual contributions of Peruvian colonial science to modern science in general, but rather through a study of pharmacy practice in Lima contribute to this discourse by providing an enhanced understanding of the complex nature of science in Peru in the early modern period revealing the importance of both local circumstances and Atlantic connections.

The book's focus on medical *practice* follows recent research in the history of science. The history of medicine and indeed science in general has until recently been written around the achievements of a few prominent individuals or small bodies of practitioners and their role in the progress and triumph of scientific medicine. In 1967 George Basalla developed a seminal model about the spread of western science, in which he envisaged non-Western societies to be recipients of scientific knowledge and practices that had diffused from Europe.[36] His model has been criticised on many grounds. Of particular relevance for this study, is the consensus that western science was not the product of a one-way process, but that colonial practices were forged through interactions and exchanges with local scientists within both the colonies and Europe, and that they varied according to different cultural, social, political, and geographical settings.[37] Most scholars now see the history of science as a product of social processes that recognise the plurality and coexistence of modes of enquiry.[38] As such, in discussing the Scientific Revolution, Steven Shapin has argued that there is a need to move beyond such "free-floating concepts" to investigate the human practices that contributed to knowledge and that these can only be understood in their particular historical and geographical

35 See Victor Navarro Brotóns and William Eamon, "Spain and the Scientific Revolution: Questions and Conjectures," in *Más allá de la Leyenda Negra: España y la revolución científica*, eds. Victor Navarro Brotons and William Eamon (Valencia: Instituto de Historia de la Ciencia y Documentación López Piñero, 2007), 27–38.

36 George Basalla, "The Spread of Western Science," *Science* 156 (1967): 611–22. Basalla's model describes the diffusion of western science as a whole but it has relevance to medicine.

37 MacLeod, "Introduction," 2–7. Many of the criticisms are summarised in Dhruv Raina, "From West to Non-West Basalla's Three-stage Model Revisited," *Science as Culture* 8 (4) (1999): 497–516.

38 Pamela H. Smith, "Science on the Move: Recent Trends in the History of Early Modern Science." *Renaissance Quarterly* 62 (2) (2009): 358–61.

contexts.[39] The importance of geography in the development of science, specifically of the Enlightenment, has also been stressed by a number of scholars.[40] Some twenty years ago, Roy Macleod reported that there were increasing attempts to "localize [sic]" science.[41] Inasmuch as this has occurred in studies of Latin American science and medicine, they have focussed on the period of the Bourbon reforms and especially the Enlightenment;[42] while it remains the case that fewer studies have been conducted on professional medical practices in the late sixteenth and seventeenth centuries.[43]

Consistent with this perspective, this book aims to situate medical practice and pharmacy in particular within the specific cultural, historical and geographical context of Lima during the early colonial period. Very little has been written on pharmacy in colonial Spanish America. Paula De Vos has pioneered work in this field through her research on late colonial Mexico; her insights have been the touchstone for this study.[44] Luz María Hernández Sáenz has also studied apothecaries as a distinct professional group in late eighteenth and early nineteenth century Mexico.[45] In many respects this book complements these studies in its focus on the early colonial period and on Peru, a region that from a colonial perspective was geographically more distant from Spain and where the natural environment and cultures of the Andes presented different opportunities and challenges for the practice of pharmacy.

Apothecaries have been selected as the focus of this book since they were the medical practitioners directly involved in the practical tasks of acquiring

39 Shapin, *Scientific Revolution*, 4.

40 See David N. Livingstone and Charles W.J. Withers, eds. *Geography and Enlightenment* (Chicago: The University of Chicago Press, 1999); David N. Livingstone, *Putting Science in its Place: Geographies of Scientific Knowledge* (Chicago: The University of Chicago Press, 2003); Charles W.J. Withers, *Placing the Enlightenment: Thinking Geographically about the Age of Reason* (Chicago: The University of Chicago Press, 2007).

41 MacLeod, "Introduction," 3.

42 Antonio Lafuente, "Enlightenment Science in an Imperial Context: Local Science in the Late-Eighteenth-Century Hispanic World," *Osiris* 15 (2001): 155–73; Juan José Saldaña, "Science and Happiness during the Latin American Enlightenment," in *Science in Latin America: A History*, ed. Juan José Saldaña (Austin: University of Texas, 2006), 51–92. See also the chapters in the same volume by Luis Carlos Abboleda and Diana Soto Arango, and by Antonio Lafuente and Leoncio Lopez-Ocón.

43 James E. McClellan III, *Colonialism and Science: Saint Domingue in the Old Regime* (Baltimore: Johns Hopkins University Press, 1992), 6.

44 De Vos, "Art of Pharmacy," and "From Herbs to Alchemy: the Introduction of Chemical Medicine to Mexican Pharmacies in the Seventeenth and Eighteenth Centuries," *Journal of Spanish Cultural Studies* 8(2)(2007): 135–68.

45 Luz María Hernández Sáenz, *Learning to Heal: The Medical Profession in Colonial Mexico, 1767–1831* (New York: Peter Lang, 1997).

materia medica as well as preparing medicines, and were therefore more likely than physicians to be innovators in medical practice. They were uniquely qualified to judge the qualities of products and in a position to experiment with different doses and combinations and assess their efficacy. Such empirical methods were intrinsic to the art of pharmacy and for this reason apothecaries have been regarded as pioneers in the development of science.[46] Indeed, it has been argued that it was from apothecaries that physicians acquired knowledge of the natural world that enabled them to challenge the prevailing natural philosophy necessary for the development of modern science.[47] Scholars recognise that it may not have been the initial intention of apothecaries to provide alternative explanations for the causes of illness, but rather provide more effective treatments, which they continued to employ within in a traditional Galenic framework.[48] Nevertheless, they argue that it was through practice rather than theoretical reasoning that medical science progressed.[49] This book will examine the extent to which apothecaries in Lima were involved in empirical and experimental methods and will demonstrate that inasmuch as they used these procedures they did not represent a change in the natural philosophy underlying medical practice.

Practitioners of Medicine

This study is not a comprehensive account of medical practice in early colonial Lima. It focuses on professional medicine and does not explore in detail what might be called the popular sector or what Lawrence Brockliss and

46 The same argument has been made for alchemists who engaged with the natural world of minerals. See: Smith, "Science on the Move," 355–56.

47 Paula Findlen, *Possessing Nature: Museums, Collecting, and Scientific Culture in Early Modern Italy* (Berkeley and Los Angeles: University of California Press, 1994), 9–10, 241–56. For the role of apothecaries in undertaking early experiments in Italy and the adoption of recipes by physicians see: William Eamon, *Science and the Secrets of Nature: Books of Secrets in Medieval and Early Modern Culture* (Princeton: Princeton University Press, 1991), 7–11, 147–51, 357–59.

48 Lorraine Daston and Katharine Park, *Wonders and the Order of Nature 1150–1750* (New York: Zone Books, 1998), 136–37.

49 Smith, *Business of Alchemy*, 4. The edited volume by Pamela H. Smith, Amy R. Meyers and Harold J. Cook, *Ways of Making and Knowing: The Material Culture of Empirical Knowledge* (Ann Arbor: University of Michigan Press, 2014)) also argues that history of science was not built on a history of concepts alone, but on a history of making and using objects to understand the world.

Colin Jones have termed "the medical penumbra."[50] While this may be regarded as a limitation, paradoxically we probably know more about the character o[f] popular medicine in terms of methods of healing and medicinal products than we do about the *daily practices* of professional practitioners.[51] This is because popular healers were sometimes charged with witchcraft and brought before the ecclesiastical courts or Inquisition. It is worth noting, however, that the accused that appear in these studies may not be representative of the bulk of popular healers, whose practices were generally tolerated unless they involved in obviously superstitious or idolatrous methods, such as magic or divination.[52] Other scholars have found evidence for the practices of popular healers in legal cases brought by slave owners claiming that they had been sold slaves who were sick or had an undisclosed ailment that popular healers had been unable to cure.[53] This evidence is relatively abundant for Lima since African slaves comprised over half of the city's population of some 27,000 in 1636.[54]

---

50 Lawrence Brockliss and Colin Jones, *The Medical World of Early Modern France* (Oxford: Clarendon Press, 1997), 8–20, 228–29.

51 See for example María Emma *Mannarelli*, "Inquisición y mujeres: las hechiceras en el Perú durante el siglo XVII," *Revista Andina* 3(1) (1985): 141–56 and *Hechiceras, beatas y expósitas: mujeres y poder inquisitorial en Lima* (Lima: Fondo Editorial del Congreso del *Perú*, 1998); Ana Sánchez, *Amancebados, hechiceros y rebeldes* (*Chancay, siglo XVII*) (Cusco: Centro de Estudios Regionales Andinos, Bartolomé de las Casas, 1991); Alejandra B. Osorio, "'El Callejón de la Soledad': Vectors of Cultural Hybridity in Seventeenth-century Lima," in *Spiritual Encounters: Interactions between Christianity and Native Religions in Colonial America*, eds. Nicholas Griffiths and Fernando Cervantes (Birmingham: University of Birmingham Press, 1999), 198–229, and "Hechicerías y curanderías en la Lima del siglo XVII: Formas femeninas de control y acción social," in *Mujeres y género en la historia del Perú*, ed. Margarita Zegarra (Lima: CENDOC-Mujer, 1999), 59–75; Leo Garofalo, "Conjuring with Coca and the Inca: the Andeanisation of Lima's Afro-Peruvian Ritual Specialists, 1580–1690," *The Americas* 63 (1)(2006): 53–80; Linda A. Newson and Susie Minchin, *From Capture to Sale: The Portuguese Slave Trade to Spanish South America in the Early Seventeenth Century* (Leiden: Brill, 2007), 248, 251–52, 264–65; Claudia Brosseder, *The Power of Huacas: Change and Resistance in the Andean World of Colonial Peru* (Austin: University of Texas Press, 2014).

52 Nicholas Griffiths, "Andean *Curanderos* and their Repressors: The Persecution of Native Healing in Late Seventeenth- and Early Eighteenth-Century Peru," in *Spiritual Encounters: Interactions Between Christianity and Native Religions in Colonial America*, eds. Nicholas Griffiths and Fernando Cervantes (Birmingham: University of Birmingham Press, 1999), 185–97.

53 Newson and Minchin, *From Capture to Sale*, 252, 264. The legal cases are to be found in the section "Causas de Negros" of the Archivo Arzobispal, Lima.

54 Frederick P. Bowser, *The African Slave in Colonial Peru, 1524–1650* (Stanford: Stanford University Press, 1974), 341.

Due to scholarly interest in popular healers, not only in Peru, but also other parts of the Spanish empire, there is an emergent view that in early modern times a form of medical pluralism existed and that medical practices were a fusion of indigenous, African, and European medical traditions.[55] The focus here on professional medical practitioners suggests that this view might need to be modified to some extent, at least in the case of early colonial Lima. This study suggests that there was not a unified free market in which medical practitioners competed for clients, but that it was segmented, with the professional sector being relatively distinct from the popular sector with which there was little exchange and from which few medicinal products were adopted. The study therefore questions the appropriateness of the concept of a "medical marketplace," as proposed by Roy Porter for early modern England, to Spanish colonial cities.[56] It also urges caution in believing that there was a free flow of medical ideas, practices and products.

Studies of the professional sector of medicine in early colonial Peru have focussed on institutional aspects of medical practice, including the *protomedicato*, the teaching of medicine in universities, and the establishment of hospitals.[57] Very little has been written about the daily practice of medicine and especially the role of apothecaries. Despite the book's ostensibly narrow focus on one group within the medical profession, it is clear that the role and status of apothecaries cannot be fully understood without reference to physicians

55 For example, Gonzalo Aguirre Beltrán, *Medicina y magia: el proceso de aculturación en la estructura colonial,* rev. ed. (México: Universidad Veracruzana, Instituto Nacional Indigenista, 1992); Noemí Quezada, *Enfermedad y maleficio: el curandero en el México colonia,* 2nd ed. (México: Universidad Nacional Autónoma de México, Instituto de Investigaciones Antropológicas, 2000); Luz Adriana Maya Restrepo, "Botánica y medicina africanas en la Nueva Granada, siglo XVII," *Historia crítica* 19 (2000): 27–47; Martha Few, *Women Who Live Evil Lives: Gender, Religion and the Politics of Power in Colonial Guatemala* (Austin: University of Texas Press, 2002); Laura Lewis, *Hall of Mirrors: Power, Witchcraft, and Caste in Colonial Mexico* (Durham, NC: Duke University Press, 2003); Pablo F. Gómez, "The Circulation of Bodily Knowledge in the Seventeenth-century Black Spanish Caribbean," *Social History of Medicine* 26:3 (2013), 383–402.

56 Roy Porter, "The Patient's View," *Theory and Society* 14(2)(1985): 175–98.

57 Key texts are: Hermilio Valdizán and Angel Maldonado, *La medicina popular peruana,* 3 vols. (Lima: Torres Aguirre, 1922); Juan B. Lastres, *Historia de la medicina peruana.* 3 vols. (Lima: Impr. Santa María, 1951); Guerra, *El hospital,* 429–75; Lanning, *Royal Protomedicato*; Miguel Rabí Chara, *Del Hospital de Santa Ana (1549 a 1924) al Hospital Nacional Arzobispo Loayza (1925 a 1999): 450 años de protección de la salud de las personas* (Lima: INDECOPI, 1999) and *El hospital de San Bartolomé de Lima: la protección y asistencia de la gente de color de 1646 a 1821 y evolución posterior: examen de un proceso histórico, social y sanitaria* (Lima: Grahuer, 2001); Warren, *Medicine and Politics.*

and surgeons, who are thus drawn into the discussion rather than excluded from it. Apothecaries warrant particular attention, however, for more than other professional medical practitioners they were pivotal in supplying Lima with medicines, interacting on the one hand with transatlantic merchants and on the other with local producers and traders of *materia medica*. They, unlike physicians, had to hand the raw materials with which to experiment and therefore had the potential to be pioneers in the development of medicine.

While the study focuses on the role of apothecaries in the practice of medicine, through concentrating on their daily practices, it also provides insight into their social standing within the city and into the manner in which professional groups in general organised their businesses and were regulated. Lima's social structure differed in some respects from other colonial cities. As capital of the Viceroyalty of Peru the city symbolised and promoted the authority of the Spanish state throughout South America and as such its social hierarchy reflected the traditional values that underpinned society in Spain.[58] Its vice-regal role also meant that the state's bureaucratic and ecclesiastical presence was more substantial than elsewhere in South America potentially providing greater opportunities for regulation and social control. However, due in part to Peru's geographical distance from Spain, in reality state control was still limited, as shown in attempts to regulate medical practice and to define social groups in law as envisaged in the *sistema de castas*.[59] In the period under study, Peru was emerging from a bloody conquest and civil wars and the colony's social hierarchy was still in the process of consolidation. It faced the challenges of incorporating diverse ethnic groups and maintaining a hierarchy when opportunities for wealth creation in trade and mining provided opportunities for social advancement, even if ultimately the parameters within which people forged their lives were defined by the colonial state.[60] In such circumstances,

---

58 For the way in which the authority of the king was promoted through ceremonies see Alejandra B. Osorio, *Inventing Lima: Baroque Modernity in Peru's South Sea Metropolis* (New York: Palgrave Macmillan, 2008).

59 For succinct accounts of the *sistema de castas* see: Magnus Mörner, *Race Mixture in the History of Latin America* (Boston: Little, Brown and Company, 1967), 53–73; R. Douglas Cope, *The Limits of Racial Domination: Plebeian Society in Colonial Mexico City, 1660–1720* (Madison: The University of Wisconsin Press, 1994), 9–26; and Ilona Katzew, *Casta Paintings* (New Haven: Yale University Press, 2004), 39–61.

60 For the development of social hierarchies and their limitations see. Lewis, *Hall of Mirrors*, 15–41; Irene Silverblatt, *Modern Inquisitions: Peru and the Colonial Origins of the Civilized World* (Durham: Duke University Press, 2004), 4–27; María Elena Martínez, *Genealogical Fictions: Limpieza de Sangre, Religion, and Gender in Colonial Mexico* (Stanford: Stanford University Press, 2008), 271–72; Andrew B. Fisher and Matthew D. O'Hara, "Introduction:

individuals resorted to different ways of signifying their social status, for example, by dress, charitable works, or group membership.[61] This study demonstrates that apothecaries sought to indicate their status by distancing themselves from popular healers and by adopting the cultural attributes of elites. The impact of their social positioning, the study argues, was generally to weaken the innovative potential of their profession, already discouraged by the Church, Inquisition, and regulation.

It is hoped that this book will be a small response to James Lockhart's call for scholars to "simply to find out what went on in the Spanish colonies"[62] and contribute to knowledge of the social history of Lima at a time when its social and political structures were still in the process of formation and idealised views of how the colonies should be governed were adapting to the reality of the New World. It illustrates how individuals and groups forged their economic and social lives in a context where Spanish laws and regulations had to adapt to local circumstances and were only partially effective.[63]

Prospectus

Through an examination of the way in which apothecaries were trained, established their businesses, acquired and prepared medicines, this book argues that apothecaries had the potential to be innovators in science, especially in the New World where they encountered new environments and diverse healing traditions. However, it shows that despite experimental tendencies among some *boticarios* in Peru, especially in the very earliest years of conquest before regulatory measures were introduced, apothecaries in Lima generally adhered to traditional humoral practices, continuing to import *materia medica* from Spain and raise Old World plants locally, rather than adopt native botanical materials or take advantage of the region's rich mineral resources. It suggests that this adherence to orthodox practices did not derive primarily from

Racial Identities and Their Interpreters in Colonial Latin America," in *Imperial Subjects: Race and Identity in Colonial Latin America*, eds. Andrew B. Fisher and Matthew D. O'Hara (Durham: Duke University Press, 2009), 12–15: Rachel S. O'Toole, *Bound Lives: Africans, Indians, and the Making of Race in Colonial Peru*. Pittsburgh PA: University of Pittsburgh Press, 2012), 4.

61 Fisher and O'Hara, "Introduction," 15–23.

62 James Lockhart, *Spanish Peru 1532–1560: A Colonial Society* (Madison: The University of Wisconsin Press, 1968), 233.

63 Tamar Herzog, *Upholding Justice: Society, State, and the Penal System in Quito (1650–1750)* (Ann Arbor: University of Michigan Press, 2004), 5–8.

effective state regulation, which was applied flexibly and inconsistently according to local circumstances, but rather reflected the extent to which humoral beliefs were entrenched in Spanish thought and had permeated popular beliefs with the support of the Church and Inquisition. It responds to Roy MacLeod's appeal for scholars of colonial science to conduct more research "from the perspective of colonial life."[64]

64 Roy Macleod, "Nature and Empire: Science and the Colonial Enterprise," *Osiris* 15 (2000): 6.

CHAPTER 2

Learning to Make Medicines

Study with learned men with many years' experience in the pharmacy, who are not immoral but virtuous.[1]

Any understanding of pharmacy methods must necessarily take account of the training and licensing of apothecaries, which was specified in law. It was the intention that laws governing medical practice in Spain, specifically Castile, should be mirrored in its colonies.[2] These laws laid down the type of training that physicians, apothecaries and surgeons were to receive, which varied according to the tasks that each was expected to perform. Whereas in theory physicians were to be university educated, for the most part surgeons learned their skills through practical training. Apothecaries fell in between. On the margins of professional medicine and of lower social status were empirics, such as bonesetters, midwives and barbers, who acquired specialist technical skills through experiential learning.

Differences in training effectively created a social hierarchy of medical professionals that was based primarily on the level of university education each had received. Since university education was only open to those who could demonstrate purity of blood or *limpieza de sangre*, the legal training requirements in theory excluded persons from certain ethnic and social groups from aspiring to become physicians or apothecaries. Even though apothecaries generally had a lower status than physicians, Spanish laws reserved for them the exclusive right to prepare medicines. Despite the existence of laws regarding the training and licensing of apothecaries, as this chapter demonstrates, the *protomédicos* and *cabildos*, which were encharged with their compliance, were

1 Archivo del Real Jardín Botánico, Madrid, [hereafter ARJBM] División 1, legajo 17 Prohemiales 3 Libro de examen de los simples medicinales Antonio de Robles Cornejo 1617. The Spanish reads "aprenda con hombres doctos y experimentados de muchos años en la botica que no sea vicioso sino virtuoso."

2 *Recopilación de las leyes de los reynos de las indias* (Madrid: Gráficas Ultra, 1943), 2: lib. 5 tit. 6 ley 2: 140.

 | DOI 10.1163/9789004351271_003

forced to interpret them flexibly in the face of a lack of funding for medical education and a shortage of personnel.

Makers of Medicines

According to Spanish law, physicians were expected to attend the sick, diagnose illnesses, and prescribe medicines, but in theory at least were not permitted to prepare medicines, which remained the preserve of apothecaries.[3] A proposal to change Castilian ordinances to permit physicians to prepare medicines where no apothecary was available had been mooted in the late fifteenth century, but it was not incorporated into legislation.[4] The separation of tasks between physicians and apothecaries appears to have been driven less by an anxiety about the physical harm that physicians might inflict on patients and more by a concern about the fraud and excessive prices that might follow, if they both prescribed and prepared their own medicines. For the same reason the Castilian ordinances banned physicians from entering into business partnerships with particular apothecaries, stipulating that patients were to be free to send their prescriptions to any *boticario* they wished.[5] A particular worry was possible collusion between practitioners who were relatives.[6] However, physicians and surgeons who contravened the ban on preparing medicines received only modest fines for the first and second offences; in theory at least the third brought a two-year ban on practising in the place where they worked.[7] While these laws had been enacted in Spain and in theory were to apply to its colonies, they were often contravened. This was particularly true during the civil wars in Peru that immediately followed Spanish arrival, when in the absence of licensed practitioners and limited regulation, medicine was practised

3 *Recopilación de las leyes, pragmáticas reales, decretos, y acuerdos del Real Proto-Medicato: hecha por encargo y dirección del mismo Real Tribunal por Don Miquel Eugenio Muñoz* (Valencia: Imprenta de la Viuda de Antonio Bordazar, 1751), cap. XIII ordinance 3: 159–60 1537.

4 José Damián González Arce, "Los proyectos de ordenanzas generales de médicos, cirujanos y boticarios de Castilla (ca.1491–1513)," *Dynamis* 31(1)(2011): 222. It was the intention that the ordinances would apply to all Castilian territories, but there were disputes between physicians, opposition from the local authorities in other cities which had jurisdiction over medical practice, and the Royal Court, which meant that it was never adopted.

5 González Arce, "Proyectos de ordenanzas," 222.

6 *Recopilación de las leyes, pragmáticas reales* (Muñoz), cap. XIV ordinance 2: 170.

7 *Recopilación de las leyes, pragmátics reales* (Muñoz) cap. XIII ordinance 2: 159. Fines for the first and second offences were 10,000 and 20,000 *maravedís* respectively, which at 272 *maravedís* for one peso, were about 37 and 74 pesos respectively.

by a multiplicity of individuals from diverse backgrounds with differing levels of skill. Even after relative political stability had been achieved, the appointment of a royal *protomédico* encharged with the regulation of medical practice did not occur in until 1568; thereafter there were often gaps in appointments, when the *cabildo* rather than the state assumed responsibility for healthcare, as it had done since the city was founded in 1535.

The earliest medical practitioners to arrive in Peru accompanied armies of conquest. Some were licensed physicians, such as Hernando de Sepúlveda who accompanied Pedro de Alvarado to Peru in 1534 and was appointed as the first *protomédico* by the *cabildo* in Lima.[8] Another was Alvaro de Torres who provided medical support for Governor Cristóbal Vaca de Castro in the Peruvian civil wars of the 1540s.[9] Both these practitioners had graduated from the University of Salamanca and operated as both physicians and surgeons. However, many others, probably the majority, went as surgeons on armies of conquest when they performed the multiple roles of diagnosing sickness, treating wounds, and prescribing and preparing medicines. A military manual published by seasoned soldier Captain Bernardo Vargas de Machuca in 1599 specified the basic medicines that surgeons should carry with them in the field and indicated the types of remedies they should apply.[10]

In the early stages of colonial rule, therefore, it was surgeons rather than *boticarios* who prepared medicines; it was only after political stability had been achieved that trained *boticarios* moved to the New World. Meanwhile some surgeons who had arrived in Lima at an early date stayed on and sought acceptance as physicians or permission to prepare medicines, sometimes claiming they had lost their titles to practise or by demonstrating they had exceptional skill. Andrés Gonzales, who was of Portuguese descent and became a wealthy *boticario* and trader of medicines in Cartagena, does not appear to have had any medical training. When he was investigated as a foreigner in 1620, he testified that he had arrived in the Indies as a soldier, but finding a shortage of *boticarios* in the city had taken over the *botica* of one who had recently

8 *Libros de cabildos de Lima*, eds. Bertram T. Lee *et al.* (Lima: Torres Aguirre, 1935–1963), 1: 141–42 Licencia a dotor [sic] Sepúlveda 27 Apr. 1537; Deza Bringas, *Testimonios del linaje médico*, 31–35.

9 Gustavo Delgado Matallana, *Historia de la enseñanza médica en el Perú* (Lima: Universidad Nacional Mayor de San Marcos, 2008), 1–6.

10 Bernardo de Vargas Machuca, *The Indian Militia and Description of the Indies*, ed. Kris Lane, trans. Timothy F. Johnson (Durham, NC: Duke University Press, 2008), 60–69. See also Chapter 6.

died.[11] The *protomédico* and *cabildo* in Lima generally resisted moves by those without formal training to become licensed,[12] but it did allow some surgeons to practise surgery without licence.

Despite efforts by the municipal authorities and the *protomédico* to draw distinctions between physicians, surgeons and *boticarios*, they were blurred in the eyes of many and even in official sources practitioners were referred to inconsistently. Hence, when Francisco de Alva was made *boticario* to the Inquisition in 1574, he was described as being a surgeon and *boticario*.[13] Similarly, at the end of the century, in a legal case pursued by Pedro de Vergara for the recovery of debts for medicines he had dispensed, he was described as both a licensed *médico* and *boticario*.[14] Any local concern there may have been about physicians and surgeons preparing medicines focussed not on the illegality of the practice or the types of medicines they dispensed, but rather on their poor quality.[15] Hence in 1538, the *cabildo's* reaction to complaints that physicians and surgeons were selling poor quality medicines and charging excessive prices was not to impose fines and ban them from dispensing drugs, but rather to send inspectors to destroy the offending medicines and regulate their prices.[16]

Education and Practical Training

Despite the fact that many medicines were prepared illegally by persons other than *boticarios*, the educational and training requirements of different types of licensed medical practitioners were clearly distinguished. Physicians first had to obtain a Bachelor of Arts degree from a recognized university, which took four years, and then study for four years in a Faculty of Medicine in order to obtain a bachelor's degree in medicine. Finally, they had to work under the

---

11 Archivo General de Indias (AGI) Escribanía de Cámara 589B Denuncia contra Andrés Gonzales, boticario, Portugués 1620.

12 *Libros de cabildos de Lima,* 1: 161–62 Mandamiento de cirugía 30 Aug. 1537.

13 *Libros de cabildos de Lima,* 7: 549–550 Título de familiar al bachiller Alba [sic] 21 Jan. 1574. This position was later taken over by Juan de Bilbao (*Libros de cabildos de Lima,* 8: 201 Familiar del santo oficio a Juan de Bilbao 24 Feb. 1576).

14 Archivo General de la Nación, Peru (hereafter AGNP) Santo Oficio Contencioso (hereafter SO CO) 8–81 Pedro de Vergara, médico, licenciado, contra Nuño Rodríguez de Acevedo 23 Dec. 1599.

15 No detailed accounts exist of inspections of private pharmacies, but those that exist for hospital pharmacies (discussed in Chapter 4) and for those conducted in Spain, suggest that some inspections may have also specified that certain products should be acquired.

16 *Libros de cabildos de Lima,* 1: 181 Sobre las medicinas 23 Jan. 1538.

supervision of recognised doctors for two years before they were allowed to practise. Despite the last requirement, physicians, unlike *boticarios* and surgeons, actually received very little practical training.[17] However, they held the highest status due to their university education. In contrast, according to Spanish regulations in 1528 and 1563, surgeons and *boticarios* were not required to attend to university before being examined, but only show that they had practised under a recognised *boticario* or surgeon for four years.[18] From 1588 it was stipulated that licensed *boticarios* had to be at least 25 years old,[19] although training often began somewhat earlier. Writing in Peru, the Salamanca-trained physician Antonio de Robles Cornejo argued that training should not begin before the age of 15, since younger scholars did not have the strength or capacity to work and learn.[20] This was echoed by Antonio de Aguilera in his guidance to *boticarios* in his *Exposición sobre las preparaciones de Mesue* (1569) where he advised that a good apothecary should have "prudence and knowledge" (prudencia y ciencia), the acquisition of which required time. As such, he judged that although training might start at age 12 or 14 to 16 or 18, it took until 22, 24, or 26 for a *boticario* to acquire the necessary skills by working alongside an expert pharmacist.[21]

All apothecaries received on-the-job training, but not all undertook academic study. Nevertheless, the latter was considered desirable, since *boticarios* had to have knowledge of Latin in order to interpret physicians' prescriptions and to read manuals written on the preparation of medicines, which in the early sixteenth century were generally published in Latin.[22] This meant that in Spain at least apothecaries, unlike most surgeons, generally had a university education.[23] In the mid-sixteenth century it was proposed that physicians

17 *Recopilación de las leyes, pragmáticas reales* (Muñoz), cap. X ordinance 1: 137–38.

18 *Novísima recopilación de las leyes de España* (Madrid, 1805) lib. 8 tit. 13 ley 1: 106–107; *Recopilación de las leyes pragmáticas reales* (Muñoz), cap. XI ordinances 1–4: 150–52, cap. XII ordinances 1 and 2: 155–56.

19 *Novísima recopilación de las leyes de España*, lib. 8 tit. 13 ley 1: 106 1588.

20 ARJBM División 1, leg. 17 Prohemiales 3 Libro de examen de los simples medicinales Antonio de Robles Cornejo 1617. It reads that at age 15 years "tendra de esta edad fuerzas para trabajar en lo que fuere necesario y entendimiento libre para los secretos del [arte de farmacia]."

21 Antonio de Aguilera, *Exposición sobre las preparaciones de Mesue* (Alcalá: Juan de Villanueva, 1569), fols.17v–18.

22 Aguilera, *Exposición*, fol. 17; Christóval Suárez de Figueroa, *Plaza universal de todas ciencias y artes* (Madrid: Luis Sánchez, 1615), 301.

23 In fact some surgeons did attend university and were examined in Latin, in which case they were known as *cirujanos latinos*. Other surgeons without a university education, who were examined in Spanish, were known as *cirujanos romancistas*.

should write prescriptions in the vernacular, obviating the need for apothecaries to have knowledge of Latin. However, this suggestion was consistently rejected by the Crown which was anxious to restrict knowledge of potential harmful medicines to literate experts.[24] Latin therefore remained a legal prerequisite for obtaining a license to practise as an apothecary.[25] It also supported the status interests of *boticarios* since it distinguished them from surgeons and other healers and sellers of drugs, and allied them with higher status physicians. While those *boticarios* trained in Spain may have possessed Latin, as will be shown below this was not always the case in Lima.[26] It is worth noting that apart from Latin, *boticarios* were also required to have knowledge of arithmetic in order to work out weights and measures.[27]

From 1593 Spanish laws forbade women from practising pharmacy or owning *boticas* even if they did not practise pharmacy themselves but employed a licensed practitioner or salaried *oficial*.[28] However, widows often inherited *boticas* from their deceased husbands and in Seville the *cabildo* often permitted them to retain ownership of a pharmacy and either employ a trained *boticario* or pass its administration to a male relative.[29] This may have also been the case in Lima, where before eventually selling her deceased husband's *botica* Marina de Alva employed a Spanish *boticario* to administer it.[30] In Mexico City in the late eighteenth century a number of *boticas* were registered as being owned by women.[31] These may have been owned without licence since the law remained in force throughout the colonial period. Nowhere is any justification provided

24 Clouse, *Medicine*, 132.

25 *Recopilación de las leyes, pragmáticas reales* (Muñoz), cap. XII ordinance 1: 155, cap. XIV ordinance 9: 179.

26 ARJBM División 1, leg. 17 Prologo. Libro de examen de los simples medicinales Antonio de Robles Cornejo 1617.

27 ARJBM División 1, legajo 17 Prohemiales 2 Libro de examen de los simples medicinales Antonio de Robles Cornejo 1617.

28 *Novísima recopilación de las leyes de España*, lib 8. tit. 13 ley 3: 107 2 Aug. 1593. This stipulation was contrary to Roman law which allowed it (Lanning, *Royal Protomedicato*, 231). This restriction was not raised in the drafting of laws to be followed by the *protomédico* in Spain in the early sixteenth century (González Arce, "Proyectos de ordenanzas reales," 220–226).

29 Mercedes Fernández-Carrión and José Luis Valverde, *Farmacia y sociedad en Sevilla en el siglo XVI* (Sevilla: Servicio de Publicaciones del Ayuntamiento de Sevilla, 1985), 20.

30 AGNP Real Audiencia. Causas Civiles leg. 16 cuad. 81 fol. 422 Pleito de ejecución promovido por Baltasar de Zamora y Pedro Tenorio, mercaderes, vecinos de la ciudad de Trujillo y por otros acreedores, contra las bienes y herederos del bachiller Francisco de Alva, boticario morador en la Ciudad de los Reyes. 1576.

31 Hernández Sáenz, *Learning to Heal*, 151; De Vos, "Art of Pharmacy," 51–52.

for the ban on women practising pharmacy,[32] though moral attitudes of the time generally militated against the participation of women in the public sphere.[33] Even though women may not have been licensed to practise, and could not legally own *boticas*, they appear to have undertaken auxiliary activities in the pharmacy. In fact, Antonio de Robles Cornejo advised *boticarios* to employ their wives in keeping clean its utensils and equipment, and suggested they might even sell medicines when the *boticario* was absent.[34] Of course, the activities that wives actually undertook in the pharmacy may have extended beyond those specified. However, it remained the case that formal medical training was not available to them.

Apothecaries from Spain

As noted above, a few unlicensed practitioners with experience of preparing medicines in the field may have stayed on to practise and sought licences to do so, but in the earliest years of the colony most *boticarios* in Lima came from Spain with the intention to setting up businesses. Commonly these apothecaries had been licensed in Spain where they had possessed a *botica* or had worked as a salaried employee; some were the sons of *boticarios* who were following in the family tradition and once established in Lima continued to trade medicines with their relatives in Spain.[35] There was a lack of employment opportunities in Spain at this time and *boticarios* may have seen greater career prospects overseas.[36] However, migrating to the Americas required a licence from the *Casa de Contratación* and acquiring one was not a simple process. Initially the

32 Lanning, *Royal Protomedicato*, 231.

33 Nancy E. Van Deusen, *Between the Sacred and the Worldly: The Institutional and Cultural Practice of Recogimiento in Colonial Lima* (Stanford: Stanford University Press, 2001), 20–24.

34 ARJBM División 1, leg. 17 Prohemiales 6 Libro de examen de los simples medicinales Antonio de Robles Cornejo 1617.

35 Fernández-Carrión and Valverde, *Farmacia y sociedad*, 64. For *boticarios* in Spain who sent their sons to the Americas see: Diego, son of Antonio Bernal (Seville), AGI Contratación 5537 L1 fol. 210v. (Image 420) Licence granted to Diego Bernal 1557; Pedro, son of Francisco García (Plasencia) AGI Contratación 5255 N1 R68 Licence granted to Pedro García 9 May 1598; Juan, son of Pedro García de Poveda (Calahorra) AGI Contratación 5222 N1 R9 Licence granted to Juan García de la Poveda 1572.

36 For the lack of opportunities for trained physicians in Spain see Kristy Wilson Bowers, *Plague and Public Health in Early Modern Seville* (Rochester: University of Rochester Press, 2013), 29.

Crown encouraged immigration, but in the wake of the turbulent years of conquest and the rebellion of Gonzalo Pizarro, it decided to control the number of migrants going to Peru, especially of single men, for whom it was judged there were insufficient rewards in the form of *encomiendas* and limited employment opportunities. Immigration therefore became restricted to those who were deemed to be productive members of society and the migration of families was favoured.[37] Hence, the licences granted to individuals were generally given for a specified number of years only, after which they were to return to Spain or, if they were married, send for their wives.[38] The rule was difficult to enforce, but prosecutions were conducted if the opportunity arose. Hence, at the end of the sixteenth century the *boticario* Cristóbal Gómez, who had left his wife in Seville, was imprisoned in Lima and ordered to pay a fine of 300 pesos before being sent back to Spain as a prisoner. There he complained that all his wealth was in Peru and he successfully petitioned the *Casa de Contratación* to allow him to return to Peru with his wife, children and two servants.[39]

Licences to travel to the Americas also stipulated where individuals were to reside and for how long.[40] They might also require them to practise their profession and no other; migrants also had to provide bonds as security, especially if there was some doubt about their intentions.[41] Hence, the *boticario* Yuste de León who received a licence to travel to Tierra Firme had to provide a bond of 200,000 *maravedís* that he would practise his profession,[42] while Luis de León, travelling to the Tierra Firme as a servant to the *boticario*, Gerónimo Luis, was similarly required to post a bond for 200,000 *maravedís*, though in this case it was to ensure that he would remain in the region and not move to another for

37 Woodrow Borah, *Early Trade and Navigation between Mexico and Peru, Ibero-Americana* 38 (Berkeley and Los Angeles: University of California, 1954), 98–101, 107; Peter Boyd-Bowman, "Spanish Patterns of Emigration to the Indies to 1600," *Hispanic American Historical Review* 56 (4)(1976): 583.

38 *Recopilación de las leyes de las Indias*, lib. 1 tit. 7 ley 14 19 Oct 1544 and lib. 7 tit. 3 ley 8 2 Dec. 1578.

39 AGI Indiferente General 2104 N135 Licence granted to Cristóbal Gómez, boticario, 1599. For another case of single men being required to return to Spain for their wives see AGI Justicia 356 no 2 ramo 1 El fiscal contra Alonso Bernal, boticario vecino de Sevilla 1562–1569.

40 *Recopilación de las leyes de las Indias*, lib. 9 tit. 26 ley 41 19 Oct. 1566, 6 Oct 1578.

41 Ibid, lib. 9 tit. 26 ley 43 17 Apr. 1553, 7 Feb 1567; Ida Altman, *Emigrants and Society: Extremadura and Spanish America in the Sixteenth Century* (Berkeley: University of California, 1989), 208, 253.

42 AGI Contratación 5537 L3 fol.303 (Image 605) Licence granted to Yuste de León 5 Jan. 1569.

eight years.[43] It seems that greater restrictions were placed on those who were unmarried or who went as servants.

Licensed apothecaries were slow to arrive. In 1538 it was said there was only one *boticario* in the city, probably Alonso de Alemán.[44] At time, he and a number of physicians and surgeons were said to be selling expensive and poor quality out-of-date medicines, while others were preparing them illegally.[45] Another early arrival was *bachiller* Francisco de Alva, who became one of the most prominent apothecaries in Lima.[46] He like many other *boticarios* travelling to Lima in the sixteenth century migrated with his family. Another immigrant *boticario* was Cristóbal Carrasco, who had been examined in Madrid by the *protomédico* and chamber physician, Doctor Juan Gutiérrez de Santander, and had been practising in Spain for fifteen years. He had owned a *botica* in Plasencia and in 1581 was licensed to travel to Peru with his wife, two children and four servants.[47] Those who owned *boticas* in Spain often took drugs and equipment from their pharmacies with them. One such apothecary was Mançio Gasco who was a licensed *boticario* and *vecino* of Seville, who accompanied the physician Doctor Castellanos to Trujillo.[48] Similarly in 1591 when Juan Sánchez sailed to Peru with his wife and three children, he took with him fifteen medical books and nearly one hundred types of medicines worth 585 reals.[49]

Not all *boticarios* travelled to Peru with the intention of setting up new businesses. Some accompanied eminent officials, particularly the Viceroy. Unlike those who established businesses, these were mainly single men. Francisco

---

43 AGI Contratación 5538 L1 fol.405 (Image 809) Licence granted to Luis de León 14 Mar. 1582.

44 *Libros de cabildos de Lima*, 2: 115 El bachiller Pacheco malquerencia Dec. 1545. He had received a licence to travel to Tierra Firme on 3 Apr. 1538 (AGI Contratación 5536 L5 fol. 103r. Image 191).

45 *Libros de cabildos de Lima*, 1: 181 Sobre las medicinas 23 Jan. 1538, 1: 254 5 [Precios excesivos] Dec. 1538, 1: 256 [visita de la botica desta ciudad] 6 Dec. 1538, 1: 387 [Curas con e[n] salmos] 13 Oct. 1539.

46 In the sources consulted for this study, Francisco de Alva is the only *boticario* referred to as a *bachiller* (AGNP Real Audiencia leg. 16 cuad. 81 Inventario de los bienes del bachiller Francisco de Alva 9 Feb. 1576). He left for Lima with his wife about 1550 (AGI Lima 566 L6 N420), so his university education would have been in Spain.

47 AGI Indiferente General 2092 N86 Licence granted to Cristóbal Carrasco, boticario, 1581.

48 AGI Indiferente General 2090 N53 Licence granted to Mançio Gasco, boticario, 1578.

49 AGI Contratación 1097 N 5 197–202 Registro del navío Santa Catalina 1592. He appears in the ship's passenger list with his wife Francisca de Ortega and their children Ana, Gabriel and Mariana (Images 905–906). He was travelling with his father Cristóbal de Salcedo, aged 52, and his mother Catalina Rodríguez, who was a former resident of Nombre de Dios but had been living in Seville for 15 years. See also: AGI Contratación 5234B N1 R36 Licence granted to Juan Sánchez 1591 and Appendix 1.

Gutiérrez accompanied Diego López de Zúñiga y Velasco, the fourth Conde de Nieva in 1560,[50] and in 1569 Gerónimo Rodríguez travelled to Peru with Francisco de Toledo.[51] Unlike most other single migrants, no restrictions were placed on them in terms of their destination, length of stay, or the occupation they were to practise. The Spanish physician Antonio de Robles Cornejo who lived in Peru for many years observed that it had excellent medical practitioners, but was critical of those who arrived in the early years of Spanish settlement. He suggested that it was the less educated and skilled in all professions that migrated at that time, such that Peru had some apothecaries and physicians who were "ignorant and lazy."[52]

University Medical Education

The professional apothecaries who migrated from Spain had generally been formally educated and trained, but over time the majority were Creoles for whom the absence of the title 'bachiller' suggests that in the early colonial period at least most *boticarios* did not attend university. Aspirant *boticarios* did not have to attend courses in medicine, but in any case this was difficult since medical education in Peru was slow to become established. The University of San Marcos was founded in 1551 and in 1569 some medical instruction started with the arrival of the royal *protomédico*, Antonio Sánchez Renedo, who taught natural philosophy and astrology.[53] However, despite various proposals to found medical chairs that would enable the University to award medical degrees, this was delayed because of the lack of funds. This reflected in part the general lack of student interest in studying medicine because of the low status of the profession compared to the law or the Church.[54] The situation

50 AGI Contratación 5537 Lib. 2 fol. 97 (Image 195) Licence granted to Francisco Gutiérrez 7 Mar. 1560.

51 AGI Contratación 5537 Lib. 3 fol. 340 (Image 679) Licence granted to Gerónimo Rodríguez 1 Feb. 1569.

52 ARJBM División 1, leg. 17 Prologo Libro de examen de los simples medicinales Antonio de Robles Cornejo 1617.

53 Luis Antonio Eguiguren, *Alma mater: origines de la Universidad de San Marcos (1551–1579)*(Lima, 1939), 257–58, 337; Lastres, *Historia de la medicina peruana*, 49–55, 87–94; Lanning, *Royal Protomedicato*, 29–30; Matallana, *Historia de la enseñanza médica*, 76.

54 Susan E. Ramírez, *Provincial Patriarchs: Land Tenure and the Economics of Power in Colonial Peru* (Albuquerque: University of New Mexico Press, 1985), 176–77, 226; Eduardo Zarate, *Inicios de la escuela de medicina de Lima* (Lima: No Publisher, 2005), 27–28, 30. In Spain students showed an equal lack of interest in studying medicine (Javier Alejo

deteriorated after 1599 when the salaries paid to the incumbents of all university chairs were significantly reduced and support for the chair of medicine and philosophy, which had commanded a salary of 800 pesos, was withdrawn. In 1619 Viceroy Esquilache considered the lack of medical education to be a pressing issue since the general lack of physicians meant that barbers and surgeons were carrying out harmful treatments and were commanding large incomes without, it was said, being able to read or write.[55] He therefore argued that two chairs of medicine should be established. However, these did not materialise until 1634, when under growing pressure from the *cabildo* and the then *protomédico*, Doctor Juan de la Vega, the governing viceroy, the Conde de Chinchón, assigned income from the sale of *solimán* (sublimate of mercury) to support two medical chairs of *prima* and *visperas* with salaries of 600 pesos and 400 pesos respectively;[56] a move that was approved by the Crown in 1638.[57] Even so, salaries were often not provided and the chairs frequently remained vacant.[58]

Inasmuch as aspirant *boticarios* attended university, they would have pursued a general degree in the arts that enabled them to learn Latin, before undertaking practical training alongside licensed *boticarios*. In reality, those

Montes and Maria Carmen Rodríguez García, "Los estudios de la facultad de medicina en la Universidad de Salamanca de finales del siglo XVI," *Espacio, tiempo y forma, Serie IV, Historia moderna* 7 (1994): 38–39.

55 Archivo Histórico 'Domingo Angulo', Universidad Nacional Mayor de San Marcos (hereafter UNMSM), Archivo Histórico Tesorería General, Libro de Caja, ano 1619 (1577–1617] no. 28 Relación del estado, rentas y cátedras de la universidad de los reyes, Virrey Príncipe de Esquilache 10 Apr. 1619. It was suggested that the two chairs could be could be funded by the Crown supplementing the salaries paid to physicians to treat patients in the hospitals of Santa Ana and San Andrés by 300 *pesos ensayados* each.

56 AGI Lima 45 N4 fols. 146–147 El Conde de Chinchón 21 Apr. 1634, Márquez de Mancera 29 May 1640; Luis Antonio Eguiguren, *Diccionario histórico cronológico de la universidad real y pontificia de San Marcos y sus colegios* (Lima: Torres Aguirre, 1940), 1: 1016–1024; Lastres, *Historia de la medicina peruana*, 2: 51, 87–92; Lanning, *Royal Protomedicato*, 327–28, 331; Luis Martín, *The Intellectual Conquest of Peru: The Jesuit College of San Pablo, 1568–1767* (New York: Fordham University Press, 1968), 98; Delgado Matallana, *Historia de la enseñanza médica* 10–25, 104–112. These salaries were under half of those paid to professors of theology, law and the arts (Lanning, *Royal Protomedicato*, 327). The first chairs were filled by the *protomédico* Juan de la Vega (*prima*) and Andrés de la Rocha (*vísperas*) (José Antonio Suardo, *Diario de Lima (1629–1639)*, ed. Rubén Vargas Ugarte (Lima: "Lumen," 1936), 2: 76–77). The latter had only graduated with a doctorate in medicine in 1630 when he was examined by Juan de la Vega (Suardo, *Diario*, 107).

57 *Recopilación de leyes de las Indias*, lib. 1 tit. 22 ley 33 7 Mar. 1638.

58 AGI Lima 337 Real cédula 19 Jun. 1689.

working in *boticas* might acquire some knowledge of Latin without attending classes. They did, however, need to be literate.

Preparatory Schooling

The educational opportunities for students in Lima varied according to their class and ethnic background. Elite parents paid for their sons to be educated at primary level by private tutors, who could be either professional teachers or members of the religious orders. Tutors were usually contracted to teach reading, writing and arithmetic on an annual basis for a specified salary. Commonly they were paid 100 to 125 pesos for this instruction, though it could be less if the tutor resided in the pupil's home or more expensive if more advanced forms of instruction were required. For example, a merchant, Juan de Cardenas, paid a tutor 300 pesos over a year and a half for instructing his son in accounting practices.[59] Private tuition was only a practical proposition for the wealthiest families. Overtime, as the number of children increased, primary schools were established. Here fees were about half the cost of private tuition. Some of the first steps in education were taken by the religious orders that often ran classes attached to their convents, but other private schools also sprang up. By the beginning of the seventeenth century there were said to be ten or twelve approved primary schools, three of which were supported by the government to teach the poor free of charge. There were said to be about one thousand pupils attending these schools.[60] With the expansion of schools, in 1594 guidelines were drawn up that specified how pupils should be taught reading, writing, and simple arithmetic, and how they should conduct themselves.[61] About 1630 there were said to be twenty-eight *escuelas públicas* run by professional teachers for children.[62]

The desirability of founding secondary schools, which were residential and would prepare students for a university education by teaching students in Latin, was recognised at an early date. In 1575 Viceroy Toledo attempted to found

59 For examples of teaching contracts see: AGNP Protocolos Siglo XVI Ramiro Bote 14 fols. 1370-1370v. Francisco Díaz y Juan de Arriaça celebran concierto 14 Oct. 1597; Eguiguren, *Diccionario histórico cronológico*, 1: CCXCII, 2: 294–300; Luis Martín and Jo Ann Geurin Pettas, *Scholars and Schools in Colonial Peru* (Dallas, TX: Southern Methodist University, 1973): 115–17.

60 Bernabé Cobo, *Obras* (Madrid: Ediciones Atlas, 1956), 2: 414; Carlos Daniel Valcarcel, *Historia de la educación colonial* (Lima: Editorial Universo, 1968), 2: 31–32.

61 The guidelines are reproduced in Martín and Pettas, *Scholars and Schools*, 118–22.

62 Fray Buenaventura de Salinas y Córdova, *Memorial de las historias del Nuevo Mundo Pirú* [sic]. Vol. 1 (Lima: Universidad Nacional Mayor de San Marcos, 1957), 257.

the secular college or *colegio* of San Felipe y San Marcos for the sons of conquistadors and *beneméritos*, but it did not materialise until 1592 and then only admitted 20 students. Its ordinances banned "gente baja" (the lower classes), Mulatos and Zambahigos from attending as well as those condemned by the Inquisition.[63] Like many other institutions whose financial support derived in part from *encomiendas*, the decline in Peru's native population severely affected the College's income.[64] By the beginning of the seventeenth century, therefore, students had to pay their own subsistence costs.[65] Meanwhile, in 1582, the Jesuits had founded the *colegio real* of San Martín for the sons of conquistadors, *vecinos* and other "gente noble" (elite persons).[66] In the early seventeenth century and in contrast to San Felipe and San Marcos, the *colegio real* of San Martín was said to be flourishing and providing a good education, specialising in teaching philosophy and theology.[67] In 1612 it had 220 students who each paid 150 to 200 *pesos de nueve reales* a year for instruction, food, lodging, and medical care.[68] Despite supposedly being a school for the elite, unlike the *colegio* of San Felipe y San Marcos, initially it seems to have admitted persons from all ethnic backgrounds for by the mid-seventeenth century the Rector had to

63 Cobo, *Obras*, 2: 438–40. For the ordinances of the colegio of San Felipe y San Marcos by the Marqués de Cañete in 1592 see: AGI Lima 323A Ordenanzas del colegio de San Felipe y San Marcos 8 Aug. 1592; Pedro Manuel Alonso Marañón, "Constituciones del colegio real de San Felipe y San Marcos de Lima," *Estudios de historia social y económica de América*, 15 (1997): 419–34 which contains a transcription of the original manuscript in the Biblioteca Nacional Madrid, Manuscript 3043.

64 Cook, *Demographic Collapse*.

65 AGI Lima 337 La universidad de San Marcos 1 May 1601; UNMSM, Archivo Histórico Tesorería General, Libro de Caja, ano 1619 (1577–1617) no. 28 Relación del estado, rentas y cátedras de la universidad de los reyes, Virrey Príncipe de Esquilache 10 Apr. 1619.

66 ARSI Perú 4 fol.7 Catalogo común de las cosas y personas de la provincia del Perú 1583; Cobo, *Obras* 2: 436–38; AGI Lima 208 N11 2 May 1586. Its foundation was approved by Viceroy Martín Enríquez in 1586.

67 AGI Lima 322 Colegio de San Felipe y San Marcos 28 May 1604; AGI Lima 35 Número 5 Libro v fol. 30v Relación de las provincias, conventos ... que tiene las ordenes en el Perú 162; UNMSM, Archivo Histórico Tesorería General, Libro de Caja, ano 1619 (1577–1617] no. 28 Relación del estado, rentas y cátedras de la universidad de los reyes, Virrey Príncipe de Esquilache 10 Apr. 1619.

68 AGI Lima 275 fol. 521v. Relación de lo que se paga de vino, aceite i medicinas ... 1612. See also Reginaldo de Lizárraga, *Descripción breve de toda la tierra del Perú, Tucumán, Río de la Plata y Chile*. Biblioteca de autores españoles 216 (Madrid: Ediciones Atlas, 1968), cap. 46: 35; Antonio Vázquez de Espinosa, *Compendio y descripción de las Indias occidentales*. Biblioteca de autores españoles 231 (Madrid: Ediciones Atlas, 1969), 306; Salinas y Córdova, *Memorial*, 182; Eguiguren, *Diccionario histórico cronológico*, 2: 302.

be reminded not to admit Mulattoes and Mestizos.[69] Finally, the *colegio* of San Toribio was founded in 1594 for those seeking ordination as secular priests and was said to have "good and virtuous students."[70] Educational provision was dogged by jurisdictional disputes between the secular authorities and the religious orders. The latter, especially the Jesuits at the College of San Pablo, ran popular classes for lay students and thereby competed with providers elsewhere, and especially the University of San Marcos. This dispute was partially resolved in 1580 after which San Pablo became the preparatory school for students wishing to study the humanities at the University. At the same time, San Pablo received the exclusive right to teach Latin and Greek, but it could not award its own degrees.[71] Henceforth the University was the only institution that could award bachelors' degrees, masters' degrees, and doctorates.

Educational Opportunities for Non-Elites

The educational opportunities for non-elites varied by ethnic group. The Crown was of two minds about the education of Indians. On the one hand it considered the education of native elites to be fundamental to its mission to Christianise and 'civilise' native peoples and to be means of facilitating their political control; on the other it was concerned that literacy and knowledge of the law might enable indigenous people to challenge the privileged position of Spaniards and Creoles.[72] Others argued that schools for native children would divert much needed financial support from the Spanish sector to Indians, who as conquered and 'uncivilised' people were less worthy of education.[73] In as much as it was thought desirable to educate Indians, state support focussed on provision for native elites. It was late in coming, however. A royal school for the sons of indigenous leaders was not established in Lima until 1618 when the Crown founded the Colegio del Príncipe in El Cercado.[74] Prior to this, the

69 Cobo, *Obras*, 2: 425; Martín, *Intellectual Conquest*, 36–38.

70 Cobo, *Obras*, 2: 440–41; UNMSM, Archivo histórico Tesorería General, Libro de Caja, ano 1619 (1577–1617) no. 28 Relación del estado, rentas y cátedras de la universidad de los reyes, Virrey Príncipe de Esquilache 10 Apr. 1619.

71 Martín, *Intellectual Conquest*, 16–33; Eguiguren, *Alma mater*, 495–98.

72 Monica Alperrine-Bouyer, *La educación de las élites indígenas en el Perú colonial* (Lima: Instituto de Estudios Peruanos, 2007), 31–33.

73 Ibid., 84–85.

74 Alcira Dueñas, *Indians and Mestizos in the "Lettered City"* (Boulder: University Press of Colorado, 2010), 16–18; Alperrine-Bouyer, *Educación de las élites indígenas*, 75, 89; John Charles, "Trained by Jesuits: Indigenous letrados in Sixteenth-Century Peru," in *Indigenous*

religious orders had offered classes to Indians, with the Jesuits establishing a school in El Cercado in 1568.[75]

Unlike Indians, who were regarded as free subjects of the Crown and therefore did not have to demonstrate *limpieza de sangre*, this requirement represented a potential obstacle to the education and later to the acquisition of a license to practise for non-elites.[76] As María Elena Martínez has shown, the concept of *limpieza de sangre* was originally framed in Spain on the basis of genealogy and religious adherence, but even there it was never clearly defined.[77] In Spanish America the presence and intermarriage of persons from different ethnic groups, made the demonstration of *limpieza de sangre* even more difficult, such that the granting or denying of the status of *limpieza de sangre* came to rely on oral testimony, reputation, or skin colour, thereby rendering it open to interpretation.[78] The University of San Marcos was modelled on the universities of Salamanca and Valladolid in Spain, where university attendance required students, at least in theory, to be legitimate and demonstrate *limpieza de sangre*,[79] but even in Spain the requirement to demonstrate purity of blood for entry into university and obtain a license to practice medicine was often overlooked.[80] Similarly, in Peru the adherence of the authorities to this legal requirement was not constant over time and was often interpreted flexibly.[81]

In Lima, initially at least, the concept of *limpeza de sangre* did not have racial connotations and there does not appear to have been any formal barrier to Indians, Blacks or persons of mixed race from attending university there.

Intellectuals: Knowledge, Power and Colonial Culture in Mexico and the Andes, eds. Gabriela Ramos and Yanna Yannakakis (Durham: Duke University Press, 2014), 61–62, 72–74.

75 Eguiguren, *Diccionario histórico cronológico*, 1: 773–74; Martín and Pettas, *Scholars and Schools*, 18.

76 John Tate Lanning, *Academic Culture in the Spanish Colonies* (Oxford: Oxford University Press, 1940), 40.

77 For the origin of the concept of *limpieza de sangre* and its incorporation into Spanish legislation see Martínez, *Genealogical Fictions*, 25–60.

78 Ibid., 168–70.

79 Stafford Poole, "The Politics of *Limpieza de Sangre*: Juan de Ovando and His Circle in the Reign of Philip II," *The Americas* 55 (1999): 363, 388.

80 José Luis Valverde and Guillermina López Andújar, "Los disposiciones legales sobre el certificado de 'limpieza de sangre' en relación al ejército profesional farmacéutico," *Boletín de la sociedad española de la historia de la farmacia* 31 (1981): 259–69; Kamen, *Spanish Inquisition*, 233–34, 241–43.

81 Lanning, John Tate, "Legitimacy and *Limpieza de Sangre* in the Practice of Medicine in the Spanish Empire," *Jahrbuch für Geschicte von Staat, Wirtschaft und Gesellschaft Lateinamerikas* 4 (1967), 40–41, 46–52, 58–60.

Indeed, in 1576 Viceroy Francisco Toledo saw the university education of Mestizos as rendering them useful citizens, who through their knowledge of native languages could be instrumental in converting the Indians to Christianity and integrating them into colonial society.[82] In the 1602 constitution of the University of San Marcos, the only social group specifically excluded under statute 238 were those who had been sentenced by the Inquisition.[83] The rather liberal stance taken by the University in the early colonial period allowed people from diverse ethnic backgrounds to attend. However, an individual's lack of purity of blood always be could be raised at any stage, perhaps by those seeking to eliminate rivals or damage reputations.[84] In the seventeenth century, there were growing concerns, often from white professionals seeking to protect their privileged position, that the influx of non-whites into the University was damaging its reputation and its degrees. This led to a harder stance being taken on admissions.[85] In 1678 a *cédula* was issued reinforcing statute 238, but this time specifying that Mestizos, Mulattoes, *Zambos* and *Quarterones* should be excluded.[86] Even so, the edict was not consistently applied.

For those wishing to progress to the University of San Marcos another significant obstacle was cost. Its 1602 constitution specified that those wishing to graduate with a bachelor's degree in law or the arts had to pay 200 reals, or in theology and medicine 300 reals. A *licenciatura* cost 310 reals a year. This did not include the chickens, sweetmeats, candles,[87] and other goods and tips paid to various university personnel, as well as the cost of a dinner for the rector,

---

82 Cobo, *Obras*, 2: 406 Viceroy Toledo 3 Oct. 1576; Van Deusen, *Between the Sacred and the Worldly*, 55, 217n120.

83 Constituciones y ordenanças de la Vniuersidad, y Studio General de la Ciudad de los Reyes del Piru, 1602 at: https://archive.org/details/constitucionesyo01univ [Accessed 10 Mar. 2016] Statute 238 p. 41. This included those whose parents or grandparents had been sentenced by the Inquisition.

84 See for example Juan Méndez Nieto, who despite calling himself licenicado, actually failed to get complete his medical studies in Spain, it is suggested due to the lack of a certificate of *limpieza de sangre* (Juan Méndez Nieto, *Discursos medicinales* (Salamanca: Universidad de Salamanca, 1989), XI–XII). See also the ridicule of the noble birth of Dr. Francisco Machuca in the poetry of Juan del Valle y Caviedes, in Juan del Valle y Caviedes, *Obra completa*, ed. Daniel R Reedy (Caracas: Biblioteca Ayacucho, 1984), 50–52.

85 Lanning, *Royal Protomedicato*, 182–87 and "Legitimacy and *Limpieza de Sangre*," 46–48; José R. Jouve Martín, *The Black Doctors of Colonial Lima: Science, Race, and Writing in Colonial and Early Republican Peru* (Montreal: McGill-Queen's University Press, 2014), 21–24.

86 *Recopilación de las leyes de las Indias*, lib. 1 tit. 22 ley 57 10 Dec. 1678.

87 Actually 'hachas de cera', which were large candles composed of four tapers with four wicks.

doctors and officials of the University on the day of the examination.[88] While this represented a considerable outlay, the University statutes did allow fees to be reduced for those of modest means.[89] Nevertheless, the cost must have been an obstacle for many since in 1601 the University itself petitioned the Crown to allow students to graduate up to the level of *licenciatura* free of charge.[90]

As will be shown in the next chapter, establishing a pharmacy was an expensive proposition, so that those who aspired to be licensed *boticarios* and own their own business invariably came from elite families whose sons were probably taught by private tutors or else attended one of the city's *colegios*. Some may have gone on to university, but others probably acquired some knowledge of Latin at one of the *colegios* where classes were often conducted in Latin.[91] Others who were employed in *boticas* or worked in hospitals or convents would have learned their trade through working alongside licensed practitioners from whom they might learn sufficient Latin to be able to read physicians' prescriptions. Nevertheless, it is clear that not all *boticarios* had knowledge of Latin, for Antonio de Robles Cornejo, after 25 years' experience in the Americas including Peru, felt compelled to write his 'Examen de los simples medicinales' in Spanish in order to address the fact that many *boticarios* were unfamiliar Latin. He argued that this lack of knowledge of how to make compound medicines, which depended on reading manuals written in Latin, resulted in them relying on imports from Spain which were often of poor quality and had lost their potency by the time they arrived.[92]

On the Job Training

The opportunities for learning the art of pharmacy through on the job training were rather limited in Lima; even in 1630 there were only twelve recognised

88 Constituciones y ordenanças de la Vniuersidad, y Studio General de la Ciudad de los Reyes del Piru, 1602 at: http://www.archive.org/details/constitucionesyo01univ [Accessed 28 Oct. 2015] Statute 191 p. 32–32v., Statute 212 fol. 36v.-37. Cobo. *Obras*, 2: 413 gives slightly different charges: bachelor of arts or law 25 pesos; bachelor of theology 35 pesos; and master of arts 1,000 pesos. Doctors of theology and law were charged 2,500 pesos and doctors of medicine 3,000 pesos, all pesos of 9 reals.

89 Constituciones y ordenanças de la Vniuersidad, Statute 242, p. 42; Lanning, "Academic Culture," 47.

90 AGI Lima 337 Universidad de San Marcos 1 May 1601.

91 Martín, *Intellectual Conquest*, 40–41; Alperrine-Bouyer, *Educación de las élites indígenas*, 194.

92 ARJBM División 1, leg. 17 Prologo, Libro de examen de los simples medicinales 1617.

boticarios in the city.[93] In some cases knowledge of pharmacy was passed from father to son. Pedro de Bilbao was undoubtedly inducted into the art by his father, Juan de Bilbao, who was an eminent *boticario* in Lima in the late sixteenth century and from whom he inherited his *botica*.[94] However, as in Spain, others sought formal apprenticeships.[95] The contractual obligations of apprentices in general were specified by the guild associated with their trade.[96] Initially, the *cabildo* in Lima tried to regulate the city's economic activities indirectly through setting prices; later it did so more directly through encouraging the establishment of guilds or *gremios* under its jurisdiction.[97] In 1552 the *cabildo* ordered different trades to nominate four candidates from their professions to serve as *alcaldes* from which the *cabildo* would then select two. Tradesmen generally resisted any form of regulation, but with the arrival of larger numbers of immigrants from Spain and the emergence of artisans from other ethnic groups, they were persuaded of the merits of forming guilds. Even though the establishment a guild signified greater scrutiny by the *cabildo*, it could function to protect the privileged position of its members.[98] Comprised mainly of *maestros*, among other things the guilds examined and licensed artisans, supervised the quality of goods they produced, and settled disputes among their members.[99] However, guild ordinances, which often excluded certain ethnic groups, had to be approved by the *cabildo*, and the elections of guild officials, the examination of apprentices, and inspections of

---

93 Salinas y Córdova, *Memorial*, 257. At the same there were nine *médicos*, ten surgeons and three Spanish barbers' shops with many *oficiales*.

94 AGNP Protocolos Siglo XVI 14 Ramiro Bote fols. 1629–1631 Juan de Bilbao dona a Pedro de Bilbao, su hijo, de una botica con todas sus botes y drogas 3 Aug. 1596. Similarly in Mexico City in the eighteenth century, pharmacy was often a family profession (Hernández Saenz, *Learning to Heal*, 147–48).

95 For fourteenth century apothecary apprenticeships in Spain see Javier Sorní and José María Suñe, "La farmacia en Barcelona desde *Alfons el Benigne* a *Pere el Ceremonios* (1327–1387)," *Boletín de la sociedad española de historia de la farmacia* 36 (1985): 70–71. At that tiem they were known as spicers rather than *boticarios*. For apprenticeships associated with various trades in Lima see: Lyn Brandon Lowry, "Forging an Indian Nation: Urban Indians Under Spanish Colonial Control, Peru 1535–1765." PhD Diss. University of California, Berkeley, 1991, 209–213; Bianca Premo, *Children of the Father King: Youth, Authority and Legal Minority in Colonial Lima* (Chapel Hill: University of North Carolina, 2005), 55.

96 Francisco Quiroz Chueca, *Gremios, razas y libertad de industria: Lima colonial* (Lima: Universidad Nacional Mayor de San Marcos, 1995), 19–20.

97 The trades to which this applied included tailors, shoemakers, silversmiths, carpenters and hosiers (Libros de cabildos 3: 55 Oficios mecánicos 21 Jan. 1549).

98 Francisco Quiroz Chueca, "Gremios en Lima," in *Lima en el siglo XVI*, ed. Laura Gutiérrez (Lima: Instituto Riva-Agüero, 2005), 495–510.

99 Lowry, "Forging an Indian Nation," 152.

work premises, while they were conducted by guild officials were overseen by an *alcalde* and the *escribano* of the *cabildo*.[100]

A guild for surgeons and barbers existed in Lima in the sixteenth century,[101] but for the sixteenth and early seventeenth centuries at least no evidence has been found of a guild or *gremio* being established for *boticarios*. Similarly, one does not appear to have existed in Mexico City.[102] Paula Ronderos has suggested that a guild for *boticarios* was established in Bogotá, but the source she cites does not specifically mention a *gremio*, but only refers to the "leyes reales" that governed the profession, which would seem to refer to Spanish laws rather than the ordinances of a guild.[103] In Lima, the licensing of *boticarios* and the inspection of pharmacies fell under the jurisdiction of the royal *protomédico*, or in his absence the *cabildo*. In many respects this paralleled institutional arrangements in Spain, where in common with other Mediterranean countries, *gremios* for *boticarios* existed in Aragon, Cataluña and Valencia, but in Castile, where the *protomedicato* was established it was the body responsible for regulating the profession.[104] Hence, the existence of the *protomedicato* in Lima coupled with the relatively small number of practitioners in the city probably rendered a guild unnecessary.

Even though there was no guild for apothecaries, apprenticeships took the same form as for other trades. A two-year apprenticeship contract between one Gerónimo de Espino and the maestro *boticario*, Graviel de España, in 1619, specified that the apprentice would receive no salary, but would be provided with a bed, food, and clothes and be looked after when he was sick.[105] This

100 Quiroz Chueca, *Gremios, razas y libertad*, 25–29, 42, 55–56 and "Gremios en Lima," 512, 519–23.

101 Lastres, *Historia de la medicina peruana*, 2: 79; Francisco Quiroz Chueca, *Gremios coloniales peruanos* (Lima: Universidad Nacional Mayor de San Marcos, 1991), 14–16.

102 De Vos, "Art of Pharmacy," 61n2 also doubts that *boticarios* in Mexico City formed a professional organisation or guild.

103 Paula Ronderos, "El arte de boticarios durante la primera mitad del siglo XVII en el Nuevo Reino de Granada," *Fronteras de historia* 12 (2007): 176.

104 Francisco Javier Puerto Sarmiento, "La farmacia renacentista española y la botica de El Escorial," in *La ciencia en el Monasterio del Escorial*, ed. Francisco Javier Campos and Fernández de Sevilla (Madrid: Real Universitario Escorial-María Cristina, 1993), 77–78, 83–84; Goodman, *Power and Penury*, 225–27; Clouse, *Medicine*, 114.

105 AGNP Protocolos Siglo XVII 233 Bustamente fols. 520v–521v. Gerónimo Espino natural del pueblo de Callao... entro a aprehender el arte de boticario con Graviel de España 2 Feb. 1619. For an apprenticeship for a surgeon see: AGNP Protocolos Siglo XVI 154 fols. 284v–285v. Alonso Luzero pone apprendiz a su hijo Diego Luzero con los cirujanos Juan Rabuelo y Martín Sánchez 30 Aug. 1547. He was apprenticed at only 12 years old. For apprenticeship contracts for other trades see Teresa C. Vergara, "Growing Up Indian: Migration, Labor, and Life in Lima (1570–1640)," in *Raising an Empire: Children in Early Modern*

contract was similar to those drawn up for apprentice apothecaries in Spain in the sixteenth century.[106] In some cases, the apprentices came from Spain. In these cases they appear to have been paid a salary and at the end of their apprenticeship would be provided with clothing that reflected their Spanish heritage. Hence, in 1591 one Francisco Salguero, a citizen of Jerez, contracted to serve the *boticario* Blas de Medina for three years as an apprentice. He was to be provided with lodging, bed, board and medical care and at the end of the contract was to be given an "outfit of Castilian cloth of a colour of his choosing, which should include a jerkin, cape and wide trousers, stockings, breeches and shoes, and a hat, two shirts and two doublets …".[107] It is not clear whether Francisco Salguero was paid a salary, but one Andrés Vázquez, who came from Villaviciosa in Spain, who also contracted to work for Blas de Medina for a year, received 120 *pesos de a nueve* as a salary.[108] The 1613 census of Lima does not record the presence of any apprentice pharmacists, whereas a number of Indians were being trained as apprentice surgeons and barbers.[109]

Apart from formal apprenticeships, other individuals might learn the art informally by working alongside licensed *boticarios*, including those practising in hospitals where most workers were African slaves or less commonly Indians. Some of them, such as Juan Mandinga a slave in the Hospital of San Andrés, even ascended to the position of *boticario*, but very few who learned their skills informally appear to have been examined and licensed.[110] This included the Dominican priest, Martín de Porres, who was the illegitimate offspring of a

Iberia and Colonial Latin America, eds. Ondina E, González and Bianca Premo (Albuquerque: University of New Mexico Press, 2007), 86, 92–95.

106 Pilar Herrera Hinojo, "Contratos de aprendizaje en farmacia en el siglo XVI," *Boletín de la sociedad española de historia de farmacia* year 19, 73 (1968): 73–79; Clouse, *Medicine*, 128–30.

107 AGNP Protocolos Siglo XVI 51 Rodrigo Gómez Baeza fols. 1113–1113v. Blas de Medina concierto con Francisco Salguero 25 Sep. 1591. It reads "un vestido de paño de castilla del color que lo quisiere el dicho Francisco Salguero que ese entren de sayo y capote y saragueles [from the Arabic word sarawīl meaning wide trousers] e medias calzas e zapatos y sombrero e dos camisas e dos jubones …"

108 AGNP Protocolos Siglo XVI 52 Rodrigo Gómez Baeza fols. 1003–1005v. Blas de Medina concierto con Andrés Vázquez 14 Oct. 1592.

109 *Padrón de los Indios de Lima en 1613*, comp. Miguel de Contreras, and ed. Noble David Cook (Lima: Universidad Nacional de San Marcos, 1968), 132, 222.

110 Archivo Histórico del Instituto Riva-Agüero (hereafter AHIRA) Maldonado A-III-306 fol. 115 Libros de egresos e ingresos del hospital de San Andrés 1612.

Spanish father and a former African slave mother. He became renowned for his healing powers and was canonised as a saint in 1962.[111]

Examinations and Licences

After working alongside licensed *boticarios*, apprentices submitted themselves to examination, during which they were questioned on both theoretical and practical aspects of pharmacy.[112] The process is exemplified by the title of *boticario* granted to the Limeño-born Bernardo Gil, who was examined by the *protomédico*, Iñigo de Hormero, and the licensed *boticario*, Luis Nieto Maldonado in 1609.[113] Gil was described as a small man about 25 years old, with a wound on the right hand and three moles on the face, who witnesses testified had been practising for six years. The examiners then asked him many and repeat questions in Latin and Spanish about the preparation of simple and complex medicines. They also required him to read a manual in Latin by Mesuë on how to make and preserve complex medicines. In theory the examination was supposed to take place in a hospital,[114] but this source provides no information on where the examination was held.

When Gil was declared to have satisfied the examiners and given the license to practise, he made the sign of the cross and swore that he would practise the art of pharmacy ("arte de boticario") skilfully and competently ("[h]abil y suficiente"). He was instructed to give alms to the poor and to pledge that he would not to put poison in medicines. The latter assurance might appear unnecessary given the commitment of the profession to healing the sick, but it reflected Spaniards' constant fear that they might be killed by non-Christians. In Spain this fear had led to Jews, Muslims and later *Conversos* and *Moriscos* being forbidden from practising pharmacy, such that *boticarios* had to present certificates of *limpieza de sangre*, as well as legitimacy before they could receive a licence to practise.[115] In Seville ordinances relating to the practice

111 See Celia Cussen, *Black Saint of the Americas: The Life and Afterlife of Martín de Porres* (Cambridge: Cambridge University Press, 2014).

112 *Recopilación de las leyes, pragmáticas reales* (Muñoz), cap. 12 art. 3: 157.

113 Archivo Histórico Municipal de Lima (hereafter AHML) Libro 4 de cédulas y provisiones, fol. 161 Título de Bernardo Gil, boticario 7 Nov. 1609.

114 *Recopilación de las* leyes, *pragmáticas reales* (Muñoz), cap. 12 art. 3: 157.

115 *Recopilación de las leyes, pragmáticas reales* (Muñoz), cap. 6 art. 2: 73–74; Goodman, *Power and Penury*, 219–20. For obvious reasons, Indian candidates were not required to demonstrate *limpieza de sangre* (Hernández Sáenz, *Learning to Heal*, 148), but there is no evidence that any sought to be licensed in Lima at this time.

of pharmacy specified that an apothecary wishing to establish a shop had to be an "Old Christian, of pure blood and not a Moor or Jew nor those recently converted to our holy Catholic faith or Morisco, Negro or Mulatto."[116] In the particular case of Bernardo Gil it was only noted that he was the legitimate son of Lope and Maria Gil and no certificate of *limpieza de sangre* appears to have been presented or required. However, it was not until five years later in 1614 that his license to practise as a *boticario* was registered by the *cabildo*.[117]

In 1588 Spanish ordinances stipulated that the cost of entry to the examination for *boticarios* was four *escudos* of gold, equivalent to eight pesos. While this was half of that paid by aspiring physicians and surgeons,[118] it was equivalent to about two to three months wages of a native labourer and therefore an obstacle for those of limited means.[119] In fact, in 1667 the fee was tripled to 12 *escudos*, though it remained half of that paid by physicians.[120] Fees were not paid directly to the examiners, who received an annual salary for conducting examinations. In 1593 the salary paid to the *protomédico* for this task was set at 100,000 *maravedís* (about 370 pesos), while other examiners were paid 60,000 *maravedís* and assessors 20,000 *maravedís*.[121] These salaries were paid out of fees paid by students, but sometimes the number of candidates was too small to generate sufficient income to pay them.[122]

The licensing of physicians, surgeons, barbers, and *boticarios*, as well as the inspection of *boticas* was supposed to be done by a *protomédico*. *Protomédicos* were normally appointed by the Crown, but in Peru there were often long gaps between appointments. This not only led to many people practising without license, but also provided opportunities for the *cabildo* to exert its control over medical practice. In 1581 in the absence of a *protomédico*, the *cabildo* appointed

116 Archivo Municipal de Sevilla (hereafter AMS) Varios Antiguos 370 Ordenanzas de boticarios 1 Mar 1591. This stipulation was not always followed for during an inspection of boticas in Seville in 1631, one belonging to Diego Gómez was continuing to operate even though he had been imprisoned by the Inquisition for two years and had received a licence to practise (AMS Varios Antiguos 370 Visita de boticas 1631).

117 *Libros de cabildos de Lima*, 17: 631 Bernardo Gil boticario presenta su título de tal boticario 18 Jul. 1614.

118 *Recopilación de las leyes, pragmáticas reales* (Muñoz), cap. 7 art.1: 91–92.

119 One *escudo* of gold was equivalent to 16 reals, while forced labourers were paid one real a day.

120 AHML Libros de cédulas y provisiones 12, fols. 284v–285 Ordenanzas de médicos, cirujanos, barberos, oculistas, arbolarios y boticarios y visitas dellos 9 Jul 1667.

121 *Recopilación de las leyes, pragmáticas reales* (Muñoz), cap. 7 art.3: 95.

122 Lanning, *Royal Protomedicato*, 77.

Alvaro de Torres, a knowledgeable and experienced doctor, to issue licences;[123] his appointment as *protomédico* was subsequently confirmed by the Viceroy.[124] The *cabildo* also asserted its control over the practice of pharmacy through periodically ordering all *boticarios* to present their titles.[125] If the examination of the titles of surgeons is anything to go by, not all those submitting their titles were automatically approved despite the fact that there was a shortage of licensed practitioners.[126] In 1552 six surgeons presented their titles to the *cabildo* for approval, but two were regarded as insufficient. One Francisco Sánchez was deemed not to have demonstrated his competence ("suficiencia"). This may have been the same Francisco Sánchez who in 1537 had attempted to obtain a licence claiming he had lost his title. On that occasion he had been allowed to practise, because he had shown himself to be "hábil y de espiriencia [skilled and experienced]," but he was not permitted to prepare medicines.[127] The other, Salvador de Figueroa, was only permitted to treat minor cases, whether or not he was accompanied by a physician. However, the shortage of surgeons meant that the *cabildo* often turned a blind eye to the existence of legal titles, in addition to which there were many people who practised without license. In 1616 the *protomédico*, Doctor Melchor de Amusco, observed that,

> many people with little fear of god and less regard for the law are practising medicine giving themselves titles and calling themselves *licenciados*, doctors and [there are] others who use the art of barbers, *boticarios*, those who treat hernias, herbalists and charmers and everything related to and concerning the said arts and trades without possessing title, license or authority to do so and without understanding.[128]

These circumstances reflected in part the shortage of licensed practitioners, but also that *boticarios* were often consulted, particularly by the popular classes, including slaves, because their services were cheaper than those of

123 *Libros de cabildos de Lima*, 9: 452–53 Por protomédico al Licenciado Torres 6 Nov. 1581.

124 Lanning, *Royal Protomedicato*, 29–30.

125 *Libros de cabildos de Lima*, 13: 185 Que ysiban [exhiban] los títulos de cirujanos y barberos y boticarios Lima 6 Nov. 1598.

126 *Libros de cabildos de Lima*, 3: 616 Cirujanos los que son suficientes al parecer del Licenciado Torres 11 Nov. 1552.

127 *Libros de cabildos de Lima*, 1: 161–62 Mandamiento de cirugía 30 Aug. 1537.

128 *Libros de cabildos de Lima*, 18: 157 Alonso Alférez de Jodar fiscal y alguacil del protomédico 30 Oct. 1616.

physicians.[129] Moreover, it demonstrates that while there was knowledge of the law, it was not effectively upheld by the *protomedicato* or *cabildo* and indeed was frequently ignored.

Female Medical Learning

As noted above, women were forbidden by law from owning *boticas* or practising pharmacy, yet it is clear that some women did acquire medical knowledge and dispense medicines. Native women, Africans, and those of mixed ethnicity were most prominent in the popular sector, but in 1616 the *cabildo* noted that many Spanish women and *Mestizas* were also practising some form of medicine, including acting as midwives.[130] Where then did women acquire such knowledge? Inasmuch as women were educated, they were taught by private tutors, later in convent schools by *beatas*, or else in lay schools. When formal schools were founded at the end of the sixteenth century they were exclusively for boys, such that girls had to be educated separately.[131] Elites esteemed schooling in convents since it was seen to enhance a girl's chances of making a good marriage, because it imparted Christian moral and spiritual values, and protected a girl's virginity. Also, the higher cost of this type of education might reflect positively on the economic and social standing of the family.[132]

At first convent education for girls not intending to take holy orders was limited. In fact only in 1575 did a papal bull permit the education of women in convents in the Americas, though it seems that in Lima some instruction had been occurring there informally prior to that time.[133] Initially students had to have a papal licence in order to study in convents, so the process of admission was often protracted and their numbers limited. However, after 1618 another papal bull enabled the local bishop to determine their admissibility.[134] In 1600 there were only three convents in Lima in 1600 – La Encarnación, Santa Clara, and

129 See the redhibitoria case in Archivo Arzobispal, Lima (hereafter AAL) Causas de Negros leg. 4 doc. 7 Hernando de Valdés, contra el licenciado don Diego de Morales 1620.

130 *Libros de cabildos de Lima*, 18: 157 Alonso Alférez de Jodar fiscal y alguacil del protomédico 30 Oct. 1617.

131 Luis Martín, *Daughters of the Conquistadores: Women of the Viceroyalty of Peru* (Albuquerque: University of New Mexico Press, 1983), 73–74.

132 Van Deusen, *Between the Sacred and the Worldly*, 102–111.

133 Martín, *Daughters*, 74; Van Deusen, *Between the Sacred and the Worldly*, 214n78.

134 Martín, *Daughters*, 77; Van Deusen, *Between the Sacred and the Worldly*, 107–108, 240n42.

La Concepción – the first two charging 100 pesos and 200 pesos a year respectively for food and lodging. Although by the mid-seventeenth century there were eight convents, together they educated only about 250 secular girls.[135] Secular students, known as *seglares* or *educandas*, were taught separately from novices. The nuns instructed them in them the basic skills of reading, writing, arithmetic, sewing, cooking, music, drama and sometimes Latin.[136] It seems likely that given the Christian responsibility to care for the sick, as in European convents, women might also informally acquire healing knowledge and skills, including the use of herbs and preparation of medicines.[137]

Convents were large institutions since in addition to the nuns, novices, and secular students they housed, they accommodated a large number of resident servants and slaves who provided services for both individuals and the institution as a whole.[138] According to Bernabé Cobo, the convent of La Encarnación had 700 residents consisting of 300 nuns and novices and 400 servants, slaves and secular students.[139] Such large convents resembled miniature towns and offered spaces for socialising and the exchange of ideas and skills between women from different social and ethnic backgrounds.[140] While those seeking holy orders sought primarily to develop their spirituality, they had access to libraries and often pursued literary and musical interests.[141] Far from being totally closed off from the outside world, the nuns also communicated with the

135 Van Deusen, *Between the Sacred and the Worldly*, 107–109, 240n47. According to Bernabé Cobo (Obras, 2: 429), La Encarnación was only licensed to admit 24 *seglares* though it is not clear what date this observation refers to. Van Deusen (pp. 172–75) provides a table of the numbers of *seglares* in convents in the seventeenth century.

136 Martín, *Daughters*, 79.

137 Monica Green, "Bodies, Gender, Health, Disease: Recent Work on Medieval Women's Medicine," *Studies in Medieval and Renaissance History*, ser. 3, 5 (2005): 13–14; Sharon T. Strochhia, "The Nun Apothecaries of Renaissance Florence: Marketing Medicines in the Convent," *Renaissance Studies* 25(5)(2011): 627–47; Gianna Pomata, "Practising Between Heaven and Earth: Women Healers in Seventeenth-century Bologna," *Dynamis* 19 (1999): 131–43.

138 Martín, *Daughters*, 174–77, 185–91, 199, 221–22.

139 Cobo, *Obras*, 2: 429. At the same time in the convent of La Concepción there were 250 nuns and novices and 250 servants and slaves (p. 431). For the numbers of residents in convents in Lima in the seventeenth century see: Van Deusen, *Between the Sacred and the Worldly*, 172–75. By 1700 it had over 1,000 residents (Asunción Lavrin, "Female Religious," in *Cities and Society in Colonial Latin America*, ed. Louisa Schell Hoberman and Susan Migden Socolow (Albuquerque: University of New Mexico Press, 1986), 175.

140 Martín, *Daughters*, 199; Susan Migden Socolow, *The Women of Colonial Latin America*. (Cambridge: Cambridge University Press, 2000), 99–102.

141 Lavrin, "Female Religious," 185–87.

convent's servants and slaves and they were visited, sometimes illicitly, by relatives living outside.[142] There were considerable opportunities for the acquisition of medical knowledge of different kinds.

The dowry for entry into the convent of La Encarnación was 6,000 pesos and double if a separate apartment and a slave servant were desired.[143] However, in certain circumstances the dowry required might be waived or reduced. In 1628 the abbess of the convent of La Concepción petitioned the bishop to allow the admission of a poor widow to the black veil without paying a dowry, because she was regarded as an asset for the convent

> … because she has the special gift of treating every kind of illness and is knowledgeable about women's illnesses […] for she has cured many nuns in this convent with licence of the precentor […] and has restored to complete health those suffering from diseases which physicians and surgeons have not managed to cure.[144]

Those who entered convents as secular students generally went on to elite marriages.[145] Others took vows of chastity, took the black veil, and lived in closed orders. Yet others sought more solitude away from the large convents or preferred to live in the world as *beatas* rather than under the stricter supervision of closed orders.[146] Some of those who became *beatas* may have been unable

---

142 Martín, *Daughters*, 219–30.

143 Boleslao Lewin, ed., *Descripción del Virreinato del Perú: crónica inédita de comienzos del siglo XVII* (Rosario, Universidad Nacional del Litoral, Facultad de Filosofía, Letras y Ciencias de la Educación, 1958), 58–59; Bowser, *African Slave*, 104–105. Writing of Spanish America in general, Lavrin ("Female Religious," 177) comments that in the sixteenth and seventeenth centuries dowries for nuns taking the black veil were generally between 1,000 and 2,000 pesos, but by the end of the seventeenth century had risen to 3,000 pesos. The figure of 6,000 pesos is quite high since the average dowry for convents in colonial Spanish America was normally between 3,000 and 4,000 pesos (Socolow, *Women*, 95–96).

144 AAL Monasterio de la Concepción leg. 4 exp. 1 Bernardina del Castillo Orihuela, abadesa 6 Sep. 1628. It reads "… porque tiene gracia particular en curar cualquiera enfermedad y sabe mucho en materia de las de mujeres […] por las muchas religiosas que ha curado a este convento con licencia del señor chantre […] le ha dado entera sanidad en enfermedades que los médicos y cirujanos no han acertado a curar …" Such waivers might also apply to women with musical abilities (Martín, *Daughters*, 181–82).

145 See Kathryn Burns, *Colonial Habits: Convents and the Spiritual Economy of Cuzco, Peru* (Durham: Duke University Press, 1999), 218–24 for the destination of those educated in the convent of Santa Clara in Cuzco in the sixteenth century.

146 Van Deusen, *Between the Sacred and the Worldly*, 119, 188; Socolow, *Women of Latin America*, 106–107.

to afford the high cost of becoming full members of closed orders. These nuns followed the rules of the Third Orders of the various religious orders, took vows of chastity, and wore habits, but lived independently or later in the seventeenth century in *beaterios*. These women taught, preached, and undertook charitable activities that included collecting alms and caring for the sick.[147] In Lima their spirituality was commonly recognised and they were widely consulted by the population at large on both religious and medical matters.[148] One example, was Isabel Medel Cansino, a *beata* of the Third Order of San Francisco, who treated as many as ten to twenty African slaves in her own house and employed two slaves, one of whom was responsible for collecting herbs and medicines for the pharmacy.[149] Her treatments were said to include:

> meat, bread, wood, wine, eggs, piedra lipes [copper sulphate], oil, cardenillo [verdigris], fish, tallow, virgin oil, alum, lavender, espingo [ishpink], pingo pingo,[150] vilcatongo,[151] mastic, chochos,[152] honey, aniseed, fat, sulphur, candles and salt.

Conclusion

The ordinances that governed the training, examination and licensing of apothecaries in Peru were the same as those that operated in Spain. However, local circumstances dictated that state control of the practise of pharmacy was more limited. These included the failure of the state to fund medical education in the universities and to support high level *protomédicos* who might

147 Van Deusen, *Between the Sacred and the Worldly*, 24–25 and "Circuits of Knowledge among Women in Early Seventeenth-Century Lima, in *Gender, Race and Religion in the Colonization of the Americas*, ed. Nora E. Jaffary (Aldershot: Ashgate, 2007), 138, 146. On *beatas* in Cuzco see: Kathryn Burns, "Andean Women in Religion: Beatas, 'Decency', and the Defence of Honour in Colonial Cuzco," in *Gender, Race and Religion in the Colonization of the Americas*, ed. Nora E. Jaffary (Aldershot: Ashgate, 2007), 81–91.

148 Van Deusen, "Circuits of Knowledge," 141.

149 AGNP SO CO Ca 40 doc 383 fols. 461–480 Doña Isabel Medel Cansino 1636; AGNP SO CO Ca 2 doc 8 fols. 621–22 Fragment of an invoice drawn up by Isabel Medel Cansino, no date.

150 Pingo pingo (*Ephedra andina*) is a native Andean herb that was used as a diuretic and depurative.

151 This was probably a native herb. It was put in chicha and used as a purgative by one, María Ynes, in Chancay, who during an ecclesiastical *visita* in 1662 was accused of being a *hechicera* (Sánchez, *Amancebados, hechiceros y rebeldes*, 27).

152 Lupin *Lupinus mutabilis* Sweet.

bring stricter compliance with the law. This left the administration of healthcare largely in the hands of the *cabildo*, which faced with a shortage of medical expertise, due in part to limited opportunities for training, often licensed individuals who did not have the requisite certificates, but displayed particular knowledge and skills that they had acquired informally. Despite Antonio de Robles Cornejo's judgement that early migrants from Spain were the least educated, some did have a university education and formal training, whereas most of those practising later had little recourse other than to acquire knowledge and skills informally.

Probably the greatest difference between Peru and Spain was the greater diversity of ethnic backgrounds from which *boticarios* were drawn in Lima. Despite legislation that restricted pharmacy practice to those who could demonstrate *limpieza de sangre*, in Lima few serious attempts were made to prevent Blacks or those of a mixed ethnic background from practising the art, reflecting in part the demographic dominance of those of African heritage in the city. Likewise there is no evidence that women were prevented by law from practising pharmacy, though in many cases they were probably restricted to work in ancillary activities rather than preparing medicines themselves. The presence of such an ethnically diverse population, where the regulation of medical practice was only partially effective, where distinctions between licensed medical practitioners were blurred, and where only a small proportion of the population had been formally trained, created an environment that should have fostered innovation. Yet, as Chapters 5 and 6 will demonstrate through an analysis of the types of medicines prepared, *boticarios* adhered to traditional humoral beliefs and practices and depended on Old World *materia medica*. How can this apparent paradox be explained? It seems clear that the prevalence of humoral medicine did not depend on state regulation or formal training. Knowledge could be acquired through working alongside licensed *boticarios* or in hospitals. It might also be gleaned through private study, where most medical books available for study in Lima were orthodox texts that had been sanctioned by the Inquisition. Perhaps more significantly, as Chapter 5 will show, humoral beliefs were entrenched in popular thought to the extent that lay people often applied treatments according to its principles.

CHAPTER 3

The Medicines Business

This profession is not for the poor.[1]

Once apothecaries had been trained, the opportunities open to them to practise their art varied largely according to the financial resources they possessed. Contemporary observations and advice given to those aspiring to be independent *boticarios* converge in the judgement that in order to establish a pharmacy one had to be a person of moderate means. Christóval Suárez de Figueroa's encyclopaedia of the qualities required of those practising different professions suggested that the pharmacy profession was not one for the poor. This view was echoed by Antonio de Robles Cornejo who with experience in Peru advised that no one should attempt to open up a *botica* "without being rich or at least with substantial funds."[2] The need for *boticarios* to have significant financial resources was underlined in the city ordinances of Seville in 1591 which specified that in order to obtain a licence, a *boticario* not only had to pass the requisite examinations, but also show that he possessed 500 *ducados* (690 pesos) in order to purchase simples for the preparation of medicines.[3] There is no evidence that a similar local ordinance was drawn up in Lima, though there was no lesser need for *boticarios* to have significant financial backing. The reason given was not so much the cost of the premises or labour, but the high cost of medicines. It was generally considered that those

1 Suárez de Figueroa, *Plaza universal*, 302. Paula De Vos, "The Apothecary in Seventeenth- and Eighteenth-Century Mexico: Historiography and Case Studies in Medical Regulation, Charity, and Science," *Colonial Latin American Historical Review* 13(3)(2004): 253 notes that this guide was based on Tomaso Garzoni's, *La piazza universale di tutte le professioni del mondo* [1587] 2 vols. eds. Paolo Cherchi and Beatrice Collina (Turin: Giulio Einaldi, 1996), but suggests that the role of apothecaries is likely to have been similar in Spain and Italy.

2 He says, "sin ser rico o al menos con gruas riquezas mucha cantidad de pesos." ARJBM División 1, leg. 17 Libro de examen de los simples medicinales 1617. These comments echo those of Antonio de Aguilera, who in his *Exposición sobre las preparaciones de Mesue*, fols. 20v.-21v. advised that *boticarios* should be "rich or at least be of sufficient means."

3 AMS Varios Antiguos 370 Ordenanzas de boticarios 1 Mar 1591; Fernández-Carrión and Valverde, *Farmacia y sociedad*, 15.

 | DOI 10.1163/9789004351271_004

of moderate means could buy good quality medicines at the time they were needed, whereas the less affluent could only afford poor quality medicines or had to buy them on credit, which meant they actually paid more for items of lesser quality. Given the high cost of establishing and maintaining a *botica*, there were relatively few in the city. Even in 1630 there were only twelve to eighteen recognised *boticas* in Lima, four of which were attached to hospitals.[4]

For many *boticarios* who acquired licences, the expense of setting up an independent business was not a realistic economic proposition. Moreover, established *boticarios* often discouraged those they had trained or who were in their employment from setting up independent businesses for fear of competition and that they would take their customers with them. In the case of surgeons and barbers, the guild persuaded the municipal authority in Lima to introduce a regulation stipulating that apprentices and newly trained journeymen known as *oficiales* could not set up shops within four blocks of their master's practice for a year and a day.[5] A similar ordinance, does not seem to have applied to *boticarios*, but there were private efforts to restrict the competition. For example, in 1618 Luis Nieto Maldonado rented a *botica* in Cuzco from one Fernando de Cartagena and his four-year contract specified that for two years following the end of the contract he could not set up a new *botica* in the city, either personally or through an intermediary, though he could purchase one of the two that already existed.[6] In any case, the establishment of any new *botica* required municipal approval.

In common with other trades, many trained *boticarios* who lacked the resources to set up independent businesses continued to work in the salaried employment of a *maestro* until they had secured sufficient capital to open up their own pharmacies.[7] In the 1630s, the apothecary to the Inquisition, Mateo Pastor, had at least two *oficiales* working in his *botica*.[8] *Licenciado* Bartolomé Díaz Cabeza de Vaca appears to have aspired to be an independent *boticario*, but he could only realise this ambition in 1605 by entering into a *compañía* or partnership with Francisco Martín Reyna to purchase a pharmacy that had formerly belonged to Diego de Tineo. In this *compañía* Díaz Cabeza de Vaca

4 Salinas y Córdova, *Memorial*, 257. At the same there were said to be nine *médicos*, ten surgeons and three Spanish barbers' shops with many *oficiales*. Juan Bromley, however, suggests there were 18 *boticas* ("La ciudad de Lima en el año 1630," *Revista histórica* 24 (1959): 286).

5 Quiroz Chueca, *Gremios coloniales peruanos*, 14–16.

6 "Un botica colonial," *Revista del archivo histórico del Cuzco* 4 (1953): 279.

7 Quiroz Chueca, *Gremios, razas y libertad*, 19–23.

8 AGNP SO CO 44–394 fols. 191–210 Prisión, secuestro e inventario de bienes de Tome Cuaresma 20 Nov. 1635.

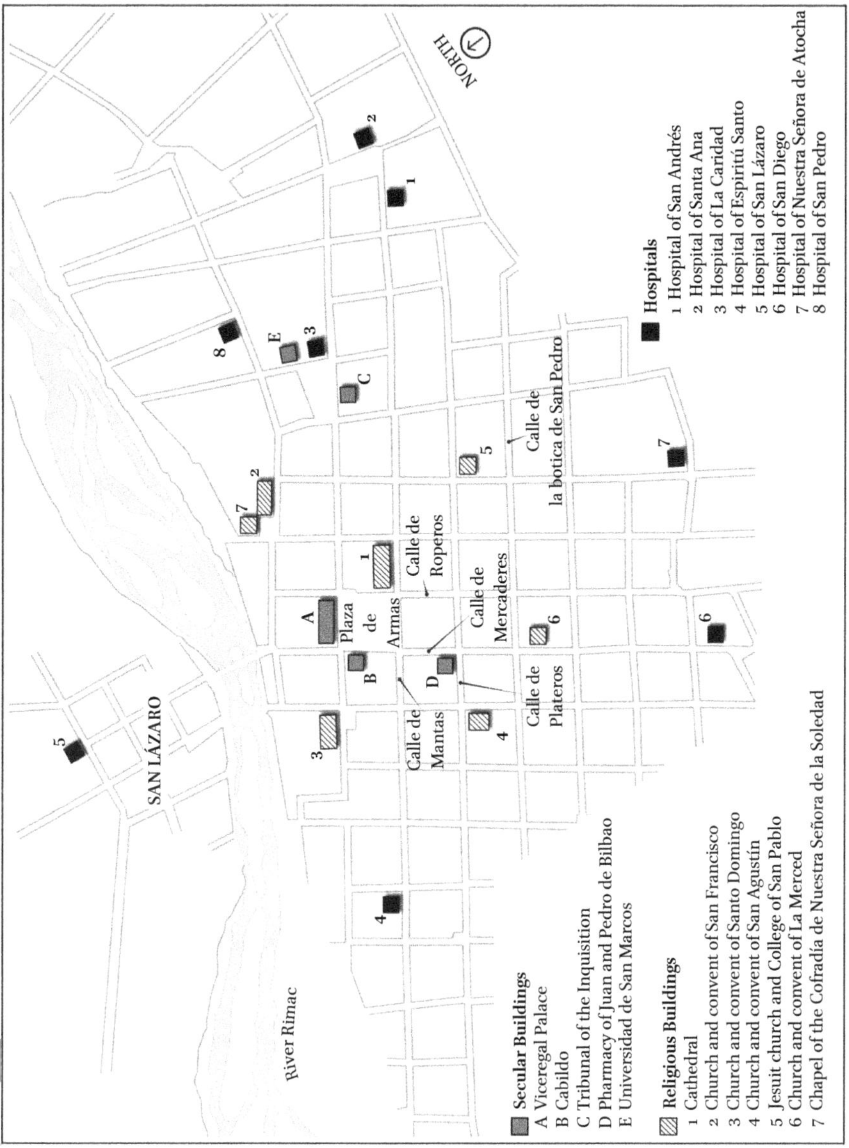

FIGURE 1 *Lima in the early seventeenth century.*

was only able to afford a one-third share.[9] Prior to this time, in 1596 he had worked under contract for Blas de Medina for the annual salary of 500 pesos.[10] This high salary probably reflected Díaz Cabeza de Vaca's experience and status as a licensed *boticario* since the annual contracts of *oficiales* working in Lima's *boticas* generally specified salaries of 200 to 250 *pesos de a nueve*.[11] These salaries were consistent with those of *oficiales* in other trades such as tailors, masons, carpenters or silkworkers, where most earned less than 250 pesos a year but skilled workers might receive as much as 500 to 600 pesos.[12] Unlike other trades, however, where *oficiales* did not normally reside in the house of the *maestro*,[13] those working in pharmacies seem to have lived on the premises and received food, lodging and clothing.

Other trained *boticarios* sought paid employment in public institutions such as hospitals, convents, or prisons.[14] (see Figure 1) Apothecaries employed in the Hospitals of Santa Ana and San Andrés were paid between 300 and 400 pesos a year, part of which might be paid in kind in the form of accommodation and food. For example, Rodrigo de Vargas, who held the post of *boticario* of the Hospital of Santa Ana for over thirty years was given a house in the hospital grounds and a ration of three pounds of beef and mutton, three loaves of bread of more than one pound, six bottles of local wine, and twelve blocks of soap from Spain.[15] This salary was only slightly less than that paid to physicians in the same hospitals and considerably more than the 200 pesos and 50 pesos paid to surgeons and barbers respectively.[16]

---

9 AAL Testamentos leg. 5 exp.1 fols. 7v–8 Testamento de Bartolomé Díaz Cabeza de Vaca 10 Apr. 1608.

10 AGNP Protocolos Siglo XVI 55 Rodrigo Gómez Baeza fols. 187–187v. Contract between Blas de Medina and Bartolomé Díaz Cabeza de Vaca 13 Aug. 1596.

11 For contracts between *boticarios* and *oficiales* see: AGNP Protocolos Siglo XVI 54 Rodrigo Gómez Baeza (1594) fols. 641–641v. Contract between Luis Nieto Maldonado and Juan de Arce 7 Jun. 1595; AGNP Protocolos Siglo XVI 55 Rodrigo Gómez Baeza fols. 980–980v. Contract between Luis Nieto Maldonado and Juan de Horosco 12 Jun. 1596.

12 Francisco Quiroz Chueca, "Artisans and Journeymen in Colonial Lima." Unpublished manuscript, 2014.

13 Quiroz Chueca, *Gremios, razas y libertad*, 22.

14 Unlike hospitals and convents, Lima's four public prisons did not seem to have salaried *boticarios* (AGI Lima 134 Cofradía de los pobres de las carceles de la ciudad de los reyes 1598; AGI Lima 131 Los hermanos de los pobres de las carceles de los reyes 27 Feb. 1593).

15 Archivo de Beneficencia Pública, Lima (hereafter ABPL) 9086 fols. 104–105 Visita al Hospital de Santa Ana fols. 104–105 no date [1588]. He was appointed to the hospital in 1567 and was still working there in 1606.

16 ABPL 9086 fols. 272–73 Visita al hospital de Santa Ana 26 May 1588; ABPL 9083 fol. 90 Libro mayor de rentas del hospital de Santa Ana desde 1593 a 1629; ABPL 9084 fols. 132, 145,

Acquiring a *Botica*

Residents of Lima who became independent *boticarios* acquired pharmacies in different ways. In the earliest years of colonial rule those apothecaries who had been licensed and practised in Spain often brought medicines and equipment with them to set up a pharmacy business, generally migrating with their families, servants or assistants. When the *boticario* Pedro de la Fuente moved to Lima in 1534, he took with him 500,000 *maravedís* (about 1,800 pesos) worth of goods, though it is not known what proportion was destined for the establishment of a *botica*.[17] Pharmacy was often a family profession such that some *boticarios* who settled in the Americas were sons of licensed practitioners in Spain.[18] Once established in the New World, pharmacies might pass from father to son, as was the case with Pedro de Bilbao in Lima who inherited his *botica* from his father, Juan de Bilbao, for whom he had worked for five years.[19] However, more evidence exists for the purchase of *boticas* either individually or as part of a joint venture.

---

162 Libro de cuentas de gastos del hospital de Santa Ana año 1598; ABPL 9086 fols. 6–7, 124 Visita al hospital de Santa Ana 1606; AGI Lima 122 fol. 38 Información del hospital de Santa Ana 1570. In 1582 the salary of the *boticario* at the hospital of San Andrés was only 150 pesos (AGI Lima 126 fols. 9v., 16v. El hospital real de los españoles de advocación San Andrés 1582), but in the early seventeenth century was 400 pesos, equivalent to that paid in the hospital of Santa Ana (Cobo, *Obras*, 2: 444). However, the ordinances for the hospital of San Andrés in 1577 made no provision for a salaried *boticario*, rather a priest took care of the *botica* which was supposed to be inspected by a physician or *protomédico* every three months (Guillermo Lohmann Villena and Maria Justina Sarabia Viejo, *Francisco de Toledo: Disposiciones gubernativas para el virreinato del Perú 1575–1580* (Seville: Escuela de Estudios Hispano-Americanos, 1989), 318. For salaries for *boticarios* in Mexico City in the eighteenth century see Hernández Sáenz, *Learning to Heal*, 162, which indicates similar differentials between different types of medical practitioner.

17 AGI Contratación 5536 L2 N167 Licence granted to Pedro de San Martín and Pedro de Fuente, boticario 21 Mar. 1534.

18 Joaquín Herrera Dávila, "Las boticas sevillanas de 1631," *Boletín de la sociedad española de historia de la farmacia* 39 (154–155) (1988): 73; Fernández-Carrión and Valverde, *Farmacia y Sociedad*, 61–64, 73.

19 AGNP Protocolos Siglo XVI 14 Ramiro Bote fols. 1629–1631 Juan de Bilbao dona a Pedro de Bilbao, su hijo, de una botica con todas sus botes y drogas 3 Aug. 1596. In fact Juan Bromley states that Juan de Bilbao inherited it from his father Francisco de Bilbao who had possessed the contract for the establishment of a pharmacy in the Hospital of Santa Ana (Juan Bromley, *Las viejas calles de Lima* (Municipalidad Metropolitana de Lima: Lima, 2005), 257–58.

The cost of establishing a *botica* was high. When a pharmacy was imported from Spain for the Hospital of Santa Ana in 1551, it was valued at 3,400 *pesos de oro*. However, details only exist for a shipment of 30 wooden chests containing medicines, equipment and books, valued at about 1,062 pesos (289,110 *maravedís*).[20] As with *boticas* in general, the medicines accounted for the most significant proportion of pharmacy assets, in this case about 65 percent.[21] The equipment, excluding medicinal books and manuals, was valued at only about 230 pesos (61,750 *maravedís*)(See Table 1). This was significantly less than the value of the equipment of a well-established private *botica*, such as that belonging to Bartolome Díaz Cabeza de Vaca. In 1608 this pharmacy contained stills (*alquitaras*), mortars, spatulas, sieves, ladles, a variety of boxes and phials, and an oven together valued at 2,217 pesos

TABLE 1 *Expenditure on the installation of the first pharmacy for the Hospital of Santa Ana, 1551.*

	Maravedís	Percentage
Materia medica	186,855	64.6
Equipment	61,750	21.4
Books	5,225	1.8
Import tax	27,204	9.4
Labour to build the furniture for the pharmacy and for the preparation and loading of goods for shipment	8,076	2.8
Total	289,110	100.0

Source: AGNP Protocolos Siglo XVI 63 Diego Gutiérrez fols. 167–88 El hospital de españoles y naturales compañía con Francisco de Bilbao 15 Oct. 1551.

20 AGNP Protocolos Siglo XVI 63 Diego Gutiérrez fols. 167–88 Hospital de los españoles y naturales compañía con Francisco de Bilbao de la botica 20 Oct. 1551; Miguel Rabí Chara, "La primera botica de los hospitales de la ciudad de Lima en el siglo XVI," *Asclepio* 52 (2000): 273–77.

21 AGNP Protocolos Siglo XVI 63 Diego Gutiérrez fols. 167–88 El hospital de los españoles y naturales con Francisco de Bilbao de la botica 9 Mar 1552. The detailed cost of individual items in the *botica* suggests it was worth 289,110 *maravedís* (1,062 pesos), of which 61,750 was spent on equipment. The figure of 289,110 *maravedís*, however, is difficult to reconcile with the stated overall cost of 3,400 *pesos de oro en plata ensayada.*

(See Table 2).[22] However, *boticarios* starting out on their pharmacy careers generally owned much more basic equipment. The weights, cooking pans, spatulas and mortars that the *boticario* Juan Sánchez took with him when he migrated to Lima in 1592 were valued at only 53 pesos.[23]

The total cost of the *botica* of the Hospital of Santa Ana of 3,400 *pesos de oro en plata ensayada*,[24] which was equivalent to 5,625 *pesos corrientes*, does not seem out of line with the value of private *boticas* in the city. The *botica*

TABLE 2 *Assets of the pharmacy belonging to Bartolomé Díaz Cabeza de Vaca, 1608.*

Pesos	**Reals**	**Percentage**	**Item**
596	6	4.4	Cash in a bag in the pharmacy
2,367	2	17.5	Simple and compound medicines
2,217		16.4	Equipment – stills (*alquitaras*), mortars, spatulas, sieves, ladles, a variety of boxes and phials, an oven and other essential tools
200		1.5	An old and infirm African slave
5,708	6	42.2	Client debts (of which 3,874 pesos were receipts for medicines supplied)
1,474		10.9	Owed by Francisco Martín Reyna part investor in the pharmacy
700		5.2	A calvary and linen
274	2.5	2.0	Furniture, including a desk (bureau) and chairs
13,538	0.5	100.0	

Source: AAL Testamentos leg. 5 exp. 1 fols. 175–178 Testamento de Bartolomé Díaz Cabeza de Vaca boticario y autos sobre su cumplimiento con el albacea Juan Manuel Carrasco, 1608–1626.

22 AAL Testamentos 5 leg. 1 fol. 165v. Memoria de las medicinas que tenía esta botica cuando la compraron... Bartolome Cabeza de Vaca 1608. The most expensive items were those made of metal – mortars, boiling pans and ladles –which were worth 250 pesos. Other items consisted of boxes, jars, pots and other receptacles containing pill, powders, syrups, cordials, oils, ointments and plasters. It is not clear whether the value of these receptacles included the medicines they contained.

23 AGI Contratación 1097 N5 fols. 199–202 Registro de Santa Catalina 1592.

24 AGNP Protocolos Siglo XVI 63 Diego Gutiérrez fols. 167–88 Hospital de los españoles y naturales compañía con Francisco de Bilbao de la botica 20 Oct. 1551; Rabí Chara, "Primera botica," 273–77. A *peso de oro* was equivalent to 450 maravedís and a *peso corriente* 272 *maravedís*.

commissioned by Diego de Tineo from Seville in 1555 cost 5,000 *pesos de buen oro*.[25] This pharmacy was designed to be exceptionally well-appointed with its installations fashioned by skilled artisans. A carpenter was instructed to create a ceiling for the pharmacy some twenty-two feet square on which were to be painted golden stars and a large sun with golden rays. Tineo indicated that the boxes to be used for the medicines were to be finely decorated with gilt and in place of labels (*medallas*) there were to be paintings of notable historical figures. One of these was to depict the legend known as "Virgil in a basket" (See Figure 2). In this legend, Virgil being enamoured with Nero's daughter, was enticed to lower himself from a window in a basket, but was suspended by her halfway thereby exposing him to public ridicule.[26] In revenge for his humiliation Virgil employed magic to extinguish the fires of Rome that could only be rekindled by holding a torch or candle to the woman's private parts. This popular legend was applied to many historical figures, including Hippocrates, and was attached to Virgil in the thirteenth century because of his association with magic and divination. Virgil was regarded as an authority by astrologers and alchemists and was even thought to possess the secret of the Philosopher's Stone.[27] The use of this image signifies the apothecary's interest in alchemy, which is further supported by his importation of six stills for use in distillation. The importance of alchemy to pharmacy practice of the time will be discussed further in Chapter 5.

Not all pharmacies were installed so extravagantly, but nevertheless, they commanded fairly high prices. In 1551 a *botica* sold to one Pero Lopes de Aguirre for 2,210 *pesos de buen oro*,[28] and in 1576, when the *botica* of Francisco de Alva was auctioned following his death, it netted a similar 2,400 pesos.[29] However, Alva's will was disputed by his children and five *boticarios* testified that it was actually worth more than 4,000 *pesos de buen oro*, because it was the best in the city and possessed very good equipment and medicines.[30] One of the

25 John Carter Brown Library (hereafter JCB) Mss codex Sp 136 Francisco Martínez y compañía obligación – Diego de Tineo y consortes 1555.

26 John Webster Spargo, *Virgil the Necromancer: Studies in Virgilian Legends* (Cambridge, Mass.: Harvard University Press, 1934), 136–55, 198–206.

27 Spargo, *Virgil the Necromancer*, 277–79.

28 AGNP Protocolos Siglo XVI 8 Simón Alzate fols. 841v–842 26 June 1551.

29 The *botica* had been purchased from Luis Núñez de Prado (AGNP Real Audiencia. Causas Civiles leg. 16 cuad. 81 fol. 7v., 16 Pleito…contra las bienes y herederos del bachiller Francisco de Alva, boticario morador en la Ciudad de los Reyes, 1576).

30 AGNP Real Audiencia. Causas Civiles leg. 16 cuad. 81 fols. 119–26, 687–715 Pleito… contra las bienes y herederos del bachiller Francisco de Alva, boticario morador en la Ciudad de los Reyes. 1576. The *boticarios* were: Guillermo Rodríguez aged 48, Francisco Velásquez aged 30, Blas de Medina aged 34, Diego de Tineo 70 and Doctor Franco, a physician.

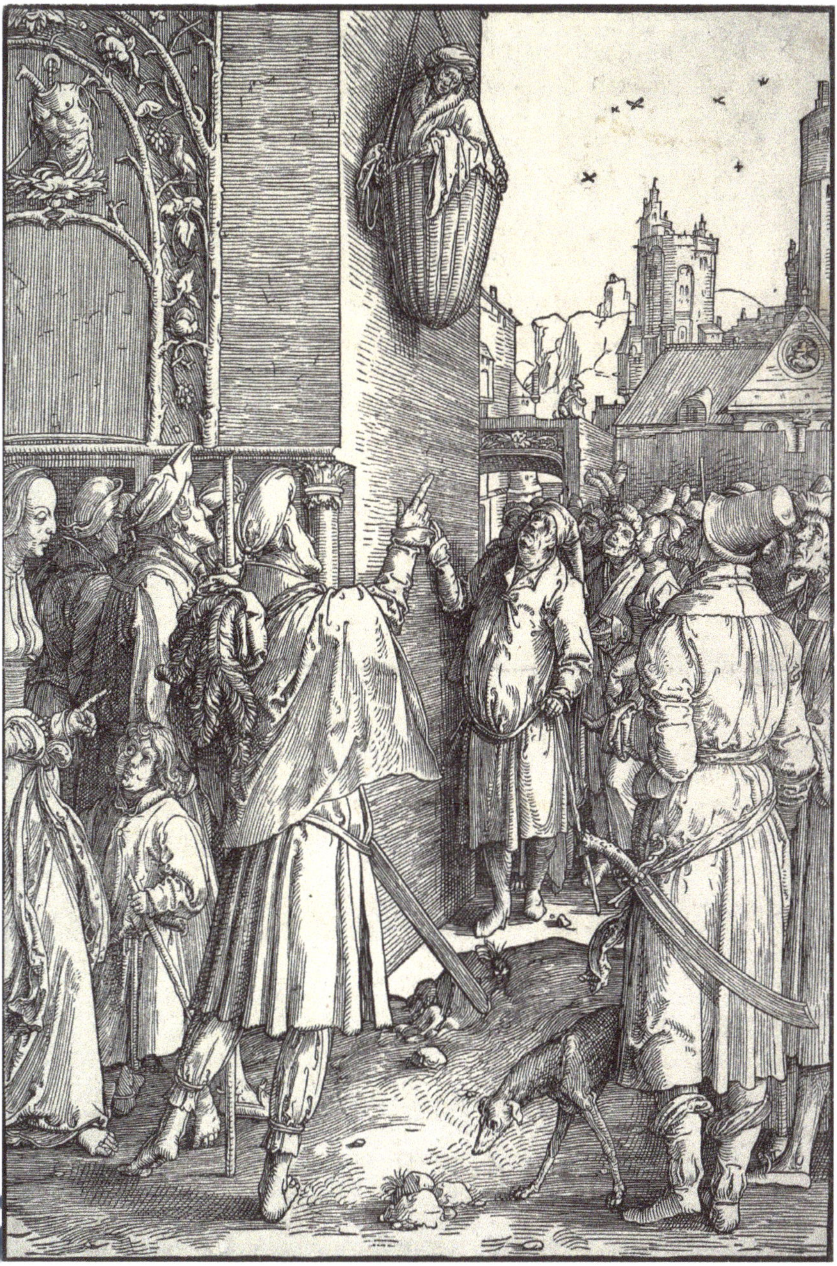

FIGURE 2 *The poet Virgil in a basket. Lucas van Leyden, Woodcut, Leiden 1512.*
COURTESY OF THE METROPOLITAN MUSEUM OF ART, NEW YORK.

witnesses was Diego de Tineo, the owner of the aforementioned costly *botica*. Francisco de Alva was *familiar* to the Inquisition and was probably the most eminent *boticario* in the city at the time.[31] He was said to be worth 50,000 pesos *ensayados* owning several houses including one on the plaza. He also owned a shop where the *botica* was located and two "shop doors" (puertas de tiendas) where presumably he sold medicines.[32] The cost of establishing a *botica* can be compared to setting up a manufacturing enterprise, where the initial investment for a craft workshop might be between only 50 to 200 pesos, and for a manufacturing workshop 500 *pesos de a nueve*.[33] Clearly the high cost of establishing a *botica* limited the number of people who could purchase one outright.[34]

Due to the high cost of establishing a *botica*, some pharmacies were set up as joint enterprises. A common way of establishing businesses in sixteenth-century Lima was to form a *compañía* of two or more investors.[35] Apothecaries were able to attract investment from non-*boticarios*, because pharmacy was considered to be a profitable business.[36] In 1605 the *boticario* Bartolomé Díaz Cabeza de Vaca entered into a *compañía* with Francisco Martín Reyna for the purchase of a *botica* from Pedro and Joan de Tineo, which was located next to the cathedral.[37] Pedro and Joan de Tineo were nephews of the *boticario*

31 *Libros de cabildos de Lima*, 7: 549 Título familiar al bachiller Alba [sic] 21 Jan. 1574, *Libros de cabildos de Lima*, 8: 201 Familiar del santo oficio a Juan de Bilbao 24 Feb. 1576.

32 AGNP Real Audiencia. Causas Civiles leg. 16 cuad. 81 fol. 7v., 687 Pleito…contra las bienes y herederos del bachiller Francisco de Alva, boticario morador en la Ciudad de los Reyes. 1576. In 1599 the *boticario* Francisco Martín Reyna was renting a house under the *portales* of the plaza from the heirs of Marina Alva (*Libros de cabildos de Lima*, 13: 516–17 Francisco Martín Reyna 21 Jul. 1600).

33 Quiroz, *Artesanos y manufactureros*, 83. For similar shared investments in pharmacies in Mexico see: Hernández Sáenz, *Learning to Heal*, 161–62.

34 In the late eighteenth and early nineteenth centuries *boticas* in Mexico City were commonly valued at between one and two thousand pesos though might be considerably more in the case of the major hospitals For a hospital *botica* it was estimated that 6,000 pesos were required for installations and equipment only, and a further 14,000 pesos to stock it (Hernández Sáenz, *Learning to Heal*, 159–162; De Vos, "Art of Pharmacy," 72–73).

35 Quiroz, *Artesanos y manufactureros*, 84, and *Gremios, razas y libertad*, 71–82.

36 For example, in 1551 an *alcalde ordinario*, Gerónimo de Silva, sold a *botica* to Pero Lopes de Aguirre, with whom he had formed a *compañía*, neither of whom were referred to as *boticarios* (AGNP Protocolos Siglo XVI 8 Simón Alzate fols. 841v–842 26 June 1551). For Mexico City see: De Vos, "Art of Pharmacy," 72–74.

37 AAL Testamentos 5–1 fols. 12v–13 Testamento de Bartolomé Díaz Cabeza de Vaca 1608.

Diego de Tineo.[38] The agreed sum of 4,000 *pesos corrientes* was to be paid in two instalments, half to Pedro de Tineo at the end of April 1605 and the other to Joan de Tineo at Christmas the same year. The first instalment of 2,000 pesos was paid in cash on 10 May 1605, while the second was to be paid from the profits from the *botica*. In fact the latter was paid on 4 February 1606. Less than three years later on 15 April 1608, Díaz Cabeza de Vaca died. At that time after deducting expenditures and debts, the *botica* was worth 7,320 pesos, of which one-third belonged to his estate and the other two-thirds to Francisco Martín Reyna, who continued to own the *tienda* after his death.[39] It is unclear at this time whether Francisco Martín Reyna was a trained *boticario*. In the list of Limeños making a donation to the Crown in 1590 he is referred to as a *pulpero* and between 1595 and 1600 was supplying the Hospital of Santa Ana with honey, resins and burlap.[40] However, sometime later, in 1615 and 1618, he was importing *materia medica* from Spain and was referred to as a *boticario*.[41] It may be that his original interest in the pharmacy business derived from being a supplier of these products. Arrangements between artisans and those who supplied them with raw materials, or who traded products on their behalf, were commonplace in other enterprises in Lima.[42] In 1624 a *botica* was sold by one Pedro de Reyna to the *boticario* Bernardo Gil for 4,000 pesos.[43] The seller's surname suggests that this may have been the same *botica* that had been owned by Francisco Martín Reyna which he had inherited as a relative. If this was the case, then its value in 1624, which did not include medicines, had not increased since 1605. When Gil died in 1662 the *botica* was still valued at 4,000 pesos.

---

38 Diego de Tineo was still practising as a *boticario* in 1590 (AGI Lima 272 fols. 94–112v. Servicio hecho al rey nuestro señor en la ciudad de los reyes 1590).

39 AAL Testamentos 5–1 fols. 175–181v. Testamento de Bartolomé Díaz Cabeza de Vaca 1608.

40 AGI Lima 272 fols. 94–112v. Servicio hecho al rey nuestro señor en la ciudad de los reyes 1590; ABPL 9084 fols. 241–242v. Libro de cuentas de gastos del hospital de Santa Ana 1599–1600; ABPL 9085 fols. 59–64 Libro de la razón que toma Bartolomé de la Cueva escribano y veedor deste hospital de Santa Ana…desde el primero del mes de agosto 1595.

41 AGI Contratación 1162 N4 43–46 Registro del navío San Pedro 1615; AGI Contratación 1166 N1 403–406 Registro del navío El Espíritu Santo 1618.

42 Quiroz Chueca, "Compañías y gremios," and *Artesanos y manufactureros*, 85; Ruth Pike, *Aristocrats and Traders: Sevillian Society in the Sixteenth Century* (Ithaca, NY: Cornell University Press, 1972), 100.

43 AAL Testamentos 52–21 fols. 8v. Testamento de Bernardo Gil, boticario 1662.

The Premises

Clearly those seeking to acquire or establish *boticas* had to have access to considerable capital resources, but in addition they had to shoulder significant running costs. The value of pharmacies recorded in historical sources generally referred to its medicines, equipment and books and not the premises where it was located, since these were generally rented. A functioning pharmacy required at least three rooms: a front room where the *boticario* met clients and dispensed medicines; a back room known as a *trastienda* or *rebotica* where the medicines were prepared, the equipment kept, and accounts drawn up; and a store room or *aposento*.[44] In the case of Díaz Cabeza de Vaca, rent for the building in which his *botica* was located was 650 pesos a year; in addition he rented an *aposento* next door, for an unspecified amount, and where in fact he lived.[45] It was the tradition in Spain, even until recently, for *boticarios* to live on the premises, very often above the pharmacy which was on the ground floor.[46] This *botica* was situated in a prime location next to the cathedral and elsewhere rents were somewhat less.[47] In 1551 the physician, Alvaro de Torres was renting out a *tienda* and *trastienda* on the road running to Callao for the much smaller sum of 120 pesos a year.[48] Even hospitals might rent extra premises. In 1574 Rodrigo de Vargas, the *boticario* of the Hospital of Santa Ana, was renting two houses in the hospital's plaza for 60 pesos and 15 pesos a year.[49] Sometimes the cost of premises was paid for in kind, as was the case with Bernardo Gil who rented an *aposento* from the widow of the former *boticario* Melchor Malo de Molina for a notional 100 pesos a year for which he paid in kind through supplying her household with medicines.[50]

As for the location of a pharmacy, wind and humidity were thought to damage drugs,[51] so the advice to aspirant *boticarios* was that it should be "situated in a healthy place, dry (ajena de humedad) and free from dust, smoke and bad

44 Hernández Sáenz, *Learning to Heal*, 152; De Vos, "Art of Pharmacy," 88–89.

45 AAL Testamentos 5–1 fols. 14v., 181r. Testamento de Bartolomé Díaz Cabeza de Vaca 1608.

46 Herrera Dávila, "Boticas sevillanas de 1631," 72.

47 For an overview of rents in Lima in the seventeenth century see María Antonia Durán Montero, *Lima en el siglo XVII: Arquitectura, urbanismo y vida cotidiana* (Sevilla: Diputación Provincial, 1994), 166–74.

48 AGNP Protocolos Siglo XVI 8 Simón Alzate fols. 924–924v. 9 Jul. 1551.

49 ABPL 9080 fol. 102 Libro de cuentas, censos y haberes que corresponden al del hospital de Santa Ana 1575 a 1585.

50 AAL Testamentos 52–21 fol. 10–10v. Testamento de Bernardo Gil, boticario 1662.

51 Aguilera, *Exposición*, fol. 24. "…not windy or humid, or least very clear where there is a lot of sunshine."

odours."[52] The climate and elevation of Lima and its immediate surroundings did not vary significantly, so climatic factors were probably not an important consideration in the siting of pharmacies; of greater concern was the need to be close to the main market for medicines, which was among elites in the city centre.

Employing Pharmacy Workers

Licensed *boticarios*, including the *oficiales* referred to above, were probably only a small proportion of the numbers that assisted or even practised pharmacy. Many other pharmacists were Blacks and Indians who worked as salaried employees or slaves in privately-owned *boticas* and hospitals. As early as 1572 the *cabildo* of Lima was concerned that Blacks and Indians working in *boticas* were threatening the lives of patients by supplying medicines that did not comply with prescriptions, sometimes substituting items with ingredients that had been banned, such as opium, or selling mercury chloride or corrosive sublimate (*solimán*). It judged that the art of being an apothecary required scientific knowledge, skill and precision, which it was impossible for Blacks and Indians to possess; it was recognised that even Spaniards trained in the art occasionally made mistakes. The *cabildo* therefore ordered that Blacks and Indians should not work in *boticas* and that apothecaries found guilty of employing them should be fined 200 pesos and the workers exiled.[53]

Despite these concerns and attempts at regulation, to be discussed more fully in Chapter 5, Indians were assigned to work in pharmacies as forced labourers, while Blacks were widely employed there. In fact, *boticarios* observed that clients often sought advice and treatment from practitioners from the same ethnic background and thus they often employed Indians and Blacks to expand their customer base.[54]

Indian Forced Labourers

When the Spanish arrived in Peru, the native population of Lima was small and subsequently most Indians who resided there came from outside the city.

52 Suárez de Figueroa, *Plaza universal*, 302.

53 *Libros de cabildos de Lima*, 7: 268 Boticarios no tengan en boticas negros 28 Apr. 1572 and 270–72 Que no den medicinas negros en las boticas ni entren en ellas 2 May 1572. The art required "mucha ciencia e abilidad e fieldad."

54 Eguiguren, *Alma mater*, 256.

The 1613 census of Lima registered only about two thousand Indian residents;[55] these included urban migrants and those from outside the city who had been assigned there to undertake labour in public service. Arriving in Lima these forced labourers settled in El Cercado from whence, under an allocation system referred to as the *mita de plaza*, they were assigned by the *corregidor* to work in the maintenance of the city's infrastructure and elite houses or were allocated for agricultural labour. The Hospital of Santa Ana regularly received forced labourers to work in its pharmacy. For example, in 1596 the *corregidor*, Alonso de Mendoza Ponce de León, assigned Hernando Quispi from Yauyos in the hinterland of Lima to work for one year under Rodrigo de Vargas, the *boticario* of the Hospital of Santa Ana.[56] What tasks such workers may have performed is uncertain, though they were probably fairly unskilled since another *mitayo*, Juan Malca Atoc from Chinchacocha in the region of Junín, who was assigned there in 1593, was only twelve years old.[57] After 1572 *mitayos* were in theory to be remunerated for their labour at the rate of one real a day.[58] Such labour had the advantage of being cheap, but since it was constantly changing employers found it difficult to develop the skills of such workers.

Those who lived permanently in the city and others who were not required for public labour service might contract themselves to employers for fixed periods and wages. These contracts were supposed to be drawn up in the presence of a *corregidor*. Apart from fixed wages, workers on contract might receive clothing, shelter and medical care, conditions that might be attractive to those lacking any alternative means of subsistence. The minimum wage for contracted workers was 12 pesos a year, often plus lodging, food, clothing and medical care, though wages varied according to their skills.[59] In the Hospital of

---

55 Salinas y Córdova, *Memorial*, 245; Cook, *Indian Population*, 151.

56 AGNP Protocolos Siglo XVI 20 Rodrigo Alonso Castillejo fols. 271v.–272 1 Jul. 1596. There are a large number of contracts for the assignment (*asiento*) of indigenous labourers for different tasks in AGNP Protocolos Siglo XVI 18, 19, 20. For the employment of Rodrigo de Vargas in the Hospital of Santa Ana see: AGI Lima 122 fol. 36–37v. Información hecha… de la parte del hospital de los naturales 30 Oct. 1577; ABPL 9086 Visita al Hospital de Santa Ana fols.104–105 no date [1588].

57 AGNP Protocolos Siglo XVI 19 Rodrigo Alonso Castillejo fol. 575v. 16 Sep. 1593.

58 Lowry, "Forging an Indian Nation," 176–80; Paul Charney, *Indian Society in the Valley of Lima, Peru, 1532–1765* (Lanham, MD: University Press of America, 2001), 20–21. In 1563 the hospital de los espanõles (San Andrés) was employing a *yanacona* at 1 real a day (AGI Lima 131 Juan de Alvear en nombre del administrador y fundador del hospital despañoles 1563).

59 For Lowry, "Forging an Indian Nation," 195, 200–203. For an example see AGNP Protocolos Siglo XVI 51 Rodrigo Gómez Baeza fols. 285–285v. Blas de Medina concierto con Juan Real 8 Mar 1591.

Santa Ana ordinary workers, gardeners, or those who worked in the hospital's *chácara* were paid between 40 and 50 pesos a year.[60] In addition, some Indians were being employed in the *botica* on a casual basis for a few days, perhaps to undertake specific or skilled tasks, for which they were paid at the higher rate of 3 reals a day. Working in a hospital environment, Indians might acquire healing skills. One Indian worker in the Hospital of Santa Ana, Pedro Capicha, acquired sufficient skills as a barber and surgeon to be assigned to work on its hacienda in the valley of Jauja in order to treat the Indians there who were suffering from scrofula and other diseases, for which he was exempted from forced labour.[61]

Black Pharmacy Workers

Blacks vastly outnumbered Indians in Lima. In 1613 there were about 10,000 Blacks in the city,[62] and they were more commonly employed in all types of *boticas* than Indians. Most *boticarios* possessed several slaves, though many probably worked in their households rather than their pharmacies.[63] The will of one eminent apothecary, Francisco de Alva, who became *boticario* to the Inquisition,[64] owned six slaves, of whom one Matheo aged 30 worked in the *botica*.[65] This slave had clearly acquired considerable pharmacy skills, because following the *boticario's* death in 1576 when most of his possessions were auctioned, the "negro boticario" who remained with his second wife became

---

60 ABPL 9084 fols. 132–70 *passim*, fols. 241–242v. Libro de cuentas de gastos del hospital de Santa Ana año 1598. Charney (*Indian Society*, 21) gives wages of between 22 and 180 pesos a year for those contracted to work in agriculture.

61 ABPL 9095 Real Provisión 31 Aug. 1617. The text is rather ambiguous since it could refer to the general treatment of Indians or to illnesses which were specific to them. It reads: "lamparones y otras enfermedades de los indios naturales."

62 Salinas y Córdova, *Memorial*, 245.

63 There is evidence for the purchase of slaves by *boticarios* in the accounts of the slave trader, Manuel Bautista Pérez. Bernardo Gil bought a male slave from him in 1618 at the high cost of 655 pesos (AGNP SO CO Ca. 2 doc. 8 Venta e rendimento de duzemtas e vimte e sete peças de escravos 1618) and in 1625 Juan Matías de Vera, at that time *boticario* to the convent de los Descalços, purchased one for 580 pesos (AGNP SO CO Ca. 20 doc. 201 Venta de 76 pieças de esclavos 1625). In addition, the records of burials in the church of Sagrario attached to the cathedral, include payments, normally of 8 pesos, for the interment of adult slaves by Lima's most prominent *boticarios*, including Diego de Tineo, Francisco de Alva and Juan de Bilbao (AAL Libro Parroquial Sagrario Difuntos libros 1–3 1567–1609).

64 *Libros de cabildos de Lima*, 7: 549–550 Título familiar al bachiller Alba 21 Jan. 1574.

65 AGNP Real Audiencia. Causas Civiles leg. 16 cuad. 81 fol. 7v.-8 Pleito...contra las bienes y herederos del bachiller Francisco de Alva, boticario morador en la Ciudad de los Reyes. 1576.

central to a law suit between her and Francisco de Alva's children by his first marriage. The slave was deemed to be worth 1,000 *pesos ensayados* and able to bring in more than 250 to 300 pesos a year through being hired out.[66] It was common practice in Lima for widows to secure an income through hiring out their slaves. At that time, the "wages" earned by slaves averaged between about 8 and 12 pesos a month.[67] The skills acquired by Matheo were perhaps exceptional, but Blacks were routinely employed in *boticas*. Another skilled *boticario* slave belonging to Bernardo Gil was also judged to be worth more than 500 pesos.[68] Similarly, Francisco Martín Reyna purchased one Luis Biafra for 516 pesos for the *botica* he jointly owned with Bartolomé Díaz Cabeza de Vaca. By the time of the *boticario's* death in 1608, the slave had also died and been replaced by a "Matheo" from Mozambique. This slave, who also worked in the *botica*, had been purchased from father Pedro de Pareja, of the Compañía de Jesús, but was described as old and judged to be worth only 200 pesos.[69] In general, however, *boticarios* were advised not to allow employees to make medicines or to sell poisonous ones, especially if they were slaves in whom, it was judged, there was "always less trust and confidence."[70]

Not only private *boticas*, but also hospitals were staffed largely by African slaves. They mainly undertook routine tasks such as cooking, cleaning and washing, but might also serve as nurses and assist in surgery. In fact, in a *visita* of the Hospital of Santa Ana in 1587 it was recommended that "gente de color" be employed as nurses and assistants in preference to Indians due to their greater dedication to work.[71] Apart from undertaking routine tasks, there is

66 AGNP Real Audiencia. Causas Civiles leg. 16 cuad. 81 fols. 343, 346, 770 Pleito…contra las bienes y herederos del bachiller Francisco de Alva, boticario morador en la Ciudad de los Reyes. 1576.

67 Bowser, *African Slave*, 102–104.

68 AAL Testamentos 52–21 fols. 88–104 Testamento de Bernardo Gil, boticario 1662.

69 AAL Testamentos 5 leg 1 fol. 13v–14, 179 Testamento de Bartolomé Díaz Cabeza de Vaca 1608. At this time the average cost of a newly-arrived slave was between 570 and 600 pesos (Newson and Minchin, *From Capture to Sale*, 228–29). In 1625 the *boticario* Bernardo Gil similarly purchased an African slave for 570 pesos (AGNP SO CO Ca. 20 doc. 201 Venta de 69 pieças de diferentes naciones que traxo Sebastian Duarte 1625). For the employment of Blacks in *boticas* in Cartagena see: Archivo General de la Nación, Colombia (hereafter AGNC) Médicos y Abogados 6 fols. 944v–945 Martín Sánchez de Velasco…informe sobre sus visitas a las boticas de Cartagena 1634.

70 ARJBM División 1, leg. 17 Prohemiales 8 Libro de examen de los simples medicinales Antonio de Robles Cornejo 1617.

71 Rabí Chara, *Hospital de Santa Ana*, 74. This is based on leg. 9086 in the ABPL, from which documents relating to this *visita* have since been lost.

some evidence that they were being trained in pharmacy. In the early seventeenth century, the post of *boticario* of the Hospital of San Andrés was held by an African slave, Juan Mandinga.[72] Somewhat later in 1639 one Antonillo Angola was working in the pharmacy of Santa Ana and despite being slave was earning 7 pesos a year.[73] Most renowned of all was Martín de Porres, a Mulatto and America's first Black saint, who combined the duties of nurse, barber-surgeon, and apothecary in the Dominican convent of El Rosario.[74]

Running a Pharmacy

Despite Lima being a particularly healthy city, life expectancy in the sixteenth century was low. Its residents were constantly preoccupied with their health which meant that they were willing to expend large sums of money on medical treatments.[75] A priest attached to the Cathedral who suffered from a long-term illness and had no financial resources was willing to take out a loan of 3,000 pesos from its *mayordomo* to pay for his treatment.[76] The high demand for medicines and willingness to pay high prices should have made pharmacy a profitable business, but a central feature of the way it was managed was that it ran largely on credit. This was problematic because often the patients died or migrated elsewhere before clearing their debts, so that *boticarios* were often owed several thousand pesos. On his death in 1636, a number of Pedro de Bilbao's clients were noted as living in Chile, Mexico, and Potosí.[77] Often relatives of the deceased or institutions had to be pursued through the law courts in order to recover the debts. This could be a protracted and costly process which meant that *boticarios* had to have significant financial backing in order to keep their businesses running on a day-to-day basis in the meantime.

Elite families generally made annual contracts with physicians and surgeons to treat their households. How much they charged varied, possibly according

72 AHIRA Maldonado A-III-306 fol. 115 Libros de egresos e ingresos del hospital de San Andrés 1612.

73 ABPL 9104 Libro de cuentas de gastos del hospital de Santa Ana 29 Aug. 1639.

74 Cussen, *Black Saint*, 55–56, 69–84.

75 For the general predisposition of Spaniards to spend large amounts of money on medicine see Lanning, *Royal Protomedicato*, 230. Colonial documents are replete with comments by officials on the state of their health.

76 AAL Causas Civiles leg. 20 exp. 5 Causa de acreedores a los bienes del padre Juan de Vargas y Mendoza que fue de la catedral de Lima 1618.

77 AGNP Protocolos Siglo XVII 1789 Sánchez Vadillo fols. 2068–2072 Inventario de bienes de Pedro de Bilbao 25 Aug. 1636.

to the number of patients they were required to attend. The New Christian surgeon, Tomé Cuaresma, charged an annual fee of thirty to forty pesos for a family, with payments occasionally paid in kind, for example in bags of wheat,[78] whereas in 1633 Licenciado Pedro Rodríguez Merchán contracted a surgeon, Luis de Molina Guzmán for the annual salary of 70 pesos to treat all persons in his household and *chácara*.[79] There is no evidence that similar contracts were made with apothecaries, but it is clear from legal cases that elite families generally acquired medicines from the same *boticario* and that bills were drawn up on an annual basis.[80] Rather than *boticarios* being contracted on a salary, the amount they were paid was dependent on the ailments they were treating and the medicines they dispensed. The slave trader, Manuel Bautista Pérez had agreements with at least two *boticarios,* namely Pedro de Bilbao and Alonso de Carrión, to treat his household and the African slaves on his *chácara*, but whether these were underpinned by legal contracts is unknown. For the year 1628 Manuel Bautista Pérez owed 1,052 pesos to Pedro de Bilbao, while in 1639 when Pérez was put to death by the Inquisition, he was in debt to Alonso de Carrión to the order of 1,710 pesos for medicines he had supplied at various times between 1635 and 1639.[81]

The procedure for charging for medicines and recovering debts was as follows. A physician would draw up a prescription (*receta*) for medicines which would then be supplied by a *boticario*. Generally the patient did not pay for the medicines immediately, but when the medicines were delivered he or she signed the prescription acknowledging that they had been received. The signed receipts or *vales*, which did not indicate the cost, were then kept by the *boticario* as evidence of the medicines he had supplied. Bartolomé Díaz Cabeza de Vaca kept his receipts for different patients and households on separate strings, which at the time of his death numbered 195. He often recorded the profession of his clients, from which it is apparent that he served a wide spectrum of individuals from the governor, members of the *cabildo*, priests,

78 AGNP SO CO Ca. 44 doc. 394 fols. 772–775 Conciertos de curar de Tomé Cuaresma 1623, 1625 and 1630.

79 AAL Causas Civiles leg. 43 exp. 2 Causa ejecutiva que sigue Luis de Molina Guzmán, cirujano, contra el Lic. Pedro Rodríguez Merchán 5 Oct. 1634.

80 AGNP SO CO Ca. 27 doc. 277 Pedro de Bilbao contra Don Juan Arévalo de Espinosa 1629). For the bills incurred by Manuel Bautista Pérez with Pedro de Bilbao and Alonso de Carrión see: AGNP SO CO Ca. 57 doc. 431 1629, 1635–1640.

81 For the bills incurred by Manuel Bautista Pérez with Pedro de Bilbao and Alonso de Carrión see: AGNP SO CO Ca. 57 doc. 431 1629, 1635–1640. When the value of the medicines was assessed by the physicians Doctors Gerónimo Andrés Rocha, Juan de la Vega and Manuel Pérez they were judged to be worth about half the amount claimed.

teachers, and merchants, to a variety of artisans, including silversmiths, a gilder, tailors, hat makers, shoemakers, a glovemaker, a confectioner, and a locksmith. Of the clients, 92 still owed him money at the time of his death. These debts averaged 43 pesos, but ten people owed over 100 pesos. While each of these debts might have been small, they totalled some 3,874 *pesos*, which together with other debts represented 42 percent of the assets of his *botica*.[82] (See Table 2).

In general large debts, that is mainly those over 100 pesos, were pursued through the courts. A significant number of legal cases relating to the recovery of sums owed to *boticarios* are to be found in the section Causas Civiles in the Archivo Arzobispal in Lima.[83] In presenting a claim a *boticario* would include a list of the medicines that he had supplied and the *vales* on which the list was based (See Figures 3 and 4). The legal procedure was that a physician or *boticario* would then be employed to assess the value of the medicines; in most cases they were valued at about half of what the *boticarios* claimed. *Boticarios* were infamous for overcharging for medicines, so that they rarely challenged the lower assessments.

Sometimes clients objected to the bills on the grounds that the *vales* had not been signed or were not authentic. They might also refuse to pay claiming collusion between the *boticario* and the witnesses who were called to testify. In response to a claim for 150 pesos brought by the *boticario* Bernardo Gil, the defendant a priest, Doctor Sebastián de Betanzos, claimed that two of the witnesses had "a close friendship and connexion with him [Gil] and are in his house and company and eat with him, and as such I think they are untrustworthy and challenge they should be witnesses or be believed."[84] Similarly, in a redhibition case brought against Manuel Bautista Pérez by one Doña Francisca de Guzmán y Quintana for the sale of a slave who was suffering from severe stomach pains and unable to work, she claimed that all the witnesses, which included two surgeons, were his "servants, compatriots, [and]

---

82 AAL Testamentos Leg 5 exp. 1 fols. 27v–35v. Testamento de Bartolomé Díaz Cabeza de Vaca 1608.

83 For seventeen cases between 1613 and 1651 see: AAL Causas Civiles leg. 14 exp. 35, leg. 17 exp. 18, leg. 20 exp. 5, leg. 32 exp 14, leg. 33 exp. 19, leg. 39 exp 5, 16, leg. 41 exp. 15, leg. 42A exp. 2, 3, 10, leg. 48A exp. 11, 20, leg. 50 exp. 6, 16, 24, 38, leg. 60 exp.6. For overcharging see also: Biblioteca del Palacio Real, Madrid II/546 fols. 119–119v. Cuaderno de algunos papeles...Marqués de Montesclaros 1 Apr. 1612.

84 AAL Causas Civiles leg. 48A exp. 20 Autos seguidos por Bernardo Gil, boticario, contra el Dr. Sebastián de Betanzos, clérigo de menores órdenes, por 150 pesos de medicinas adquiridas en su botica. 20 Oct. 1639.

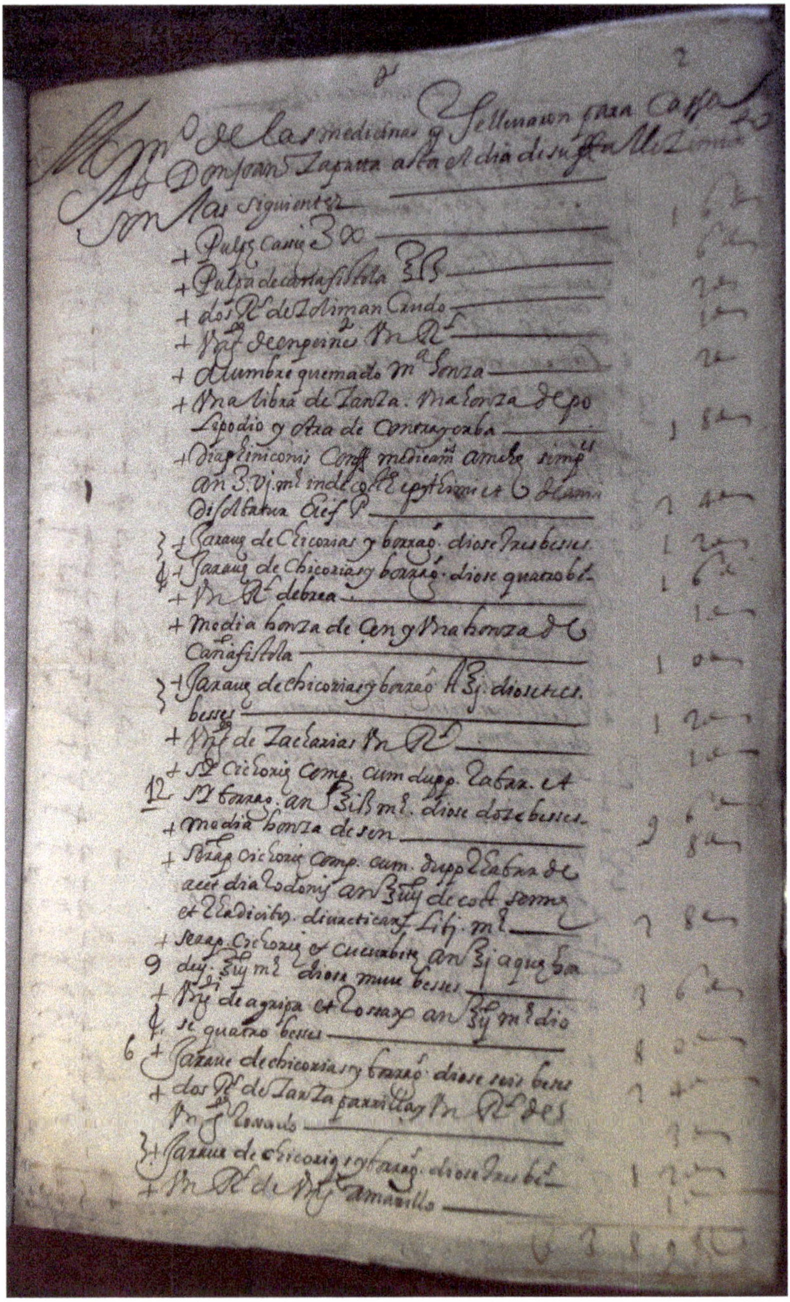

FIGURE 3 *List of medicines supplied by Bernardo Gil to Don Juan Zapata 1640.*
Source: AAL Causas Civiles legajo 50 exp. 16 Autos seguidos por Bernardo Gil, boticario, contra los bienes y albacea del Lic. Don Juan Zapata, clérigo presbítero. 1640.
COURTESY ARCHIVO ARZOBISPAL, LIMA. PHOTO: AUTHOR.

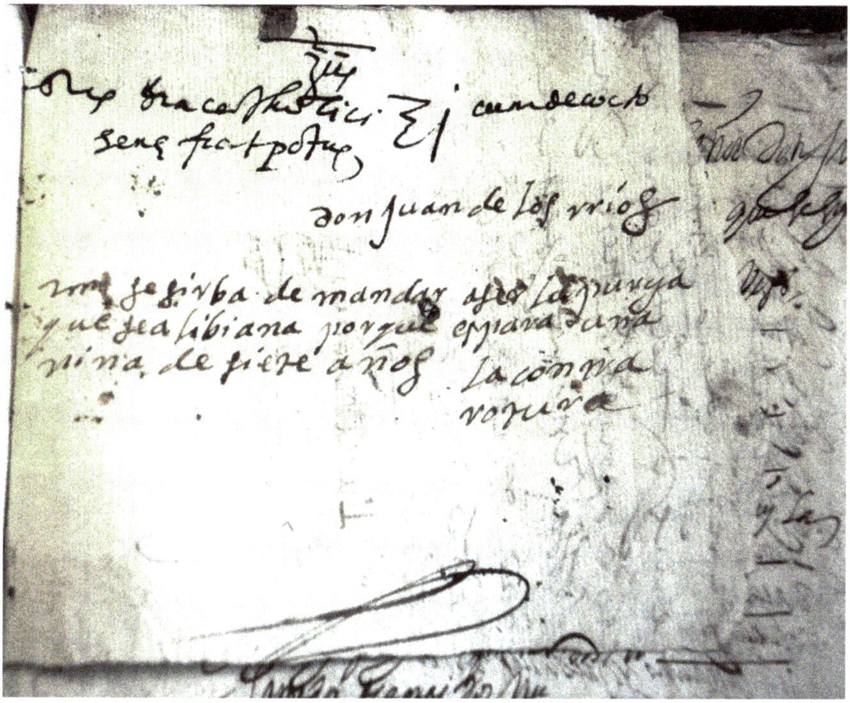

FIGURE 4 *Receipt for medicines supplied to Don Juan de los Ríos by Bernardo Gil, 1633.*
... diacatholici ʒi cumdecocto sene fiat potus
[one ounce of diacatolicon with a decoction of senna to make a potion].
don juan de los rríos
... se sirva de mandar aser [hacer] la purga que sea libiana [liviana] porque es para una niña de siete años. La contrarotura.
[...it serves to order to make a purgative which should be light because it is for a girl of seven years old. The plaster.]
Source: AAL Causas Civiles Leg. 42A, exp. 2 Causa seguida por Bernardo Gil, dueño de botica, contra el bachiller Don Juan de los Ríos, clérigo presbítero. 1633.
COURTESY ARCHIVO ARZOBISPAL, LIMA. PHOTO: AUTHOR.

close relatives."[85] Clients occasionally asserted that the *boticario* had supplied the medicines free of charge. Hence, Doña Beatriz de Garay stated that even though she had signed the *vales* presented by the *boticario* Mateo Pastor, this was only to eliminate fraud and that he had not charged for medicines, indeed she claimed that she could even request medicines by word of mouth. She said this was because he was a "paysano" of her mother and he treated her as family because "in this kingdom those who are from the same place in Spain regard

85 AGNP Real Audiencia Causas Civiles leg. 70 cuad. 263 Autos seguidos por Doña Francisca de Guzmán y Quintana contra Manuel Bautista Pérez sobre la redhibitoria de un esclavo 1626.

each other as *parientes* (relatives)."[86] In other cases, the prebend and teacher of the Cathedral claimed he was unable to pay because of the high cost of living in Lima and because due to a long illness he had run up bills with three doctors, a surgeon and a *boticario*.[87] On the other hand, *boticarios* or their executors defended their right to include unsigned *vales* or those signed by a relative because the patients were too ill to sign or had sent their slaves to the *botica* to collect the medicines on their behalf, explanations that were often accepted.[88] Clearly in many cases debts could not be recovered, though there is evidence of relatively small amounts being pursued over several decades.

The largest debts were incurred by monasteries, convents, hospitals, and the Inquisition. It was practice for the *cabildo* to make contracts with specific *boticarios* to supply medicines to all the city's monasteries and from the outset it had to tackle the issue of overcharging.[89] Up to the beginning of the seventeenth century this contract, while substantial, was never worth more than 5,000 *pesos corrientes* and it was handled by one *boticario*. However, in 1604 the contract was divided between two *boticarios* and by 1606 the cost had risen to 13,015.5 pesos, a figure that the *cabildo* considered unacceptable. In order to reduce the cost, the contract was put out to tender and in 1610 it was split between two other *boticarios*: Gerónimo Pujadas, who was to supply the Dominican, Franciscan, and Jesuit monasteries, and Pedro de Bilbao the Augustinian. Pujadas's pharmacy and contract were later taken over by Francisco de Sandoval about whom there were constant complaints. It was claimed he committed many frauds, altering and adding to prescriptions, such that one claim that he submitted for supplying medicines between 1619 and 1620 was reduced significantly

---

86 AGNP SO CO 132–1199 Don Diego Laurencio Valenzuela administrador del patronato de Mateo Pastor de Velasco contra doña Beatriz de Garay 14 Jun. 1663.

87 AAL Causas Civiles leg. 20 exp. 5 Causa de acreedores a los bienes del padre Juan de Vargas y Mendoza que fue de la catedral de Lima 1618.

88 See for example, AAL Causas Civiles leg. 41 exp. 15 Autos ejecutivos seguidos por Gabriel de España, boticario, contra el Lic. Diego Cabrera albacea y tenedor de bienes del Lic. Francisco Juárez Salgado 1632; AAL Causas Civiles leg. 42A exp. 3 Lima. Causa seguida por Bernardo Gil, contra los bienes que quedaron por fin y muerte del padre Luis Nieto Palomino 1632/1633; AAL Causas Civiles leg. 31 exp. 14 Causa ejecutiva seguida por Antolín Reynoso, boticario, contra Alonso Martínez Pastrana, contador mayor, albacea y tenedor de bienes de don Juan Velásquez 1627. In this case they were signed by his sister or niece, witnesses differ, but the argument was that in his will he indicated in detail the debts he owed. See also AGNP SO CO 125–1091 Gaspar de Calderón sobre medicinas que dio a Juan de Turiçes difunto 18 Sep. 1656.

89 AGI Lima 112 Tristán Sánchez, contador, 1588.

by the assessor to 1,840 pesos. Aware that fraud had also been perpetrated for four years previously, receipts for this period, which amounted to some 13,025 pesos, were also reviewed and assessed by the *boticarios*, *licenciado* Antonio de Robles and Antolín Reynoso, who valued them at 3,511 pesos, an amount to which Sandoval agreed.[90] Subsequently, it was suggested that a limit should be placed on the amount that a *boticario* could claim; both 3,500 and 2,200 pesos were suggested. It was noted that there were other more suitable *boticarios*, who had demonstrated "more satisfaction and knowledge" who could undertake the commission.

Francisco de Sandoval not only supplied several monasteries, but also the female Convent of La Concepción. In 1625 he initiated a legal case against the Convent on behalf of the widow of Gerónimo Pujadas from whom he had assumed charge of the *botica*. This was over the payment of 10,087 pesos relating to medicines that had been supplied between 1619 and 1622.[91] However, the claim was disputed by the Convent on the grounds that not all the *vales* for items listed had been presented and others were unsigned. It also asserted that some of the items had not been claimed for within three years, as was apparently required by law, and were therefore invalid. In addition the Convent argued that the assessment by the *boticario*, Juan Ximénez Villayzan, had included many invalid *recetas* and a number of arithmetic errors. The assessor himself acknowledged that the task of reviewing some 5,912 *recetas* had been daunting and had been hard work over two months. The Convent then raised the question of whether the widow of Gerónimo Pujadas had a legal claim. In attempting to resolve the issue, a reassessment was ordered on the basis of 3,987 agreed receipts and in the end, in 1629, a value of 5,788 pesos 2 reales was imposed by the physician and later *protomédico*, Juan de la Vega. The latter amount appears to have been paid, but there were ongoing disputes between Sandoval and the Convent over medicines that he had supplied on his own account.[92] As late as 1650, the legitimate son of Gerónimo Pujadas

90 AGI Lima 97 Consulta a la Real Audiencia sobre las medicinas donadas a los conventos 12 May 1621; Carta de la Real Audiencia al rey sobre limosna de medicinas a los conventos 6 May 1622. Most likely Antonio de Robles was the physician Antonio de Robles Cornejo, who was the author of several manuscripts on the use of medicinal simples to be discussed in Chapter 5.

91 AAL Monasterio de la Concepción leg. 2 exp.18 Causa seguida por Francisco de Sandoval, boticario de Lima, contra el Monasterio de la Concepción 1626–1629.

92 AAL Monasterio de la Concepción leg. 3 exp. 19 Causa seguida por Francisco de Sandoval, boticario de Lima, contra el Monasterio de la Concepción por las medicinas que sacaron de su botica 1627.

was still trying to claim for the *recetas* on which agreement had not been reached.[93]

Even if claims were valid, often clients lacked the resources to meet them. The Convent of La Concepción claimed that it was poor and did not receive government support, unlike male monasteries. Although in theory it received substantial dowries for the entry of women into the Convent, very often they were paid from *censos*. These were annuities paid from the income of a house or other property, usually of five percent, which were pledged for a number of years or in perpetuity.[94] The problem from the perspective of the Convent was that often householders could not afford repairs to their properties so that many fell into disrepair such that the income they generated declined.[95] Apart from the *censos*, the only other source of income was from an *obraje* producing serges and rope and this was deemed insufficient to pay for medicines and for the service of medical practitioners. The Convent admitted that it owed "a large amount of pesos" which it was unable to pay.[96]

Francisco de Sandoval may have been running a particularly fraudulent business, but supplying medicines to convents required substantial financial resources and incurred some risk for anyone accepting the contract. When Pedro de Bilbao died in 1636, he was not only owed 8,211 pesos for prescriptions supplied to 156 individuals, plus 76 pesos supplied to the Inquisition's prison, but also for medicines supplied over nine years to the Convent of La Merced and for four years to the Convent of San Agustín.[97] In addition he was owed 28,000 pesos worth for medicines he had supplied to the Convent of Nuestra Señora de la Encarnación, which was subject to a law suit.[98] This was not all,

93 AAL Monasterio de la Concepción leg. 9 exp. 60 Causa seguida por Ignacio de Pujadas, hijo legítimo de Gerónimo de Pujadas, contra el Monasterio de la Concepción por 11,000 pesos de medicinas que le dio de su de su botica y le han quedado debiendo 1651.

94 Arnold J. Bauer, "The Church in the Economy of Spanish America: Censos and Depósitos in the Eighteenth and Nineteenth Centuries," *Hispanic American Historical Review* 63(4) (1983): 715–17; Brian R. Hamnett, "Church Wealth in Peru: Estates and Loans in the Archdiocese of Lima in the Seventeenth Century," *Jahrbuch für Geschichte Lateinamerikas* 10 (1973): 115–16.

95 AGI Lima 215 N 6 R 1 fol. 3 Informaciones del monasterio de la Concepción de Lima 18 Mar 1603.

96 AGI Lima 215 N 6 R 1 fol. 11v. Informaciones del monasterio de la Concepción de Lima 18 Mar 1603.

97 This excluded the cost of other medicines that had been supplied previously.

98 AGNP Protocolos Siglo XVII 1789 Sánchez Vadillo fols. 2068–2072 Inventario de bienes de Pedro de Bilbao 25 Aug. 1636.

because another *boticario*, Alonso de Carrión who was not listed amongst his debtors, also certified that he owed Pedro de Bilbao 650 pesos.[99]

One may wonder why *boticarios* allowed clients to run up such large debts, even if they were exaggerated. It suggests that their businesses were sufficiently profitable to bear the debts and that the amounts that they were owed did not affect the day-to-day operation of their pharmacies. There are no instances of *boticarios* being made bankrupt or evidence of them complaining of being poor. Such debts were common in many businesses at this time.

In the early modern period, business success depended on reputation and trust.[100] In Europe the largest debts were incurred by elites, such as government officials and lawyers. Apothecaries felt obliged to treat them even if they anticipated that they would not be paid, since they feared that refusal would damage their reputations.[101] Debts, though incurring a cost, might actually bring some benefits. They could be used to develop or maintain relations of patronage-clientage that could ensure continued custom. Large contracts with major public and charitable institutions could only be fulfilled by *boticarios* with considerable financial backing and a good reputation. Although as shown above a good reputation was not always justified, the award of such contracts served as an indicator of their high economic status. Supplying medicines on credit to charitable institutions might also reflect on the religious piety and social standing of a *boticario*. For this reason, Paula De Vos argues that *boticarios* in Mexico City allowed charitable institutions to run up debts and rarely called them in.[102] The evidence for Lima indicates that convents were similarly allowed to build up debts over considerable periods of time, but in contrast to Mexico some *boticarios* in Lima did pursue some convents through the courts, as was the case of Pedro de Bilbao against the Convent of La Encarnación. Furthermore, in common with other *boticarios* he did not demure from overcharging charitable institutions. It suggests that there were limits to the support that *boticarios* gave to charitable causes in the form of reduced prices for medicines. After all, as will be shown in Chapter 7, they could demonstrate their

99 AGNP Protocolos Siglo XVII 1789 Sánchez Vadillo fols. 1375–1378v Alonso de Carrión to Juan de Sanmillán 28 Jul. 1636.

100 Daviken Studnicki-Gizbert, *A Nation upon the Ocean Sea: Portugal's Atlantic Diaspora and the Crisis of the Spanish Empire, 1492–1640* (Oxford: Oxford University Press, 2007), 84–86.

101 Brockliss and Jones, *Medical World*, 324; Robert Ralley, "Medical Economies in Fifteenth Century England," in *Medicine and the Market in England and its Colonies, c.1450–1850*, eds. Mark Jenner and Patrick Wallis (New York: Palgrave Macmillian, 2007), 29–30.

102 De Vos, "Art of Pharmacy," 185–86.

charity and piety in other ways, such as through membership of *cofradías*, private donations, and charitable works.[103]

Conclusion

The manner in which *boticas* were established and apothecaries and ran their businesses did not differ significantly from those in Spain. However, the personnel they employed and their interaction with charitable institutions seems to have differed. In Lima as in Spain, it was the case that *boticarios* had to have substantial financial resources to own a *botica*. Although detailed financial accounts kept by *boticarios* are lacking, the fact that pharmacy could attract non-*boticario* investors suggests that it was regarded as a profitable business. As will be shown in Chapter 7, the most prominent apothecaries amassed significant personal fortunes and could pay large dowries for their daughters. While *boticarios* in Lima were certainly interested in making profits, at the same time they were not entirely capitalistic for they did not invest their gains in expanding their businesses, but rather expended them on charitable activities that confirmed their social standing and assured them of an advantageous position in the afterlife.

Because substantial financial resources were needed to establish a *botica*, few were established in the city. Yet there were many others who were practising pharmacy as salaried employees, forced labourers, or slaves in both private pharmacies and hospitals. While the *cabildo* issued ordinances against *boticarios* employing non-licensed workers, especially Blacks and those of mixed race, they were not vigorously enforced. While this reflected in part the predominance of African slaves in the city's population, the seeming preference for the employment of slave labour may also have derived from their status of permanent servitude that enabled *boticarios* to invest in developing the pharmacy knowledge and skills of these workers in a way that was not possible with Indian forced labourers who were generally assigned for short periods and were constantly changing.

The ethnic diversity of those employed in *boticas* provided opportunities for the exchange of medicinal knowledge. However, the hierarchical structure of employment in *boticas* and the slave status of many employees would have discouraged a two-way exchange. Employees would have been taught how to prepare medicines by a licensed *boticario*, who invariably had been trained in humoral medicine and on whom they depended for their job, livelihood, and

103 For Mexico City see De Vos, "Art of Pharmacy," 171–81.

treatment. Nevertheless, there is evidence that Blacks and Indians were altering prescriptions, as attested by *cabildo* attempts to control their employment in pharmacies. Whether such changes to prescriptions were the result of error, insufficient guidance, or deliberate changes based on experience is unknown. However, the general absence of native botanical materials in pharmacy inventories and prescriptions, to be discussed in Chapter 6, suggests that the exchange of knowledge between ethnic groups with different healing traditions with the context of a functioning pharmacy was limited.

Pharmacies whether established in hospitals or run as private businesses did not operate as independent enterprises. They were subject to regulation by the *protomedicato* and municipal authorities, which among other things arranged for the inspection of pharmacies. This was primarily to ensure that out-of-date and dangerous drugs were not being prescribed and to prevent overcharging. However, they also paid attention to the types of medicines they contained, so that as will be shown, the inspections served to promote orthodox humoral practice. The regulation of pharmacies will be explored in Chapter 5 where competing approaches to medical practice are considered. Since considerable insight into medical practices in Peru can be gleaned from an analysis of the cargoes of *materia medica* and books imported from Spain and traded locally, the study turns first to an analysis of the transatlantic and local trading networks through which these commodities moved.

CHAPTER 4

Trading Medicines and *Materia Medica*

> The Indies have been rewarded better with respect to plants than other goods: for those that have come to Spain are few and do not grow well: those that have passed from Spain are many and they yield well.[1]

Materia medica represented the most significant ongoing cost for apothecaries. The medicinal products prescribed by physicians in the New World emanated from geographically diverse sources and were handled by an equally broad range of traders that included large scale merchants, local producers and sellers, and even *boticarios* themselves. Consistent with Spanish humoral beliefs and with state policies controlling medical practice in the early modern period, many medicinal products employed in Peru were imported from Spain many having been acquired from merchants based in Lisbon, Antwerp or Venice.[2] However, as will be shown, these imports were unable to meet local demand and were often of poor quality and expensive. Hospitals and *boticarios* alike therefore purchased simple medicinal products in local markets, while hospitals and convents also established their own herb gardens and sometimes their own pharmacies for the preparation of compound medicines. This chapter therefore examines the extent of the dependency of medical practice in Lima on the transatlantic trade, showing how inadequacies in provision should have fostered an interest in local *materia medica* and encouraged innovation.

1 José de Acosta, *Historia natural y moral de las Indias* in *Obras del Padre José de Acosta*. Biblioteca de autores españoles 73 (Madrid: Ediciones Atlas, 1954), lib. 4 cap. 31: 125. ["Mejor han sido pagadas las Indias en lo que toca a plantas que en otra mercaderías: porque las que han venido a España son pocas y danse mal: las que han pasado de España son muchas y danse bien."].

2 Francisco Guerra, "Drugs from the Indies," 44–48; Mercedes Fernández-Carrión and José Luis Valverde, "Research Notes on Spanish American Drug Trade," *Pharmacy in History* 30–31(1988–1989): 29–30; De Vos, "Art of Pharmacy," 90–101; Stefan Halikowski-Smith, "'Profits Sprout Like Tropical Plants': A Fresh Look at What Went Wrong with the Eurasian Spice Trade c. 1550–1800," *Journal of Global History* 3(2008): 390–409.

 | DOI 10.1163/9789004351271_005

Organisation of the Transatlantic Trade

In order understand the availability of *materia medica* from Spain it is necessary to have knowledge of the way that the transatlantic trade was organised. To ensure that Spain and its citizens enjoyed the economic benefits that derived from the acquisition of its American colonies, the Crown instituted a monopolistic trading system. This involved the establishment of the *Casa de Contratación* (Board of Trade) in Seville in 1503, which among other things registered all out going cargoes and levied appropriate taxes. For their protection, from 1526 ships were not permitted to sail to the Americas alone but were required to travel in convoys; from the 1560s a fleet system was established with each fleet operating on a two-year cycle and focused on a limited number of ports in both Spain and the Americas. One fleet – the *Flota* – was destined for New Spain and Central America, and the other – the *Galeones* – focussed on the South American mainland and the ports of Cartagena and Nombre de Dios (later Portobello). All goods, including medicines, destined for Peru passed through the latter ports.[3] The fleets were protected by *armadas* – armed vessels – which were paid for by a tax known as the *avería* which was based on the value of the cargo being shipped. The fleet system reached its apogee in the 1580s when the *Galeones* fleet comprised over 90 vessels, after which sailings became less regular and the number of ships comprising each fleet declined.

Consistent with Spain's policy of retaining its monopoly of trade with the Indies, all ships and their cargoes sailing to the New World had to be registered in Seville where bonds had to be provided. All merchandise, which included medicines and books, was subject to the same procedures of registration and inspection, while cargoes of books were additionally scrutinised by officials of the Inquisition to ensure that they did not include any heretical or banned works. The ships themselves were inspected three times: first, to ensure that ships were seaworthy and possessed the necessary equipment, including arms and artillery for their defence; and on the second and third occasions, to ensure they possessed sufficient crew and provisions for the journey.[4]

Each vessel carried a bewildering variety of goods ranging from domestic and foreign cloth and clothing, hardware, furniture, bedspreads, books,

3 For the operation of the fleet system see: Clarence H. Haring, *Trade and Navigation between Spain and the Indies* (Cambridge, Mass.: Harvard University Press, 1918), 201–30; John Lynch, *Spain under the Habsburgs* (Oxford: Blackwell, 1965) 1: 147–66.

4 Enriqueta Vila Vilar, *Hispanoamérica y el comercio de esclavos: los asientos Portugueses* (Seville: Escuela de Estudios Hispanoamericanos, 1977): 143–44; Newson and Minchin, *From Capture to Sale*, 23–25.

medicines, wine and oil among other things, all contained in array of boxes, chests, sacks, bundles, flasks, and bottles. Items were registered by both generalist and specialised traders, as well as by passengers travelling with the vessel. An itemised list of all goods contained in each box or bale needed to be presented to officials of the *Casa de Contratación* for tax evaluation purposes. Medicines destined for the Americas were for the most part subject to the same taxes as other commodities, and these taxes were considerable. First there was a customs duty known as the *almojarifazgo*. Initially this *ad valorem* tax was set 7.5 percent, with 2.5 percent levied in Seville and 5 percent in the Americas, but in 1566 both were doubled and a further 2.5 percent was collected on arrival in American ports, thereby giving a total tax of 17.5 percent.[5] Duties exacted in the Americas were based on prices there rather than in Spain, so that goods destined for Peru first paid *almojarifazgo* in Panama, and then on arrival in Callao a further 5 percent based on the increase in the value of the commodity between the isthmus and Peru.[6] In addition, all cargoes were subject to the *avería* which was a tax imposed to pay the cost of convoying and defending the fleets. This tax, which was collected in Seville, varied between 1 and 12 percent according to the perceived foreign threat at the time and therefore the need for defence.[7] Books were subject to the *avería*, but they were exempt from the *almojarifazgo*. It was observed that merchants were making a good profit from trading books since there was a growing demand from schools and universities and it was suggested that in order to raise revenue the Crown might impose the *almojarifazgo* on all books, except those destined for churches, convents, and monasteries. Nevertheless, the exemption remained in force.[8]

From 1553 all goods destined for the support of hospitals and convents, which included medicines, while being subject to the *avería*, were exempt

5 Rafael Antúnez y Acevedo, *Memorias históricas sobre la legislación y gobierno del comercio de los españoles con sus colonias en las Indias occidentales* (Madrid: Imprenta de Sancha, 1797), 211–18; Haring, *Trade and Navigation*, 84. This level of duty continued to 1660.

6 See AGNP Cajas Reales: Lima H-3 leg. 4 lib. 24-a fols. 1–30 Aranceles para cálculo del almojarifazgo (1617). *Almojarifazgo* was also collected in Lima on intercolonial trade, but at the lower rate of one percent (Borah, *Early Trade and Navigation*, 112–13).

7 Haring, *Trade and Navigation*, 67–82.

8 AGI Lima 143 fol. 35 Memorial y apuntamiento sumario de las cosas muy importantes 1612; *Recopilación* lib.8 tit. 15 ley 27 4 Nov 1548; Antúnez y Acevedo, *Memorias históricas*, 218; Irving A. Leonard, *Books of the Brave: Being an Account of Books and of Men in the Spanish Conquest and Settlement of the Sixteenth-century New World* (Berkeley and Los Angeles: University of California, 1992), 133; Carlos A. González Sánchez, *New World Literacy: Written Culture across the Atlantic, 1500–1700*, trans. Tristan Platt (Lewisburg: Bucknell University Press, 2011), 49–50.

from the *almojarifazgo*.[9] However, this exemption does not appear to have been applied consistently. The fleet of Juan Flores Rabanal dispatched in 1618 contained four cargoes of medicines, one for each of the three hospitals of Santa Ana, San Andrés and La Caridad in Lima, and the other for the royal hospital in Potosí.[10] While the *avería* was levied on all four cargoes, at the rate of about 1.1 percent, only the consignment for the hospital in Potosí appears to have been exempt from *almojarifazgo*. This seems to have been because the *boticario* in Seville who was remitting the medicines had previously paid this duty. As for the other three consignments, taxes were levied on rounded values of cargoes resulting rates varying between 5.8 and 8.0 percent.[11] In some cases officials did not exempt the cargoes of medicines for hospitals, but reduced their value and levied the regular duty on the lesser amount.[12] In contrast to medicines destined for hospitals, which in theory should have been exempt from the *almojarifazgo*, the shipping records of the *Casa de Contratación* in Seville suggest that at the end of the sixteenth century private merchants were paying *almojarifazgo* at 5 percent.[13] In order to avoid paying taxes, therefore, it was said that *boticarios* resorted to hospital pharmacies to acquire medicines at cheaper prices, despite the fact that hospital ordinances specifically forbade them to sell medicines on pain of a fine of twenty pesos and for the second offence forty pesos and loss of office. It was the intention that the *materia medica* destined for hospitals should be used to treat the poor and sick.[14] Nevertheless,

9 *Recopilación* lib.8 tit. 15 ley 28 15 Dec. 1553. When the first *botica* for the hospital of Santa Ana was shipped to Lima in 1551, 5,829 *maravedís* were paid in *averías*, which at this time was calculated on the basis of tonnage, calculated to be 7 and 9.5 twelfths tons. A further 4,500 *maravedís* customs duty ("aduana de indias") were levied (AGNP Protocolos Siglo XVI 63 Diego Gutiérrez fols. 185–186 Hospital de los españoles y naturales compañía con Francisco de Bilbao de la botica 20 Oct. 1551).

10 AGI Contratación 1166 N4 277–80, 297–298 Registro del navío San Francisco 1618; AGI Contratación 1166 lib.10 fols. 353–56 Registro del navío San Pedro 1618; AGI Contratación 1166 lib. 1 fols. 459–65 Registro del navío El Espíritu Santo 1618.

11 It is not clear why different levels of taxes were imposed, especially since they were all assigned to hospitals and assessed for tax by the same officials.

12 AGI Contratación 1126 lib. 1 fols. 323–24 Registro del navío Nuestra Señora de las Angustias 1597–1598. In this consignment to the hospital of Portobello, the assessed value of the medicines was reduced by 25,000 maravedís from 103, 989 *maravedís* and 5 percent *almojarifazgo* paid on 78,989.

13 See for example, AGI Contratación 1127 lib. 2 fols. 91–94, 263–64, 433–36 Registro del navío San Cristóbal 1597–1598.

14 AGNP Protocolos Siglo XVI 63 Diego Gutiérrez fol. 186 Hospital de los españoles y naturales compañía con Francisco de Bilbao de la botica 20 Oct. 1551; Ordenanzas y constituciones del hospital real de Santa Ana, Lima 28 Feb. 1609 (Ordinance 45).

in the early seventeenth century officials of the royal exchequer in Lima grew concerned that the Crown was losing tax revenue because hospitals were selling medicines to private *boticarios*, while apothecaries were making large profits and paying their *oficiales* high salaries.[15] Although, as will be shown below, there is evidence that on occasions physicians acquired medicines from hospitals, these were generally not imported products but rather botanical materials that were produced by the hospitals themselves in their gardens and on their haciendas.

As with many financial transactions at the time, there was considerable scope for fraud in the assessment of taxes. With the exception of boxes containing books, the cargoes themselves were not inspected, rather those registering them attested on oath to the nature, quantity, and value of their contents. It was common practice for merchants to undervalue cargoes, it was said by as much as a fifth or a quarter, in order to reduce the taxes payable. As a consequence, taxes were generally based on a total figure that was marginally higher than the total value of items given on the registration list. On other occasions a corrupt official might be bribed to lower the valuation. Another source of fraud was that passengers' personal effects were exempt from *almojarifazgo*, so that immigrants often took large quantities of merchandise for sale, even though they were specifically forbidden to do so.[16] The Crown realised that the lack of detailed inspections of cargoes left the way open for fraud, but the cursory procedure that was adopted minimised delays in dispatching ships and facilitated the acquisition of profits for merchants on whom it depended to generate revenue for its exchequer.[17]

Although individual boxes of merchandise were not inspected, detailed lists of their contents had to be presented to officials. These lists contain information on the amount and value of each individual medicinal product contained in the shipment. Such detailed lists survive for cargoes sent with the fleets between 1583 and 1624.[18] After that date detailed cargo lists for each box were not required, rather just a general description of their contents using generic names, such as "medicinas," with taxes assessed by weight rather than value.[19]

15 AGI 143 Memorial y apuntamiento sumario de algunas cosas muy importantes al reparo y aumento de las rentas de Su Magestad 1612.

16 Antúnez y Acevedo, *Memorias históricas*, 211, 236; Lutgardo García Fuentes, *Los peruleros y el comercio de Sevilla con las Indias, 1580–1630* (Sevilla: Universidad de Sevilla, 1997), 56.

17 Haring, *Trade and Navigation*, 90–91; Lynch, *Spain under the Habsburgs*, 2: 181.

18 AGI Contratación 1080 to 1174. These legajos also include the *armadas* destined for New Spain.

19 Joseph de Veitia Linage, *Norte de la contratación de las Indias Occidentales* (Sevilla: Imprenta de Francisco de Blas, 1672), lib. 1 cap. 18, para 6, pp. 118–19; Haring, *Trade and Navigation*, 91.

Since details of individual consignments are not generally available for shipments after 1624, the analysis here focuses primarily on the period prior to this date, though it includes some information for a few boxes dispatched up to 1640.[20]

In addition to providing exceptional insight into the nature and value of the *materia medica* being exported from Spain, these registrations reveal information about the merchants, factors, and other individuals involved in the trade. The preamble to the registration of each cargo gives the name of the person registering it, often their residence, and occasionally their occupation. It goes on to provide the name of the ship, shipmaster, and fleet with which it is to travel and its destination. It then specifies the person to whom the goods are to be delivered. Normally more than one person is named in the event that the specified recipient should be absent. This was a common occurrence since merchants and factors were often on the move and slow communications between Spain and the Indies meant that knowledge of people who had moved or died was often imperfect. Sometimes the final recipient of the goods was a named *boticario* in Lima or Cartagena, but in other cases it was a factor who would ensure their onward transmission or alternatively a merchant who was to arrange their sale. Sometimes traders entrusted boxes of medicines to passengers travelling on ship and even to the shipmaster or another member of the crew, with instructions about their delivery. The precise ownership of the goods and who would bear the risk in the event of loss were also specified (Figure 5). Thus, the cargo registrations make it possible to identify who was trading medicines and therefore reconstruct trading networks not only between Spain and the Americas, but to some extent within the colonies.

Apothecaries, Pepperers and Spicers

The medicine trade in Spanish America is best understood in the context of changes occurring in the structure of the trade in Europe. In the thirteenth century pharmacy began to split from medicine, encouraged by the specialisation of the two sciences and by the emergence of professionals who were more involved in trading drugs and preparing medicines than practicing medicine *per se*. Those trading medicines included apothecaries, pepperers and spicers. These traders initially handled similar products, namely drugs, spices and other commodities such as sugar and dried fruit, but later began to specialise. In England the pepperers tended to be wholesale merchants and shippers, such

20 Of the 249 shipments, only 13 fall in the period 1624 to 1634.

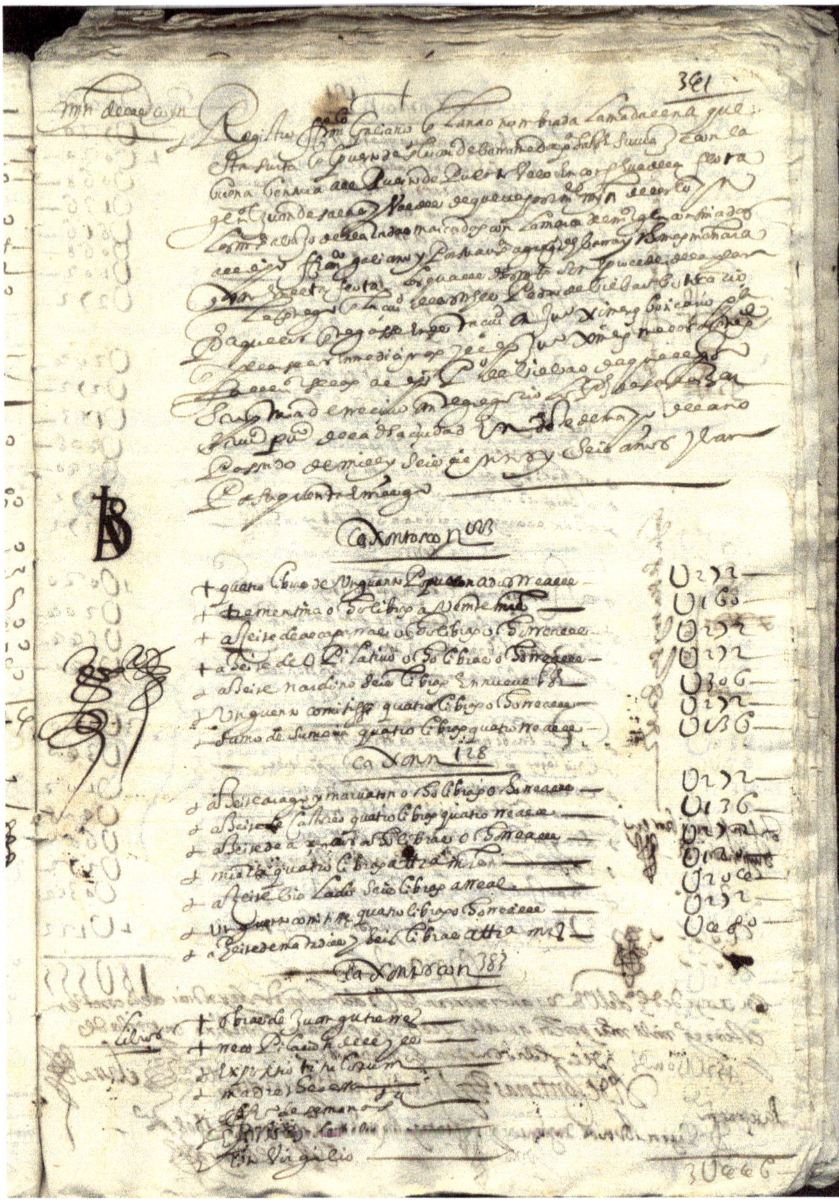

FIGURE 5 *Register of cargoes shipped by Francisco Galiano to Pedro de Bilbao, 1607.* Source: AGI Contratación 1151B N1 Image 683 Registro del navío La Magdalena 1607.

Francisco Galiano registers in the ship called La Magdalena, which is anchored in the port of Sanlúcar de Barrameda to make the journey with good fortune to Puerto Belo in company of the fleet of general Juan de Salas y Valdés, of which the shipmaster is Martín de Lazcoain, the goods declared below marked with the mark in the margin consigned to Francisco Galiano and in his absence to Gregorio de Ibarra and Thomas Manara who travel with this fleet, which are those goods which are and proceed from the silver that the apothecary Pedro de Bilbao gave him in the city of the kings [Lima] to deliver to the apothecary Juan Ximénez in this city [Seville] for medicines and the said Juan Ximénez has given them to me to take to the said Pedro de Bilbao from whom he presents a notarised receipt before Gregorio López de Salazar public notary of the city on the twelfth of May last year of 1606 and they are carried on his account and risk.

Large Rough Box Number 123

Four pounds of *populeón* [complex] ointment at two reals	272 [maravedís]
Turpentine eight pounds at 20 maravedís [a pound]	160
Oil of capers eight pounds eight reals	272
Opilativo oil [to remove obstruction] eight pounds eight reals	272
Oil of spikenard six pounds nine reals	306
Comitisse ointment [unidentified] four pounds eight reals	272
Fumitory syrup four pounds four reals	136

Large Box Number 128

Aragon and marciaton [complex] oil eight pounds 8 reals	272
Oil of castoreum four pounds four reals	136
Oil of wormwood eight pounds eight reals	272
Juniper oil four pounds at thirty maravedís [a pound]	120
Violet oil six pounds at one real [a pound]	204
Comitisse ointment [unidentified] four pounds eight reals	272
Oil of *mata* [unidentified shrub] sixteen pounds at thirty maravedís	480

Large Rough Box Number 383

Books
Works of Juan Gutiérrez
Recopilación de leyes
Expósitio titulorum
Mother Theresa
Service for Holy Week [*Oficio de semana santa*]
Letters of [Marco] Tulio
A Virgil

that they came to be known as grocers, that is selling goods *en gros* (in gross amounts). Spicers on the other hand worked in the retail trade and like apothecaries prepared medicines. In medieval England the distinction between apothecaries and spice merchants was practically non-existent; both belonged to the grocer's company or guild until 1617 when the apothecaries broke away and formed a separate company.[21] In Italy the apothecaries formed separate guilds from about 1300,[22] but in France, as in England, the apothecaries, spicers, druggists, herbalists, and wax chandlers formed a single guild.

In Spain, early legislation regulating the activities of spicers (*especieros*) and *boticarios* often referred to them together.[23] Hence inspections of *boticas* and spice shops were conducted on a similar basis and at the same time every two years, primarily with the objective of ensuring that poor quality medicines

21 T.D. Whittet, "Pepperers, Spicers and Grocers – Forerunners of the Apothecaries," *Proceedings of the Royal Society of Medicine* 61 (1968): 25–26; Paul Freedman, *Out of the East: Spices and the Medieval Imagination* (New Haven: Yale 2008), 61–62, 116–22.

22 *Kremers and Urdang's History of Pharmacy* (Madison WI: American Institute for the History of Pharmacy, 1986), 56–58, 67–90; David Gentilcore, *Healers and Healing in Early Modern Italy* (Manchester: Manchester University Press), 60–61.

23 In the fourteenth and fifteenth centuries pharmacists in the Barcelona region were at different times known as spicers and apothecaries and sometimes the same person was referred to by both titles (Javier Sorní and José María Suñe, "Barcelona. Baja edad media. Especieros o boticarios?" *Boletín de la sociedad española de historia de la farmacia* 34 (Number 136) (1983): 139–46). Like physicians, surgeons and *boticarios*, in the fifteenth century Spain *especieros* were also supposed to demonstrate *limpieza de sangre* before being allowed to conduct their business (Valverde and López Andújar, "Disposiciones legales," 257), but possibly because of the growing distinction between the two professions and the increased control over the training of *boticarios* and preparation of medicines, the requirement for spicers to demonstrate *limpieza de sangre* does not appear in later legislation (*Recopilación de las leyes, pragmáticas reales* (Muñoz), cap. VI ordinance 1: 71–72).

and spices were not being sold.[24] *Boticarios* and *especieros* were, however, distinguished from *drogueros*. From 1588, *boticarios* were ordered not to sell *drogas*, except those that might contain opium or *confecciones de alquermes* or *jacintos*.[25] At that time *especieros* were making medicines such as syrups and electuaries,[26] but from the end of the fifteenth century draft ordinances for the medical profession began to distinguish between the responsibilities of *boticarios* and *especieros*, suggesting that medicines such as canafistula, rose and violet oil, *carne de membrillo* (quince cheese), rose sugar and waters made through distillation were to be the preserve of *boticarios*.[27] Nevertheless, the specific medicines that could be prepared by apothecaries and spicers do not appear to have been included in general legislation but rather left to city ordinances and the judgement of inspectors. In the early seventeenth century, *especieros* in Antequera in Spain were being fined for selling senna (*sen*), polypody (*polipodio*) and poppy (*adormideras*),[28] but generally they expressed more concern about the quality of goods they dispensed than their type. While spicers did prepare medicines, they became primarily traders of spices, wax, honey, grain, fat, tallow, pitch, among other products.[29] Spicers included confectioners (*confiteros*) who focused on products made of sugar

24 *Novísima recopilación de las leyes de España*, lib. 8 tit. 13, ley 2: 107 3 Mar. 1477 and 4: 108–109 7 Nov. 1617; *Recopilación de las leyes, pragmáticas reales* (Muñoz), cap. XV ordinance 1: 187. In 1527 the city ordinances of Seville referred to *boticarios* and *especieros* together. Those found guilty of selling poor quality drugs would have them confiscated on the first occasion, pay double on the second, and suffer one hundred lashes on the third (*Recopilación de los ordenamientos de Sevilla* (Sevilla: Juan Varela de Salamanca, 1527), p. 237v. Online at: http://fondotesis.us.es/fondos/libros/332/13/ordenancas-de-sevilla/ [Accessed 2 Jul. 2016].

25 *Recopilación de las leyes, pragmáticas reales* (Muñoz), cap. XIV ordinance 16: 184 1588. *Confecciones de alquermes* or *jacintos* were complex medicines. The former was based on the Kermes insect (Luis de Oviedo, *Methodo de la colección, y reposición de las medicinas simples, de su corrección, y preparación* (Madrid: Luis Sánchez, 1622), 153) and the latter on a variety of precious and semi-precious stones (Oviedo, *Methodo*, 163).

26 *Recopilación de las leyes, pragmáticas reales* (Muñoz), cap. XIV ordinance 17: 184 1588. See also, González Arce, "Proyectos de ordenanzas," 224.

27 Archivo de Simancas, Cámara de Castilla, Diversos de Castilla leg. 1 doc. 56 fols. 1–11 Ordenanzas que sus altezas deben mandar ordenar acerca de los físicos, boticarios y especieros [1498] Online at: http://pares.mcu.es/ParesBusquedas/servlets/Control_servlet?accion=3&txt_id_desc_ud=2224592&fromagenda=N [Accessed 2 Nov. 2015].

28 Mercedes Fernández-Carrión and José Antonio Pérez Romero, "Visitas de inspección sanitaria en especierías, confiterías, cererías y aguardenterías de Antequera durante el siglo XVII," *Baética* 8 (1985): 444.

29 See the city ordinances of Seville: Recopilación de los ordenamientos de Sevilla, 1527, p. 237v.

and flour, but who along with the wax chandlers (*cereros*) also traded wax.[30] A similar pattern of specialisation was evident in Lima in the sixteenth century where *confiteros* sold spices, sugar, dried fruit and honey, and *cereros* wax and candlewicks.[31] The guild of *cereros* was one of the first guilds to be established in Lima in 1551. At that time, it included *confiteros*, of which there were 18 in the city in the 1630s.[32] However, towards the end of the colonial period the *cereros* allied with the tallow-chandlers (*veleros*), who not only made candles, but also traded oils, wax and ointments.[33] As will be seen later in this chapter, the trade in products required for the preparation of medicines in Lima shows some degree of specialisation, though *boticarios* also traded some raw medicinal products, such as wax.

The Transatlantic Trade in *Materia Medica*

The analysis of the transatlantic shipment of *materia medica* presented here is based on an examination of the cargoes of 350 ships sailing with the galleon fleets to Tierra Firme that were destined for Panama (Nombre de Dios, Portobello, and Panama), as well as to Cartagena de Indias, and Peru (Lima, Potosí and Cuzco) between 1583 and 1640.[34] These vessels contained 249 consignments exclusively of medicines, of which 61 were specified as being destined for Peru, the majority to Lima (53).[35] However, it is likely that a good proportion of the goods arriving with the Tierra Firme galleons, especially those destined for Nombre de Dios, or after 1597 Portobello, would have found their way to Lima.[36] Only cargoes composed wholly of medicines and medical equipment

---

30 Fernández-Carrión and Pérez Romero, "Visitas de inspección," 438–39.

31 Quiroz Chueca, *Artesanos y manufactureros*, 85.

32 Salinas y Córdova, *Memorial*, 257; Bromley, "Ciudad de Lima," 285. Earlier in the sixteenth century there were nine workshops of *cereros* (wax workers), *confiteros* (confectioners) and *candeleros* (candle makers) together, and seven of *pasteleros* (pastry-cooks) and *molineros* (millers) (Quiroz Chueca, *Artesanos y manufactureros*, 95).

33 Quiroz Chueca, "Gremios en Lima," 506–507, 511–12.

34 AGI Contratación leg. 1094–1172, 1180 *passim*.

35 The value of eight of these cargoes is not specified, so they are not included in calculations here, which are based on the value of 241 cargoes.

36 The terminus of the Tierra Firme fleet was moved from Nombre de Dios to Portobello in 1597 due to the shallow nature of the bay, difficult navigation, and the unhealthy climate (Haring, *Trade and Navigation*, 184–85; Enriqueta Vila Vilar, "Las ferias de Portobelo: apariencia y realidad del comercio con Indias," *Anuario de estudios americanos* 39 (1982): 279–80; Christopher Ward, *Imperial Panama: Commerce and Conflict in Isthmian America, 1550–1800* (Albuquerque: University of New Mexico Press, 1994), 103–37.

have been analysed here. Most ships contained only one or two consignments exclusively of medicines, while many had none. These consignments were destined primarily for hospitals, *boticarios* or large scale merchants. However, small quantities of medicines were often included in mixed cargoes, since many merchants were generalist traders.[37] These have not been included in the analysis, neither have the small quantities of medicines that passengers took with them for their personal use. Finally, the analysis excludes certain categories of *materia medica* that were generally handled by other traders. They include oil, spices, notably saffron, pepper, cumin, clove, and cinnamon, which could be used for culinary purposes as well as medicines, though small amounts of these products were sometimes included in consignments of medicines as well. The organisation of the trade thus reflects the growing, but still blurred, distinction between spice merchants and *boticarios* in Spain at the time.

The largest cargoes of medicines were destined for hospitals or prominent *boticarios*. Responsibility for the supply of medicines for hospitals lay with their *mayordomos*, who were themselves normally traders rather than persons with medical expertise.[38] Rodrigo Arias de Buiça, who was *mayordomo* of the Hospital of Santa Ana in the mid-1590s,[39] was also a prominent merchant. Born in Salamanca, he settled in Lima and made at least two journeys to Spain trading in other commodities as well as medicines.[40] According to Ordinance 30 of the Hospital of Santa Ana, the *mayordomo* was permitted to send 500 pesos a year to Spain for the purchase of medicines. For this purpose a list of medicines had to be drawn up and signed by the hospital's physician, surgeon and *boticario*, who were then to check off the medicines when they arrived ensuring that they were of good quality.[41] There were criticisms that merchants and *boticarios* in Spain often sent medicines that were past their best.[42] In fact

37 Lockhart, *Spanish Peru*, 79–80.

38 Ibid. 91.

39 ABPL 9085 Libro de la razón que toma Bartolomé de la Cueva, escribano veedor del hospital de Santa Ana, 1595–1596. While *mayordomo* his slaves were treated in the hospital (fols. 10–11).

40 Garcia Fuentes, *Los peruleros*, 111, 114–15. He also supplied the hospital of San Andrés with medicines (AGI Contratación 1145A Registro del navío San Vicente y San Juan 1605; AGI Contratación 1145B Registro del navío San Pedro 1605). For his petition to travel to Peru see AGI Contratación 5233 N23 Expediente de información y licencia de pasajero a indias de Rodrigo Arias de Buiça 14 Jul. 1590. Arias de Buiça died in Lima 1609. For his estate see: AGI Contratación 518 N1 R2 Autos sobre los bienes de Rodrigo Arias de Buiça 1617).

41 *Constituciones y ordenanzas del hospital real de Santa Ana*, Lima.

42 ARJBM División 1, legajo 17 Prologo. Libro de examen de los simples medicinales Antonio de Robles Cornejo 1617.

not all consignments reached the permitted value of 500 pesos. For example, the cargoes of medicines registered for the Hospitals of San Andrés and Santa Ana by the Peruvian merchants Alonso González de la Canal y Juan Bautista Crespo in 1618 were valued at only 91 pesos and 31 pesos respectively.[43]

The procedure followed by hospitals in acquiring medicines was that the *mayordomo* would entrust a quantity of pesos, normally in the form of silver bars, to a merchant or other individual, generally a resident of Peru, who would travel to Spain and arrange for the purchase of medicines.[44] The purchased medicines would then be shipped back to Lima with the next fleet.[45] The same process of remitting silver with a factor was employed by private *boticarios* in Lima. Sometimes, the contract specified the particular person from whom the medicines were to be purchased.[46] The cost of transport and the taxes imposed meant that the value of medicines that arrived was often considerably below the value of the silver that had been remitted. Hence, although in 1633 the Hospital of Santa Ana sent 585 pesos of silver to Spain for the purchase of medicines, those purchased were valued at only 250 pesos, the rest being absorbed in unspecified "gastos."[47] Such a shortfall was not unusual. In 1639 the *mayordomo* of the same hospital similarly entrusted 600 pesos to Francisco de Arano to acquire a list of specified medicines through Pedro de Roças in Spain, but the medicines he obtained were valued at only 438 pesos, the remainder being consumed by taxes and expenses.[48] A partial explanation for the reduced value of the medicines is that they were undervalued in order to reduce tax liabilities, but the costs of shipping were also high. Commonly transport costs and taxes on silver and other goods shipped to Spain were about 10 percent of

43 AGI Contratación 1166 N4: 277–78, 297–98 Registro del navío San Francisco 1618. There was also a consignment for Juan de Bilbao as well as for a *boticario* in Panama. Alonso González de la Canal was one of the most prominent merchants in Lima who in 1630 was Prior of the Consulado de Mercaderes in Lima (Bromley, "Ciudad de Lima," 280, 284). He was also responsible for funding the reconstruction of the church of Nuestra Señora de Montserrat and its opening ceremony (Suárez, *Desafíos transatlánticos*, 190). He died on 3 June 1635 having been given a purgative by a doctor (Suardo, *Diario de Lima* 2: 82).

44 For example, ABPL 9083 Libro mayor de rentas del hospital de Santa Ana fol. 75v. 1615; ABPL 9104 no folio Escritura de recibo de Francisco de Arana 27 May 1637.

45 See also, the registration of cargoes for the hospitals of San Andrés and Santa Ana respectively by the Peruvian traders Alonso González de la Canal and Juan Bautista Crespo (AGI Contratación 1166 N4: 277–78 and 297–98 San Francisco 1618).

46 For example, AGI Contratación 1151B N6: 429–30 Registro del navío Santa Cruz 1607 and 1163 N1 R2 81–3 Registro del navío La Visitación de Nuestra Señora 1615.

47 AGI Contratación 1180 N2 R7 fols. 217–18 Registro del navío Nuestra Señora de la Concepción 1634.

48 ABPL 9104 no folio Escritura de recibo de Francisco de Arana 27 May 1637; AGI Contratación 1184 N2 R2 fols. 51–52 Registro del navío Nuestra Señora de la Candelaria 1640.

their value.[49] The cost of transport of only six boxes of medicines from Portobello to Lima in 1650 was an exorbitant 125 pesos.[50] In addition, payments to factors could reach 30 percent of the value of the goods they handled.[51] It is perhaps not surprising that Gaspar de Perales, who among his other trading activities supplied the Hospital of San Andrés with medicines, was described in 1595 as one of the richest merchants in Peru.[52]

Temporally the volume of the medicine trade peaked in the 1590s and early 1600s after which it declined (Figure 6). This reflected trends in the galleon trade in general which shrank in the early seventeenth century as Spain's inability to supply its colonies with merchandise led first to the fleets sailing every two years rather than annually, and later from the 1620s to becoming even more irregular.[53] The increase in the volume of medicines being shipped to Peru probably reflected the general penetration of *peruleros* into the galleon

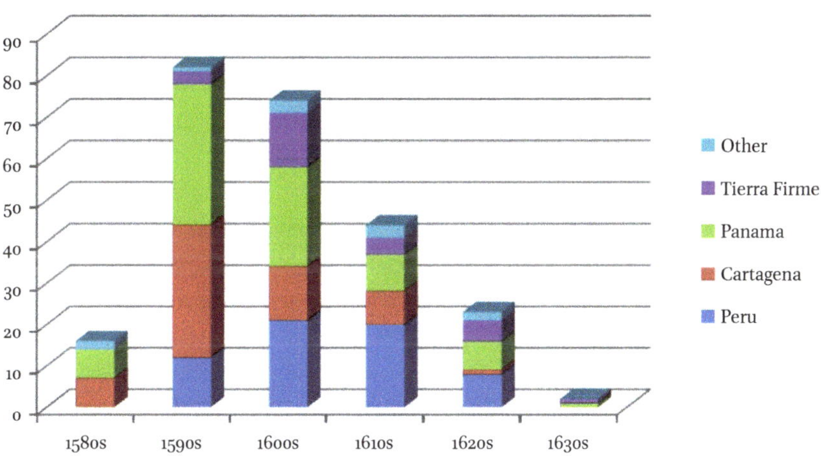

FIGURE 6 *Number of consignments of medicines to different destinations, 1580s to 1630s.*
SOURCES: AGI CONTRATACIÓN LEG. 1094–1172, 1180.

49 García Fuentes, *Los peruleros*, 41–43.

50 ABPL 9100 Libro de cuentas del hospital de Santa Ana 1649–1651 Juan de Valverde 5 Mar. 1650.

51 Margarita Suárez, *Comercio y fraude el en Perú colonial: las estrategias mercantiles de un banquero* (Lima: Banco Central de Reserva del Perú, Fondo Editorial: Instituto de Estudios Peruanos, 1995), 58.

52 AGI Indiferente General 2102 N100 (Image 2) Información de Gaspar de Perales 12 Sep. 1595; AGI Contratación 1115 N4 676–77 Registro del navío la Magdalena 1596 and 1116 N6: 348–49 Registro del navío San Gregorio 1596.

53 Haring, *Trade and Navigation*, 208; Huguette and Pierre Chaunu. *Séville et l'Atlantique, 1450–1650* (Paris: A. Colin, 1956), 6_2: 586–587; Lynch, *Spain under the Habsburgs*, 2: 200–206; Suárez, *Comercio y fraude*, 28–40.

trade.[54] *Peruleros* were traders who had been born or resided in Peru who acted as factors for local residents, travelling to Spain taking with them silver bars entrusted to them for the purchase of specific goods.[55] Initially, merchants in Spain often sent their sons to the New World, where they became partners and factors.[56] While many of these early traders may have aspired to return to Spain in fact they often stayed and a second generation of merchants emerged who were based in Peru. Their involvement in the galleon trade reached its peak in the 1590s.[57]

Of the 249 shipments of medicines from Spain with the Tierra Firme fleets between 1583 and 1640, about one quarter were destined specifically for Peru. Of the 61 Peruvian cargoes, 34 were registered by *peruleros*, 8 by merchants, and 10 by *boticarios* based in Seville.[58] Merchants were always on the move so that although the ships' registers recorded the domicile of the trader it was not always the case that this was their place of birth. Equally an individual might be described on different occasions as being a resident of different places. Hence the merchant, Pedro de Avendaño, was at times described as a *vecino* of Seville having lived there for some time, when in fact he had been born in Peru. The registers therefore constitute an imperfect guide to the birth place of merchants and should be used in conjunction with other documentary and published sources.[59]

Keeping this limitation in mind, an analysis of 61 consignments of medicines to Peru suggests that those remitted by *peruleros* averaged 150 pesos and were substantially smaller than those dispatched by merchants and *boticarios* based in Seville whose shipments averaged nearly 400 pesos and 250 pesos respectively (See Table 3). Of the thirteen *boticarios* in Seville who were involved in the galleon trade to the Tierra Firme between 1583 and 1622, only four were involved in shipping medicines direct to Peru (See Table 4), though they, and the other nine, may also have supplied medicines in small quantities to merchants who included them as part of their general cargoes.[60] Those *boticarios*

54 García Fuentes, *Los peruleros.*

55 García Fuentes, *Los peruleros*; Guillermo Lohmann Villena, *Plata del Perú, riqueza de Europa: los mercaderes peruanos y el comercio con la metropolí en el siglo XVII* (Lima, Fondo Editorial del Congreso del Perú, 2004); Suárez, *Comercio y fraude*, 33–40.

56 Lockhart, *Spanish Peru*, 88–91.

57 García Fuentes, *Los peruleros*, 56.

58 The residences of the remaining nine are unknown.

59 See especially García Fuentes, *Los peruleros.*

60 In addition to the thirteen listed in Table 4, Fernández-Carrión and Valverde (*Farmacia y sociedad*, 71) name another four *boticarios* who were trading with the Indies between 1580 and 1584.

TABLE 3 *Consignments of medicines to Peru by trader type, 1591–1622.*

Registered by	Number of consignments from Seville	Total value in pesos	Average value in pesos
Sevillian merchants	18	5,676	315
Apothecaries	*10*	*2,499*	*250*
Non-apothecaries	*8*	*3,177*	*397*
Peruleros	34	5,100	150
Unknown	9	665	74
Total	61	11,441	188

Sources: AGI Contratación legs. 1094–1172.

in Seville who were involved in the Atlantic trade represented only a quarter of the total number in Seville, where according to official inspections of *boticas* conducted in 1594 and 1631 there were only 42 and 49 respectively.[61]

The two most important *apothecaries* in Seville who registered medicines for Peru were Juan Sánchez and Juan Martínez de Ortuçar. In 1618 Juan Sánchez dispatched one large cargo worth 244,664 *maravedís* (900 pesos) for the royal hospital of Potosí and three years later sent a much smaller consignment worth 30 pesos to the Hospital of San Andrés in Lima.[62] He also supplied a number of *boticarios* in Lima, namely Juan de Bilbao, Francisco Martín Reyna, and Gerónimo Pujadas, while he also shipped medicines to Panama for sale through intermediaries. Juan Sánchez possessed a *botica* in the Cathedral district of Seville[63] and his appointment as an inspector of the city's *boticas* in 1614 suggests he was a *boticario* of some standing.[64] Juan Martínez de Ortuçar seems to have traded mainly with *boticarios*. He was a major supplier not only to Juan de Bilbao in Lima, but also to *boticarios* in Cartagena and Nombre de Dios.[65] Cristóbal de Castro and Francisco Marroquín also sent small quantities to Lima for sale.[66]

61 AMS Sección 13 Siglo XVI Tomo 1 documento 114. Sevilla 20 June 1594; AMS Varios Antiguos 370 Visitas de boticas 1631; Herrera Dávila, "Boticas sevillanas," 63–81.

62 AGI Contratación 1166 N1: 459–65 Registro del navío El Espíritu Santo 1615; AGI Contratación 1171 N13: 181–82 Registro del navío Nuestra Señora de la Candelaria 1621.

63 Herrera Dávila, "Boticas sevillanas," 79.

64 AMS Varios Antiguos 414 Visita de las boticas 12 Apr. 1614.

65 They were the *boticarios* Andrés Gonzales and Francisco Suarez in Cartagena and Agustín de Bonilla in Nombre de Dios.

66 AGI Contratación 1127 N2: 91, 263 Registro del navío San Cristóbal 1598.

TABLE 4 *Apothecaries in Seville trading with the Tierra Firme and Peru, 1583–1634.*

Registered by apothecary in Seville	Dates of dispatch of cargoes	Number of fleets with medicines	Total number of consignments of medicines
Cristóbal de Castro	1583–1600	4	7
Pedro del Castillo	1586–1593/4	2	0
Juan Martínez de Ortuçar	1586–1601	5	9
Francisco de Ribera	1586–1601	7	16
Francisco Rocha Araña	1593–1615	6	6
Hernando de Medina	1593–1594	1	1
Francisco Marroquín	1597–1598	1	1
Cristóbal Gómez	1601	1	1
Francisco Galán Ramírez	1604–1619	6	8
Francisco de Ortega	1609–1622	4	7
Gerónimo Méndez	1612	1	1
Francisco Meléndez	1615–1618	2	0
Juan Sánchez	1615–1622	5	10
Miguel Fernández	1634	1	1
Francisco Ramírez Galán	1634	1	1
Total		47	69

Sources: AGI Contratación legs. 1080–1172, 1180, 1184.

Those *boticarios* and merchants based in Seville who wished to sell medicines on their own account rather than fulfil orders sent by American clients, generally sent them to Panama or Cartagena, since their closer geographical location meant that sales could be effected and the profit remitted to Spain more promptly. Hence, Francisco de Ribera, who sent large quantities of medicines to Tierra Firme on several occasions, generally registered them for Cartagena, specifying that they should be entrusted to the merchant, Luis de Espliega, and the *boticario*, Andrés Gonzales, who were to sell them for the best prices for cash and not on credit. He further instructed that they were to remit the revenue to Spain in the form of "gold, assayed silver or reals" and not in any other merchandise.[67] It is worth noting that Doctor Melchor de Amusco, a

67 For example, AGI Contratación 1094 N4: 175 Registro del navío San Pedro 1591, AGI Contratación 1095 N1: 465 Registro del navío Santa Catalina Mártir 1592. The gold, silver or pesos were to be remitted in ships that were carrying silver to Spain, presumably because

Number of boxes consigned to Lima	Total value of medicines dispatched in pesos	Value of medicines dispatched to Lima in pesos
1	255	45
0	296	0
2	2,534	852
0	5,548	0
0	386	0
0	33	0
1	121	121
0	255	0
0	798	0
0	276	0
0	268	0
0	89	0
6	2,146	1,482
0	45	0
0	36	0
10	13,086	2,500

priest as well as physician who became *protomédico* in Lima in 1616, similarly acted as an agent for the *boticario* Cristóbal de Castro and the merchant Juan Bautista Dorta when he was based in Panama.[68]

they would be guarded by the *armadas*. Andrés Gonzales was a prominent *boticario* in Cartagena, who in 1620 was accused of settling in Cartagena without license and trading illegally (AGI Escribanía de Cámara 589B Denuncia contra Andrés Gonzales, boticario, Portugués 1620).

68 A citizen of Toledo, Melchor de Amusco graduated with a doctorate in medicine from the University of Seville in 1583. In the same year, he also petitioned for licence to travel to Tierra Firme with his wife, children and servants, his medical credentials being certified by the king's chamber physician, Andrés Zamudio de Alfaro (AGI IG 2093 N177 Expediente de concesión de licencia para pasar a Tierra Firme, a favor del doctor Melchor de Amusco 1583; AGI IG 1952 lib.2 fol. 166v. Real Cédula…para que dejen pasar a Tierra Firme al doctor Melchor de Amusco 28 Dec. 1583).

TABLE 5 *Apothecaries in lima receiving consignments of medicines from Spain, 1583–1640.*

Apothecaries in Lima receiving consignments	Value of medicines in pesos	Dates of dispatch of medicines	Number of consignments	Percentage of total medicines dispatched by value
Juan de Bilbao	1,532	1591–1601	4	38.1
Pedro de Bilbao	849	1607–22	7	21.1
Gerónimo Pujadas	457	1618–19	2	11.4
Blas de Medina	286	1601	1	7.1
Luis de Alfaro	278	1597–98	1	6.9
Francisco Martín Reyna	202	1615–18	2	5.0
Francisco Crespo	180	1601	1	4.5
Bartolomé Díaz Cabeza de Vaca	164	1597–98	1	4.1
Juan Sánchez	73	1592	1	1.8
Graviel de España	unspecified	1640	1	
	4,021	1597–98	21	

Sources: AGI Contratación legs. 1080–1172, 1180, 1184.

Of the medicines sent to Peru, about ten percent went to hospitals and half to *boticarios*. Only ten *boticarios* are named as recipients of medicines, of whom Juan de Bilbao and his son, Pedro de Bilbao, together accounted for about 60 percent of the total value of medicines received by *boticarios* in Lima (Table 5). Only a few *boticarios* in Lima seem to have had the financial resources to become involved directly in the Atlantic trade; most probably acquired their medicines from these few *boticarios*, merchants or other local sources. Given their prominence as apothecaries in Lima, it is worth describing in detail how Juan de Bilbao and Pedro de Bilbao arranged one shipment. In April 1599, they entrusted six bars of silver valued at 1,771 pesos ensayados to the *perulero*, Pedro de Avendaño. He was instructed to acquire a list of specified medicines from Juan Martínez de Ortuçar, a *boticario* in Seville, who lived in the parish of Santa Catalina, or in his absence from Juan Gutiérrez, a *boticario* who resided in the barrio of Alfalfa, or else from Pedro or Rodrigo del Castillo, who were also *boticarios*.[69] Avendaño was to be paid 30 pesos for the service. That year, Avendaño sailed to Spain with the *flota* of General Don Luis Fajardo. In February 1601 Juan Martínez de Ortuçar registered two cargoes of medicines on the Nuestra Señora de la Concepción and San Nicólas, which sailed in the fleet commanded by Don Francisco del Corral y Toledo. Martínez de Ortuçar specified that on arrival in America the medicines were to be entrusted to Pedro de Avendaño, who was probably travelling with one of the vessels, and who was to arrange for their transfer to Lima. The medicines were valued at 852 pesos on which taxes of 5 percent *almojarifazgo* and 2 percent *avería*, amounting to 67 pesos together, were paid. The value of the medicines was thus significantly lower than the amount of silver indicated in the contract between Bilbao and Avendaño, yet in 1602 Bilbao declared himself satisfied that the contract had been fulfilled. It is perhaps worth noting that these medicines represented less than five percent of the total value of all the cargoes registered for that fleet by Pedro de Avendaño in Seville, calculated at 19,140 pesos *ensayados*.[70]

The total value of 241 consignments of medicines carried to Tierra Firme in fleets between 1583 and 1634 was about 46,379 pesos, of which 11,441 pesos worth were destined specifically for Peru (Table 6).[71] These figures probably underestimate the true value of the medicines slightly, since as indicated above they tended to be undervalued in order to minimise the amount of tax paid. However, it suggests that imports of medicines only averaged about two to three hundred pesos a year and as such accounted for only a small proportion of the medicines actually consumed in Lima. In 1570 the Hospital of Santa Ana was treating 80 to 90 Indians and claimed it was spending 3,000 pesos a year on medicines.[72] The annual accounts and more general reports for the hospital suggest it spent a rather more modest sum of about 500 to 800 pesos a year,[73] such that the figure of 3,000 pesos was probably exaggerated to obtain some

69 AGNP Protocolos Siglo XVI 15 Ramiro Bote fols. 2239–2239v. Juan de Bilbao da poder a Juan Martínez de Ortuçar, boticario de la ciudad de Sevilla 16.4.1599; AGNP Protocolos Siglo XVI 15 Ramiro Bote fols. 3006v-3008 Pedro de Avendaño, residente en Lima entrega recibo a Juan y Pedro de Bilbao 27.4.1599.

70 García Fuentes, *Los peruleros*, 111.

71 The value of eight of the 249 consignments is not given in the sources.

72 AGI Lima 122 fols. 19v., 37v. Del hospital de los naturales de la ciudad de los reyes sobre que se haga alguna merced con que los yndios se puedan curar atento a su pobreza 16 Jan. 1570.

73 ABPL 9080 fols. 254–57 Libro de cuentas del Hospital de Santa Ana 1575 a 1585; ABPL 9083 fols. 73–74, 122–23 Libro mayor de rentas del hospital de Santa Ana desde 1593 a 1629; ABPL 9084 fols. 167–68, 241–242v. Libro de cuentas de gastos del hospital de Santa Ana 1598; ABPL 9085 fols. 59–64 Libro de la razón…deste hospital de Santa Ana de los gastos que

TABLE 6 *Destination and value of cargoes of medicines by trader type, 1583–1634.*

Destination	Value of *materia medica* in pesos registered by		Total value of consignments in pesos	Percent registered by apothecaries	Total number of consignments
	Merchant/ passenger	Apothecary in Seville			
Lima	6311	1600	7911	20.2	53
Potosí	160	899	1059	84.9	3
Cuzco	2471	0	2471	0	5
Cartagena	9130	7451	16581	44.9	61
Nombre de Dios	4052	1076	5128	21.0	33
Portobello	4477	1096	5572	19.7	32
Panama	2353	379	2732	13.9	17
Tierra Firme	3184	513	3697	13.9	26
Other	1192	37	1229	3.0	11
Total	33330	13049	46379	28.1	241

Sources: AGI Contratación legs. 1094–1172, 1180.

charitable funding from the Crown. Meanwhile in 1563 the Hospital of San Andrés for Spaniards was spending two pesos a day for about half that number of patients;[74] by 1600 the expenditure had risen to over 1,000 pesos a year.[75] As for the prison, the annual expenditure on medicines was judged to be 50 pesos a year.[76] Apart from public institutions, the large debts that were run

hace Rodrigo Arias de Buyca [Buiça] mayordomo…desde el primero del mes de agosto 1595.

74 AGI Lima 131 Juan de Alvear en nombre del administrador y fundador del hospital despañoles 1563. At that time the hospital had 44 Spanish sick patients and 7 who were mentally ill. In 1619 it was said that the hospital was treating 1,800 people a year (AGI Lima 301 Relación de las ciudades, villas y lugares, parrochias y doctrinas que ay en este Arçobispado de Lima 20 Apr. 1619).

75 ABPL 8427 Libro de cuentas que llevo el Licenciado Don Sebastián Clemente, mayordomo del hospital real de San Andrés, que corre desde el día 15 de abril del año 1600. In 1619 it was said that the hospital was treating 2,000 people a year (AGI Lima 301 Relación de las ciudades, villas y lugares, parrochias y doctrinas que ay en este Arçobispado de Lima 20 Apr. 1619).

76 AGI Lima 134 Cofradía de los pobres de las cárceles de la ciudad de los reyes 1598.

up by some private clients, which have been discussed in Chapter 3, indicate the high consumption of medicines in the city. Even though more medicines would have been imported than is evident from the analysis above, it is reasonable to conclude that imports of *materia medica* from Spain failed to meet the demand in Lima. As such products had to be acquired from alternative and more local sources.

The Intercolonial Trade in *Materia Medica*

The discussion hitherto has focused on the importation of medicinal products from Spain, however, some were imported from other American regions. Perhaps the most notable source was Mexico from which the most important imports were resins, balsams, and oils, which were generally unavailable on the coast of Peru. They included liquidambar, *copal, tacamahaca*[77] and *sangre de drago*. Other products imported were mechoacan, *guaiacum* (lignum-vitae), cacao, tobacco, and Mexican pepper.[78] The fact that all these products appear in the schedule of taxes to be paid on goods coming from New Spain, and that the resins in particular are common in pharmacy inventories and prescriptions, suggests they were traded on a significant scale.

In the 1590s, between thirty five and forty vessels were plying the South Sea.[79] Although in the early seventeenth century the Crown ramped up restrictions on trade between Mexico and Peru, largely to control the outflow of silver through Mexico to China and the influx of silk to Peru, the number of vessels involved in intercolonial expanded and contraband trade flourished.[80] Apart from ships trading directly with Mexico, other smaller vessels plied the Pacific coast, with some delivering sarsaparilla from Ecuador.[81] It is impossible to ascertain the overall volume of medicines imported to Lima from American regions, but it was probably significant in the case of the resins and oils.

---

77 De Vos, "Art of Pharmacy," 101–10. Tacamahaca was an American gum-resin extracted from a variety of trees whose name derived from the Aztec term, tecomahiyac (Francisco Hernández, *Quatro libros* (Mexico: Casa de la viuda de Diego Lopez Daualos, 1615) parte 1 lib. 2 cap. 16 fol. 16v.; Monardes, *Historia medicinal*, fols. 2–3.

78 See AGNP Cajas Reales: Lima H-3 Leg. 4 Libro 24-a fols. 34–39 Tasación de las mercaderías que vienen a esta ciudad de los reyes de las provincias de México (1617).

79 Lawrence A. Clayton, "Trade and Navigation in the Seventeenth-Century Viceroyalty of Peru, Journal of Latin American Studies 7 (1): 6–7.

80 John Lynch, *Spain Under the Habsburgs. Volume Two: Spain and America 1598–1700* (Oxford: Basil Blackwell, 1981), 225–26.

81 Marie Hellmer, "LeCallao (1617–1815)," *Jahrbuch für Geschicte von Staat, Wirtschaft und Gesellschaft Lateinamerikas* 2 (1965): 181.

However, evidence from medicinal products found in pharmacies and contained in prescriptions, to be discussed in Chapter 6, suggests that the *range* of products imported was limited. Thus inadequacies in the Spanish trading system do not seem to have stimulated a flourishing interregional exchange of products, knowledge and practices, though the evidence is limited. Such exchanges that existed probably occurred though the personal contacts of *boticarios* and by Jesuits travelling through the network of Colleges they had established in the Viceroyalty.[82]

Acquiring *Materia Medica* Locally

Apart from imports from Spain, the sources from which *materia medica* were acquired were diverse. A few substitutes were sought in native plant assemblages and local mineral resources, while European plants were grown in local gardens, especially those belonging to the hospitals and religious orders. Ordinances for the Hospital of Santa Ana in 1609 clearly show how the authorities tried to ensure that it was supplied with fresh medicines at moderate prices. However, it seems that in the first instance hospitals relied on imports from Spain and only when the expected cargoes did not arrive or when there were shortages did they acquire *materia medica* locally.[83] The *mayordomo* of the Hospital of Santa Ana was exhorted to buy medicines in bulk when they were available rather than in small quantities when the need arose and prices were higher.[84]

The account books of the Hospitals of Santa Ana and San Andrés provide some insight into the suppliers of *materia medica*, since they often indicate the persons from whom purchases were made, though unfortunately not on a consistent basis.[85] About one third (150) of the 460 entries found in hospital

82 Martín, *Intellectual Conquest*, 97–118.

83 In 1641 the surgeon of the Hospital of Santa Ana reported that he had been forced to buy some medicines from Graviel de España because the expected shipment from Spain had not arrived (ABPL 9127 fol. 95v. Pedro Garcia Capicha 8 Jul. 1641).

84 *Constituciones y ordenanzas del hospital real de Santa Ana*, Lima.

85 For the Hospital of Santa Ana see: ABPL 9080 Libro de cuentas, censos y haberes que corresponden al hospital de Santa Ana, 1575–1584; ABPL 9083 Libro Mayor de rentas del Hospital de Santa Ana, 1575–1633; ABPL 9084 Libro de cuentas de gastos del hospital de Santa Ana, 1597–1599; ABPL 9084 Libro de cuentas de gastos del hospital de Santa Ana, 1597–1599; ABPL 9085 Libro de la razón que toma Bartolomé de la Cueva, escribano veedor del hospital de Santa Ana, 1595–1596; ABPL 9127 Protocolo de cuentas del hospital de Santa Ana, 1640–1736. For the Hospital of San Andrés accounts indicating the source

TABLE 7 *Sources of* materia medica *supplied to the hospital of Santa Ana 1575–1600 and 1640–1641.*

	Number of entries	Total value in pesos	Percentage of value	Percentage of total entries
Apothecary (*boticario*)	70	9,476.5	42.6	46.7
Merchant (*mercader*)	23	5,617.5	25.2	15.3
Physician (*médico*)	7	1,906	8.6	4.7
Shop (*tienda*)	21	1,680	7.5	14.0
Indian (*indio*)	3	976	4.4	2.0
Shopkeeper (*pulpero*)	6	588	2.6	4.0
Farm (*chácara*)	7	580	2.6	4.7
Keeper of cellar or tavern (*bodeguero*)	1	384	1.7	0.7
Kitchen garden (*huerta*)	4	333	1.5	2.7
Store (*casa*)	1	248	1.1	0.7
Confectioner (*confitero*)	2	240	1.1	1.3
Surgeon (*cirjuano*)	2	151	0.7	1.3
Auction (almoneda)	1	36	0.2	0.7
Barber (*barbero*)	1	20	0.1	0.7
Native market (*tianguez*)	1	18	0.1	0.7
	150	22,254	100.00	100

Sources: ABPL 9080 Libro de cuentas, censos y haberes que corresponden al hospital de Santa Ana, 1575–1584; ABPL 9083 Libro mayor de rentas del hospital de Santa Ana, 1575–1633; ABPL 9084 Libro de cuentas de gastos del hospital de Santa Ana, 1597–1599; ABPL 9085 Libro de la razón que toma Bartolomé de la Cueva, escribano veedor del hospital de Santa Ana, 1595–1596; ABPL 9086 Protocolo de expedientes del hospital de Santa Ana, 1599–1607; ABPL 9127 Protocolo de cuentas del hospital de Santa Ana, 1640–1736.

accounts kept irregularly between 1575 and 1600 and from 1640 and 1641 indicate the name and occupation of the supplier or the location of the source of supply (See Table 7). As might be expected, the more detailed entries tend to relate to bulk purchases of goods. Over eighty other persons are named in the accounts but unfortunately no further details are given.

---

of medicines are only available for 1600 (ABPL 8427 Libro de las cuentas que llevó el licenciado don Sebastián Clemente mayordomo del hospital de San Andrés, 1600).

What is striking is the variety of types of traders and producers from whom the hospitals acquired *materia medica* and the degree to which the suppliers specialised in particular products (Figure 7). Thirteen *boticarios* based in Lima at different times sold medicines to the Hospital of Santa Ana. Francisco de Alva, Juan de Bilbao, Francisco Martín Reyna, Pedro de Bilbao, Graviel de España and Juan Matías de Vera all supplied medicines to the hospital over several years, following each other chronologically rather than supplying them simultaneously.[86] Apart from the items purchased from Juan de Bilbao that were recorded only as "medicinas," the products most commonly supplied by *boticarios* were senna, rhubarb, scammony and a number of complex electuaries, most commonly *diafinicón* and *diacatolicón*.[87] However, it seems that *boticarios* were sometimes unwilling or reluctant to supply hospitals because they feared that because of their limited resources they would not be paid.[88]

Large quantities of unspecified medicines were also supplied by several individuals referred to only as "mercaderes," including Francisco Rodríguez Soria and Alonso de Paz. Apart from unspecified medicines, the only items that were consistently traded by merchants were spices – saffron, clove and cinnamon – and some mineral products, namely *cardenillo* (verdigris or acetate of copper), *alumbre* (alum or potassium aluminium sulphate) and *solimán* (mercury chloride). Merchants also acted as agents for other suppliers. So for example, although physicians were explicitly forbidden to prepare medicines,[89] in 1600 one Doctor Figueroa, supplied the Hospital of San Andrés with 680 pesos worth of unspecified medicines, through the merchant, Juan López de Altopica.[90] In most cases, physicians seem to have been supplying simples, mainly purgatives such as rhubarb, scammony and canafistula rather than complex medicines.[91]

Hospitals acquired similar products from "tiendas." *Tiendas*, such as the "tienda de Anaya", were probably retail outlets for goods imported by

86 Others were Francisco Crespo, Francisco Cano, Mateo Pastor, Blas de Medina, Gerónimo Pujadas, Juan Bécquer Cantero, Juan Matías de Vera, and Alonso de Carrión.

87 For the composition of diafinicón and diacatolicón see Oviedo, *Methodo*, 88, 122. The former was based on dates and the latter on senna, canafistula and tamarind.

88 AGI Lima 214 N19 R1 fol. 14v. Información…del hospital de San Andrés 1602.

89 *Recopilación de las leyes, pragmáticas reales* (Muñoz), cap. XIII ordinance 3: 159–60 1537.

90 ABPL 8427 Libro de las cuentas que llevó el licenciado don Sebastián Clemente mayordomo del hospital de San Andrés, 1600.

91 ABPL 9080 Libro de cuentas, censos y haberes que corresponden al hospital de Santa Ana, 1575–1584; ABPL 9084 Libro de cuentas de gastos del hospital de Santa Ana, 1597–1599. The physicians supplying the Hospital of Santa Ana were Licenciados Hidalgo and Pedro de Vergara. Lic. Hidalgo also supplied some unspecified medicines.

peruleros.[92] They supplied similar items to merchants, but normally in smaller quantities. One supplier was the "casa de Valladolid", which specialised in the supply of wax for making ointments. This store probably belonged to the Valladolid family of wax chandlers whose shop was located on the Calle de Valladolid.[93] In addition to these specialised suppliers of wax, it was also traded by *boticarios*. The testament of the *boticario* Juan Matías de Vera indicated that he possessed barrels, blocks, and boxes of white wax from Castile which were worth 1,400 pesos, which was almost equivalent to the value of all the *materia medica* he owned, which was estimated at 1,500 pesos. Although the *boticario* may have been using some wax for ointments himself, the large quantity suggests that he may have been trading it as a simple product,[94] as well as

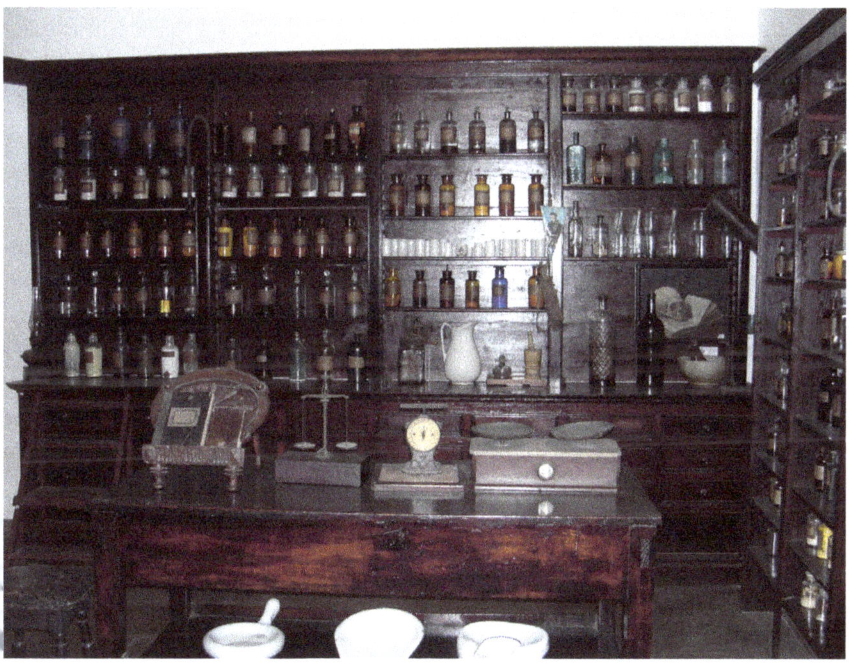

FIGURE 7 *Pharmacy of the convent of Los Descalzos, Lima.*
PHOTO AUTHOR

92 See AGI Contratación 1145B N4: 303–11 Registro del navío Santa Maria del Juncal 1605 for imports by one Juan Núñez de Anaya. See also, García Fuentes, *Los peruleros*, 84.

93 Bromley, *Viejas Calles de Lima*, 316.

94 AAL Testamentos 25–1 fol. 6 Testamento de Juan Matías de Vera, boticario, 1641.

making it into wax-based medicines such as ointments and plasters for sale, including to the Hospital of Santa Ana.[95]

Other specialist suppliers were confectioners, who sold honey, and a *bodeguero* who supplied oil. Only five sellers referred to as *pulperos* appear in the hospital accounts and they were mainly trading gums and resins – *almaciga* and *incensio* – and some canafistula. In addition the hospital purchased some items in the marketplace, occasionally from Indians or Africans. For example, it acquired large quantities of canafistula from one Jaime Canpi.[96] It is likely many other purchases were made from unnamed persons, but in quantities too small to warrant entry into the pharmacy accounts. In the 1650s at least the hospital was buying large quantities of sugar direct from the Jesuits,[97] most likely from their haciendas at Surco located just southwest of Lima or from their estates to the north in the Huara Valley.[98] Finally, most of the named persons whose occupation is not specified appear only once or twice in the accounts. The exceptions are four persons who were trading almost exclusively in gums, resins, honey, and saffron,[99] suggesting that there was some specialisation amongst traders. It is worth noting that of the 150 named entries, only four were women, including one African and one Indian. While this probably underestimates the number of local people supplying the hospital with *materia medica*, it may not apply to Andean traders, especially native women, who tended to specialise in the supply of food, drink or clothing rather than unprocessed products.[100]

Despite the diverse range of sources from which hospitals acquired *materia medica*, because of difficulties of timely supply, the poor quality of medicines, and probably cost, most hospitals and monasteries established their own herb gardens. When the Hospital of Santa Ana was inspected in the 1588, it possessed no gardener, only an Indian who it was said knew nothing about gardening, which resulted in it having to acquire herbs from outside at considerable

95 ABPL 9127 fol. 63 Memoria de lo gastado en la botica [hospital de Santa Ana] 1640–1641.

96 ABPL 9080 Libro de cuentas del hospital de Santa Ana 1575 a 1585 for accounts for 1575.

97 ABPL 9100 Libro de cuentas del hospital de Santa Ana, 1625–1690.

98 Nicholas P. Cushner, *Lords of the Land: Sugar, Wine, and Jesuit Estates of Coastal Peru, 1600–1767* (New York: SUNY Press, 1980), 29–38, 63–68.

99 These were: Juan de Guevara (12 entries), Antonio Herrera (7), Bartolomé Rodríguez (6) and Pedro Marqués (5).

100 Jane E. Mangan, *Trading Roles: Gender, Ethnicity and the Urban Economy in Colonial Potosí* (Durham, NC: Duke University Press, 2005), 76–105, 139; Ilana Aragón Noriega, "El pan, el vino, y otros negocios: aspectos laborales de la mujer," in *Lima en el siglo XIV*, ed. Laura Gutiérrez Arbulú (Lima: Pontificia Universidad Católica del Perú, Instituto Riva-Agüero, 2005), 265.

expense. The *mayordomo* was therefore ordered to ensure that "lettuces, cabbages, borage, parsley, and other herbs" were always available for the treatment of the sick.[101] A decade later the hospital was employing two native gardeners and others in its *chácara*,[102] In 1599 the *mayordomo*, then the *perulero* Rodrigo Arias de Buiça, was able to report that he had overseen the cultivation of

> ...lettuces, cabbages, radishes, aubergines, aval and other vegetables as well as medicinal plants such as borage, mallow, manzanilla, and others for the pharmacy and treatment of the poor.[103]

Even so, an inspection of the hospital in 1607 found that many of the drugs in the pharmacy were in a poor state.[104] Worth mentioning here, but discussed more fully in Chapter 6, is the substantial garden and pharmacy of the Jesuit College of San Pablo, which became a wholesale centre for other pharmacies in Lima and received orders from all over the Viceroyalty.[105]

The local trade in medicines was not one-way. Hospitals were forbidden to sell medicines,[106] but they did so in small quantities along with larger quantities of certain products, such as roses and fat, which were produced in their gardens and *chácaras*.[107] In 1575, the Hospital of Santa Ana was supplying huge quantities of roses from its *chácara* to three of Lima's eminent *boticarios*, Juan de Bilbao, [Juan de] Alva and [Diego de] Tineo, as well as to three doctors and the Hospital of San Andrés.[108] Juan de Bilbao purchased about half of the 834 pounds of roses that were sold by the hospital that year.[109] Not insignificant

101 ABPL 9806 fol. 271v. Visita al hospital de Santa Ana 26 May 1588.

102 ABPL 9084 fols. 132–68 Libro de cuentas de gastos del hospital de Santa Ana, 1597–1599.

103 ABPL 9086 fols. 321–23 *Visita* al hospital de Santa Ana 22 Oct. 1599 in Protocolo de expedientes del hospital de Santa Ana, 1599–1607. Part of this volume (fols. 271–74) which relates to an important *visita* conducted on 26 May 1588 is no longer in the archive.

104 ABPL 9806 fols. 320–23 Visita al Hospital de Santa Ana, cargos que resultan contra el bachiller Juan Manuel Carrasco mayordomo del hospital de los naturales 17 Jan. 1607.

105 Martín, *Intellectual Conquest*, 102.

106 Ordinance 45 Constituciones y ordenanzas y del hospital real de Santa Ana, Lima 28 Feb. 1609.

107 See for example, AAL Hospitales leg. 2 exp. 3 Solicitud presentada por Francisco López de Cepeda, mayordomo y administrador del hospital de los naturales de Santa Ana [1622]; ABPL 9127 Memoria de lo gastado en la botica [hospital de Santa Ana] 1640–1641.

108 ABPL 9080 Libro de cuentas del hospital de Santa Ana 1575 a 1585 fols. 60–71 Cargo de lo que ha de haver este hospital de lo que procede de la chácara 1575.

109 In 1627 the hospital of San Andrés similarly purchased 382 pounds roses: see BNL 1577 Cuentas que da Hernando de Herrera mayordomo que fue deste hospital de San Andrés Agosto 1627.

quantities were also sold to African women who traded them in the city. Roses were valued for their astringent properties and were used to prepare different types of medicines, such as rose water, rose oil, rose honey, rose conserve, and rose syrup.[110] Notwithstanding the widespread use of roses in pharmacy, the quantity purchased by Bilbao seems enormous and it maybe that he sold them on to other *boticarios* or used them to manufacture products for sale in his pharmacy. In any case, it suggests the large scale of his business.

Hospitals not only sold simple products, but on occasions also provided medicines for private individuals. This is evident from a claim made in 1622 by the *mayordomo* of the Hospital of Santa Ana, Francisco López de Çepeda, on the estate of the physician, Doctor Diego Ramírez, for 652 pesos worth of medicines it had supplied.[111] These medicines included syrups, electuaries and ointments, but also a purge for a female African slave.

Much less in known about the way in which owners of private phramacies obtained *materia medica* locally. Probably most was acquired from small retailers or in the market. In Spain *boticarios* often possessed their own private gardens where they experimented with new plants from overseas. Well known are the botanical gardens of Nicólas Monardes and Simón de Tovar in Seville.[112] There is no evidence for apothecary gardens in Lima, though it is known that private gardens existed. However, contemporary observations suggest that these gardens were dominated by plants imported from Europe. The anonymous *Descripción del Virreinato* written at the beginning of the seventeenth century recorded that most gardens were watered by canals and were filled with flower pots with carnations (*claveles*), stocks or wallflowers (*alhelies*), bay (*albahaca*) and common cress (*mastuerzos*).[113] Of course, such observations need to be viewed with caution for they were generally made by Europeans who may have been unfamiliar with native plants.

110 Enrique Laval, *Botica de los Jesuitas de Santiago* (Santiago: Asociación Chilena de Asistencia Social, 1953), 172.

111 AAL Hospitales leg. 2 exp. 3 Solicitud presentada por Francisco López de Cepeda, mayordomo y administrador del hospital de los naturales de Santa Ana, sobre los 652 pesos quedo debiendo Doctor Diego Ramírez, difunto, al dicho hospital 1622. See also the sale of *polvos de coloquíntidas* to Doctor Don Luis Çegarra (ABPL 9127 fol. 45 Memoria de lo gastado en la botica [hospital de Santa Ana] 1640–1641).

112 Barrera-Osorio, *Experiencing Nature*, 212–26. Findlen, *Possessing Nature*, 256–61 makes the same general observation.

113 Lewin, *Descripción*, 38. It is generally recognised that the author of this was a Jewish "spy" Pedro de León Portocarrero.

Conclusion

The transatlantic trade in medicines was dominated by merchants and prominent *boticarios* in Seville, who controlled their prices. Apart from the high cost of the products themselves, the price of imported medicines in Peru was inflated by high state-imposed taxes and transport costs, and the profit that *boticarios* expected to make. Not only did the high cost of imported medicines restrict access to them, but weaknesses in Spain's monopolistic trading system meant that over time the supply declined and became unpredictable. Increasingly imported medicines were criticised as being not only expensive but also of poor quality. Hence, the trading system failed to support the type of medical practice that regulation and the Church promoted, reducing colonial dependency on Spain and encouraging the emergence of other sources of supply. This did not result, however, in an active search for alternative products that might have encouraged experimentation and the adoption of native *materia media*, which might ultimately have challenged humoral practices. It has been shown that local sources of supply, for example, hospital gardens, focused on the cultivation of Old World plants, and as Chapter 6 will demonstrate, the few native products that were adopted were substitutes for those that were central to the practice of humoral medicine.

In order to explain why there was limited experimentation, the following chapter examines the changing nature of medical practice in Spain and Europe more broadly, including debates about the efficacy of local versus imported medicinal products. In particular, it explores the effectiveness of the Inquisition and system of regulation in supporting orthodox humoral practices.

CHAPTER 5

Selecting *Materia Medica*

> The New World laid bare the limitations of classical texts, but those texts continued to provide necessary models for the intellectual and actual appropriation of the New World.[1]

The *materia medica* that were imported from Spain and traded locally clearly reflected the natural philosophy that underpinned medical practice at the time. In sixteenth and seventeenth centuries healing practices in Europe were dominated by humoral beliefs based on the study of classical texts, but new experimental methods were emerging that challenged this approach and focused on new *materia medica*, notably chemicals. This was therefore a period when different approaches to medical practice existed. This chapter will show how orthodox medical practice was promoted by the regulatory framework that the Spanish were developing for medical practice and by the Inquisition, though these had their limitations and may even have had potentially counterintuitive effects. Moreover, the two approaches were not always opposed, but could be combined or work in parallel. Hence, a number of *protomédicos* such as Antonio Sánchez Renedo and Antonio de Robles Cornejo, while generally promoting humoral practices, also possessed an interest in native medicinal plants, an approach that was inherently empirical, and even experimental. Nevertheless, it will be shown how orthodox medical practices generally prevailed, though it will be argued that their prevalence cannot be attributed solely to effective regulation and control. It will demonstrate that where empirical methods were employed, the aim was primarily to find solutions to old problems rather than challenge the natural philosophy that underlay medical practice.

Humoralism

Medical practice in sixteenth-century Spain was dominated by the views of Galen and Hippocrates, which during the Renaissance attracted renewed

1 Nieto Olarte, "Scientific Practices," 147.

 | DOI 10.1163/9789004351271_006

interest as humanist scholars turned back to Ancient Greece for their inspiration and began to examine the original Greek texts. Galen and Hippocrates saw illness as a function of an imbalance in the humours or bodily fluids – blood, phlegm, black bile and yellow bile – which, like all substances, were regarded as hot or cold, moist or dry.[2] Hence blood was hot and wet, phlegm cold and wet, yellow bile hot and dry, and black bile cold and dry. Humoral medicine thus sought to correct any humoral imbalance, which it did through diet, purging, vomiting, and bleeding. Imbalances might derive from inappropriate behaviour, such exhaustion or excessive consumption, or from particular temperature, air or water conditions that could upset a body's hydraulics. Treatments were personalised according to an individual's complexion or temperament, as well as their gender and age.[3] However, they were applied on the general principle that an imbalance in the humours could be restored through prescribing medicines or foods that possessed properties contrary to those being displayed by the patient. A person with a phlegmatic complexion might therefore be treated with substances deemed to be "hot." Humoral beliefs were entrenched in popular thought to the extent that in the absence of doctors lay people often applied treatments according to these principles. Soldiers on military campaigns, for example, might make and administer purgatives, and even let blood.[4]

Astrology, or the movement of the planets and stars, was believed to influence the four elements – earth, fire, water and air – which in turn affected the humours, and consequentially human complexions and temperaments. Such beliefs were held by Christians, Jews, and Muslims alike.[5] The cosmos was

2 Foster, *Hippocrates' Latin American Legacy*, 2–4; George Foster, "Relationship between Spanish and Spanish-American Folk Medicine," *Journal of American Folklore*, 66 (1953): 201–02; Siraisi, *Medieval and Early Renaissance Medicine*, 102–09; Roy Porter, *The Greatest Benefit to Mankind: The Medical History of Humanity from Antiquity to the Present* (London: HarperCollins, 1997), 55–62, 73–77, 168–86; Lindemann, *Medicine and Society*, 12–15, 68–69.

3 John Henry, "Doctors and Healers: Popular Culture and the Medical Profession," in *Science, Culture and Popular Belief in Renaissance Europe*, ed. Stephen Pumfrey, Paolo L. Rossi and Maurice Slawinski (Manchester: Manchester University Press, 1991), 199–200; Brockliss and Jones, *Medical World*, 111; Lindemann, *Medicine and Society*, 12, 15; Luis García Ballester, *La búsqueda de la salud: sanadores y enfermos en la España medieval* (Barcelona: Ediciones Peninsula, 2001), 129–33, 145, 176–80. For a recent succinct introduction to humoral medicine in Spain and Spanish America see Earle, *Body of the Conquistador*, 19–41.

4 Vargas Machuca, *Indian Militia*, 64–65.

5 Siraisi, *Medieval and Early Renaissance Medicine*, 97–114; Jorge Cañizares-Esguerra, "New World, New Stars: Patriotic Astrology and the Invention of Indian and Creole Bodies in Colonial Spanish America, 1600–1650," *The American Historical Review* 104(1) (1999): 36–37, 50; García Ballester, *Búsqueda de la salud*, 176–80; Monica Azzolini, "Reading Health in the Stars: Politics and Medical Astrology in Renaissance Milan, *Horoscopes and Public Spheres: Essays*

thought to influence not only human bodies, but all natural things. Hence, the virtues of plants found in particular places were considered to be the most appropriate for the treatment of people and diseases to be found there; some even argued that they had been placed there by God to meet local needs.[6] Not only were the movements of the planets and stars seen to affect the humours, but also indicate the specific times or critical days that plants should be collected and therapies applied.[7]

Views on the suitability of local versus imported medicines varied, however. Arguments in favour of employing local plants often stressed the excessive cost and often poor quality of imported medicines. Sometimes these arguments were imbued with patriotic sentiments that took pride in local remedies. Others, such as Paracelsus, who objected to the universalism of Galenic theory and promoted the employment of empirical methods, also advocated the use of local plants. Conversely, merchants who saw any preference for local *materia medica* as a potential threat to their business expressed more sceptical views, as did Galenic physicians who generally focussed on fitting newly-discovered *materia medica* into a humoral framework. The arguments became more complex as a debate emerged as to whether imported plants grown in a new environment were as effective as when they were raised in their place of origin.[8] Much of this debate was conducted at an intellectual level in Spain. The issue does not appear to have been widely discussed in Lima. In Peru, there was an overriding belief in the therapeutic value of plants of Old World origin, but there is no evidence of a discussion from the perspective of cosmological influences

---

in the History of Astrology, eds. Günter Oestmann, H. Dareel Rytkin, and Kocku von Stukrad (Berlin: Walter de Gruyter, 2005), 187–89.

6 Andrew Wear, "The Early Modern Debate about Foreign Drugs: Localism versus Universalism in Medicine," *The Lancet* 354 (1999): 150; Richard Drayton, *Nature's Government: Science, Imperial Britain and the 'Improvement' of the World* (New Haven: Yale University Press, 2000), 12–13.

7 Siraisi, *Medieval and Early Renaissance Medicine*, 135–36; Anthony Grafton and Nancy Siraisi, "Between the Election and My Hopes; Girolamo Cardano and Medical Astrology," in *Secrets of Nature: Astrology and Alchemy in Early Modern Europe*, eds. William R. Newman and Anthony Grafton (Cambridge, MA: MIT Press, 2001), 78–86; Azzolini, "Reading Health in the Stars," 197–201.

8 Cañizares-Esguerra, "New World, New Stars," 49–53; Cooper, *Inventing the Indigenous*, 21–50; Wear, "Early Modern Debate," 150–51 and *Knowledge and Practice in English Medicine, 1550–1680* (Cambridge University Press, Cambridge, 2000), 72–77, 86–92. For the case of sarsaparilla and see Anne E Winterbottom, "Of the China Root: a Case Study of the Early Modern Circulation of *Materia Medica*," *Social History of Medicine* 28 (1)(2015): 34–36.

of the relative merits of growing them in Europe as opposed to raising them locally. The main concern was with the quality of medicines with imports being deemed inferior due to their long journey from Spain. The predominant belief in the efficacy of plants of Old World origin was evident in the approach that naturalists and medical practitioners took to native *materia medica* where their emphasis was on finding products with the same healing qualities that could act as effective substitutes for those that were generally used in Europe.

Scholarly Scientific Explorations

Whatever views were held at the time, they demonstrated a general interest in acquiring *materia medica* from the New World. This quest was driven in part by commercial interests, though actually very few American plants were adopted in Europe in the early modern period. At the same time a genuine intellectual curiosity prevailed about the lands and peoples of the New World, knowledge of which was deemed important for "good government." Thus, Philip II himself sponsored the well-researched scientific expedition to Mexico by the physician, Francisco Hernández. He also initiated an empire-wide enquiry into the nature of its peoples, their environments, and history, a task that was overseen by the Spanish cosmographer Juan López de Velasco and produced responses known collectively as the *relaciones geográficas*.[9] In this survey local officials were instructed to inquire about the medicinal and poisonous plants to be found their jurisdiction and on their use by the local people to treat the sick.

The Crown did not sponsor a scientific expedition to Peru that was comparable to that of Hernández, but Antonio Sánchez Renedo, who arrived in Lima as royal *protomédico* in 1569, took a particular interest in local herbs and plants.[10] His research in this area was known to López de Velasco in Spain, who reported to the Crown that Sánchez Renedo was writing a "Historia natural de la yervas y plantas y cosas notables de aquellas partes" and recommended

9 Goodman, *Power and Penury*, 68–71, 234–38; Barrera-Osorio, "Knowledge and Empiricism," 231–32. For the text and context of Francisco Hernández' expedition see Simon Varey, ed., *The Mexican Treasury: The Writings of Dr. Francisco Hernández*, trans. Cynthia L Chamberlain and Simon Varey (Stanford: Stanford University Press, 2000) and Varey, Chabrán and Weiner, eds., *Searching for the Secrets of Nature*. For the *relaciones geográficas* of Peru see: *Relaciones geográficas de Indias. Peru*, ed. Marcos Jiménez de la Espada. Biblioteca de autores españoles 183–85. 3 vols. (Madrid: Ediciones Atlas, 1965).

10 Lanning, *Royal Protomedicato*, 29–30; Matallana, *Historia de la enseñanza médica*, 76.

that he should be rewarded to encourage his labours. Unfortunately no copies of this text have been found.[11] Shortly after in 1587, the Salamancan physician Antonio de Robles Cornejo, who had met Hernández in Madrid, migrated to Peru. He was generally supported by wealthy relatives, but in 1594 he was provided with a large salary by the city of La Paz that enabled him to live there for a year.[12] By the beginning of the seventeenth century Robles Cornejo had travelled extensively in Peru and was a good friend of Andrés Gonzales the rich and experienced *boticario* in Cartagena referred to in the last chapter as one of that city's main traders in medicines.[13] His experience formed the basis of a manuscript he wrote entitled, "Simples medicinales indianos." Its publication was approved by the Crown in 1617, when he was given license to take four printers to Peru to publish and sell the book.[14] However, the Crown declined to provide him with a salary or with financial assistance to publish the work, as had been the case with Francisco Hernández. In compensation he made him *protomédico* of Tierra Firme, with which he remained dissatisfied. During the return journey to Peru, his manuscript and the printing equipment, which he had paid for at his own expense, were seemingly lost in a shipwreck off Panama. Reporting on the disaster, he claimed that he possessed no copy and had lost 25 years work.[15] However, a manuscript of 709 pages entitled "Examen de los simples medicinales," which was similarly approved for publication

11 AGI IG 1086 Lib. 6 fol. 200v. (Image 405) Juan López de Velasco 28 May 1578; Matallana, *Historia de la enseñaza médica*, 27, 76. On Juan López de Velasco see: María M. Portuondo, *Secret Science: Spanish Cosmography and the New World* (Chicago: University of Chicago Press, 2009).

12 AGI IG 2096 N 94 Expediente de concesión de licencia para pasar a Perú a favor de Antonio de Robles Cornejo, 1586; ARJBM División 1, leg. 17 fol. 197 Libro de examen de los simples medicinales Antonio de Robles Cornejo 1617; Miguel Colmeiro, "Noticias acerca de un manuscrito perteneciente al licenciado Antonio Robles Cornejo," *Revista de los progresos de las ciencias exactas, físicas y naturales* 9 (7) (Madrid, 1859): 440–44.

13 ARJBM División 1, leg. 17 fol. 263 Libro de examen de los simples medicinales Antonio de Robles Cornejo 1617; Quintín Chiarlone and Carlos Mallaína, *Historia de la farmacia* (Madrid: Imp. José M. Ducazcal, 1865), 292. For the shipment of medicines to Andrés Gonzales see: Contratación 1080–1163 *passim* 1583–1612. Between 1582 and 1612 he handled 18 of 54 cargoes destined for Cartagena, which were worth about one-third of the value of all medicines imported through Cartagena.

14 AGI IG 428 Lib. 35 fols. 15v.–16 Licencia al Licenciado Antonio de Robles Cornejo 4 Nov. 1617; AGI Contratación 5363 N10 fols. 17, 52–52v. Informaciones de pasajeros a Indias 23 Apr. 1618.

15 AGI Panama 17 R3 N34 Antonio de Robles Cornejo 24 Jun. 1619; Mar Rey Bueno, "Concordias medicinales de entrambos mundos." *Revista de Indias* 66 (no. 237) (2006): 349.

in Madrid in 1617, survives in archive of the Real Jardín Botánico in Madrid.[16] (Figure 8) Clearly written by Robles Cornejo it is not clear what relationship this manuscript may have had to the one that was lost, though it would appear that several decades later a manuscript by him was in the hands of the Sevillian physician Gaspar Caldera de Heredia.[17]

Even though some intellectuals showed an interest in native plants, they often viewed them through the lens of humoralism and attempted to fit them within a humoral framework. In his manuscript Robles Cornejo considered the characteristics of each plant in turn, discussing their origins, names, where they were to be found, and what had been written about them by other authors. In outlining his approach to describing flowers and fruits he recorded that he took advice from living and past masters and consulted diligently books by the most esteemed ancient and modern authors.[18] In the text he refers mainly to traditional authors including Dioscorides, Galen, Mesüe, Avicenna, Laguna, Serapion, Platearius and Pliny, though not without some criticism, but also to the contemporary naturalists Nicólas Monardes, Cristóbal de Acosta, Garcia de Orta, and Carolus Clusius. He also refers to these authors in the marginalia. Both the illustrations and marginalia are entered in a different coloured ink from the text and they appear to have been inserted by a different hand; in fact blank spaces for illustrations are left above the description of some plants suggesting that the manuscript was probably incomplete. Although Robles Cornejo mainly cites traditional texts, he sometimes refers to "los modernos" who were experimenting with plants, though often to criticise them. His criticisms were largely about the procedures used in the preparation and application of particular medicines; he did not reject the employment of empirical methods *per se*. In fact it is clear from the text that he himself was conducting experiments

16 ARJBM División 1, leg. 17 Libro de examen de los simples medicinales Antonio de Robles Cornejo 1617. For notes on the biography of Robles Cornejo see: Chirlone and Mallaína, *Historia de la farmacia*,, 292–300; Colmeiro, "Noticias," 440–44; Mar Rey Bueno, "Los proyectos sobre materia médica peruana de Antonio de Robles Cornejo y Matías de Porres (1617–1621)," in *Rotas da Natureza: Cientistas, vaigens, expedições, instituições*, eds. Ana Leonor Pereira and João Pita (Coimbra: Universidade de Coimbra, 2006), 27–31. For a summary account of the contents of the manuscript see: Quintín Chirlone and Carlos Mallaína, "Biografía Antonio Robles Cornejo," *El restaurador farmacéutico*, ano 11 no. 8 20 Mar. 1855. On line at: http://bibliotecavirtual.ranf.com/es/catalogo_imagenes/grupo.cmd?path=2010122 [Accessed 11 May 2016].

17 Rey Bueno, "Los proyectos," 29–30.

18 ARJBM División 1, leg. 17 fol. 260 Libro de examen de los simples medicinales Antonio de Robles Cornejo 1617.

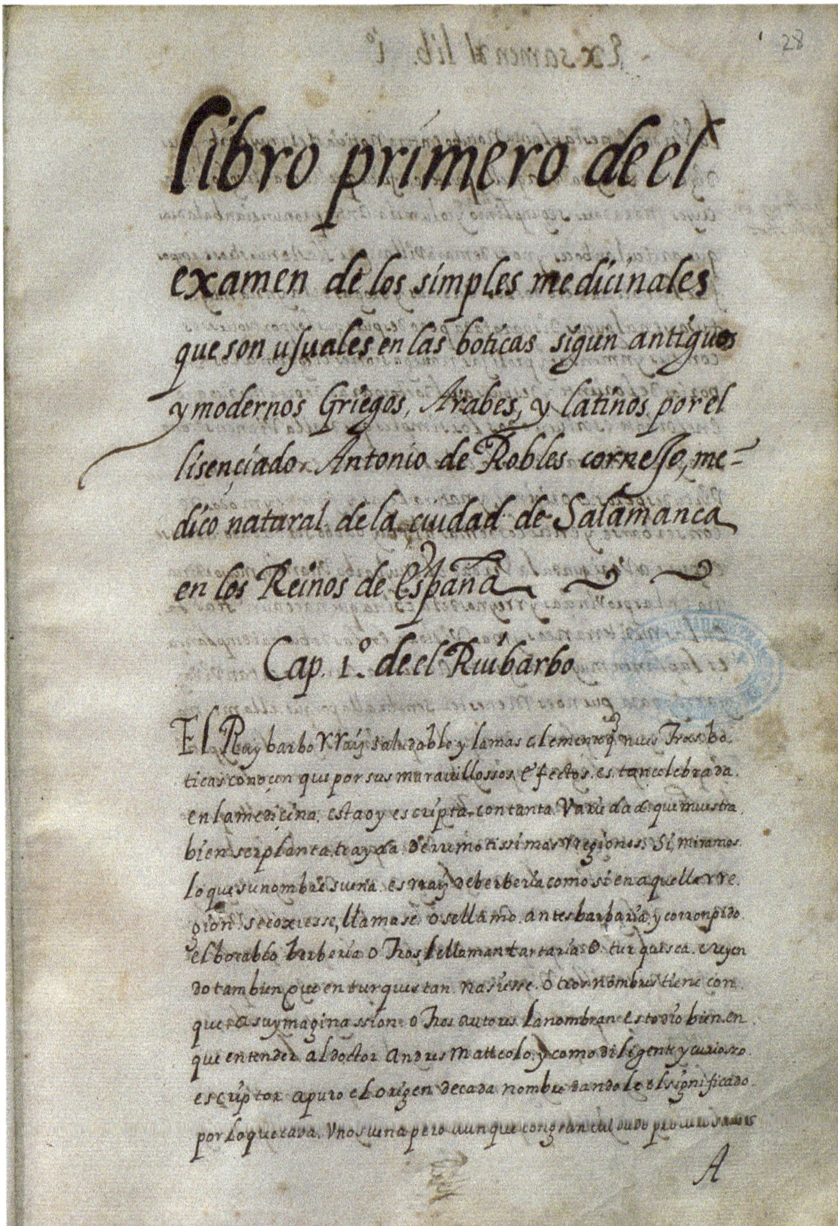
Libro primero deel examen de los simples medicinales que son usuales en las boticas segun antiguos y modernos Griegos, Arabes, y latinos por el lisenciado Antonio de Robles cornesso, medico natural de la ciudad de Salamanca en los Reinos de España

Cap. 1.º deel Ruibarbo

FIGURE 8 *Front page of Antonio de Robles Cornejo's "Examen de los simples medicinales," 1617.* COURTESY SPAIN. MINISTERIO DE CULTURA. ARCHIVO DEL REAL JARDÍN BOTÁNICO, MADRID. DIVISIÓN 1, LEG. 17 FOL. 1.

with a number of native plants.[19] Robles Cornejo does not name specific "modernos" or modern authors, but in his exposition on minerals he indicates an awareness of the writings of Paracelsus.[20]

Scholars were interested in nature from the perspective of demonstrating the magnificence of God and his works. Paradoxically, however, this Christian spur to reveal the secrets of nature led to observations in the New World that sometimes challenged prevailing scientific and cosmological beliefs derived from biblical texts.[21] Among the scholar/naturalists who travelled extensively in Peru were the Jesuits José de Acosta and Bernabé Cobo, who were at different times at the College of San Pablo.[22] José de Acosta's *Historia natural y moral de las Indias* was published in 1590 and Bernabé Cobo's *Historia del Nuevo Mundo* followed in 1653, although it was based largely on his observations in Peru and the southern Andes in the first three decades of the seventeenth century.[23] Cobo based his account on direct observations and his descriptions of plants and animals are exceptional in their exactitude. Acosta, however, wrote much of his *Historia* in Spain and paid relatively little attention to medicinal plants. His *Historia* was essentially a natural philosophy that focussed on the principles and causes of natural phenomena.[24] Cobo underlined differences

19 See for example his comparison of use of *juncia* (Gencian root) by traditional and modern *boticarios* in ARJBM División 1, leg. 17 fol. 94 Libro de examen de los simples medicinales Antonio de Robles Cornejo 1617.

20 Ibid., fols. 589, 591.

21 Barrera-Osorio, *Experiencing Nature*, 103. For Acosta see Barrera-Osorio, *Experiencing Nature*, 114–20; Saul Jarcho, "Origin of the American Indian as Suggested by Fray Joseph de Acosta (1589)," *Isis* 50 (4) (1959): 430–38; Thayne R. Ford, "Stranger in a Foreign Land: José de Acosta's Scientific Realisations in Sixteenth-century Peru," *Sixteenth Century Journal* 29 (1) (1998): 19–33; Sabine McCormack, *On the Wings of Time: Rome, the Incas, Spain and Peru* (Princeton: Princeton University Press, 2009), 153–65; Andrés I. Prieto, *Missionary Scientists: Jesuit Science in Spanish South America 1570–1810* (Nashville: Vanderbilt University Press, 2011), 143–68. For Cobo see: Luis Millones-Figueroa, "La historia natural del padre Bernabé Cobo: algunas claves para su lectura," *Colonial Latin American Review* 12 (1) (2003): 85–97 and Prieto, *Missionary Scientists*, 99–115. For a comparison of their approaches and methods see Prieto, *Missionary Scientists*, 8, 102 05, 169 94.

22 Acosta went to Peru in 1571 and he returned to Spain via Mexico in 1587, where he died in 1600. Cobo arrived in Peru in 1599 and stayed in the Andean region until 1630, when he went to Mexico. He subsequently returned to Peru in 1650 where he died in 1657.

23 Acosta, *Historia natural y moral*, 1–247; Cobo, *Obras*.

24 Acosta, *Historia natural y moral*, 3–4; Barrera-Osorio, *Experiencing Nature*, 115. See also, Sabine Anagnostou, "Jesuits in Spanish America: Contributions to the Exploration of the American Materia Medica," *Pharmacy in History* 47 (1) (2005): 5–10.

between the New World and the Old seeing them as evidence of the God's omnipotence, whereas Acosta adopted an Aristotelian approach which encouraged him to focus on their similarities and on the general principles underlying natural phenomena. Often scholars struggled to reconcile their observations with prevailing cosmological thought, sometimes leading them into convoluted reasoning. When this failed, they were often forced to resort to divine intervention or miracles for an explanation.

Other scholars in Peru who had a particular interest in the influence of the stars and planets on healing practices included the Creole Augustinian Antonio de la Calancha. Calancha argued that being located in the southern hemisphere and coming under a different constellation from the north, Peru was particularly blessed.[25] However, another non-medical resident of Peru, Juan de Figueroa, who among other things served on Lima's *cabildo* and was *familiar* to the Inquisition, disagreed. He had a passionate interest in astrology and argued against the specificity of the southern stars. In his *Opusculo de astrología en medicina* (1660) he contended that the influence of the stars was universal and he adopted a more traditional approach paying particular attention to the identification of the critical days for treatments, including the letting of blood.[26] Although his book was published in Lima and medical astrology was taught in the university,[27] Claudia Brosseder argues that by the time his book was published the discourse on astrology had shifted towards astronomy and as such his work had little impact on medical practice or treatises.[28]

Knowledge of critical days was also seen as essential to the Mercedarian historian, Martín de Murúa, who worked for a period as a missionary in Peru and in 1611 published his *Historia General del Perú*. While he was impressed by native healers' knowledge of the virtues of medicinal plants, he was concerned that they did not know "the necessary methods to apply them, and further the

25 Antonio de la Calancha, *Corónica moralizada del orden de San Agustín en el Perú* (Barcelona: Pedro Lacavalleria, 1639); Cañizares-Esguerra, "New World, New Stars," 50–51, 59; Claudia Brosseder, "Astrology in Seventeenth-century Peru," *Studies in History and Philosophy of Biological and Biomedical Sciences* 41(2) (2010): 147.

26 Juan de Figueroa, *Opusculo de astrología en medicina* (Lima: No Publisher, 1660), 101–92; Pedro M. Guibovich Pérez, *Censura, libros e inquisición en el Perú colonial, 1570–1754* (Seville: Universidad de Sevilla, Secretariado de publicaciones, 2004), 259–61; Brosseder "Astrology," 147–50.

27 Eguiguren, *Alma mater*, 257; Matallana, *Historia de la enseñanza médica*, 76.

28 Brosseder, "Astrology," 151, 155.

most advantageous times."[29] The extent to which physicians used astrology in their individual treatments probably varied, but the influence of the stars and cosmos was embedded in early modern thought from the elite to the popular level. It was, in Jorge Cañizares-Esguerra's words something that "everybody took for granted."[30]

Initially the development of science was driven by the desire of scholars to find new answers to old problems rather than to challenge the existing natural philosophy.[31] Hence, native plants were placed within a Galenic framework and were classified as being hot, cold, dry, or humid to different degrees. This involved testing them for their smell and taste, and in assessing their therapeutic function and efficacy.[32] The process of assessment was a major undertaking given the number of native plants that needed to be observed and categorised and, as the following chapter will demonstrate, it often produced conflicting outcomes. Indeed the difficulties of agreeing on how the American plants fitted into the existing humoral framework was a significant factor delaying their adoption in Europe.[33] What is significant, however, is that the procedures that were being used clearly embodied inherently contradictory approaches. While the aim was to support a humoral approach to medical practice, at the same time the empirical methods of observation and experiment that were being employed were key features of the scientific approach to medicine that was being advocated in Europe by Paracelsus among others.

29 Martín de Murúa, *Historia general del* Perú (Madrid: Instituto Gonzalo Fernández de Oviedo, 1964 [1616]), 103 "por no aplicarse por el modo necesario, ni aun en los tiempos convenientes."

30 García Ballester, *Búsqueda de la salud*, 177; Goodman, *Power and Penury*, 28. Cañizares-Esguerra, "New World, New Stars," 37. On p. 45 he notes that Franciscan friar Bernardino de Sahagún, the physician, Francisco Hernández, and Philip II himself were firm believers in the influence of the constellations on peoples and their environments. See also: Henry, "Doctors and Healers," 201–03.

31 Edward Grant, "When Did Modern Science Begin?" *The American Scholar* 66 (1997): 111.

32 Guenter B. Risse, "Transcending Cultural Barriers: the European Reception of Medicinal Plants from the Americas," in *Botanical Drugs of the Americas in the Old and New Worlds: Invitational Symposium at the Washington-Congress, 1983*, ed. by Wolfgang-Hagen Hein (Stuttgart: Wissenschaftliche Verlagsgesellschaft, 1984), 32, 34–35; Paula Ronderos, *El dilema de los rótulos: Lectura del inventario de una botica santafereña de comienzos del siglo XVII* (Bogotá: Pontificia Universidad Javeriana, 2007), 131. For native plants classified according to Galenic principles, such as wet or dry, hot or cold see: RGI 2: 7–9 Relación de la ciudad de Cuzco, Vasco de Contreras y Valverde 1 Jan. 1650, and ARJBM División 1, legajo 17 Libro de examen de los simples medicinales 1617 *passim*.

33 Estes, "European Reception," 11–13.

Paracelsianism

Paracelsus argued for an experimental approach to the diagnosis and treatment of illness and advocated the employment of chemical methods that were being used by alchemists. Alchemists were concerned with the search for the legendary Philosopher's Stone, which it was thought could turn base metals into gold and prolong life. In the search for this substance they focussed on the transformation of minerals containing mercury and sulphur using methods of distillation, calcination and sublimation. By the late thirteenth and early fourteenth centuries these processes had produced the discoveries of alcohol and mineral acids, notably sulphuric acid (oil of vitriol) and nitric acid (*aqua fortis*).[34] These methods were also applied to other *materia medica*, particularly herbs. Distillation and mineral acid dissolution aimed to produce purer forms of waters or oils – "fifth essences" or quintessences – that were seen to have healing properties.[35] However, these medicines, like simple herbal remedies, were applied within a Galenic humoral framework. Even so, the experimental methods by which they were produced began to challenge the existing natural philosophy based on scholasticism. They questioned the humoral interpretation of illness and saw body malfunctioning to be the result of a chemical reaction caused by an external agent.[36] Chemistry was seen to be the key to understanding nature and central to medical treatments. As such Paracelsus promoted the *internal* application of chemically prepared medicines. Traditionally such medicines had been used quite extensively, but because of their

---

34 Allen G. Debus, *The Chemical Philosophy: Paracelsian Science and Medicine in the Sixteenth and Seventeenth Centuries* vol. 1 (New York: Science History Publication, 1977), 20–23; Robert P. Multhauf, "The Significance of Distillation in Renaissance Medical Chemistry," *Bulletin of the History of Medicine* 30 (1956): 330–33 and *Chemistry, and the Scientific Revolution* (Cambridge, Mass.: Harvard University Press, 2005), 12–25. For the relationship between alchemy and chemistry see: William R. Newman, "From Alchemy to 'Chymistry'," in *The Cambridge History of Science*, eds. Katharine Park and Lorraine Daston (Cambridge: Cambridge University Press, 2006), 3: 497–517.

35 Robert P. Multhauf, "Significance of Distillation," 333–36 and "John of Rupescissa and the Origin of Medical Chemistry," *Isis* 45(2)(1954): 359–61; Mar Rey Bueno and Maria Esther Alegre Pérez, "Renovación en la terapéutica real: los destiladores de su magestad, maestros simplicistas y médicos herbolarios de Felipe II," *Asclepio* 53 (1)(2001): 33.

36 Debus, *Chemical Philosophy,* 51–61; Allen G. Debus, *The English Paracelsians* (New York: Franklin Watts, Inc., 1968), 26–29 and "Chemists, Physicians and the Changing Perspectives on the Scientific Revolution," *Isis* 89 (1) (1998): 71–74; Bruce T. Moran, "The *Herbarius* of Paracelsus," *Pharmacy in History* 35(3) (1993): 99–127 and *Distilling Knowledge. Alchemy, Chemistry, and the Scientific Revolution* (Cambridge, Mass.: Harvard University Press, 2005), 71–79.

toxic properties had only been employed *externally*.[37] While distillation was still essential to their experiments, the Paracelsians, if not Paracelsus himself, became more interested in precipitates and residues.[38] Inorganic salts, often based on mercury, sulphur and antimony, and spirits (vitriol, laudanum and tartar), which had traditionally been used by alchemists to prepare quintessences, thus began to feature more prominently in medicines.[39]

José María López Piñero has argued that the adoption of chemical methods in Spain did not necessarily involve the acceptance of a new natural philosophy.[40] Indeed, Phillip II himself was interested in the process of distillation and established three distilleries, the first at Aranjuez in 1564. However, the medicines they produced were simple waters and oils that were based on botanical materials in which he had a special interest.[41] In fact Paracelsus's work was not well known in Spain, where the chemical methods that were employed developed more directly from the alchemic tradition embodied in the works of Ramón Llull, Arnau de Villanova, and John of Rupescissa, which had an influence beyond Spain in the fifteenth and sixteenth centuries.[42] In fact knowledge of distillation methods dated back to classical times having

37 Multhauf, "Significance of Distillation," 340–41; George Urdang, "How Chemicals Entered the Official Pharmacopoeias," *Archives internationales d'histoire des sciences* 7 (1954): 304. Paracelsus added salt to mercury and sulphur as the three essential material and symbolic components of matter.

38 Robert P. Multhauf, "Medical Chemistry and 'the Paracelsians'," *Bulletin of the History of Medicine* 28(1954): 125–26; Multhauf, "Significance of Distillation," 344–46; Debus, "Changing Perspectives on the Scientific Revolution," 73–74; Debus, *Chemical Philosophy* 1: 112–17. While vitriol was used by both Paracelsus and the Paracelsians, the former used it as a medicine itself, while his followers were more interested in it as a reactant to make other products.

39 Multhauf, "Medical Chemistry and the 'Paracelsians'," 110–20; De Vos, "From Herbs to Alchemy," 154–60.

40 José M. López Piñero and Francesc Bujosa Homar, "Tradición y renovación en la medicina española del siglo XVI," Asclepio vol. 30–31 (1978–1979): 285–306.

41 Francisco Javier Puerto Sarmiento, "Alquimia aúrea: alquimia y destilación en la corte de Felipe II (1527–1598)," *Dynamis* 17 (1997):118–26; Mar Rey Bueno and María Esther Alegre Pérez, "Los distiladores de Su Magestad: distilación, espagiria y paracelsismo en la corte de Felipe II," *Dynamis* 21 (2001): 331–47 and "Renovación," 27–55. In fact Philip II' s interest in chemical processes was inconsistent with orthodox Catholic beliefs which linked alchemy to witchcraft. This may help explain why the Inquisition was inconsistent in its approach to these practices (Puerto Sarmiento, "La farmacia renacentista española," 126).

42 Miguel López Pérez, "La influencia de la alquimia medieval hispana en la Europa moderna," *Asclepio* 54 (2002): 211–29; López Piñero, "Paracelsus and his Work," 113–41; Debus, "Paracelsus and the Delayed Scientific Revolution," 148–50.

been described by Dioscorides and Mesuë, whose texts were among the most commonly consulted by apothecaries in the early modern period.[43]

It has been argued that the development of Paracelsian medicine in Spain was delayed by the Counter Reformation. Following the Reformation, many countries in Europe began to censor the publication of heretical books and control the introduction of foreign literature. Some controls were introduced in Castile in 1502, but the main impetus came in 1558 when the Inquisition in Spain was ordered to compile an Index of prohibited books.[44] It included sections of Paracelsus's work, which being based on chemical principles were linked to witchcraft. This censorship coupled with the ban a year later on Spaniards studying abroad has traditionally been seen as having a detrimental impact on the development of medicine, and indeed science in general, delaying the Scientific Revolution in Spain until the late seventeenth century, behind that in England, France, and Italy.[45] However, recent research has questioned the efficacy of these controls, showing that few Spaniards sought training abroad and the law was often circumvented or ignored.[46] It has also demonstrated that chemical methods were being employed quite widely having developed from the practices used by alchemists, though generally within a Galenic framework, while works by Paracelsus and his followers circulated in Spain despite the prohibitions.[47] Furthermore, it has been noted that medical knowledge need not depend on the diffusion of printed texts, but might be disseminated in more informal ways.

43 Richard Palmer, "Pharmacy in the Republic of Venice in the Sixteenth Century," in *The Medical Renaissance of the Sixteenth Century*, eds. A. Wear, R.K. French and I.M. Lonie (Cambridge: Cambridge University Press, 1985), 114–15.

44 Kamen, *Spanish Inquisition*, 103–34.

45 López Piñero, *Ciencia y técnica*, 141–44; López Piñero, "Paracelsus and his Work," 119–21; Debus, "Paracelsus and the Delayed Scientific Revolution," 148, 160–61; Jonathan I. Israel, "Counter Reformation, Economic Decline, and the Delayed Impact of the Medical Revolution in Catholic Europe," in *Health Care and Relief in Counter-Reformation Europe*, eds. Ole Peter Grell, Andrew Cunningham, with Jon Arrizabalaga (London: Routledge, 1999), 40–55.

46 Goodman, "Philip II's Patronage," 50–53 and *Power and Penury*, 220–21; Kamen, *Spanish Inquisition*, 104–08. López Piñero, *Ciencia y técnica*, 121–22 notes that many works by Paracelsus and his followers circulated in Spain despite prohibitions at the end of the sixteenth century.

47 Rey Bueno, "Paracelsistas," 41–55. For recent evaluations of the impact of Paracelsus in Spain see: Rodríguez Guerrero, "Censura y Paracelsismo"; López Pérez, "Spanish Paracelsus Revisited."

Maintaining Medical Orthodoxy

During the sixteenth and early seventeenth centuries traditional humoral explanations for illness and their treatments were therefore being challenged in Europe, but what about Spanish America and specifically Peru? In the New World several procedures operated to maintain orthodox medical practice. Spain regulated medicine more than any other nation in the early modern period and it sought to transfer the regulatory framework that it was developing in Castile to the New World. This endeavored to regulate the training and licensing of medical practitioners, in part through the founding chairs in universities for teaching medicine and by establishing medical boards, the *tribunales del protomedicato*, under the authority of the Crown (See Chapter 2).[48] Even though the Crown did not regulate the trade in medicines, some official guidance was given on the products that a well-stocked pharmacy should possess that was based on the needs of humoral medical practice.[49] Furthermore, the Crown introduced a system of inspections to ensure that poor quality and dangerous drugs were not being sold.[50] In some regions of Europe the regulation of pharmacies was supported by physicians who sought to maintain their authority within the medical profession by limiting the activities of apothecaries to the preparation of only those medicines that were composed of ingredients specified in official pharmacopeia.[51]

Crown attempts to regulate medical practice in the New World were supported by the Inquisition which discouraged progressive developments through the censorship of books deemed to be heretical and through controls on the introduction of foreign literature. While these activities promoted orthodox medical practice, in fact they might have been counter-productive in creating a conservative intellectual environment in Spain that might encourage

48 Risse, "Medicine in New Spain," 15; Lanning, *Royal Protomedicato passim*; De Vos, "Art of Pharmacy," 6.

49 Charles Davis and María Luz López Terrada, "Protomedicato y farmacia en Castilla a finales del siglo XVI: edición crítica del *Catálogo de las cosas que los boticarios han de tener en sus boticas*, de Zamudio de Alfaro, protomédico general (1592–1599), *Asclepio* 62 (2) (2010): 579–626. In fact new medicines could be added, if they were judged to be effective within the context of Galenic medicine (Clouse, *Medicine*, 75–90).

50 *Novísima recopilación*, lib. 8 tit. 13, ley 2: 107 3 Mar. 1477 and ley 3: 107 2 Aug. 1593; *Recopilación de las leyes, pragmáticas (Muñoz)*, cap. 15 art. 2: 188; Clouse, *Medicine, Government and Public Health*, 114–17.

51 Harold J. Cook, "Physicians and Natural History," in *Cultures of Natural History*, eds. Nicholas Jardine, James A. Secord and Emma C. Spary (Cambridge: Cambridge University Press, 2008), 96–97.

some practitioners of a more progressive persuasion to develop their careers in the New World where surveillance was more limited. The remainder of this chapter therefore explores the successes and failures of official attempts to regulate medical practice, in particular the activities of *boticarios*, first directly through regulation and second indirectly through the actions of the Inquisition. The particular influences that these procedures may have had on medical practice will be viewed and assessed in the following chapter through an examination of the medicines that were actually prepared and employed in treatments in Lima.

The Regulation of Pharmacies

In Spain the regulation of apothecaries and their pharmacies originally lay with the municipal authorities. However, with the establishment of the *protomedicato* in 1477 control over the training, examining, and licensing of medical practitioners, that included *boticarios*, passed to specially appointed *protomédicos*, thereby reducing the role of municipalities in the regulation and inspection of *boticas*.[52] According to the Pragmatic of 1593, inspections were to be conducted annually by *corregidores* accompanied by two *regidores* and an approved physician; those conducted in Seville also included *boticarios*.[53] These *visitas* scrutinised the titles of *boticarios* and inspected the pharmacies' medicines, weights, and measures. The inspections often resulted in fines and the destruction of poor quality and potentially dangerous drugs; in extreme cases a *botica* could be closed down.[54] A city-wide inspection of *boticas* in

52 José Luis Valverde, "Regulaciones de farmacia contenidas en las ordenanzas municipales de las ciudades españolas," *Sonderdruck aus Veröffentlichungen der Internationalen Gesellschaft für Geschichte der Pharmazie* [*Die Vörträge der Hauptversammlung in Luxemburg*]: 36: 135–57. Stuttgart, 1970.

53 *Recopilación de las leyes, pragmáticas* (Muñoz), cap. 15 art. 2: 188; *Novísima recopilación*, lib. 8 tit. 13 ley 9: 107 a Aug. 1593. For sixteenth and early seventeenth century inspections in Seville see: AMS Varios Antiguos 414 Visitas de boticas 12 Apr. 1614, 1625, 1631; AMS Sección 13 siglo XVII vol. 2 doc. 6 fols. 50–51v. 1631; Fernández-Carrión and Valverde, *Farmacia y sociedad*, 21–28; M. Fernández-Carrión and D. Martín-Castilla, "Francisco de Ortega y la profesión farmacéutica sevillana en el primer tercio del siglo XVII," *Boletín de la Sociedad Española de Historia de la Farmacia* 37 (148) (1986): 293–99; Herrera Dávila, "Boticas sevillanas," 73–78.

54 Lanning, *Royal Protomedicato*, 243–44. Accounts of Sevillan *visitas* do not describe the contents of *boticas*, but refer to items as being absent or in a bad state.

Seville in 1631 resulted in over half of its 49 *boticarios* being fined.[55] It was an imperfect system that was open to fraud, bribery, and favouritism.[56] During an earlier inspection of the Seville's *boticas* in 1594 by the Madrileño *boticario*, Juan Pérez de Prado, several *boticarios* had complained that he had levied illegal payments for the inspection and imposed arbitrary and excessive fines, noting that he had dined in the houses of several *boticarios*, which was against the law.[57]

Not only were the inspectors required to ensure the quality of the medicines, but also that pharmacies contained particular essential *materia medica*. Although several pharmacopoeias were published in Spain in the early sixteenth century,[58] it was not until 1593 that the Crown ordered that a "general pharmacopeia" should be drawn up by Spain's *protomédicos*, three physicians, and three *boticarios* that would serve as guidance for apothecaries and pharmacy inspectors.[59] It was previously thought that a pharmacopeia such as this was not produced until the eighteenth century.[60] However, a list entitled "Catálogo de las cosas que los boticarios han de tener en sus boticas," that was drawn up in the late 1590s by Andrés Zamudio de Alfaro who was *protomédico general* in Spain, has recently been uncovered by Charles Davis and María Luz López Terrada.[61] The *materia medica* included in his extensive list of over 400 items is contained in Appendix B. The extent to which inspectors, or indeed *boticarios* in Spain, used this list is not known. Nevertheless, there were other similar guides, such the *Directorio de boticarios* produced by the *boticario* Francisco de Ortega who inspected *boticas* in his home city of Seville in 1625.[62] Probably more commonly used, including in Peru, were pharmacy manuals written by

---

55 Herrera Dávila, "Boticas sevillanas," 76, 78–81. Actually 53 percent.

56 Lanning, *Royal Protomedicato*, 248–49.

57 AMS Sección 13 Siglo XVI vol. 1 doc. 114. Sevilla 20 Jun. 1594. See also Herrera Dávila, "Boticas sevillanas," 76–77 for a case brought against Francisco de Ortega.

58 Davis and López Terrada, "Protomedicato y farmacia," 589. See Chapter 6 for a discussion of pharmacopeias.

59 *Novísima recopilación de las leyes de España*, lib. 8 tit. 13, ley 3: 107 2 Aug. 1593.

60 Lanning, *Royal Protomedicato*, 233; Clouse, *Medicine*, 140.

61 This list was found among the papers of a *boticario*, Pedro de Brines, in the Archivo Histórico de Protocolos de Madrid 1744 fol. 793–94 and has been studied by Davis and López Terrada, "Protomedicato y farmacia."

62 Francisco de Ortega, *Directorio de boticarios, en que se ponen ocho advertencies…* (Sevilla: Matías Clavijo), 625. For the activities of Francisco de Ortega in Seville see: M. Fernández-Carrion and D. Martín-Castilla, "Francisco de Ortega," 289–301.

the Arabic scholar Mesuë (Yūhannā ibn Māsawayh),[63] or those based on his writings such as the Franciscan Bernardino de Laredo's, *Modus faciendi* (1527) and Luis de Oviedo's *Methodo de la colección, y reposición de las medicinas simples* (1581).[64] In any case, evidence from the contents of six *boticas* in Seville in the sixteenth and early seventeenth centuries shows a very clear correspondence between the types of products recommended by Zamudio de Alfaro and those kept in pharmacies in both Spain and Lima.[65]

The regulation of *boticas* in Peru followed the same procedures as in Spain and similarly included the inspection of hospital pharmacies.[66] The Pragmatics issued in 1477, 1491 and 1498 governing the operation of *protomedicatos* in Spain formed the basis for the regulation of medicine in America,[67] but their establishment in the New World was slow and incomplete. Initially the *cabildo* of Lima appointed *protomédicos* with the authority to licence doctors and inspect *boticas*[68] and when the Crown appointed Antonio Sánchez Renedo as *protomédico general* and president of the *Tribunal* in Lima in 1568,[69] it was reluctant to cede responsibility to him. It complained that Sánchez Renedo

63 For a study and revaluation of the importance of Mesuë see: Paula S. De Vos, "The 'Prince of Medicine': Yūhannā ibn Māsawayh and the Foundations of the Western Pharmaceutical Tradition," *Isis* 104 (4) (2013): 667–712.

64 Bernardino de Laredo, *Modus faciendi: cum ordine medicandi* (Seville: Jacobo Cromberger, 1527); Oviedo, *Methodo*. See also Chapter 6.

65 Fernández-Carrión and Valverde, *Farmacia y sociedad*, 80–96. See Appendix B.

66 Lanning, *Royal Protomedicato*, 52, 245–51.

67 In the mid-eighteenth century, Miguel Eugenio Muñoz, an *oidor* of the *audiencia* of Valencia and deputy of the *protomedicato* was appointed by the Crown to bring together the laws and decrees that had been issued in Spain relating to the *protomedicato*, which included these early pragmatics. Miguel Eugenio Muñoz, *Recopilación de las leyes, pragmáticas, reales decretos, y acuerdos del Proto-medicato* (Valencia: Imp. De la Viuda de Antonio de Bordazar, 1751). Online at: https://books.google.co.uk/books/about/Recopilacion_de_las_leyes_pragmaticas_re.html?id=JRe_Ab6MzzoC&redir_esc=y [Accessed 1 Mar. 2017]. The legislation is also found in *Novísima recopilación de las leyes de España* (Madrid, 1805) on line at: http://fama2.us.es/fde//ocr/2006/novisimaRecopilacionT1.pdf [Accessed 1 Mar. 2017].

68 See for example, the appointment of Lic. Hernando de Sepúlveda in 1537 (*Libros de cabildos de Lima,* 1: 141–42 Licenica al dotor [sic] Sepúlveda 27 Apr. 1537), Lic. Alvaro de Torres in 1551 (*Libros de cabildos de Lima,* 4: 371 Médicos 17 Apr. 1551), and Lic. Francisco Gutiérrez in 1556 (*Libros de cabildos de Lima,* 5: 520 El hospital despañoles médico y concierto con el 4 Sep. 1556).

69 Lastres, *Historia de la medicina peruana*, 2: 29–38, 57–58; Lanning, *Royal Protomedicato*, 29–30, 62. The municipality exerted control over the appointment of *protomédicos* for longer in Mexico City where a Tribunal was not established until 1646.

had not presented his title to the *cabildo* and should do so on pain of payment of the considerable fine of 1,000 pesos.[70] The *cabildo* was still complaining in 1576 when it suggested that even though Sánchez Renedo had inspected the *boticas*, *visitas* should follow the "custom [costumbre]" and be undertaken by members of the *cabildo* (*alcalde ordinario*, *regidor* and *fiel ejecutor*) with a physician of their choice.[71] Following the death of Sánchez Renedo in 1579, the *cabildo* reasserted its authority commissioning the *fiel ejecutor* (its officer for weights and measures) to conduct pharmacy inspections with a physician and *boticario*.[72]

Inspections in Lima do not appear to have been undertaken on the regular and systematic basis that was specified in the Pragmatics, but rather intermittently in response to complaints.[73] In 1581 it was said that the Lima's *boticas* had not been visited for "a long time" and that there were "great irregularities because the medicines that were being sold were corrupted and damaged and many of them [the *boticas*] lacked the principal ingredients from which complex medicines had to be made..."[74] In response, the *cabildo* appointed the interim *protomédicos* Doctors Alvaro de Torres and Enríque Méndez to conduct an inspection. Again in 1598 the *cabildo* observed that because it had been a long time since the city's pharmacies had been inspected, they contained many "corrupt medicines" which were "of no value." On this occasion it ordered all *boticas* to be closed and for them to be inspected by the *alcalde* and *fiel ejector* in company with the then royal *protomédico*, Iñigo de Hormero, who was ordered to take remedial action.[75] The exercise was repeated for the same reason five years later.[76]

---

70 *Libros de cabildos de Lima*, 7: 9 Que el protomédico mostrase en el cabildo el título, en ínterin no usase el dicho oficio 5 May 1570.

71 *Libros de cabildos de Lima*, 8: 226 Lo que toca a la visita de las boticas que le guarda la costumbre 9 Apr. 1576.

72 *Libros de cabildos de Lima*, 9: 73 Que se visiten las boticas 3 Aug. 1579.

73 Lanning, *Royal Protomedicato*, 52. See for example, the reaction of the *cabildo* to criticism of the *botica* belonging to Alonso de Alemán (*Libros de cabildos de Lima*, 2: 115 El bachiller Pacheco malquerencia 1 Dec. 1545).

74 AHML Libro 2 de cédulas y provisiones fol. 15v–16 and *Libros de cabildos de Lima*, 9: 408 Al señor licenciado Torres para lo de las boticas 14 Jul. 1581.

75 *Libros de cabildos de Lima* 13: 185–86 Que ysiban [exhiban] los títulos de cirujanos y barberos y boticarios 6 Nov 1598. Lanning (*Royal Protomedicato*, 53) suggests that overnight closure of all *boticas* was to prevent spoiled medicines being hidden or transferred between *boticas*.

76 *Libros de cabildos de Lima*, 14: 561–62 Sobre visitar los boticas 10 Nov. 1603.

From the earliest days, there were complaints about the poor quality of medicines available and the high prices that *boticarios* charged. The *cabildo* generally responded to these complaints by sending a doctor to investigate. In 1538, when Lima possessed only one *boticario*, Doctor Hernando de Sepúlveda was appointed to carry out an inspection and establish a list of prices.[77] However, less than a year later this *botica* still contained many medicines that were described as "muy dañadas," which the physician, Bachiller Juan de Castro was ordered to inspect and destroy.[78] Commonly inspections involved the posting of a list of prices.[79] This was regarded as particularly important for the poor, who often resorted to pharmacies and paid with "silver in hand" rather than getting a prescription from a physician.[80]

The regulation and inspection of pharmacies extended to hospitals, convents, and prisons. At the time the pharmacy of the Hospital of Santa Ana was established in 1551,[81] its *boticario* Francisco de Bilbao was contracted to supply it with medicines for a period of six years. However, this contract was dissolved two years later and in 1554 a new one was made with Pedro López to supply the Hospital, which at that time operated in conjunction with the hospital for Spaniards; two years later he was failing to meet his obligations.[82] Subsequently responsibility for ensuring that hospitals were supplied with medicines lay with their *mayordomos*.[83] The purchase of medicines constituted a significant proportion of the limited expenditure of hospitals, which depended largely on Crown disbursements, income from lands, donations, or charity. Typically the expenditure of hospitals exceeded their income. In 1570 the cost of running the Hospital of Santa Ana was estimated to be 8,000 pesos when its income was only 2,500 pesos; the cost of the medicines alone was estimated to be 3,000

---

77 *Libros de cabildos de Lima*, 1: 254 Visita de la botica desta ciudad 6 Dec. 1538. Unfortunately no records of the *arancel* have been found.

78 *Libros de cabildos de Lima*, 1: 387 [Curas con e[n]salmos] 16 Oct. 1539.

79 *Libros de cabildos de Lima*, 5: 108–09 Arancel de boticarios 17 Nov. 1553; *Libros de cabildos de Lima*, 5: 393 Para que hiciese arancel de boticarios 7 Feb. 1556.

80 *Libros de cabildos de Lima*, 5 108–09 Arancel de boticarios 17 Nov. 1553; *Libros de cabildos de Lima*, 5: 425 Boticarios 28 Mar. 1556.

81 AGNP Protocolos Siglo XVI 63 Diego Gutiérrez fols. 167–88 Hospital de los españoles y naturales compañía con Francisco de Bilbao de la botica 20 Oct. 1551; Cobo, *Obras*, 2:444; Rabí Chara, "Primera botica," 273–77. The initial construction of the Hospital of Santa Ana was made possible by the assignment of land by the Dominican, Archbishop, Jerónimo de Loayza, and several donations from the Crown (Guerra, *El hospital,* 433–34).

82 *Libros de cabildos de Lima*, 4: 511 El hospital que es tome la cuenta 18 Aug. 1556.

83 See Chapter 4.

pesos.[84] Similarly, in 1602 the *mayordomo* of San Andrés complained that the building was in ruins and that there were insufficient funds to pay the salaries of its employees or buy items for the pharmacy. At that time the Hospital's income was 12,000 pesos, while its running costs were estimated at 26,000 pesos a year.[85] The high cost of medicines reflected in part the large number of people being treated in the hospitals; the two main hospitals of Santa Ana and San Andrés were caring for about 2,000 patients each a year.[86] Meanwhile the basic income of the hospitals, which had initially derived from the tribute income from *encomiendas*, had declined significantly with the demographic collapse of the native population.[87] Not surprisingly, the archival sources are replete with petitions to the Crown for donations.

The *mayordomos* of the Hospitals of Santa Ana and San Andrés, who were appointed by the archbishop and *cabildo*, were required by hospital ordinances to ensure that their *boticas* were inspected by a physician every three to four months to ensure they were well stocked and that the medicines were not damaged.[88] Inspections of hospitals as a whole occurred less regularly, though they also included the pharmacy. Some, inspections such as those conducted of the Hospital of Santa Ana in 1606 and 1620, were conducted by the *protomédico* at the time, and the cost of these constituted an added burden on already stretched hospital finances.[89] The *visita* by the *protomédico* Melchor de Amusco in 1620 cost 52 pesos.[90] More often, however, inspections were undertaken by a member of a religious order and representatives of the *cabildo*.[91]

---

84 AGI Lima 122 Del hospital de los naturales de la ciudad de los reyes 16 Jan. 1570.

85 AGI Lima 214 no. 19 doc. 1 Don Fernando de Cordóva y Figueroa, mayordomo of San Andrés 6 Oct. 1602.

86 AGI Lima 301 Relación de las ciudades, villas y lugares, parrochias y doctrinas que ay en este Arzobispado de Lima 20 Apr. 1619.

87 AGI Lima 125 Juan Manuel Carrasco, mayordomo del hospital de Santa Ana 15 May 1604.

88 ABPL 9086 Cargos que resultan contra el bachiller Juan Manuel Carrasco, mayordomo del hospital de los naturales 17 Jan 1607; *Constituciones y ordenanzas del hospital de Santa Ana de Lima* art. 27 and 45 28 Feb. 1609; Lohmann Villena and Sarabia Viejo, *Francisco de Toledo*, 318 Ordenanzas para el hospital de San Andrés de Lima, 9 Oct. 1577.

89 The *visita* by the *protomédico* Melchor de Amusco in 1620 cost 52 pesos (ABPL 9097 Libro de cuentas de gastos del hospital de Santa Ana 1620 y 1621).

90 ABPL 9097 Libro de cuentas de gastos del hospital de Santa Ana 1620 y 1621.

91 For visitas see: ABPL 9086 fols. 65–92 Visita al hospital de Santa Ana 4 Dec. 1590, fols. 271–74 1588, fols. 118–23 1606, fols. 320–23 1607; ABPL 9097 Libro de cuentas de gastos del hospital de Santa Ana 1620 y 1621.

Formal responsibility for the supply of medicines to hospitals lay with their *mayordomos*. In 1607 when the mayordomo of the Hospital of Santa Ana, Bachiller Juan Manuel Carrasco, was accused with not having ensured that the *botica* was supplied with medicines, he claimed that neither the hospital's physician nor *boticario* had informed him that they were required.[92] Nevertheless, the medicines inspected during the 1606 *visita* were generally found to be in good condition. Only one item – bladder cherry (*trociscos de alquequenje*) – was to be destroyed, while the violets and polypody (*trociscos de polipodio*) were described as damp and were to be dried in the sun. An ointment with litharge (*unguento de almartaga*) was to be softened with Castilian oil (*aceite de Castilla*) and four of the syrups (*jarabes*) were to be perfected (*suba al punto*). Finally the senna was to be cleaned of dust and stems (*palillos*). The *visita* also noted that the pharmacy lacked chebulic myrobalan (*mirabolanos chebulos*). There is no evidence that *boticarios* were fined for not possessing particular types of medicines, though as will be shown in the next chapter, the general approach encouraged the use of Old World plant materials rather than native ones.

The Impact of the Counter Reformation and Inquisition

Just as it is difficult to be precise about the impact of the Counter Reformation and Inquisition on medical practice in Spain, so it is for Peru. In Spain the actions of the Inquisition served to create a conservative intellectual climate which, even if they did not result in the imprisonment or confiscation of goods of offenders, may have encouraged medical practitioners of a more progressive persuasion to migrate to Spanish America. One clear example, though for Cartagena rather than Lima, is Pedro López de León who arrived in the city in 1590 as surgeon to its hospital, garrison and the galleons that visited the port.[93] López de León spent more than twenty-five years in Cartagena and published a notable manual entitled *Práctica y teórica de las apostemas en general y particular. Questión y prácticas de cirugía, de heridas, llagas y otras cosas nuevos y particulares* (1628). He was a student of the progressive surgeon, Bartolomé Hidalgo de Agüero at the Hospital del Cardenal in Seville, who as a result of

92 ABPL 9086 Cargos que resultan contra el bachiller Juan Manuel Carrasco, mayordomo del hospital de los naturales 17 Jan. 1607.

93 Jairo Solano Alonso, *Salud, cultura y sociedad en Cartagena de Indias siglos XVI y XVII* (Universidad del Atlántico: Barranquilla, 1998), 127–29.

experimentation had come to oppose trepanation and periosteotomy and favour the drying and closing wounds to prevent contamination.[94]

In theory the greater distance of Peru from the metropolis should have made it an attractive destination for medical practitioners seeking to escape the surveillance of the Inquisition, even though a tribunal of the Inquisition was established in Lima in 1570.[95] *Conversos* were particularly vulnerable to being charged with heresy, as were those who employed chemical methods who might be accused of witchcraft. However, from the limited evidence available, it seems that the licenced medical practitioners that arrived in Peru generally had a conservative training at a Spanish university, very often at the University of Salamanca. One progressive physician and surgeon was Pedro Gago de Vadillo. He worked in hospitals in Huamanga and the mining district of Castrovirreyna, and ultimately in the Hospital of San Andrés in Lima. Although not a student of Hidalgo de Agüero, he similarly advocated the drying of wounds, a procedure that challenged traditional Galenic methods that used unguents and kept wounds open.[96] In his book, *Discurso de la verdadera cirujía y discursos de censura de ambas vías* (1632) he described various cures he had undertaken in the Hospital of San Andrés. Prior to 1640 only two physicians and two surgeons were brought before the Inquisition in Lima and it was for judaizing or promoting heretical beliefs rather than unorthodox medical practices.[97] One surgeon was Alexandre Pérez who came from Flanders. When his possessions were seized by the Inquisition in 1612, his library contained a mixture of traditional and progressive medical texts, including books on surgery by Doctor León,[98] Doctor Hidalgo,[99] Doctor Francisco Díaz,[100] and

94 Ibid., 110–11. On Bartolomé Hidalgo de Agüero see Kristy Wilson Bowers, "Tradition and Innovation in Spanish Medicine: Bartolomé Hidalgo de Agüero and the Vía Particular," *The Sixteenth Century Journal* 41(1)(2010): 29–47.

95 Kamen, *Spanish Inquisition*, 103–34; José T. Medina, *Historia del tribunal del Santo Oficio de la Inquisición de Lima* (Santiago, Chile: 1956), 1: 1–18.

96 Bowers, "Tradition and Innovation," 46–47. The full title is *Discursos de verdadera cirugía, y censura de ambas vías, y elección de la primera intención curativa, y unicion de las heridas* (Madrid: Juan Gonçalez, 1632).

97 Medina, *Historia del tribunal del Santo Oficio*, 1: 39, 310, 319; 2: 137. The two physicians, Juan Álvarez and Álvaro Nuñez, and the surgeon Tomé Cuaresma were all accused of judaizing. On Tomé Cuaresma see Newson and Minchin, *From Capture to Sale*, 264.

98 This would not have been the book by Pedro López de León which was not published until 1628. Possibly it was Andrés de León's *Tratados de medicina, cirugía, y anatomía* (Valladolid: Luis Sánchez, 1605).

99 Probably Bartolomé Hidalgo de Agüero, *Thesoro de la verdadera cirugía* (Seville, 1604).

100 Possibly Francisco Díaz, *Tratado nuevamente impresso, de todas las enfermedades de los riñones, vexiga, y carnosidades de la verga, y urina* (Madrid. F. Sánchez, 1588).

Doctor Murillo.[101] Other healers brought before the Inquisition included a priest and an *oidor* who were using herbs.[102] Another priest from Genoa was deported as an illegal immigrant, but not without some of his medical books being seized.[103]

Even though there may be little evidence of progressive medical practitioners migrating to Peru, this does not mean that all those who arrived were ignorant of modern methods. It is significant that in his manuscript Antonio de Robles Cornejo while referring most frequently to traditional texts such as those by Galen, Dioscorides, Avicenna, Mesüe and others, in discussing the qualities of minerals particularly also revealed knowledge of the methods that Paracelsus was advocating.[104] Neither does the limited evidence for progressive texts mean that medical practice lacked innovation. The absence of facilities for training and examining doctors in Spanish America meant that during the sixteenth century Creole practitioners often had little option but to work by trial and error, the experience of which led some to the conclusion that formal training was unnecessary. Moreover, they might be preferred as doctors. One surgeon in Santa Fe de Bogotá in the 1620s noted how new medical graduates arriving from Spain made many mistakes because the country was "a different region [with] a different climate, different medicines, different complexions, different foods, and as such different subjects."[105]

The Circulation of Medical Texts

Very little is known about the educational background of *boticarios* practising in Lima, but it seems likely that most acquired knowledge of the properties of different products and how to prepare them through a combination of on-the-job training, as described in Chapter 2, and consulting medical tracts and manuals that were available locally.[106] In this context the Inquisition through its scrutiny of books sent to the New World as well as those published

101 AGNP SO CO ca. 16 doc. 194 fols. 1–8 Secuestro de Alexandre Pérez, cirujano, de Flandes, en el pueblo de Yllimo (Saña) 1612. Other items confiscated were two books of remedies, part in Spanish and in Flemish, several boxes containing drugs wrapped in paper, a small chest with pharmacists' weights, two blistering jars and their covers, a bag of surgical instruments and some jars of medicinal cream. Murillo probably referred to Jerónimo Murillo, *Therapeutica, método de Galeno en lo que toca a cirugía* (Zaragoza, 1561).

102 Medina, *Historia del tribunal del Santo Oficio*, 109–10, 257–59.

103 Ibid., 138.

104 ARJBM División 1, legajo 17 fols. 588–91 Libro de examen de los simples medicinales Antonio de Robles Cornejo 1617.

105 AGNC Colonia Médicos y Abogados 11 fol. 853 Miguel de Çepeda Santa Cruz [1626].

106 See Chapter 6 on how medicines were prepared.

or circulating in Lima had the potential to influence the types of medicines prescribed. It is recognised, however, that this was not the only way in which knowledge of medicine and medical practice was diffused.

In general medical texts and manuals were not easy to acquire. At first the Crown banned the establishment of a printing press in Lima fearing that it might facilitate the spread of heretical literature. However, this policy became untenable in the face of the demand for catechisms to facilitate native conversion and the growing needs of the university.[107] In 1580 an Italian printer, Antonio Ricardo, having set up a printing press in Mexico City, was encouraged to move to Lima and four years later was given permission to establish one under the supervision of the Jesuits at the College of San Pablo. The first book to be printed there was the *Doctrina cristiana y catecismo para la instrucción de los indios* (1584).[108]

Any text to be printed in Lima had to be licensed by the viceroy or *audiencia*; ecclesiastical authors in addition had to obtain permission from their superiors. These bureaucratic obstacles were probably less significant barriers to publication than the practical difficulties that authors and printers faced. These included the cost of printing, shortages of paper, and poor quality typefaces that generally resulted in physically inferior books. Moreover, before 1630 there were only three printing presses in the city. These limitations meant that relatively few texts were produced in Lima, print runs were short, and authors commonly sought publication in Europe.[109] Those books that were published were predominantly theological, though legal texts also figured significantly, while some books on poetry and the history and culture of Peru and Europe were also printed.[110] Pedro Guibovich has calculated that only seven percent of over a thousand books published in Lima before 1700 were in the field of

---

107 AGI Lima 126 Vecinos of Lima 12 Aug. 1581, Doctores de la universidad 13 Aug. 1581.

108 Rubén Vargas Ugarte, *Impresos peruanos (1584–1650)* (Lima: Universidad Nacional San Marcos, 1953), 1: 6–10; José Toribio de Medina, *La imprenta en Lima,* 1584–1824 (Santiago: Impreso y grabado en casa del autor, 1904), xx–xxx; Pedro M. Guibovich Pérez, "Printing Press in Colonial Peru: Production Process and Literary Categories in Lima," *Colonial Latin American Review* 10 (2) (2001):168–69. For the testament of Antonio Ricardo see: "Testamento de Don Antonio Ricardo," *Revista del Archivo Nacional del Perú* 19 (1955): 293–306.

109 Salinas y Córdova, *Memorial,* 1: 257; Guibovich Pérez, "Printing Press," 168–73; Catalina Romero Romero, "Libros, cultura y sociedad en el Perú virreinal: Las bibliotecas de los colegios jesuitas de Arequipa, Potosí y las misiones de Moxos en el siglo XVIII." PhD diss., Universidad de Complutense de Madrid, 1992. Vol 1: 4–21.

110 Antonio Rodríguez-Buckingham, "Change and the Printing Press in Sixteenth-Century Spanish America," in *Agent of Change: Print Culture Studies after Elizabeth L. Einstein,* eds. Sabrina Alcorn Baron, Eric N Lindquist and Eleanor F. Shevlin (Amherst and Boston: University of Massachusetts Press, 2007), 228–30.

applied sciences, and of those only ten were on medicine.[111] The first medical text to be published in Lima was Matías de Porres's book, *Breve advertencies para beber frío con nieve*, which was published in 1621.[112]

With few books being printed locally, the majority of those circulating in Lima either accompanied their immigrant owners to Peru or were brought by merchants for booksellers on commission or for sale on their own account. Many professionals, including medical practitioners, who migrated to the New World took books with them, no doubt forewarned that they were harder to come by and more expensive than in Spain. The high cost of books derived in part from transport costs, taxes, and the higher cost of living,[113] but also from the significant profits expected by merchants involved in the book trade.[114] Cheaper second-hand books might be sold in the marketplace when their owners died and undoubtedly others were inherited.[115]

In theory all books that arrived in the New World had been inspected and approved by the Inquisition. In 1558 the Spanish Inquisition was ordered to compile an Index of prohibited books and between 1559 and 1784 the Spanish crown published eight Indexes of banned books. All books written by Paracelsus were banned.[116] Other texts were permitted but with certain sections expurgated. These included the writings of the physician and alchemist Arnau de Vilanova, who employed experimental methods that included distillation and the preparation of alcohol and mineral acids.[117] Books on the banned list

111 Guibovich Pérez, "Printing Press," 179.

112 Vargas Ugarte, *Impresos peruanos*, 1: 90. For a discussion of Porres and his work see: Mar Rey Bueno, "Concordias," 347–62.

113 Guillermo Aulet Sastre, "Precios autorizados de libros españoles en Indias," *Revista de Indias* 24 (1946): 311–12; Teodoro Hampe-Martínez, "The Diffusion of Books and Ideas in Colonial Peru: A Study of Private Libraries in the Sixteenth and Seventeenth Centuries," *Hispanic American Historical Review* 273(2)(1993): 220–21; Romero Romero, "Libros, cultura y sociedad," 20; Pedro Guibovich Pérez, "Bibliotecas de médicos en Lima colonial," in *Del autor al lector*, ed. Carmen Castañeda (Mexico City: CIESAS, 2002), 296. Prices were even higher in Cuzco (Leonard, *Books of the Brave*, 299–300).

114 AGI Lima 143 fol. 35 Memorial y apuntamiento sumario de las cosas muy importantes 1612. For the import taxes paid on books see Chapter 4.

115 Guibvoich, "Bibliotecas de médicos," 303.

116 *Index et catalogus librorum prohibitorum* (Madrid: Apud Alphonsum Gomezium, 1583), 60; José Pardo-Tomás, *Ciencia y censura: la Inquisición española y los libros científicos en los siglos XVI y XVII* (Madrid: CSIC, 1991), 220–27.

117 *Index et catalogus librorum prohibitorum*, 10; Debus, *Chemical Philosophy*, 20–21, 24. For other medical texts banned by the Inquisition in the sixteenth century see: José Pardo-Tomás, "Autores médicos en los índices inquisitoriales españoles del siglo XVI," *Dynamis* 5–6 (1985–1986): 201–14.

did not remain constant over time. Books that had been previously sanctioned might later be expurgated or banned. For example, Andrés Laguna's interpretation of Dioscorides, which had been widely used in the sixteenth century, was expurgated in 1632 to make it more faithful to the original classical text and to remove any hypothetical superstitions, for example the supposed abortifacient properties of cardamom. From 1612 some of the philosophical writings of Francisco Valles who had been *protomédico* in Spain, were also expurgated.[118] In general, censorship was most intense in the first part of the seventeenth century.[119]

All books that were imported, whether they were carried by individuals or merchants, were examined when they were loaded onto ships in Seville and again when they arrived in Callao, whilst in Lima printing presses, bookshops and public and private libraries, including the extensive ones owned by the religious orders, were all subject to inspection.[120] While the focus of the Inquisition was on books of a heretical nature, there were areas where medical texts might be interpreted to fall in this category. These were the fields of alchemy and astrology, especially judicial astrology, where practices were often associated with magic and witchcraft.[121] It was in these areas that the inquisitors focussed their attention.[122]

Pedro Guibovich argues that in Lima the impact of Inquisition was greater on the circulation of books than on their production, since authors often self-censured to ensure that their works did not attract Inquisitorial attention. Hence, when Juan de Figueroa, himself apothecary to the Inquisition, argued in his *Opúsculo de astrología de medicina* (1660) that astrology and knowledge of the heavens was essential for curing sickness, he was at pains to point out that the text did not contradict orthodox Christian beliefs and indeed he

118 Pardo-Tómas, *Ciencia y censura*, 217–19, 252.

119 Guibovich Pérez, *Censura*, 346.

120 Eguiguren, *Diccionario histórico cronológico*, 1: 664; Guibovich, *Censura*, 99–132. For the process in Spain see: Pardo-Tomás, *Ciencia y censura*, 29–45; Gonzalez Sánchez, *New World Literacy*, 50–54. The AGI contains the records of all cargoes sent to the Americas in individual ships. The titles of all books are included, whether or not they belonged to private individuals or were being shipped to booksellers. For the period under study see AGI Contratación 1080–1184 Registros de navíos 1583–1640.

121 Pardo-Tomás, *Ciencia y censura*, 154–82, 248–64; Guibovich, *Censura*, 219–20.

122 Medina, *Historia del tribunal del Santo Oficio*, 2: 35–41. A decree issued by the Inquisition in Lima in 1629 specified the activities that fell under "astrología judiciaria" and "arte mágica" were to be regarded as heretical, including the use of hallucinogenic drinks made of achuma (*Trichocereus bridgesii* Britton & Rose), chamico (*Datura ferox* L.) and coca.

dedicated the volume to the Viceroy.[123] Others avoided censure by circulating their writings in manuscript form rather than through publication.[124] Pedro Guibovich has also argued that Juan Gerónimo Navarro's *Sangrar y purgar en días de convención* (1645) which employed empirical methods to challenge prevailing ideas about bloodletting on particular days, escaped censure because he was part of Lima's small elite that included the Jesuits who scrutinised his work.[125]

As was recognised at the time, the inquisitorial process was imperfect. Books might be hidden in other cargoes of merchandise or bound in with other works, while often there were insufficient personnel to conduct inspections, which were often cursory.[126] In 1583 Inquisitor Ulloa was concerned that cargoes destined for Lima were being unloaded in the ports of Guayaquil, Manta, and Paita where there were no commissioners to carry out inspections. He recommended that priests who lived in the vicinity should arrange for all books to be returned to the ships and brought to Lima.[127] Even where books were inspected, it has been argued in the case Mexico that most examinations were conducted by theologians with little knowledge of science and medicine, so that unless books were obviously related to magic or witchcraft banned items might easily slip through the inquisitorial net.[128] Among the belongings of one Pedro Durango de Espinosa, a deceased Spanish bookseller who became domiciled in Lima, were two copies of the Koran![129] One shipment of books to two booksellers of Cuzco, Rodrigo de Fajardo and Bartolomé Arias contained a text entitled "fisonomía natural."[130] This might be *Libro de phisonomia natural y varios secretos de naturaleza* by Jerónimo Cortés, a scientist and astrologist, which was published in Valencia in 1598. Although this volume was not

---

123 Guibovich, *Censura*, 249, 258–60, 268. He comments that the three copies he consulted had a lot of marginalia indicating that it was widely consulted.

124 Guibovich, *Censura*, 274.

125 Pedro Guibovich, "Autores, censores y producción de libros en el virreinato peruano" (2015), 7–8. Unpublished manuscript at: https://escriturasvirreinales.files.wordpress.com/2015/05/guibovich-autores_y_censores-u-c.pdf [Accessed 11 Nov. 2015].

126 Leonard, *Books of the Brave*, 174–79; Guibovich, *Censura*, 266–67.

127 Archivo Histórico Nacional, Madrid. Inquisición 1034 fol. 355 Licenciado Antonio Gutiérrez de Ulloa 1 Feb. 1583.

128 Guibovich, *Censura*, 263.

129 AGI Contratación 273 R3 N73 (fol.37) Bienes de difuntos de Pedro Durango de Espinosa 1606; Carlos A. González Sánchez, "Consideraciones sobre el comercio de libros en Lima a principios del siglo XVII," *Anuario de Estudios Americanos* 54 (2) (1997): 681.

130 AGI Contratación 1138B N8: 366 Registro del navío Nuestra Señora del Rosario 1601.

censured, a popular almanac by the same author entitled *Lunario y pronostico perpetuo*, first published in Valencia in 1594, was expurgated in 1632.[131]

A wealth of evidence exists for the texts that were available for use by medical practitioners in early colonial Lima. These take the form of inventories of books accompanying imported cargoes and handled by booksellers, as well as lists included in the testaments of apothecaries. Studies using these sources have revealed that they were dominated by theological and legal titles, though chronicles, histories, novels, and poetry also figured.[132] Booksellers generally possessed only a few titles related to medicine and pharmacy, but this might be expected given the small size of the market for books of this kind.[133] The titles in circulation were overwhelmingly traditional texts, such as those by Galen, Hippocrates, Dioscorides, Mesuë, or their interpreters. The field of surgery was dominated by Juan Fragoso's *Chirugía universal* (1581) and that of pharmacy by Bernardino de Laredo's *Modus faciendi* (1527). There were a number of other texts, however, which figured quite often and reveal an interest in the medicinal use of plants recently encountered in both the Americas and Far East.[134] These included the Seville-based physician-trader-botanist, Nicólas Monardes', *Dos libros, el uno que trata de todas las cosas que se traen de nuestras Indias Occidentales que sirven al uso de la medicina* (Seville, 1565) and the Sevillan physician, Simón de Tovar's *De compositorum medicamentorum examine, nova methodus* (Antwerp, 1586). Also represented was Cristóbal de Acosta's, *Tratado*

131 López Piñero, *Ciencia y técnica*, 195; Pardo-Tomás, *Ciencia y censura*, 282.

132 Irving A. Leonard, "Best Sellers of the Lima Book Trade," *Hispanic American Historical Review* 22(1) (1942): 5–33; Irving A. Leonard, "On the Lima Book Trade, 1591," *Hispanic American Historical Review* 33(4)(1953): 515–19; Carlos A. González Sánchez, "El libro y la carrera de Indias: registro de ida de navíos," *Archivo hispalense* 72 (1989): 96–97; Hampe-Martínez, "Diffusion of books"; Carlos A. González Sánchez, "Los libros de los españoles el virreinato del Perú. Siglos XVI y XVI," *Revista de Indias* 56 (no. 206) (1996), 7–47; González Sánchez, "Consideraciones sobre el comercio," 665–92. Several of Leonard's articles have been revised and published as, *Books of the Brave*. Even though these are scholarly studies, they have only used a fraction of the documentary sources available.

133 Leonard, "Best Sellers," 5–33; Eguiguren, *Diccionario histórico cronológico*, 697–722; Guibovich, "Bibliotecas de médicos," 302. For the development of the Lima book trade see Leonard, "On the Lima Book Trade," 515–19; Guibovich, *Censura*, 265–67.

134 For books published that showed an interest in newly-discovered plants see: Puerto Sarmiento, "Farmacia renacentista," 105–11, 116–18. For Nicolás Monardes see: Barrera-Osorio, *Experiencing Nature*, 122–23; J. López Piñero, "Las 'nuevas medicinas' americanos en la obra (1565–1574) de Nicolás Monardes," *Asclepio* 42 (1)(1990): 3–67; for the biography of Monardes see: Francisco Guerra, *Nicolás Bautista Monardes: Su vida y su obra (ca. 1493–1588)* (Mexico: Fundidora, 1961).

de las drogas y medicinas de la indias orientales (Burgos, 1578), which contained descriptions of plants found in the Far East, based on Garcia de Orta's *Colóquios dos simples e drogas da India* (Goa, 1563).[135]

Experimental tendencies are suggested by the work entitled "esperimentos médicos" which was imported by the booksellers of Cuzco, Rodrigo de Fajardo and Bartolomé Arias.[136] This was probably Jerónimo Soriano's, *Libro de experimentos médicos, fáciles y verdaderos* (Zaragoza, 1598). It was a collection of "experiments" or remedies assembled for use by the public at large. It included those that had been proposed by eminent medical experts to which the author suggested modifications that he had gleaned from his own experience.[137] From a different, but potentially experimental perspective, there is evidence for the possession of texts dealing with minerals. This is perhaps not surprising given the abundance of minerals that the Spanish encountered in Peru. One text found in many cargoes of books was Gaspar de Morales's, *Libro de las virtudes y propiedades maravillosas de las piedras preciosas* (1605), which was eventually banned by the Inquisition.[138] In fact in 1606, one Juan de Sarria, a book seller in Lima, certified that he had received nineteen copies of the book from Spain.[139]

In understanding what the Spanish authorities perceived to be best pharmacy practice, the list of books imported for the establishment of the first *botica* for the Hospital of Santa Ana in 1551 is instructive (Appendix B). It is worth noting that it pre-dates policies emanating from the Council of Trent.[140] Of the eleven books shipped for the pharmacy, the overwhelming majority were written in the Galenic tradition.[141] There was no copy of Galen's *De Simplicibus*,

---

135 AGI Contratación 1127 N2 fol. 94 Registro de Francisco Marroquín 1598. For Simón de Tovar see: Miguel López Pérez y Mar Rey Bueno, "Simón de Tovar (1528–1596): redes familiares, naturaleza Americana y comercio de maravillas en la Sevilla del XVI," *Dynamis* 26 (2006): 69–91.

136 AGI Contratación 1138B N8: 366 Registro del navío Nuestra Señora del Rosario 1601.

137 Michael Solomon, *Fictions of Well-Being: Sickly Readers and Vernacular Medical Writing in Late Medieval and Early Modern Spain* (Philadelphia: University of Pennsylvania Press, 2010), 54–55, 58–60.

138 González Sánchez, "Consideraciones sobre el comercio," 683, 689; Pardo-Tomás, *Ciencia y censura*, 361; Guibovich, *Censura*, 339. Guibovich gives the date of the ban as 1649, whereas Pardo-Tomás gives it as 1707.

139 Leonard, *Libros del conquistador*, 343.

140 AGNP Protocolos Siglo XVI 63 Diego Gutiérrez fols. 177v.–178 Quenta de la botica 20 Oct. 1551. See also: Rabí Chara, "Primera botica," 276–77.

141 For an account of medical texts produced and circulating in Spain in the sixteenth century see López-Piñero, *Ciencia y técnica*, 339–70.

but various Arab treatises based on his works, such as those by Avicenna, Mesuë, and Serapion, the last being the author of a twelfth century herbal.[142] It also included Luis Lobera Ávila's *Banquete de los nobles caballeros* (Augsburg, 1530). Lobera de Ávila was *protomedico* to Charles I and his text focussed on ailments commonly found among the privileged. Books on pharmacy included Bernardino de Laredo's *Modus faciendi* (Seville, 1527), which followed the Galenic-Arab tradition, but incorporated his own experiences; it was the first to be written in the Spanish language.[143] On surgery, there was a volume by the Italian Juanes de Vigo (Giovanni da Vigo), possibly *Practica in arte chirurgica copiosa* (Rome, 1514). He was noted for his powders of red precipitate of mercury which were used to treat skin diseases and syphilitic ulcers.[144] Noteworthy for this discussion was the inclusion of "un arnaldo," which almost certainly referred to a text written by the physician and alchemist, Arnau de Vilanova, based in Montpellier. Although Vilanova wrote within the Galenic tradition, his works contained accounts of distillation and the preparation of alcohol and mineral acids.[145] He has traditionally been described as an alchemist, but more recent scholarship suggests that such methods were widely known at the time and has questioned whether Vilanova was the innovator in the field that he is often held up to be.[146] There is evidence that his work was also owned by the two *boticarios* in Lima, Bartolomé Díaz Cabeza de Vaca[147] and Francisco Martín Reyna.[148] For the aid of pharmacists there was also a copy of the "vocabulario de Antonio," the first Latin vocabulary in Spanish published in Salamanca in 1492. Other unspecified titles included "un guido,"[149] probably one of the texts of the fourteenth-century French physician and surgeon,

142 These works were recommended for *boticarios* by the fifteenth century Italian pharmacist Saladino d'Ascoli, whose *Compendio de los boticarios* was translated into Spanish by Alonso Rodríguez de Tudela in 1515 (Saladino de Ascoli, *Compendio de los boticarios* (Valladolid: Arnao Guillén de Brocar, 1515)). See also Pastor Frechoso, *Boticas,* 38 n. 3.

143 López Piñero and Bujosa Homar, "Tradición y renovación," 293.

144 Laval, *Botica*, 139.

145 Debus, *Chemical Philosophy,* 20–21, 24.

146 See Michael McVaugh, "Chemical Medicine in the Medical Writings of Arnau de Vilanova." II *Trobada Internacional d'Estudis sobre Arnau de Vilanova. Arxiu de Textos Catalans Antics* 23–24: (2004–2005): 239–264.

147 AGNP Protocolos Siglo XVI 819 Hernández Francisco fol. 176v. Testamento de Bartolomé Díaz Cabeza de Vaca boticario 1608.

148 AGI Contratación 1097 N5 fol. 197 Registro de Santa Catalina 1592.

149 Probably a reference to *Cirugía magna* by the fourteenth-century French physician and surgeon Guy de Chauliac (Guido de Cauliaco), whose treatise relied heavily on Galen and Avicenna (Garciá Ballester, *Búsqueda de la salud*, 550).

Guido de Cauliaco (Guy de Chauliac); "un pandeta,"[150] an encyclopaedia, probably that compiled by Matthaeus Silvaticus; and "un luminaria mayor." The last was probably *Luminare maius, seu Interpretatio antidotarii et practicae Johannis Mesue* (Venice, 1496). This interpretation of Mesuë by Giovanni Giacomo Manlio was one of the earliest books on pharmacy to be written by an apothecary.

The largest library relating to pharmacy in Lima was in the hands of the Jesuit College of San Pablo.[151] In the early seventeenth century Bernabé Cobo recorded that it possessed 40,000 books and that "it is rare that there is a book it doesn't possess."[152] At that time its library of medical books was dominated by those from Spain, but it also included a significant number of texts on different branches of medicine published in Italy and France. On pharmacy it included the great pharmacopoeias of Luis de Oviedo and Juan de Castillo that were widely used in Spain at the time,[153] and Girolamo Mercuriale's *De compositione medicamentorum* published in Venice in 1590. The last, and maybe many other books published in Italy, may have been brought by the Italian Jesuit pharmacist, Augustino Salumbrino, who arrived at the College in 1605 with the intention of establishing a pharmacy that would supply Jesuit colleges and haciendas throughout the Viceroyalty.[154] Other medical texts included books on surgery such as *Thesoro de la verdadera cirugía y via particular contra la común* (Seville, 1604) written by the progressive surgeon Bartolomé Hidalgo de Agüero, referred to above, as well as Juan Calvo's *Primera y segunda parte de la cirugía universal del cuerpo humano* (Seville, 1580). Italian authors included Giovanni Battista Cortesi, an anatomist from Bologna, Gabrielle Falopio from Padua, and Michele Mercati from Milan, and there were also writings by the Parisian anatomist, Jean Riolan, an ardent defender of Galen, and the sixteenth century Italian mathematician, physician, and astrologer, Girolamo

150 Probably *Liber pandectarum medicinae*, completed by Matthaeus Silvaticus in 1317 and published in number of editions from the fourteenth century.

151 Martín, *Intellectual Conquest*, 106–08; Luis Martin, La biblioteca del Colegio de San Pablo (1568–1767), antecedente de la Biblioteca Nacional pp. 24–29 http://www.comunidadandina.org/bda/docs/PE-CA-0015.pdf [Accessed 16 Nov. 2015]; Guibovich, "Bibliotecas de médicos," 302.

152 Cobo, *Obras*, 2: 425.

153 Oviedo, *Methodo* and Juan de Castillo, *Pharmacopoea, universa medicamenta in officinis pharmaceuticis usitata complectens, et explicans* (Cádiz: Gadibus: Apud Joannem de Borja, 1622).

154 Martín, *Intellectual Conquest*, 99–100, 106; Martín, "Biblioteca del Colegio de San Pablo," 29; Rocco, *Miraculous Fever-Tree*, 69–71.

Cardano, who defended the Hippocratic tradition.[155] Many of these volumes may have been brought by members of the clergy who came from different parts of Europe. Medical practitioners in Lima may have been aware of these texts since they were allowed to borrow books from the College's library.[156] In 1647 the physician Juan Gerónimo Navarro had in his possession some eighty books belonging to the library which he ordered to be returned on his death.[157] Progressive texts may not have been exclusive to the College, either. While Navarro's personal library of some 400 books contained many medical volumes by interpreters of Galen and Hippocrates, including Laguna, Avicenna, and Mesuë, and even duplicate copies of some of them, he also owned a significant number of volumes on meteorology and astronomy in which he had a particular interest. These were no doubt sources for his book *Sangrar y purgar en días de conjunción* (Lima, 1645), which challenged some prevailing humoral beliefs.[158]

Focussing on the volumes possessed by private individuals one of the largest cargoes of medical books was sent from one Licenciado Pedro Colorado in Spain to the physician Doctor Melchor de Amusco in 1584. At that time Amusco was resident in Nombre de Dios, but he was to become *protomédico* in Peru.[159] The whole consignment contained over seventy books (See Appendix C). It is not possible to identify all the titles and not all were medical texts, but traditional Galenic medical titles figured prominently.[160] Most cargoes of medical books, as well as those owned by *boticarios* themselves, contained far fewer titles, generally only ten or twelve. Commonly they included copies of Mesuë, Dioscorides, Arnau de Vilanova, Serapion, and Laredo, all practical manuals rather than medical texts, but occasionally books by Italian doctors, all of a conservative persuasion, such as Antonio Musa[161] and Giovanni

155 Martín, *Intellectual Conquest*, 107. On Girolamo Cardano see: Girolamo Cardano, *Book of My Life*, trans. Jean Stoner (New York: New York Review Books, 2002) and Guido Giglioni, "Girolamo Cardano: University Student and Professor," *Renaissance Studies* 27 (4) (2013): 517–32.

156 Guibovich, "Bibliotecas de médicos," 302.

157 AAL Testamentos 28A-1 fols. 81v.–82, 207v.–208 Testamento de Juan Gerónimo Navarro 1648.

158 AAL Testamentos 28A-1 fols. 127–47 Testamento de Juan Gerónimo Navarro 1648.

159 According to the Jesuit annual letter of 1632 Melchor de Amusco left a thorn from the Christ's crown of thorns and other holy relics in his will (ARSI Peru 15 fol. 32v. Carta annua [1632 sic] Antonio Vázquez 28 May 1635).

160 AGI Contratación 1081 N2 R1 fols. 67–68 Registro de Juan Bautista de Olarte 1584.

161 He published a number of texts on pharmacy: *Examen omnium simplicium medicamentorum, quorum in officinis usus est. Jean & François Frellon* (Lyon, 1537); *In octo libros*

Battista Susio,[162] and the orthodox Italian Franciscan, Bernardino de Siena.[163] Apart from using the texts themselves, it seems that *boticarios* may also have been selling books of a medical nature. The testament of Bartolomé Díaz Cabeza de Vaca indicated that one Licenciado Alvaro owed him for an "Arnaldo" and five large copies of "Galen,"[164] while in 1610 the *boticario* Pedro de Bilbao imported three copies of "Oviedo," one "Laguna sobre Dioscórides," and one of "Fragoso de botica" from Spain.[165] This emphasis on traditional Galenic texts parallels the findings of Germán Somolinos for Mexico where in the sixteenth and first half of the seventeenth century the libraries of physicians were dominated by traditional texts.[166]

Conclusion

The Spanish authorities clearly took steps to encourage orthodox medical practices, among other things through the regulation of pharmacies and by restricting the medical texts available. Specifying the types of products pharmacists were to stock and instituting inspections clearly encouraged the adherence to humoral medical practice, even if the inspections were not conducted regularly or systematically. Also influential was the fact that medicines

aphorismorum Hippocratis & Galeni commentaria & annotationes (Basel, 1541); *In libros de ratione victus in morbis acutis Hippocratis & Galeni commentaria & annotationes* (Venice, 1546); *Examen omnium electuariorum* (Venice, 1548).

162 Possibly *Liber de sanguinis mittendi ratione* (Basel, 1558) or *Libro del conoscere la pestilenza* (Mantova, 1576).

163 For examples of the books imported and contained in pharmacies see: John Carter Brown Library Mss Codex Sp. 136 Francisco Martínez y compañía, obligación 1555; AGI Contratación 1097 N5 fol. 197 Registro del navío Santa Catalina 1592; AGI Contratación 1127 lib. 2: 94 Registro del navío San Cristóbal 1598; AGI Contratación 1155B N8: 463, 703 Registro del navío Nuestra Señora de la Concepción 1610; AGNP Protocolos Siglo XVII 819 Francisco Hernández fol. 176v. Testamento de Bartolomé Díaz Cabeza de Vaca boticario 1608.

164 AGNP Protocolos Siglo XVI 819 Francisco Hernández fol. 176v. Testamento de Bartolomé Díaz Cabeza de Vaca boticario 1608.

165 AGI Contratación 1155B N8 463, 703 Registro del navío Nuestra Señora de la Concepción. This could be *Discursos de las cosas aromáticas, árboles y frutales, y de otras muchas medicinas simples, que se traen de la India oriental y sirven al uso de medicina* (Madrid, 1572), which was based on the works of Monardes and Garcia da Orta. *See* José Luis Fresquet Febrer, ed., *Juan Fragoso y los "Discursos de las cosas aromáticas, árboles y frutales…"(1572)* (CSIC – Universidad de Valencia: Valencia, 2001), 10–111. Alternatively it could have been *Catalogus simplicium medicamentorum* (Alcalá, 1566).

166 Cited in Guibovich, "Bibliotecas de médicos," 303–04.

were being prescribed by trained physicians who had received a conservative medical education and who were discouraged from acquiring knowledge of progressive practices by the actions of Inquisition. There is no evidence for "progressive" medical practitioners seeking refuge in Lima. At the same time, the range of books imported and used in *boticas* suggests that *boticarios* were working within a humoral tradition. Whether or not this reflected the success of Inquisition in suppressing "progressive" texts or the general scarcity of books of this kind in Europe at the time is less clear. In any case, this did not necessarily mean that *boticarios* did not develop innovative methods or experiment with new *materia medica*. In fact knowledge about new preparations and treatments might be circulated in other ways, in manuscript form or by word of mouth. Further insight into *boticario* practices can be gained from an analysis of the medicines they actually prepared and employed, which is explored in the following chapter.

CHAPTER 6

Making Medicines

> Having medicines as safe as is known and with good effects, why is it necessary to use exotic foreign medicines?[1]

The *materia medica* that were actually employed by *boticarios* reflected a wide range of interwoven factors that among other things included the prevailing natural philosophy, healing traditions, the knowledge, experience and preferences of particular *boticarios*, and the availability and demand for particular medicinal products. Spain's attempt to regulate medical practice extended only partially into the realm of *materia medica*, where the primary aim was to ensure the *quality* of medicines being employed rather than their *type*. Nevertheless, as the previous chapter has shown, *boticarios* and inspectors were given guidance on the types of products that a well-stocked *botica* should possess and, in Spain at least, *boticarios* whose pharmacies lacked certain items might be fined and required to acquire them. However, medicinal imports from Spain failed to meet the demand in Peru and as such at least some *materia medica* had to be acquired locally. At the same time, changes in medical practice in Europe were beginning to influence the types of medicines being employed. In the sixteenth century humoral beliefs dominated, such that the treatments prescribed consisted primarily of purgatives and emetics, based largely on plant materials, which were aimed at correcting imbalances in the humours. Overtime, however, with the development of chemical methods, minerals and chemicals began to feature more frequently in prescriptions. The widespread availability of minerals in the Andes should, in theory, have facilitated their adoption in Peru at an early date.

1 "Teniendo pues medicamentos tan seguros como conocidos, y experimentados felizmente, porque avemos de usar medicamentos tan exóticos, y tan peregrinos…" José Colmenero, *Reprobación de pernicioso abuso de los polvos de la corteza de quarango o China china* (Salamanca: Eugenio Antonio Garcia, 1697) cited in Slater, "Green Gold Fallacies," 107. This view was expressed by a Spanish physician about the adoption of plants from the New World, but might apply equally to those practising in the Americas.

 | DOI 10.1163/9789004351271_007

It might be expected that these new influences on medical practice might be reflected in the medicines that were prepared by apothecaries in Lima. However, this chapter will demonstrate that contrary to what might be expected, apothecaries in Lima prepared medicines according to humoral principles and focussed on Old World botanical materials, while making little use of native plants and minerals. Even where native plants were adopted they were placed and applied within a Galenic framework. Thus the chapter shows that there was little cross-over in Old and New World healing traditions and practices and that, despite the putative pioneering role of apothecaries in developing new practices, they remained largely separate from other healers. The chapter explores the multiple reasons why the medical marketplace in Lima was segmented and why professional *boticarios* adopted so few native products.

Types of Medicines

Most medicines were prepared from the dried parts of plants – roots, seeds, and flower heads – and less commonly incorporated minerals, as well as precious and semi-precious stones. These simple raw ingredients were mixed with water, oil, sugar, honey, vinegar or wax, or were dried and ground to a powder; in other cases they were pressed to extract an oil, pulp or juice.[2] These *materia medica* would be incorporated into syrups, waters or electuaries that were taken internally or they would be applied externally in ointments or plasters. Not surprisingly medicinal imports were dominated by unprocessed simples from which medicines might be composed. Complex medicines or *compuestos* that combined ingredients were mainly prepared in the New World and as such they figured more commonly in pharmacy inventories and prescriptions. The cargoes destined for hospitals and *boticarios* in Lima were dominated by three broad types of simples: plant and animal simples; resins, gums and oils; and minerals. These simple products accounted for over eighty percent of medicinal imports in terms of their total value and the total number of entries (Table 8). Resins, gums and oils were important as binders for ointments and plasters,[3] and their importance among imports (about 30 percent) can probably be explained by their relative absence on the treeless coast of Peru. Minerals accounted for only a small proportion of the imports (about 10 percent by

2 De Vos, "Art of Pharmacy," 125.

3 Paula S. De Vos, "Apothecaries, Artists and Artisans: Early Industrial Material Culture in the Biological Old Regime," *Journal of Interdisciplinary History* 45 (3) (2015): 307–08.

TABLE 8 *Percentage of types of medicines in cargoes destined for hospitals and private apothecaries, 1596–1622.*

	Apothecaries percent	Hospitals percent	Percentage dif
Plant simples (excluding seeds and roots)	32.9	36.1	3.20
Seeds	0.8	1.8	1.0
Roots	1	2.2	-1.20
Spices	0.6	0.3	0.30
Minerals	11.4	8.7	2.70
Stones	0.4	1	-0.60
Oils	16.7	20.9	-4.20
Gums and resins	11.5	13.1	-1.60
Animal	1.6	0.1	1.50
Wax	6.3	0.6	5.70
Syrups	1.2	0.2	1.00
Conserves	2.1	3.4	-1.30
Electuaries	5.5	1.5	4.00
Plasters	4	0.8	3.20
Ointments	2	5.8	-3.80
Chemicals	1	0	1.00
Miscellaneous	1.1	3.6	-2.50
Total percentage	100.0	100.0	
Number cargoes	15	8	
Total number entries	1,062	348	
Total value in maravedís	870,116.5	212,159	
Average value of cargo in maravedís	58,007.5	26,519.9	
Average number of entries per cargo	70.8	43.5	

Sources: For hospitals: AGI Contratación 1115 N4 676–77 Registro del navío La Magdalena and AGI Contratación 1116 N6 349–50 Registro del navío San Gregorio, Gaspar de Perales, 1596; AGI Contratación 1145A N2 341 Registro del navío San Vicente y San Juan Bautista and AGI Contratación 1145B N8 403–05 Registro del navío San Pedro, Rodrigo Arias de Buiça, 1605; AGI Contratación 1158 N1 R2 423–25 Registro del navío Nuestra Señora de Gracia, Ambrosio Villaza, 1612; AGI Contratación 1166 N4 277–80 Registro del navío San Francisco, Alonso González de la Canal, 1618; AGI Contratación 1166 N10 353–56 Registro del navío San Pedro, Adriano Legasso, 1618; AGI Contratación 1166 N4 297–98 Registro del navío San Francisco, Alonso González de la Canal, 1618. For *boticarios*: For Juan de Bilbao: AGI Contratación 1094 N4: 332–35 1591; 1107 N6: 197–99 1593–94; 1138A 3: 113–16 1601; 1138B 6: 101–04 1601; for Francisco Crespo: AGI Contratación 1138B N9: 137–40 Registro del navío San Ignacio 1601; for Gerónimo Pujadas: AGI Contratación 1166 N10: 425–30 1618; 1168 N1: 191–96 1619; for Francisco Martín Reyna: AGI Contratación 1162 N4: 43–46 1615; 1166 N1: 403–06 1618; for Pedro de Bilbao: AGI Contratación 1151B N1: 683–84 Registro del navío La Magdalena 1607; AGI Contratación 1151B N6: 429–30 Registro del navío Santa Cruz 1607; AGI Contratación 1155B N8: 445–48 Registro del navío Nuestra Señora de la Concepción 1609; AGI Contratación 1163 N1 R2: 81–83 Registro del navío La Visitación de Nuestra Señora 1615; AGI Contratación 1164 N4: 295–96 Registro del navío San Francisco 1618; AGI Contratación 1172 N2 R7: 281–82 Registro del navío Nuestra Señora de la Candelaria 1622.

value), but even this low figure is rather larger than might be expected given their local availability. Meanwhile, prepared medicines, including ointments, electuaries, plasters, and syrups, figured less prominently among imports since many would have lost their potency during transport. These products, which were often more expensive, were more common among cargoes destined for *boticarios* than for hospital pharmacies.

The hospitals of Santa Ana, San Andrés and La Caridad treated patients from largely distinct social and ethnic groups. The Hospital of Santa Ana for Indians was founded in 1549.[4] It possessed two wards for men and women, and another for contagious diseases. It was described by Bernabé Cobo as the richest in the kingdom.[5] African slaves were not supposed to be treated in there, but it seems that the Viceroy permitted this if their owners were poor.[6] The Hospital of San Andrés was founded in 1538 and treated about two thousand people a year, most of whom were Spaniards but some were free Blacks and Mulattoes, in addition to which it ordinarily housed about sixteen to twenty mentally ill patients.[7] The Hospital of La Caridad cared for fifty to sixty poor women and housed female orphans who were provided with dowries. Although it catered for women of all ethnic backgrounds, Spanish women lived in a separate section of the hospital.[8] Despite these broad differences in the ethnicity of the patients cared for in these three hospitals, there is little evidence to suggest that different types of medicinal products were being used in their treatments (Table 9).[9]

---

4 For the establishment of hospitals in Lima see Guerra, *El hospital*, 429–75.

5 AGI Lima 301 Relación de los hospitales que ay en esta ciudad de los Reies…20 Apr. 1619; Cobo, *Obras*, 2: 445–47.

6 ABPL 9806 fols.313–16, fol. 345 Visita al Hospital de Santa Ana [1588], ABPL 9085 fols.10–11 Libro de cuentas del hospital de Santa Ana 1595–1597.

7 AGI Lima 301 Relación de los hospitales que ay en esta ciudad de los Reies…20 Apr.1619; BNP Manuscritos B1563 Libro en que se escriben y asientan los enfermos…Hospital Real de San Andrés…desde 1 Mayo 1609.

8 AGI Lima 301 Relación de los hospitales que ay en esta ciudad de los Reies…20 Apr. 1619; AGI Lima 154 Autos sobre el Hospital de la Caridad de Lima 1622; Cobo, *Obras*, 2: 449.

9 AGI Contratación 1115 N4 676–77 Cargo of La Magdalena 1596; AGI Contratación 1116 N6 348–50 Registro del navío San Gregorio 1596; AGI Contratación 1145B N8 403–05 Registro del navío San Pedro 1605; AGI Contratación 1145A N2 341 Registro del navío San Vicente y San Juan Bautista 1605; AGI Contratación 1145B N8 403–05 Registro del navío San Pedro 1605; AGI Contratación 1158 N1 R2 423–25 Registro del navío Nuestra Señora de la Gracia 1612; AGI Contratación 1166 N4 277–80, 297–98 Registro del navío San Francisco 1618; AGI Contratación 1166 N10 353–56 Registro del navío San Pedro 1618; AGI Contratación 1166 N 1 459–65 Registro del navío El Espíritu Santo 1618.

In general pharmacies contained between 200 and 300 types of *materia medica*.[10] When the *botica* of the Hospital of Santa Ana was installed in 1552 it contained 251 types of medicinal product, but over time the range it possessed declined such that when it was inspected by the physician Doctor Melchor Romero in 1606 it possessed only 146 different varieties.[11] This decline probably reflected the limited number and range of products being shipped for hospital pharmacies in general, deficiencies that were not made good by the adoption of local products. The accounts kept by the Hospital of Santa Ana indicate that between 1595 and 1600 only 62 types of *materia medica* were acquired. It is worth noting that not only do these figures fall far short of the 429 products that were recommended by the *protomédico general,* Andrés Zamudio de Alfaro, in Spain, but only about half of them were those specified in his list (Table 10 and Appendix B).[12]

Preparing Medicines

How then were medicines prepared? Evidence from the books used by *boticarios* in early colonial Lima suggests that they were guided by the classical writings of Galen and Arabic treatises written in the Galenic tradition, while for practical advice they referred to the first-century herbal of Dioscorides interpreted by Andrés Laguna or to manuals based on the writings of the Arabic scholar Mesuë (Yūhannā ibn Māsawayh).[13] That Dioscorides was widely used is evident from the large number of copies of his work imported in comparison to other medical texts. In 1591 the merchant Francisco de Butrón acquired 22 copies of Andrés Laguna's interpretation of Dioscorides.[14] However, it was a

10 The private *botica* belonging to Pedro de Bilbao contained only 94 items, the majority being simples, but this was probably an underestimate since it was visited and assessed nearly two years after his death when many of the prepared and complex medicines would have been out of date and worthless. Pedro de Bilbao died on 4 September 1634 (AGNP Protocolos Siglo XVII 1791 Diego Sánchez Vadillo fol. 3519), but the assessment of this *botica* by the *boticario*, Alonso de Carrión, was not conducted until 28 Jul. 1636 (AGNP Protocolos Siglo XVII 1789 Diego Sanchez Vadillo fol. 1312v.).

11 ABPL 9086 fols.118–23 Visita al Hospital de Santa Ana por Doctor Melchor Romero Oct. 1606.

12 De Vos, "From Herbs to Alchemy," 140–48 notes that the majority of products found in Mexican pharmacies were those specified in traditional texts.

13 For a study and re-evaluation of the importance of Mesuë see: De Vos, "'Prince of Medicine'."

14 Leonard, "On the Lima Book Trade," 514, 521.

volume by Mesuë that was used in apothecary examinations in Lima.[15] Copies of Bernardino de Laredo's, *Modus faciendi* (1527) based on Mesuë were inventoried in a number of *boticas* and cargoes of medicines, while Antonio de Aguilera's *Exposición sobre las preparaciones de Mesuë* was owned by the *boticario*, Juan Sánchez.[16] In fact up to the end of the seventeenth century in Europe, there was no pharmaceutical book of formulas that did not rely on Mesuë.[17] All these authors were Galenists and it was not until the seventeenth century that European pharmacopoeias included chemicals.

Initially the use of published texts was limited to *boticarios* who could understand Latin. Many of these texts were later translated into Spanish, but in the sixteenth century very few translations were available. In the early seventeenth century Antonio de Robles Cornejo observed that many *boticarios* in Peru did not know Latin and were therefore preparing medicines on the basis of training and experience, producing medicines that were often ineffective and relying on poor quality and expensive imports.[18] It was these circumstances that persuaded him to produce a manual on how to prepare medicines in Spanish.[19] In contrast to scholastic medical works that were structured around ailments, entries in Robles Cornejo's work in common with the writings of Mesuë and his followers were ordered alphabetically by medicinal product or recipe.[20] These included Bernardino Laredo's *Modus faciendi*, which was that most commonly used in Lima at the time. Luis de Oviedo's *Methodo de la colección y reposición de las medicinas simples* (1581), which was widely used in Spain and the Americas, possessed a similar format.

The format used in pharmacopeias reflected the growing interest of apothecaries in the qualities and therapeutic value of individual medicinal products and remedies that were often contested. While there might be a general consensus over whether a medicinal product was hot or cold, there were often differences of view about its healing properties. There was also growing concern that the life of patients was being endangered by the employment of medicines that had been prepared inappropriately or applied in the wrong

15 AHML Libro 4 de cédulas y provisiones. Título de Bernardo Gil, boticario fol. 161 7 Nov. 1609. See Chapter 2.

16 Aguilera's *Exposición*, fols. 16v–25. For the discussion of books used in Lima see Chapter 5.

17 George Urdang, "The Development of Pharmacopoeias," *Bulletin of the World Health Organisation* 4 (4) (1951): 580, 588.

18 ARJBM División 1, leg. 17 Prologo. Libro de examen de los simples medicinales Antonio de Robles Cornejo 1617.

19 See Chapter 5 for a more detailed discussion of the history of Antonio de Robles Cornejo's texts.

20 Urdang, "Development of Pharmacopoeias," 581; De Vos, "'Prince of Medicine'," 691.

TABLE 9 *Cargoes of medicines for hospitals in Lima by value and product type, 1596–1618.*

Hospital	San Andrés[a]	San Andrés[b]	San Andrés[c]
Trader	Gaspar de Perales	Rodrigo Arias de Buiça	Ambrosio Villaza
	1596	1605	1612
Plant simples	26.0	46.9	40.9
Seeds	0.2	1.6	4.5
Roots	0.5	1.5	3.0
Spices	0.2	0.0	1.7
Minerals	13.0	4.9	4.6
Stones	0.1	2.5	1.1
Oils	23.2	7.6	24.1
Gums and resins	19.0	12.0	6.8
Animal	0.2	0.0	0.0
Wax	0.0	2.2	1.3
Syrups	0.0	0.0	0.0
Conserves	8.1	3.0	4.9
Electuaries	4.5	3.0	1.5
Plasters	0.0	0.0	0.0
Ointments	3.7	14.8	2.9
Miscellaneous	1.4	0.0	2.6
Value in maravedís	66,947	55,182	30,791
Number of entries	90	62	71
	100.0	100.0	100.0

a AGI Contratación 1115 N4 676–77 Registro del navío La Magdalena and AGI Contratación 1116 N6 349–50 Registro del navío San Gregorio, Gaspar de Perales, 1596.

b AGI Contratación 1145A N2 341 Registro del navío San Vicente y San Juan Bautista and AGI Contratación 1145B N8 403–05 Registro del navío San Pedro, Rodrigo Arias de Buiça, 1605.

c AGI Contratación 1158 N1 R2 423–25 Registro del navío Nuestra Señora de Gracia, Ambrosio Villaza, 1612.

d AGI Contratación 1166 N4 277–80 Registro del navío San Francisco, Alonso González de la Canal, 1618.

e AGI Contratación 1166 N10 353–56 Registro del navío San Pedro, Adriano Legasso, 1618.

f AGI Contratación 1166 N4 297–98 Registro del navío San Francisco, Alonso González de la Canal, 1618.

San Andrés[d]	La Caridad[e]	Santa Ana[f]	Average percent by value	Total number of entries
Alonso González de la Canal	Adriano Legasso	Alonso González de la Canal		
1618	1618	1618		
22.7	30.5	49.6	36.1	104
1.1	3.3	0.0	1.8	18
2.7	0.3	4.8	2.2	16
0.0	0.0	0.0	0.3	3
9.8	12.3	7.3	8.7	25
0.5	1.6	0.0	1.0	6
12.3	38.6	19.4	20.9	71
25.8	7.7	7.1	13.1	42
0.0	0.4	0.0	0.1	2
0.0	0.0	0.0	0.6	2
0.0	1.3	0.0	0.2	4
1.9	2.7	0.0	3.4	11
0.0	0.0	0.0	1.5	3
4.4	0.3	0.0	0.8	6
7.7	1.0	4.8	5.8	20
10.9	0.0	6.9	3.6	15
24,866	25,959	8,414	35,360	
37	67	21		348
100.0	100.0	100.0		

TABLE 10 *Types of* materia medica *recommended by Andrés Zamudio de Alfaro and found in pharmacies in Lima.*

Apothecary or pharmacy	Andrés Zamudio de Alfaro 1590s	First *botica* of Hospital of Santa Ana 1551	Diego de Tineo 1555
Plant simples	28	63	91
Seeds	46	18	34
Roots	30	11	13
Flowers	11	10	8
Herbs	24	6	15
Pieces/fragments	16	5	1
Minerals	10	11	19
Stones	11	6	14
Oils	35	29	42
Gums	19	25	27
Animal	11	5	8
Cordials	16	1	4
Syrups	47	4	22
Juices	14	4	10
Waters	12	15	9
Conserves	10	4	11
Electuaries	12	3	17
Opiates	11	4	5
Pills	17	0	2
Powders	0	0	2
Plasters	19	8	16
Ointments	26	10	16
Flour	4	2	2
Chemicals	0	4	1
Miscellaneous	0	3	5
Total	429	251	304
Number and percent in Alfaro's list		125 (49.8)	192 (48.7)

Sources: Charles Davis and María Luz López Terrada, "Protomedicato y farmacia en Castilla a finales del siglo XVI: edición crítica del Catálogo de las cosas que los boticarios han de tener en sus boticas, de Andrés Zamudio de Alfaro, protomedicato general (1592–1599)," *Asclepio* 53(2)(2010): 579–626; JCB Mss Codex Sp. 136 Memoria de la botica 1555; AGNP Protocolos Siglo XVI 63 Diego Gutiérrez fols. 167–88 Hospital de los españoles y naturales compañía con Francisco de Bilbao de la botica 20 Oct. 1551; AGNP Real Audiencia. Causas Civiles legajo 16 cuad. 81 fols. 119–26, 687–715 Pleito… contra los bienes y herederos del bachiller Francisco de Alba, boticario morador en la Ciudad de los Reyes. 1576; AAL Testamentos 5-1 fols. 44–49v. Testamento de Bartolomé Díaz Cabeza de Vaca 1608; AGNP Protocolos Siglo XVII 1789 Sánchez Vadillo fols. 1372v.-1374v. Inventario de bienes de Pedro de Bilbao 25 Aug. 1636.

Francisco de Alva 1576	Bartolomé Díaz Cabeza de Vaca 1608	Pedro de Bilbao 1636
42	59	30
12	30	11
10	11	5
3	4	1
0	5	3
0	7	0
8	19	4
11	9	5
22	19	8
19	18	13
5	6	4
6	9	2
22	33	4
10	10	0
13	11	0
1	1	1
7	7	0
3	5	1
1	9	0
0	14	0
2	18	0
14	15	1
0	0	0
0	2	0
3	2	1
214	323	94
127(59.3)	170 (53.6)	52 (55.3)

Note: To make the figures comparable medicinal products are classified according to the list drawn up Andrés Zamudio de Alfaro. They are classified differently in different inventories.

quantities.[21] It was argued that the only way that the correct treatments could be applied was through trial and error, or as the Jesuit priest in Peru, Martín Vitillejos stated succinctly by referring to the Latin aphorism – *juvantibus et nocentibus sumi indicia* (evidence comes from help and harm).[22] The focus on the medicines themselves and the use of experimental methods, which began to emerge in the thirteenth century, signalled the increasing specialisation and professionalisation of pharmacy within medical practice.[23]

Even though *boticarios* might be guided by particular manuals, they often annotated them in the margins, perhaps varying the quantity or combination of ingredients specified in the text according to their own experience. They might also compose their own hand-written recipes, as might members of religious orders who also compiled *recetarios*, some for use by the population at large. The latter included those by Agustín Farfán, *Tratado breve de anothomía y chirugía* (1579), Juan de Esteyneffer's popular *Florilegio medicinal* (1712), and the hermit Gregorio López's *Tesoro de medicinas* (1672, but compiled in the 1580s).[24] These texts all followed the Galenic tradition but occasionally incorporated some local medicinal products.[25] These books were published in Mexico and as yet there is no evidence that Farfán's work or a similar volume was either used or published in Peru before the eighteenth century. However, the Jesuits in sending *materia medica* to outlying colleges in Peru might include brief notes on how to utilise particular products. For example, one despatch of medicines from the Jesuit College of San Pablo to its College at Nazca included a handwritten note as follows:

> For rose sugar it is sufficient for a light purgative to use one ounce and if you want a strong purgative one and a half ounces
> The plaster for treating dysentery it is necessary to place it on the stomach
> The rest of the ointments you already know how to use them.[26]

---

21 Michael McVaugh, "The 'Experience-Based Medicine' of the Thirteenth Century," *Early Science and Medicine* 14 (2009): 105–30.

22 ARSI Perú 1a Epistolae Generalium cartas originales fol. 170 Martín Vitillejos 20 Sep. 1620.

23 Urdang, "Development of Pharmacopoeias," 581; De Vos, "'Prince of Medicine'," 694.

24 Francisco Guerra, *El Tesoro de Medicinas de Gregorio López* 1542–1596 (Madrid: Ediciones Cultura Hispánica del Instituto de Cooperación Iberoamericana, 1982).

25 Saul Jarcho, "Medicine in Sixteenth Century New Spain as Illustrated by the Writings of Bravo, Farfán and Vargas Machuca," *Bulletin of the History of Medicine* 31 (1957): 431–39; Foster, *Hippocrates' Latin American Legacy*, 155–56.

26 AGNP Compañía de Jesús, Colegio San Pablo, Cuentas leg. 119 fol. 136v. Libro de viáticos y almacén 1628–1631. The medicines sent were rose sugar, *polvos de juanes*, Zacarias

Pharmacy Methods and Equipment

Prior to the late seventeenth century most pharmacy processes were fairly simple. They involved mixing and/or heating on a stove or in an oven, and the employment of skimmers, sieves, funnels, or presses to remove impurities.[27] Paula De Vos argues that the preparation of medicines at this time did not require a distillation laboratory.[28] However, evidence from the inventories of equipment found in pharmacies in Lima suggests that there distillation methods were widely employed. This does not necessarily mean, however, that they were being used for the processing of minerals or the production of mineral salts. Distillation methods were used to produce purer forms or "fifth essences" or quintessences of other *materia medica*, particularly herbs. Indeed Mesuë was familiar with distillation methods.[29] Nevertheless, the fact that texts by Arnau de Vilanova, which described some chemical processes, were commonly found in pharmacies in Lima suggests that distillation methods may have also been employed to prepare chemical medicines. (Figure 9)

The consignment of equipment destined for the establishment of the Hospital of Santa Ana in 1552 is indicative of the type and range of apparatus employed in hospital pharmacies of the time.[30] The shipment consisted of two *alquitaras* (metal stills) and two tin-plated boilers with four ladles and two skimmers. Other items included a measuring bowl, a balance, various weights and measures, brass funnels, golden spatulas, sieves, baskets, syrup jars and a large numbers of jars, pots, vases and boxes of different sizes.[31] *Alquitaras* were essential for the functioning of a hospital pharmacy and as such were

ointment, *basilicón* ointment, *sanalatodo* (*Gnaphalium attenuatum* DC) (an American herb), *diapalma* and *diafinicón* (plasters), some pigeons and turpentine.

27 For an account of the processes used to make medicines, see Oviedo, *Methodo*, and for a brief summary based on Oviedo see: De Vos, "Art of Pharmacy," 111–55.

28 De Vos, "Art of Pharmacy," 128 and "From Herbs to Alchemy," 145–48.

29 Palmer, "Pharmacy in the Republic of Venice," 115–17.

30 AGNP Protocolos Siglo XVI 63 Diego Gutiérrez fols. 167–88 El hospital de los españoles y naturales con Francisco de Bilbao de la botica 9 Mar. 1552. The detailed cost of individual items in the *botica* suggests it was worth 289,110 *maravedís*, of which 61,750 was spent on equipment. As noted above, the figure of 289,110 *maravedís* is difficult to reconcile with the stated total cost of 3,400 *pesos de oro en plata ensayado*.

31 AGNP Protocolos Siglo XVI 63 Diego Gutiérrez fols. 167–88 El hospital de los españoles [sic] compañía con Francisco de Bilbao 9 Mar. 1552. For the use of *alquitaras* in the Hospital of San Andrés see AGI Lima 131 Petition from Francisco Molina, mayordomo of the hospital de los españoles [San Andrés] 9 Mar. 1563.

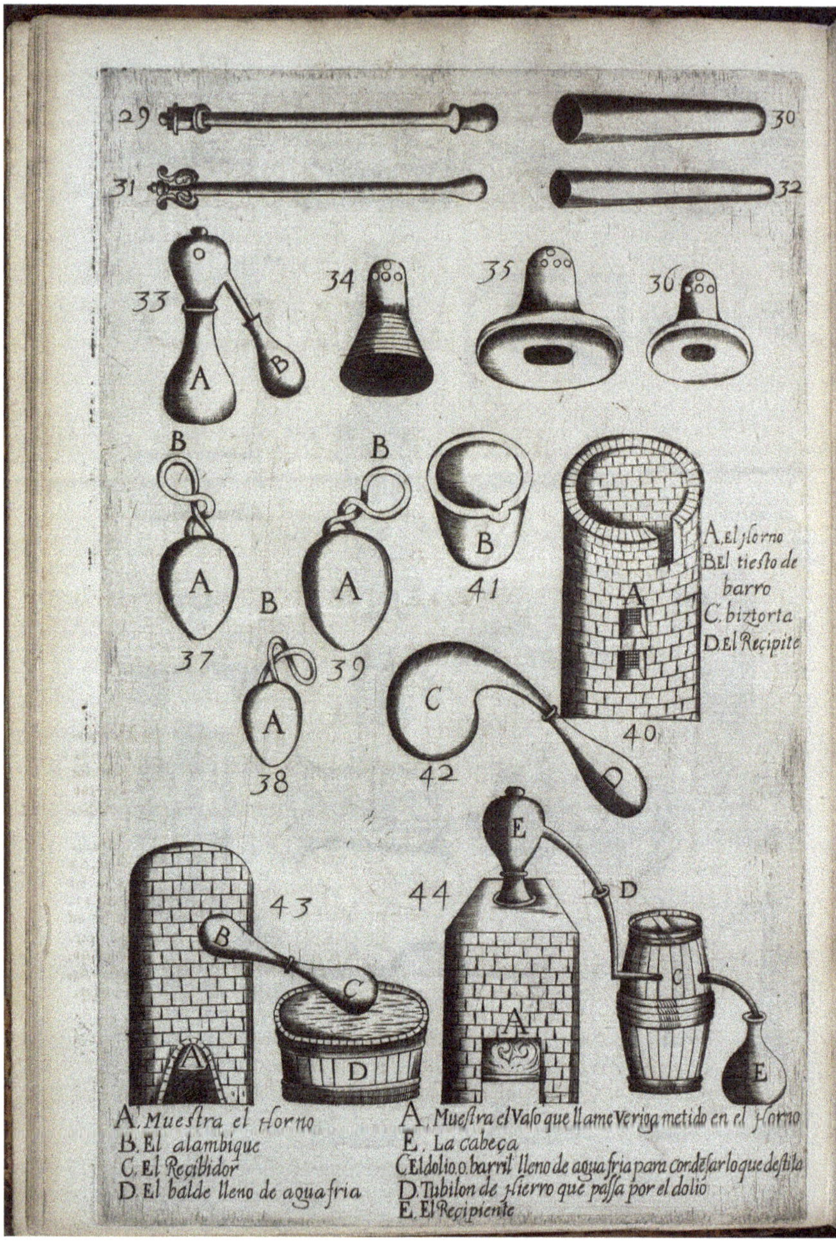

FIGURE 9 *Distillation equipment depicted by Licenciado Pedro López de León, 1628. Source: Licenciado Pedro López de León,* Prática [sic] y teórica de las apostemas en general y particular: questiones y prácticas de cirugía, de heridas, llagas, y otras cosas nuevas, y particulares. *Seville: Oficina de Luys Estupiñan, 1628.*
COURTESY BRITISH LIBRARY.

regularly repaired or replaced.[32] Some mortars were imported but others were manufactured locally.[33] The emphasis on bloodletting in treatments meant that smaller pieces of equipment such as cupping-glasses and lancets were also purchased by hospitals on a regular basis, but for use by barber-surgeons rather than *boticarios*.

Distillation equipment was not confined to hospitals. The inventory of the well-endowed *botica* of Francisco de Alva drawn up in 1576 listed four *alquitaras*, six mortars, including one each of lead and marble, three boiling pans, three ladles, two funnels, a press, and eight spatulas, of which three were of silver.[34] Similarly, in 1608 the private *botica* belonging to Bartolomé Díaz Cabeza de Vaca possessed an unspecified number of *alquitaras*, along with mortars, spatulas, sieves, ladles, a variety of boxes and phials, an oven and other essential tools.[35] The range of equipment found in pharmacies in Lima was not dissimilar to that found in *boticas* in Spain.[36]

It is worth noting that the stills were *alquitaras* rather than *alambiques*. In 1589 the *Protomédico* in Madrid, Francisco Valles, ordered that all distilled waters that were to be drunk, including syrups, should be produced using a glass *alambique* in a *bain marie* rather than a copper *alquitara*.[37] This view was also held by Antonio de Robles Cornejo, who advised *boticarios* in Peru that the best essences were distilled using a double *bain marie*.[38] *Alambiques* were said to produce better quality extracts, while *alquitaras* were believed to result in contamination by verdigris. However, not everyone agreed. *Boticarios* in Madrid argued that distillation using a *bain marie* was suitable for delicate plants, such as violets, but not for extracting the essences of other plants which

32 AGI Lima 131 Hospital de los españoles de la ciudad de los Reyes 13 Jan. 1564; ABPL 9085 Libro de la razón que toma Bartolomé de la Cueva 1595–1597 Accounts of the botica of the Hospital of Santa Ana, include expenditure on the repair of *alquitaras*.

33 ABPL 9084 Libro de cuentas de gastos del hospital de Santa Ana Ano 1598 fols. 169–70. The hospital of Santa Ana was buying mortars from one Diego Rajel, a *calderero* (a boiler maker or coppersmith).

34 AGNP Real Audiencia leg. 16 cuad. 81 fols. 14v–15 Inventario de los bienes del bachiller Francisco de Alva 9 Feb. 1576.

35 AAL Testamentos 5 leg 1 fol. 165v. Memoria de las medicinas que tenía esta botica cuando la compraron… Bartolomé Díaz Cabeza de Vaca 1608.

36 Pastor Frechoso, *Boticas*, 171–201.

37 Francisco de Valles, *Tratado de las aguas destilladas, pesos y medidas* (Madrid: Luis Sánchez 1592); Mar Rey Bueno, "El informes Valles: Los desdibujados límites del arte de boticarios a finales del siglo XVI (1589–1594),"*Asclepio* 56 (2) (2004): 245–68.

38 ARJBM División 1, leg. 17 cap. 2 del arte del boticario, Libro de examen de los simples medicinales Antonio de Robles Cornejo 1617.

required more heat.[39] It was also claimed that the waters (*aguas*) produced in a *bain marie* were not as effective for as long and that glass was more expensive than copper, a factor which may have been of greater consideration in Peru than in Spain. The belief that metal stills resulted in the contamination of distilled waters ultimately prevailed and the requirement to use glass *alambiques* for waters that were to be drunk was incorporated into legislation in Spain.[40] However, there is little evidence that *alambiques* were used in Lima at this time, whereas *alquitaras* were widely employed.[41] It is worth noting in the context of the running costs of a *botica* that the use of stills and the preparation of medicines in general required some form of heating or cooking, which consumed significant quantities of charcoal that was in particularly short supply on the coast of Lima.

Categories of Medicines

The range of equipment from simple to sophisticated was used to prepare an equally wide variety of simple and complex medicines ranging from simple waters and syrups to complex compound medicines that might be composed of more than twenty ingredients.[42] Simple syrups, as well as plasters and ointments, cost between two and three reals an application, whereas the fee for more complex purgatives could be between sixteen and twenty-four reals.

Simple syrups were made from honey or sugar with a plant ingredient of some kind. No less than sixty-six types of syrups were found in the four *boticas* examined here, the most prominent being violet, rose, verjuice (*agraz*), quince, borage and myrtle. Most of these syrups were used as general tonics and to treat diarrhoea and vomiting.[43] Sometimes similar ingredients were employed in very thick syrups called *lamedores*. Electuaries were more complex syrups that were very sugary to disguise the unpleasant taste of other ingredients, often purgatives. The most common were *diacatolicón* (a light purgative based on senna and rhubarb), *diafinicón* (a purgative based on dates and

39 Today *alambiques* are considered preferable because they enable the separation of the processes of vaporisation and condensation better and allow greater control of the process.

40 *Recopilación de las leyes, pragmáticas* (Muñoz) cap. XIV ordinance 5: 177.

41 For example, RGI 2: 7–8 Relación de la ciudad de Cuzco, Vasco de Contreras y Valverde 1 Jan. 1650.

42 This section is a modified version of Newson and Minchin, *From Capture to Sale*, 273–77.

43 Laval, *Botica*, 40, 138, 172, 202.

quince), *diamargaritón* (a compound including powder of ground pearls) and *girapliega* (based on a variety of ingredients that might include balsam wood, aloeswood, mastic and cinnamon), while *bol arménico* (Armenian bole) and powder of the myrobalan plant were also common components. These were all used as purgatives and laxatives.[44]

Other treatments for both internal and external afflictions took the form of plasters (poultices), which were placed on the outside of the body. Containing either "hot" or "cold" substances they were used to restore the balance in the humours.[45] Commonly used plasters were *diapalma*, which contained litharge and white and red vitriol and was employed to heal ulcers, wounds, dislocations and fractures, and *diaquilón*, which also contained litharge and was used as an emollient and to treat tumours.[46] Like electuaries, plasters contained a variety of ingredients.

Ointments were made of wax, animal fat, or resins with vegetable or mineral ingredients. They were primarily used to treat ailments of the skin, such as scabies (*sarna*), and less commonly for venereal disease and muscle strain.[47] These disorders commonly afflicted African slaves in Lima who were generally treated with yellow ointment, Zacarías ointment, and white ointment.[48] Yellow ointment was made of yellow wax, fat, oil, and resins and was used as a suppurative. Zacarías ointment was also made of yellow wax, but contained beef, pork and chicken fat, linseed oil and fenugreek and was used as an expectorant and to soften hard parts of the skin. White ointment served a variety of purposes, but was commonly used for the treatment of burns and skin infections.[49] The ointments used to treat non-African patients differed somewhat since their ailments were not dominated by skin infections. They included relatively simple ones based on rose, sandalwood, and in the case of *unguento basilicón*, the vegetable resin, *pez negra*. Other popular ointments were those composed of an assortment of ingredients, such as *unguento apostolorum* and

44 For electuaries see Oviedo, *Methodo*, 88–199 (for *diacatolicón* 122–29, *diamargaritón* 171–72, *diafenicón* 88–98); Laval, *Botica*, 105, 106, 141; Pilar Arrebola Nacle and Guillermina López Andújar, "Suministro de medicamentos a la gente de mar y guerra de la Real Armada (1636)," *Boletin de la sociedad española de historia de la farmacia* 27 (1986): 46.

45 Virginia Gutierrez de Pineda, *Medicina tradicional de Colombia: El triple llegado*, Vol. 1 (Bogotá: Universidad Nacional de Colombia, 1985), 94.

46 Oviedo, *Methodo*, 454–70; Laval, *Botica*, 108.

47 Anastasio Rojo Vega, *Enfermos y sanadores en la Castilla del siglo XVI* (Valladolid: Universidad De Valladolid, 1993), 75; Laval, *Botica*, 189–97.

48 Newson and Minchin, *From Capture to Sale*, 278–81.

49 Laval, *Botica*, 189–90, 195.

populeón,[50] as well as *unguentos opilativos* which were applied to remove obstructions of the liver, stomach or spleen,[51] as was *unguento agripa*, a recipe based on bryony and other roots supposedly invented by an unspecified king Agrippa.[52]

Using Purgatives and Emetics

Humoral medicine generally involved purging and vomiting to dispel malignant humours and restore bodily balance. The dominance of purgatives both among imports of *materia medica* and contained in pharmacies suggests that humoral medicine dominated in the sixteenth and early seventeenth centuries. It is significant that Robles Cornejo in his guide to the use of medicinal plants listed the purgatives first: rhubarb, rhapontic, agaric, turpeth and polypody in that order (See Figure 8).[53]

Of the 128 types of botanical simples, flowers and herbs, excluding roots and seeds, contained in the original *botica* of the Hospital of Santa Ana in 1551 and in three private *boticas*, only eight products were found in all four pharmacies: scammony, agaric, myrobalans (yellow and emblic), linaloe, colocynth, long pepper and red sandalwood, the first six of which were valued for their purgative qualities (Appendix B).[54] Among the seeds the only product found in all four pharmacies was cardamom, but its prevalence may relate to its culinary rather than medicinal use. The dominance of purgatives is also seen in the composition of cargoes of medicines sent to Lima in the late sixteenth and early seventeenth centuries (See Table 11), where senna and scammony alone accounted for about 40 percent of the value of simples dispatched to hospitals and only slightly less in the case of those destined for *boticarios*. The lower proportion imported by *boticarios* may be explained by the fact that they acquired more expensive purgatives in the form of complex electuaries.[55] Other important purgatives were myrobalans, aloe, and the fungus agaric. Aloe was said to be abundant in Peru, so the fact that it featured highly among imports

50 Oviedo, *Methodo*, 389, 410.

51 Ibid. 413.

52 Felix Palacios, *Palestra pharmaceutica chymico-galenica* (Madrid: Juan Garcia Infançon, 1706), 300; Laval, *Botica*, 191.

53 ARJBM División 1, leg. 17 fols. 1–21 Libro de examen de los simples medicinales Antonio de Robles Cornejo 1617.

54 All eight were also in Diego de Tineo's list of plant materials requested from Spain for his *botica* in Lima (JCB Mss codex Sp 136 Francisco Martínez y compañía obligación – Diego de Tineo y consortes 1555.

55 Electuaries accounted for 5.5 percent of the total value of imports in the case of private boticarios and 1.5 percent in the case of the Hospital of Santa Ana (see Table 8).

is perhaps surprising.[56] However, there were different varieties of aloe. The variety found abundant locally was probably the American aloe or agave,[57] while imported one was probably the true aloe which is native to Arabia and North Africa.[58]

Rhubarb was imported when the pharmacy was established in the Hospital of Santa Ana in 1551, but thereafter no cargoes destined directly for hospitals that are examined here contained rhubarb; small amounts were shipped to private *boticarios*, however. Even so, in the early years of its establishment the Hospital of Santa Ana was acquiring quite large quantities of rhubarb indirectly from merchants and from the *boticarios* Francisco de Alva and Juan de Bilbao.[59] Rhubarb was expensive. Cargo lists and purchases made by hospitals suggest that it was worth between 60–80 reals a pound, when other effective purgatives notably scammony could be purchased for 20–25 reals a pound and senna for only 4–6 reals. Rhubarb was highly esteemed as a mild but effective purgative so that when it was shipped fresh to Lima for the establishment of the pharmacy of the Hospital of Santa Ana, it was wrapped in an oil cloth and transported in a separate bag.[60] The special treatment afforded to rhubarb on this occasion suggests that it was probably the true rhubarb from China (*Reum rhabarbarum* L.). Writing in 1617 Antonio de Robles Cornejo, referring to Garcia de Orta, maintained that there was little rhubarb in Spain and that it was not known in the Indies. He claimed that in Peru it was substituted for by rhapontic (another type of rhubarb – *Reum rhaponticum* L.), which was native to the area around the Bosphorus,[61] or by myrobalans, or better still mechoacan or jalap (*Ipomoaea purga* Wender. Hayne).[62] However, it seems that rhubarb may have been better known in Spain than Robles Cornejo realised because as early as 1555 Diego de Tineo made a clear distinction between the two plants when he ordered eight pounds of rhubarb and two pounds of rhapontic from Seville for the establishment of his opulent pharmacy.[63] It is worth noting that

56 Lewin, *Descripción,* 77.

57 http://www.theplantlist.org/tpl/record/kew-293578 [Accessed 17 June 2016].

58 http://apps.kew.org/wcsp/namedetail.do?name_id=298116 [Accessed 17 June 2016].

59 ABPL 9080 fols.176–236, 254–57 Libro de cuentas del hospital de Santa Ana 1575 a 1585.

60 AGNP Protocolos Siglo XVI 63 Diego Gutiérrez fols. 167–88 Hospital de los españoles y naturales compañía con Francisco de Bilbao de la botica 20 Oct. 1551.

61 Clifford M. Foust, *Rhubarb: The Wondrous Drug* (Princeton: Princeton University Press, 1992), 12.

62 ARJBM División 1, leg. 17 fol. 5 Libro de examen de los simples medicinales Antonio de Robles Cornejo 1617.

63 JCB Mss codex Sp 136 fol. 864v. Francisco Martínez y compañía obligación – Diego de Tineo y consortes 1555.

TABLE 11 *Purgatives in pharmacies and in cargoes shipped to hospitals and apothecaries in Lima.*

	Cargoes for hospitals						
	Santa Ana[a]	San Andrés[b]	San Andrés[c]	San Andrés[d]	San Andrés[e]	Convento de la Caridad[f]	Santa Ana[g]
	1551	1596	1605	1612	1618	1618	1618
Senna	1.5	4.7	26.3	64.8	94.4	42.9	54.1
Scammony	19.9	34.5	14.5	0.0	0.0	0.0	0.0
Myrobalans	2.6	0.0	0.0	0.0	0.0	0.0	0.0
Aloe	1.8	5.9	0.0	9.7	0.0	6.9	0.0
Agaric	11.3	0.6	1.1	6.5	0.0	7.3	6.5
Rhubarb	2.9	0.0	0.0	0.0	0.0	0.0	0.0
Total percentage	39.9	45.6	41.8	81.0	94.4	57.1	60.6
Total value of simples (maravedís)	60,132	17,414	25,874	12,600	5,402	7,922	4,716
Number of types of simples (includes roots and seeds)	105	32	29	27	10	30	9

Sources

a AGNP Protocolos Siglo XVI 63 Diego Gutiérrez fols. 167–88 Hospital de los españoles y naturales compañía con Francisco de Bilbao de la botica 20 Oct. 1551. See also: Miguel Rabí Chara, "La primera botica de los hospitales de la ciudad de Lima en el siglo XVI," *Asclepio* 52 (2000): 276–77.

b AGI Contratación 1115 N4 676–77 Registro del navío La Magdalena and AGI Contratación 1116 N6 349–50 Registro del navío San Gregorio, Gaspar de Perales, 1596.

c AGI Contratación 1145A N2 341 Registro del navío San Vicente y San Juan Bautista and AGI Contratación 1145B N8 403–05 Registro del navío San Pedro, Rodrigo Arias de Buiça, 1605.

d AGI Contratación 1158 N1 R2 423–25 Registro del navío Nuestra Señora de Gracia, Ambrosio Villaza, 1612.

e AGI Contratación 1166 N4 277–80 Registro del navío San Francisco, Alonso González de la Canal, 1618.

f AGI Contratación 1166 N10 353–56 Registro del navío San Pedro, Adriano Legasso, 1618.

g AGI Contratación 1166 N4 297–98 Registro del navío San Francisco, Alonso González de la Canal, 1618.

Cargoes for apothecaries					Contents of *boticas*	
Juan de Bilbao[h]	**Pedro de Bilbao**[i]	**Francisco Crespo**[j]	**Francisco Martín Reyna**[k]	**Gerónimo Pujadas**[l]	**Bartolomé Díaz Cabeza de Vaca**[m]	**Pedro de Bilbao**[n]
1591–1601	1607–1621	1601	1615–1618	1618–1619	1608	1636
12.9	39.9	29.2	29.2	23.6	2.0	0.0
19.6	3.7	16.7	0.0	5.7	28.4	27.1
1.6	1.2	6.7	5.4	7.0	3.5	17.6
10.1	0.0	0.0	0.0	3.1	14.7	13.3
2.9	1.6	3.1	3.3	0.0	1.4	4.8
1.8	1.7	0.0	0.0	3.5	4.8	0.0
47.0	46.4	55.6	38.0	39.2	54.9	62.7
143,091	73,243	24,448	16,285	28,848	151,606	64,073
85	73	39	66	74	117	55

h AGI Contratación 1094: 332–35 Registro de San Pedro 1591; AGI Contratación 1107 N6: 197–99 Registro del navío Santa Catalina 1593–94; AGI Contratación 1138A 3: 113–16 Registro del navío San Nicolás 1601; AGI Contratación 1138B 6: 101–04 Registro del navío Nuestra Señora de la Concepción 1601.

i AGI Contratación 1151B N1: 683–84 Registro del navío La Magdalena 1607, AGI Contratación 1151B N6: 429–30 Registro del navío Santa Cruz 1607; AGI Contratación 1155B N8: 445–48 Registro del navío Nuestra Señora de la Concepción 1609; AGI Contratación 1163 N1 R2: 81–83 Registro del navío La Visitación de Nuestra Señora 1615; AGI Contratación 1164 N4: 295–96 Registro del navío San Francisco 1618; AGI Contratación 1172 N2 R7: 281–82 Registro del navío Nuestra Señora de la Candelaria 1622.

j AGI Contratación 1138B N9: 137–40 Registro del navío San Ignacio 1601.

k AGI Contratación 1162 N4: 43–46 Registro del navío San Pedro 1615; AGI Contratación 1166 N1: 403–06 Registro del navío El Espíritu Santo 1618.

l AGI Contratación 1166 N10: 425–30 Registro del navío San Pedro 1618; AGI Contratación 1168 N1: 191–96 Registro del navío San Salvador 1619.

m AAL Testamentos 5-1 fols. 44–49v Testamento de Bartolomé Díaz Cabeza de Vaca 1608.

n AGNP Protocolos Siglo XVII 1789 Sánchez Vadillo fols. 1372v–1374v Inventario de bienes de Pedro de Bilbao 25 Aug. 1636.

rhapontic was essentially an astringent rather than purgative.[64] The rhubarb found in *boticas* in Lima would not have been acquired locally being unsuited to the warm dry climate of the Peruvian coast; even in Europe early attempts to cultivate the plant were unsuccessful. While it could be grown in gardens and produce flowers and seeds, it did not yield roots of equivalent medicinal value to that produced in Asia.[65] The question remains open as to whether some of the rhubarb being used in Peru was in fact rhapontic. In any case it was less commonly used than other purgatives. Although mechoacan (Figure 10), a native of Mexico but known in Spain at an early date, was called the "rhubarb of the Indies" and on occasions was used as a substitute for rhubarb,[66] it was not employed as a purgative as extensively in Lima as other products such as senna and canafistula.

Using Native Plants

As noted in Chapter 4 the Spanish were interested in native plants and other natural resources from the perspective of finding profitable substitutes for the medicinal products they normally used, but which were either expensive or unavailable; at the same time there was a genuine curiosity about the natural world of the Americas that often came, though not exclusively, from members of the religious orders. While these commercial and intellectual considerations figured among those in the Americas, there practical considerations featured more prominently in the selection of *materia medica* employed. This was especially so in the early years of conquest, when pragmatism generally overrode any concern there may have been about the religious significance of particular native medicines, which often preoccupied missionaries and

64 ARJBM División 1, leg. 17 fol. 6v. Libro de examen de los simples medicinales Antonio de Robles Cornejo 1617; Oviedo, *Methodo*, 283.

65 Foust, *Rhubarb*, 179.

66 Nicólas Monardes, *Primera y segunda y tercera parte de la historia medicinal de las cosas que se traen de nuestras Indias Occidentales, que sirven en medicina* (Seville: Alonso Escriuano, 1574), 1 fols. 28v–37v; ARJBM División 1, leg. 17 fols. 204–11 Libro de examen de los simples medicinales Antonio de Robles Cornejo 1617. For Spanish adoption of mechoacan see: Barrera-Osorio, "Knowledge and Empiricism," 229–32. The *Protomédico general* Andrés Zamudio de Alfaro was recommending it to *boticarios* in Spain in the 1590s (Davis and López Terrada, "Protomedicato y farmacia en Castilla," 595) and it was found in pharmacies in Seville in the late sixteenth century (Fernández-Carrión and Valverde, *Farmacia y Sociedad*, 70, 81).

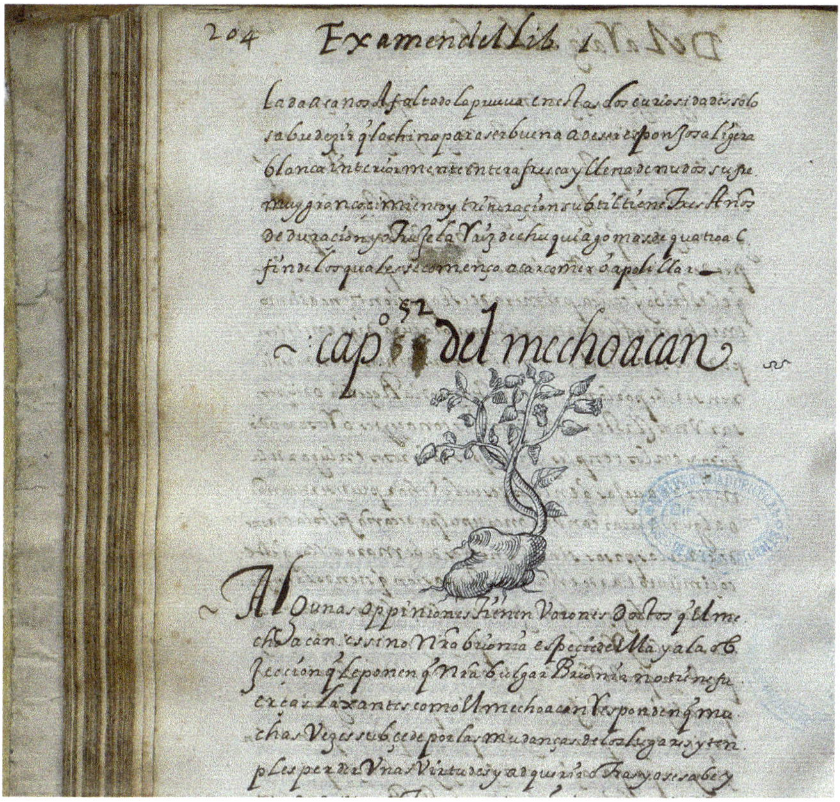

FIGURE 10 *Drawing of mechoacan in Antonio de Robles Cornejo's "Examen de los simples medicinales," 1617.*
COURTESY SPAIN. MINISTERIO DE CULTURA. ARCHIVO DEL REAL JARDÍN BOTÁNICO, MADRID. DIVISIÓN 1, LEG. 17 FOL. 204.

philosophers who were anxious about their role in indigenous rituals and witchcraft.[67]

Military personnel on expeditions and medical practitioners distant from sources of imports would have had little choice but to make use of local products. Hence, Captain Bernardo de Vargas Machuca, a seasoned soldier in the Indies, especially in present-day Colombia, wrote in his training manual for would-be conquistadores published in 1599:

---

67 Daniela Bleichmar, "Books, Bodies, and Fields: Sixteenth-Century Transatlantic Encounters with New World *Materia Medica*," in *Colonial Botany: Science, Commerce, and Politics in the Early Modern World*, eds. Londa Schiebinger and Claudia Swan (Philadelphia, PA: University of Pennsylvania Press, 2004), 98.

> In my experience I have made extraordinary cures and have tried out all these medicines, some learned from the Indians, great herbalists that they are. And I have acquired others through experience, as each one may do [in the field], discovering new medicines, being a new inventor of them through experiment as well as with good philosophy, for the health of his soldiers. Where there are no doctors, we must all make a choice. And even where there are this calls for careful study because of the simplicity of the medicines we apply, using no compounds.[68]

Vargas Machuca also provided a brief list of plants he recommended that soldiers should carry with them, which included a significant number of native products, including the resins *anime* and *caraña*, mechoacan, tobacco, bezoar stones, and *solimán crudo* (corrosive sublimate or mercury chloride).[69] In a non-military context where medicines from Spain were unavailable, Spaniards might similarly be forced to turn to native *materia medica*. Antonio de Robles Cornejo reported how Indians in the *yungas* had given a plant root to their *encomendero*, Don Diego Dávalos, a noble from Ecija in Spain, to treat his wife who was suffering from *flaquezas de cabeza* (weakness in the head) and was nearly blind.[70] Also, in 1610 when an Indian, Francisco García Julcapuma who had been working in the monastery of San Augustín in Trujillo, was found with herbs in his pocket and brought before the ecclesiastical court, he claimed that a priest had taught him to collect native herbs. It seems likely that the priest's interest in native plants was an attempt to find substitutes for familiar Old World ones that were unavailable. The plants included *tumbi* for dysentery, *pilpi* for abscesses, *tinti* for dropsy and *tulti* for use as anti-venom.[71]

---

68 Vargas Machuca, *Indian Militia*, 69. The Spanish version of the last two sentences reads, "adonde no hay médicos todos podemos tener voto y aún donde los hay, por ser simples los medicamentos que aplicamos, sin usar de compuestos, que es cosa que requiere particular estudio" (Vargas Machuca, *Milicia,* 140). This is better translated as "where there are no doctors everyone can have a say, because the medicines we apply are simples, not compounds, which is something that requires special study." On this work see also: Benjamín Flores Hernández, "Medicina de los conquistadores, en la *Milicia Indiana* de Bernardo de Vargas Machuca," *Boletín Mexicano de Historia y Filosofía de la Médicina* 6(1) (2003): 5–10.

69 Vargas Machuca, *Indian Militia*, 61.

70 ARJBM División 1, leg. 17 fol. 197 Libro de examen de los simples medicinales Antonio de Robles Cornejo 1617.

71 AAL Hechicerías 1: 17 fol. 1 Interrogatorio hecho a Francisco García Julcapuma 1610. It has not been possible to identify these native plants.

As constant complaints from hospitals attest, shortages of medicines were not unique to military campaigns or to rural areas, but also prevailed in major cities including Lima. As Chapter 4 has shown, the quantity of medicines imported failed to meet local demand by some margin such that apothecaries had to acquire *materia medica* from alternative sources. Resins and oils in particular were in short supply.

The presence of the cold Humboldt Current means that the coast of Peru receives little rain and is therefore dry and treeless. The demand for gums, resins and oils for the preparation of medicines, notably for ointments and plasters, was therefore particularly high in Lima, though shortages of these products were also common in other parts of the Americas.[72] In 1641 the surgeon of the Hospital of Santa Ana complained to the *mayordomo* that it was impossible to make yellow ointment (*unguento amarillo*), the most basic of ointments, since there was no "pine resin [pez] and virgin wax and resin [cera virgen y resina]."[73] As Table 8 shows, resins and oils figured significantly among imports from Spain. Some American resins and oils were also imported from regions further north. A schedule of import taxes on goods entering Callao from Mexico and Central America, included liquidambar, *copal, tacamahaca*[74] and *sangre de drago*, as well as mechoacan, *guaiacum* (lignum-vitae), tobacco, and pepper from Chiapas.[75] Liquidambar, *caraña, tacamahaca, anime, copal,* and *higuerilla*, were all known to Nicolás Monardes in Seville[76] and the first three were sufficiently well known in Spain to be officially recommended to pharmacists by the *Protomédico general* in the 1590s.[77] Even so, American resins and oils, indeed American *materia medica* in general, figured only rarely in *boticas* in Spain in the sixteenth century.[78]

---

72 Ronderos, *El dilema*, 104.

73 ABPL 9127 fol. 165 Don Pedro Garcia Capicha, cirujano, to Pedro Ramírez mayordomo of the hospital of Santa Ana 8 Jul. 1641.

74 De Vos, "Art of Pharmacy," 101–10. Tacamahaca was an American gum-resin extracted from a variety of trees whose name derived from the Aztec term, tecomahiyac (Francisco Hernández, *Quatro libros* (Mexico: Casa de la viuda de Diego Lopez Daualos, 1615), parte 1 lib. 2 cap. 16 fol. 16v.); Monardes, *Historia medicinal*, fols. 2–3.

75 See AGNP Cajas Reales: Lima H-3 Leg. 4 Libro 24-a fols. 34–39 Tasación de las mercaderías que vienen a esta ciudad de los reyes de las provincias de México (1617).

76 Monardes, *Historia medicinal*, fols. 2–7; Nicolás Monardes, *Joyfull Newes out of the New Found World* [1580], ed. John Frampton (London: William Norton, 1580), fols. 2–7v. See also Acosta, *Historia natural y moral*, lib. 4 cap. 29: 123–24.

77 Davis and López Terrada, "Protomedicato y farmacia," 594.

78 AMS Varios antiguos 370 Memoria de las medicinas yo Gaspar de Herrera…he dado para los presos probes [sic] de la cárcel..[Sevilla] 1562–1563; Estes, "European Reception," 13–14;

Apart from the American resins and oils, there is little evidence that licensed medical practitioners in Peru acquired or used native botanical materials. Evidence from hospital account books and from the medicines apothecaries used to treat patients shows that the only American plants being employed regularly were canafistula (*Cassia spp.*), which was used as a purgative, and sarsaparilla (*Smilax* spp.) which was used as a general tonic and to treat skin disorders, especially syphilis. There were two types of canafistula. One originated in India (*Cassia fistula* L.) and was known in Europe from the later Middle Ages; the other was native to the Americas (*Cassia grandis* L.f.) and was first encountered by the Spanish in the Caribbean. Already in the sixteenth century Santo Domingo and Puerto Rico were exporting large quantities of canafistula to Spain, where it was able to compete with that from Asia; the Asian variety was more delicate and often arrived in Europe in a deteriorated state.[79] By the beginning of the seventeenth century the American variety, which was thicker than the European, was being growing profitably in many parts of Spanish America, including around Lima and Paita on the coast of Peru.[80] In the 1590s the Hospital of Santa Ana was regularly acquiring canafistula in large quantities from sources as diverse as Indians, physicians, barbers, and the *boticario* Juan de Bilbao.[81] Bernabé Cobo suggested that the canafistula that was being used in pharmacies was generally imported rather than grown locally;[82] some of the canafistula acquired by the hospitals from *boticarios*, including from Juan de Bilbao, may have been the Asian variety. However, there is no evidence from the cargoes examined in this study that Juan de Bilbao or any other *boticario* in Lima was importing canafistula. On the other hand they

---

Risse, "Transcending Cultural Barriers," 32–33, 37–38. For some examples of Spanish pharmacy inventories see: Pastor Frechoso, *Boticas*, 114, 152, 164; Fernández-Carrión, *Farmacia y sociedad*, 80–96.

79 Monardes, *Historia medicinal*, fol. 20; Chaunu, *Seville et l'Atlantique*, vol. 6²: 1025–26; López Piñero, "Las 'Nuevas medicinas'," 28. As such the canafistula being used in Seville in the sixteenth century may have been the American variety. See: AMS Varios antiguos 370 Memoria de las medicinas yo Gaspar de Herrera…he dado para los presos probes [sic] de la cárcel..[Sevilla] 1562–1563; Fernández-Carrión, *Farmacia y sociedad*, 95, 97.

80 ARJBM División 1, leg. 17 fols. 416–17 Libro de examen de los simples medicinales 1617.

81 ABPL 9085 Libro de la razón…deste hospital de Santa Ana de los gastos que hace Rodrigo Arias de Buyca [Buiça] mayordomo…desde el primero del mes de agosto 1595 and fols. 59–64 1597; ABPL 9084 fols. 169–170 Libro de cuentas de gastos del hospital de Santa Ana año 1598; ABPL 9084 fols. 241–242v Libro de cuentas de gastos del hospital de Santa Ana año 1598 [1599–1600].

82 Cobo, *Obras*, 1: 252; Real Jardín Botánico, Madrid División 1, leg. 17 fols. 416–17 Libro de examen de los simples medicinales 1617.

were importing large quantities of senna (*Cassia senna* L.), another species of cassia. Probably most of the canafistula being used in Lima at that time was the American variety. Luis de Oviedo describes five ways in which canafistula could be employed either in syrups, often of fumitory (*Fumaria officinalis* L.), or in different types of electuary.[83]

Sarsaparilla was grown widely in the Americas, with different species being grown in Mexico, Honduras and Guayaquil.[84] Sarsaparilla (Figure 11) was particularly abundant in the Guayas Basin where according to Nicólas Monardes Indians employed it as a panacea and had taught Spaniards how to make it into a syrup, powder and water.[85] Robles Cornejo claimed that the sarsaparilla found around Guayaquil was not exported to Spain, but was employed in large quantities to treat syphilis (*bubas*) in Peru, where "because of the ease and freedom, vices are more serious."[86] In fact in the nineteenth century the sarsaparilla emanating from Ecuador was known as *Smilax syphilitica* Kunth., taking its name from the disease it was used to treat.[87] In the early colonial period the Hospital of Santa Ana in Lima was purchasing large quantities of sarsaparilla, very often from Indians.[88] Meanwhile the large cargoes of sarsaparilla that were exported to Spain in the sixteenth century did not come from Guayaquil, but rather from the Vice-Royalty of New Spain and especially from Honduras which was said to produce sarsaparilla of superior quality.[89] In Spain it was used as a substitute for the China root (*Smilax china* L.) which was similarly used to treat syphilis.[90]

Another item commonly used in medical treatments, foremost as antivenom, was the bezoar stone (*piedra bezar*), which is a calcareous concretion developed in the stomach of ruminants (See Figure 12). The use of such calcareous concretions developed in Asia and they were being employed in

83 Oviedo, *Methodo*, 118.

84 López Piñero, "Las 'nuevas medicinas'," 33.

85 Monardes, *Historia medicinal*, fols. 14–17, 46, 72. See also Acosta, *Historia natural y moral*, lib. 4 cap. 29: 123; Pedro Cieza de León, *Obras completas* (Madrid: Consejo Superior de Investigaciones Científicas, 1984), 1: 78–79.

86 ARJBM División 1, leg. 17 fols. 194 Libro de examen de los simples medicinales Antonio de Robles Cornejo 1617.

87 López Piñero, "Las 'nuevas medicinas'," 33.

88 ABPL 9080 fols.176–236, 254–57 Libro de cuentas del Hospital de Santa Ana 1575 a 1585; ABPL 9083 fols. 122–23 Libro mayor de rentas del hospital de Santa Ana desde 1593 a 1629 [1609].

89 Hernández, *Quatro libros*, parte 2 lib. 3 cap. 41 fol. 165v; Monardes, *Historia medicinal*, fol. 72; Cobo, *Obras*, 1: 193; ARJBM División 1, leg. 17 fols. 194 Libro de examen de los simples medicinales Antonio Robles de Cornejo 1617; Chaunu, *Seville et l'Atlantique*, 6^2: 1022–25.

90 Winterbottom, "Of the China Root," 33–41.

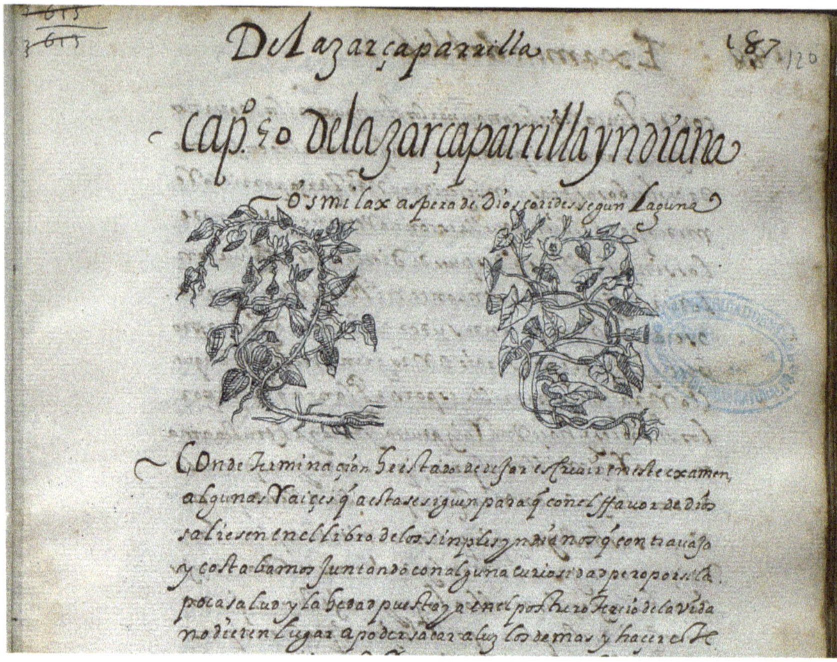

FIGURE 11 *Drawing of sarsaparilla in Antonio de Robles Cornejo's "Examen de los simples medicinales," 1617.*
COURTESY SPAIN. MINISTERIO DE CULTURA. ARCHIVO DEL REAL JARDÍN BOTÁNICO, MADRID. DIVISIÓN 1, LEG. 17 FOL. 187.

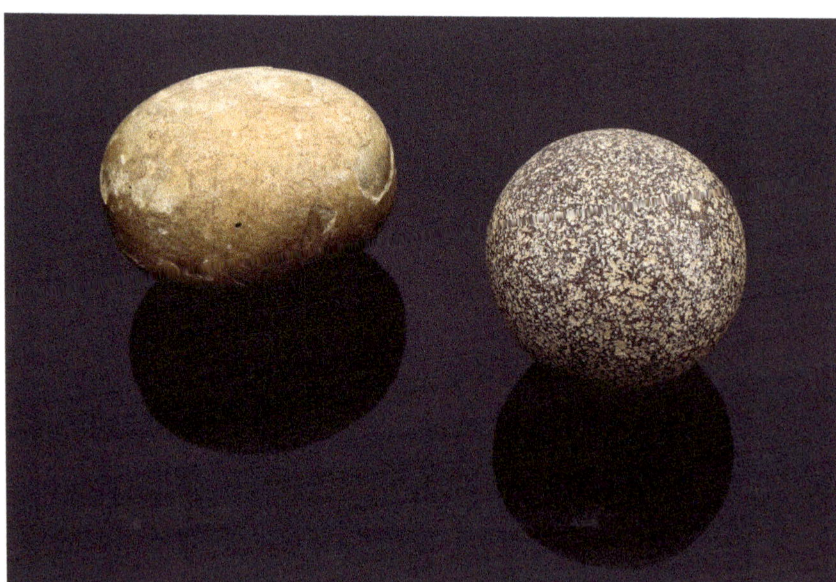

FIGURE 12 *Spherical bezoar stone from unknown animal, 1551–1750.*
COURTESY SCIENCE MUSEUM, LONDON, WELLCOME IMAGES.

Europe in the sixteenth century, though they were expensive. Nicolás Monardes dedicated a whole section of his *Historia medicinal* to the bezoar stones that were produced in Andean alpacas, guanacos and vicuñas, amongst which he indicated the last were the most esteemed.[91] His knowledge was based on information and samples provided by one Pedro de Osma, a soldier and resident in Peru in 1568.[92] Those from the Andes had been used as anti-venom by the local population in pre-Spanish times[93] and local bezoar stones were rapidly adopted by Spaniards in Peru as a welcome substitute for those imported. In the late sixteenth century they were given to the Peruvian Viceroy, the Conde del Villar, whose chamber physician examined them favourably and found them to be quick acting and healthful.[94] Bernabé Cobo also relates the story of the Governor of Chucuito, the Conde de la Gomera, who in 1610 experimented with bezoar stones by feeding two chickens mercury (*solimán*) and then giving powdered bezoar stone to one and not the other. The result was that the former lived thereby demonstrating the product's beneficial anti-venom properties.[95] This account is interesting not only from the perspective of the use of bezoar stone, but also from the fact that Spaniards were employing some rudimentary scientific methods.

Apart from these few products, the sources examined in this study contain virtually no evidence for the adoption of other native plants especially herbs. One might speculate that this reflected their low value, but other low-priced items were included in the accounts. An examination of sixteen legal claims for payments for medicines supplied by *boticarios*, which include detailed lists of medicines prescribed, including the ingredients of *compuestos* and sometimes the individual *recetas* on which they were based, also suggest that the range of native plants employed was very restricted.[96] The sixteen claims list about 30,000 medicines, but native products only figured in about seven

---

91 ARJBM División 1, leg. 17 fols. 460–62 Libro de examen de los simples medicinales Antonio de Robles Cornejo 1617; Cobo, *Obras*, 1: 128; Acosta, *Historia natural y moral*, lib. 4 cap. 42: 137–39; RGI 2: 11 Relación de la ciudad de Cuzco, Vasco de Contreras y Valverde 1 Jan. 1650. For early Spanish observations on the bezoar stone see Marcia Stephenson, "From Marvelous Antidote to the Poison of Idolatry: The Transatlantic Role of Andean Bezoar Stones during the Late Sixteenth and Early Seventeenth Centuries," *Hispanic American Historical Review* 90 (1): 3–39.

92 Monardes, *Historia medicinal*, fols. 575–62v.

93 Acosta, *Historia natural y moral*, lib. 4 cap. 42: 137–38.

94 ARJBM División 1, leg. 17 fols. 641–42 Libro de examen de los simples medicinales 1617.

95 Cobo, *Obras*, 1: 130.

96 See AAL Causas Civiles leg. 17 exp. 18 (1616); leg. 20 exp. 5 (1618); leg. 32 exp. 14 (1627); leg. 33 exp. 19 (1628); leg. 39 exp. 16 (1631), leg. 41 exp. 15 (1632), leg. 42A exp. 2 (1633), leg. 48A

percent of them and similarly accounted for a small proportion of their total value.[97] Apart from the inclusion of canafistula, sarsaparilla, mechoacan, and the resins and oils, liquidambar, *higuerilla*, *tacamahaca* and *anime*, discussed above,[98] the only other noteworthy native botanical products found in the medicines were the Peruvian balsam quina quina (*Myroxylum periferum* L.), which was used to clean and heal wounds, and the oil of the mangrove root – *cativo de mangle* (*Prioria copaifera* Griesb.), which was used for respiratory and urinary infections.[99] *Cativo de mangle* was also found in the pharmacy belonging to Bartolomé Díaz Cabeza de Vaca.[100] Also represented was the calabash (*Cucurbita* sp.) which was frequently used to make ointments or thick syrups (*lamedores*) that were prescribed to treat worms and chest infections.[101] Although calabashes (squashes) are not exclusive to the New World, they were one of the main staples on the coast of Peru and therefore are likely to have been American varieties.[102]

The prescriptions described above were all for individuals associated with the Church who might be regarded as elites. However, an analysis of the prescriptions drawn up for claims against Manuel Bautista Pérez, which were primarily for the treatment of his African slaves, contain only slightly more evidence for the use of native botanical *materia medica*.[103] Of about 2,300 medicines prescribed only about 9 percent contained products of identifiable American origin and these accounted for only about 12 percent by value.[104] Like the medicines prescribed for elites, the native products used to treat slaves

---

exp. 11 (1639), 20 (1636), leg. 50 exp. 16 (1640), 24 (1640), 38 (1640), leg. 65 exp. 6 (1651); AAL Testamentos 6 exp. 1 (1594); Hospitales 2 exp. 3 (1622); AAL AGNP SO CO 125–1091 (1656).

97 The total number of entries in the sixteen claims was 29,421 of which 2,238 were native products and the total value was 2,984 reals, of which 209 reals were for native products.

98 Canafistula figured in eleven claims, sarsaparilla in eight and mechoacan in seven. Among the oils and resins liquidambar was present in six, higuerilla in three, tacamahaca in two and anime in one.

99 Laval, *Botica*, 92.

100 AAL Testamentos 5-1 fol. 45v, Testamento de Bartolomé Díaz Cabeza de Vaca 1608.

101 Laval, *Botica*, 78.

102 Newson and Minchin, *From Capture to Sale*, 203, 215, 303.

103 The contracts that Manuel Bautista Pérez had with the apothecaries Pedro de Bilbao and Alonso de Carrión were for the treatment of his household as well as his slaves, so some persons of non-African origin were probably also treated with the listed medicines. See Newson and Minchin, *From Capture to Sale*, 259–60, 272, 305.

104 Medicines of American origin accounted for 211 entries out of 2,238 and cost 2,683 reals out of a total of 22,216. These figures are indicative rather than definitive.

were dominated by a very small number of plants. The purgatives – canafistula, cassia, and mechoacan – accounted for 36 percent of native products, and resins and oils – *higuerilla*, liquidambar, and turpentine – a further 44 percent. The only other items which appear more than five times were sarsaparilla and bezoar stones. Altogether, only eleven other items of American origin were recorded.[105]

These figures probably overestimate the importance of native *materia medica* marginally, since complex medicines, especially electuaries and syrups, contained several ingredients. Since it is impossible to disaggregate the value of different ingredients in these medicines, the medicine and its total value have been attributed to the item of American origin. In addition, in some cases it is not certain that the item was native to the Americas. This is the case with cassia and turpentine, which could have been imported from Europe.[106] Unlike hospital records, where only canafistula is mentioned, treatments for private patients indicate that at least some *boticarios* were distinguishing between canafistula, cassia, and senna (*Cassia senna* L.), all three species of *Cassia*. On what basis this distinction was made is not clear, particularly since there was no significant difference in price, even though the last, which was imported, would probably have been more expensive. Most of the claims associated with private patients date from the early seventeenth century and it is possible that the name cassia was later used to refer to the American variety of canafistula, though neither Antonio de Robles Cornejo nor Bernabé Cobo made this distinction.

A Few Experiments

Inasmuch as American botanical materials were employed by apothecaries in Lima, probably most were acquired in the market place. There is no evidence that *boticarios* possessed extensive private gardens where they experimented with native plants, though there is some evidence that some were conducting experiments. For example, the *protomédico* Doctor Iñigo de Homero was said to have experimented with papillas, a type of mechoacan, while Robles Cornejo, tried to make a sweeter version of a bitter native purgative, putallanco

105 Sarsaparilla appeared in the accounts eleven times and the bezoar stone in six. The other items were cera de Nicaragua, copal, resina de puna, caraña, quina quina, paico, suelda con suelda, ishpink, plantain, calabash, and palo santo (guaiacum).

106 In six cases cassia and mechoacan are listed together, but the medicine and its value have been counted only once under cassia.

(*Sicyos bryoniaefolius* Chod.).[107] Perhaps more interesting, due to the considerable scholarly attention it has attracted, is evidence for experiments with cinchona bark being undertaken in Lima at an early date. The Sevillian physician Gaspar Caldera de Heredia in his treatise *Acerca del polvo febrifugo de la india occidental* (1663) claimed that Jesuits from the province of Quito took the bark of the "quarango" to the apothecary Gabriel de España in Lima, who made it into a powder to treat fevers. Caldera de Heredia also noted that Gabriel de España, whose pharmacy was located next to the bridge over the river Rimac in Lima, was distributing it widely in the city for the treatment of fevers.[108] This information probably came from Spaniards returning to Seville and must refer to the early seventeenth century since Gabriel de España was described as a master apothecary in 1619.[109] At the same time the Jesuits were preparing the bark of the cinchona for distribution throughout the viceroyalty and eventually to Europe.[110] What interaction there might have been between the Jesuits and apothecaries in Lima is not known.

Native plants were no more common in hospital herb gardens. *Mayordomos* were exhorted to establish gardens to overcome shortages of imported medicines and to ensure that the *materia medica* available were fresh and cheap. Ordinance 45 of the Hospital of Santa Ana in 1609 required the *boticario* to make use of "drugs that are grown locally" (drogas que se dan en la tierra).[111] But this did not necessarily mean native plants for, as indicated in Chapter 4, inspectors instructed *mayordomos* to grow those with which they were familiar in Spain rather than those that were native to the region.

The gardens of Lima's monasteries may have contained a greater variety of native plants. The establishment of monastery gardens served both symbolic and practical functions.[112] Gardens symbolised the coming of civilisation and represented a Garden of Eden in a wilderness. Hence, even prior to the formal

---

107 RGI 2: 7–9 Relación de la ciudad de Cuzco, Vasco de Contreras y Valverde 1 Jan. 1650.

108 José María López Piñero and Francisco Calero (ed.s), *De pulvere febrifugo Occidentalis Indiae* (1663) de Gaspar Caldera de Heredia y la introducción de la quina en Europa (Valencia: Instituto de Estudios Documentales e Históricos sobre la Ciencia, Universidad de Valencia-C.S.I.C., 1992), 19,35–36: Rocco, *Miraculous Fever-Tree*, 60–61.

109 See Chapter 2, where he is called Graviel de España.

110 Rocco, *Miraculous Fever-Tree*, 76–79.

111 *Constituciones y ordenanzas*, 1609.

112 Meredith Beck Sayre, "Cultivating Soils and Souls: The Jesuit Garden in the Americas." MA diss., Simon Fraser University, 2005, 1–4; Andrew Cunningham, "The Culture of Gardens," in *Cultures of Natural History*, eds. Nicholas Jardine, James A. Secord and Emma C. Spary (Cambridge: Cambridge University Press, 2008), 38–47.

establishment of the College of San Pablo in 1568, the Jesuits had established a patio with orange trees and a kitchen garden some 400 feet long by 200 feet wide.[113] Later in 1605 when the Italian Jesuit and trained apothecary Agustino Salumbrino arrived at the College he set about establishing a pharmacy and herb garden.[114] However, with the exception of canafistula, relatively few native plants appear to have been grown the College's gardens. The inventory of its pharmacy when the Jesuits were expelled in 1767 suggests that native plants were still not being used extensively.[115] The College was, however, a major source of *materia medica* for the Viceroyalty supplying large quantities of canafistula to the Hospital of San Andrés,[116] and in the 1630s it was exporting bezoar stones and cinchona to Europe.[117]

The extent to which native plants appear to have been absent in professional medical practice is an unexpected finding, particularly given that visitors and residents in Peru, especially the Jesuit, Bernabé Cobo, observed and commented on the wide range of native plants to be found in the region and on their use by indigenous peoples for medicinal purposes.[118] Antonio de Robles Cornejo observed that *boticarios* showed little curiosity about native plants and were content to rely on imports from Spain, even though they were often of poor quality.[119] In the 1630s Antonio de la Calancha also observed that,

> This land produces innumerable beneficial medicinal herbs and roots, some known, which are the Indians' pharmacy and are used to treat Spaniards where there are no pharmacies, and many are used in cities where physicians use them, and hopefully they [the Spaniards] will try to

113 ARSI Peru Cartas anuas 12 fol. 1 Carta anua [1568] Diego de Bracamonte 21 Jan, 1569.

114 Martín, *Intellectual Conquest*, 99–100; Rocco, *Miraculous Fever-Tree*, 69–80.

115 AGNP Temporalidades. Inventarios leg. 2 cuad. 28 fols. 1–68 Inventario de la botica del Colegio de San Pablos, hecho a raíz de la expatriación de los PP. de la Compañía de Jesús 1768; Rocco, *Miraculous Fever-Tree*, 70–71.

116 AHIRA Maldonado A-III-310 fol. 31 Hospital Real de naturales de Santa Ana. Cuentas que dieron Francisco de Estrada y Fernando de Carvajal año 1645 y 1646.

117 AGNP Compañía de Jesús, Colegio San Pablo, Cuentas leg. 119 fols. 24, 107v–108v. Libro de viáticos y almacén 1628–1631; Martín, *Intellectual Conquest*, 99–102; Rocco, *Miraculous Fever-Tree*, 69–78; Anagnoustou, "Jesuits in Spanish America," 13–14.

118 Cobo, *Obras*, 1: 154–284; RGI 2: 9–11 Relación de la ciudad de Cuzco, Vasco de Contreras y Valverde 1 Jan. 1650.

119 ARJBM División 1, leg. 17 Prologo Libro de examen de los simples medicinales Antonio de Robles Cornejo 1617.

> understand those that have not been tried and will study to be herbalists, so that health might not be put in so much danger, nor simple medicines cause so much harm.[120]

The implication of this statement is that while some experimentation was taking place, native plants were not being widely employed a century after the Spanish had arrived in Peru.

Explaining the Failure to Adopt Native Botanical Materia Medica

The absence of native botanical *materia medica* in remedies prescribed by professional medical practitioners in early colonial Lima is not unique in Spanish America. Paula Ronderos in her study of a *botica* in Bogotá similarly found a lack of native products.[121] What can explain why professional medical practitioners appear to have shown so little interest in native products?

A limited explanation is that plants were sometimes misnamed. It was noted at the time that Spanish observers had the propensity to give native plants Spanish names if they possessed the same physical attributes as those found in Spain. This criticism has been levelled at Antonio de Robles Cornejo himself, who it was said followed Dioscorides and thus identified a number of plants as being of Old World in origin when in fact they were distinct indigenous ones. For example, he reported that in Peru there was an abundance of *cebollas albarranas* (maritime squill – Urginea maritima(L.) Stearn.), when it is argued that more likely it was the Caribbean spiderlily (*Hymenocallis caribaea (L.) Herb.*). Other plants might be labelled as indigenous, when in fact they were native to Africa or Asia, because they had been introduced and spread at an early date thereby giving the impression that they were native to the region.[122] More broadly, as noted above, it is not clear whether entries for canafistula referred to the American variety or to the true canafistula (*Cassia fistula L.*) of Asian origin, while some balsams, resins, and turpentine registered in pharmacy inventories and treatments were referred to generically making it impossible to know whether they derived from Old World or New World trees or plants. The acute observer Bernabé Cobo, who knew both Quechua and Aymara, recognised that many native plants had been misnamed on the basis of their similarities to European ones and was anxious to distinguish between

120 Calancha, *Crónica moralizada*, lib. 1 cap. 9: 59.

121 Ronderos, *El dilema*.

122 Colmeiro, "Noticias," 442–43. Colmeiro provides a list of other examples where Robles Cornejo may have mistaken the origin of plants. See also Anagnoustou, "Jesuits in Spanish America," 12.

them.[123] Hence in his *Historia del Nuevo Mundo* he set about describing the local plants in precise detail and devoted a whole section to explaining how he distinguished native species from foreign ones. His methods involved examining the origin of the names applied to plants and in interviewing old native informants as well as Spaniards who had been in Peru in the earliest years of colonial rule.[124]

While misnaming is likely to have contributed to an underestimation of the use of native plants, other obstacles to their adoption were probably more significant. Perhaps the most important impediment from the perspective of Spanish trained practitioners was that any new product had to be placed within the prevailing Galenic framework. Each new plant needed to be tested for smell, taste, and therapeutic function, for example, as a purgative, emollient, or sudorific medicine, as well as assessed for its efficacy.[125] Hence, the Spanish physician Matías de Porres claimed that in preparation for an uncompleted study entitled "Concordancias medicinales de entrambos mundos," he had studied native plants with "particular care and curiosity" obtaining information from old native informants who had learned by experience how to use them. Porres was educated at the University of Salamanca and became chamber physician to Francisco de Borja, Principe de Esquilache, when he was Viceroy of Peru. His arrival in Lima was facilitated by the *protomédico* at the time, Doctor Melchor de Amusco. Part of Porres's aim in writing his treatise was to demonstrate that it was unnecessary to import medicines from Spain since Peru possessed all the necessary things to support human life.[126]

Apothecaries who might be interested in using native products had few sources to turn to for guidance. Manuals imported from Europe sometimes included comments on the few American plants that had been studied in Spain, but often their humoral qualities were disputed. For example, sarsaparilla was described by Nicólas Monardes as hot and dry in the second degree

123 Prieto, *Missionary Scientists*, 189–94; Emmanuelle Moreau, "Le Père Bernabé Cobo et la nomenclature botanique," *Caravelle* 82 (2004): 195–204.

124 Cobo, *Obras*, 1: 154–58; Prieto, *Missionary Scientists*, 106.

125 Risse, "Transcending Cultural Barriers," 32, 34–35; Ronderos, *El dilema*, 131; Xavier Lozoya, "Natural History and Herbal Medicine in Sixteenth-century America, in *Science in Latin America: A History*, edited by Juan José Saldaña (Austin: University of Texas Press, 2006), 44–45. For native plants classified according to Galenic principles, such as wet or dry, hot or cold see: RGI 2: 7–9 Relación de la ciudad de Cuzco, Vasco de Contreras y Valverde 1 Jan. 1650, and ARJBM División 1, leg. 17 Libro de examen de los simples medicinales Antonio de Robles Cornejo 1617 *passim*.

126 Matías de Porres, *Breve advertencias para beber frío con nieve* (Lima, 1621), 32–32v; Rey Bueno, "Concordias," 351–52, 358.

and by Francisco Hernández as cold and dry.[127] Discrepancies in the qualities and application of different medicines were quite common at the time and they contributed to a general wariness in the use of American products for fear of the harm they might inflict.[128] As such Spaniards generally preferred to be treated with those medicines with which they were familiar.[129] Such uncertainties surrounding native plants also contributed to their delayed adoption in Europe, which was further discouraged by the low efficacy of imports that had to survive the Atlantic journey and by the existence of already effective medicines in Europe, as well as by pure prejudice against foreign products.[130]

The process of acquiring knowledge of the qualities and use of native plants might have been easier had Spaniards shown more interest in the way that indigenous peoples employed them. However, even the best ethnographic studies, such as that of Bernabé Cobo, focus on finding substitutes for products employed in Europe rather than on learning from indigenous people how they might be used. Reluctance to adopt native *materia medica*, particularly from the clergy, was based in part on the perception that native products were potentially harmful and probably more important were associated with indigenous ritual and heretical beliefs.[131] Hence, if native products were to be used in medical treatments they needed to be stripped of their cultural meaning.[132] The Jesuit, Pablo José de Arriaga, who was involved in the programme to suppress idolatry in the Andes in the early seventeenth century advised that priests should instruct popular healers, so that "removing what is superstitious and bad, advantage can be taken of what is good: as is the knowledge and use of some herbs, and other simples, which they use in their illnesses."[133] Nature thus became a "quarry" from which medicinal products could be extracted, placed within a Galenic framework, and fresh medicines made more widely

127 Monardes, *Historial medicinal*, f.22; Hernández, *Quatro libros*, parte 2 lib. 3 cap. 41 fol. 165v; Risse, "Transcending Cultural Barriers," 37–38.

128 McVaugh, "'Experience-Based Medicine'," 113–14.

129 Mauricio Sánchez-Menchero, "From Where They Are Now to Whence They Came From": News About Health and Disease in New Spain (1550–1615)," in *Medical Cultures of the Early Modern Spanish Empire*, eds. John Slater, María Luz López Terrada and José Pardo-Tomás (Farnham: Ashgate, 2014), 100–01.

130 Estes, "European Reception," 11–13; Slater, "Green Gold Fallacies," 106–112.

131 Brosseder, *Power of Huacas*, 193–98, 263–64; Prieto, *Missionary Scientists*, 6, 81–84.

132 Calancha, *Crónica moralizada* lib. 3 cap. 2 Section 12: 556; Bleichmar, "Books, Bodies, and Fields," 97–99; Crawford, *Andean Wonder Drug*, 34–39.

133 Pablo Joseph de Arriaga, *La extirpación de idolatrías del Perú* (Lima: Geronymo de Contreras, 1621), 74.

available at cheaper cost.[134] This approach was consistent with Christian world views of the time that saw nature as having been placed there by God to serve human needs.[135] Thus, as Paula De Vos shows for eighteenth century Mexico, even when indigenous medicines did penetrate pharmacies, apothecaries did not involve themselves in the healing practices that went with them.[136]

Even though there might be concern about the potential harm that native treatments might cause and their ritual significance, Spaniards often acknowledged that some Indians were great herbalists and were respected as "licenciados" within their communities. Hence bishops convened for the Second Council of Lima in 1567–1568 agreed that native healers might be given written licence to practise using herbs and roots as long as their healing practices had been examined by the bishop and any superstitious words and ceremonies removed.[137] Indigenous healing skills were also respected by Martín de Murúa who was equally concerned about the superstitious practices that accompanied them as well as their lack of knowledge of when and how to apply treatments for different ailments, circumstances that would encourage experimentation, sometimes with disastrous consequences.[138] Spanish recognition of the superior knowledge and experience of local plants possessed by indigenous people may have persuaded professional medical practitioners to leave the field to them.[139] This may have been especially true of *Conversos* who may have been more hesitant to employ native products since they were more vulnerable to charges of heresy and being brought before the Inquisition.[140] There

134 José Pardo-Tomás, "Two Glimpses of America from a Distance: Carolus Clusius and Nicolás Monardes," in Carolus Clusius: Towards a Cultural History of a Renaissance Naturalist, eds. Florike Egmond, Paul Hoftijzer and Robert Visser (Amsterdam: Edita, 2007), 179, 183, 192–93.

135 Robin Attfield, "Christian Attitudes to Nature," *Journal of the History of Ideas* 44 (3) (1983): 369–86; Per Binde, "Nature in Roman Catholic Tradition," *Anthropological Quarterly* 74(1) (2001): 16–18; Sayre, "Cultivating Soils and Souls," 3–4; Steven J. Harris, "Jesuit Scientific Activity in the Overseas Missions, 1540–1773," *Isis* 96 (1) (2005): 75.

136 De Vos, "From Herbs to Alchemy," 139.

137 Rubén Vargas Ugarte, *Concilios limenses (1551–1772)* (Lima: Imp. Juan Cardenal Guevara, 1951), 1: 255.

138 Murúa, *Historia general*, 2: 102–103. See also ARJBM División 1, leg. 17 Prologo. Libro de examen de los simples medicinales Antonio de Robles Cornejo 1617.

139 Ronderos, *El dilema*, 130.

140 For a detailed example of the influence of the Inquisition on the investigations conducted by a New Christian naturalist/medical practitioner see the case of the Portuguese physician Garcia de Orta in Hugh Cagle, "Cultures of Inquiry, Myths of Empire: Natural History

were also social status advantages for professional practitioners in distancing themselves from popular healers.[141] Timothy Walker has observed a similar process of separation between the professional and popular sectors during the Enlightenment in Portugal, when the former sought to associate themselves with ideas of rationalism and distanced themselves from popular healers who came under the increased scrutiny of the Inquisition.[142]

Not only were medical practitioners disinclined to adopt native plants, but indigenous healers were also reluctant to reveal their healing practices to them.[143] When Robles Cornejo was in La Paz he was anxious to ascertain the name and qualities of the root that some local people had given their *encomendero*, Don Diego Dávalos, to cure his wife, but was unable to extract more information from them despite offering gifts, money, and clothing.[144] For native healers their medical knowledge was often essential to their power and status within their community.[145] Such cultural resistance to the disclosure of methods of healing would have been reinforced by the experience of conquest, colonial rule, and fear of persecution. This was especially so in the late sixteenth and early seventeenth centuries Andes when the slow pace of Christian conversion led to large scale programmes to eradicate idolatrous practices.[146] While the unwillingness of native peoples to disclose knowledge of medicinal plants may have been a hindrance to their adoption by professional medical

in Colonial Goa," in *Medicine, Trade and Empire: Garcia de Orta's Colloquies on the Simples and Drugs of India (1563)*, ed. Palmira Fontes da Costa (Farnham: Ashgate, 2015), 107–128.

141 For this argument in the context of food see: Rebecca Earle, "'If You Eat Their Food': Diets and Bodies in Early Colonial Spanish America," *American Historical Review* 115 (3), 710–12.

142 Timothy D. Walker, *Doctors, Folk Medicine and the Inquisition: the Repression of Magical Healing in Portugal during the Enlightenment* (Leiden: Brill, 2005).

143 Schiebinger, *Plants and Empire*, 90–92, 104; Heidi V. Scott, *Contested Territory: Mapping Peru in the Sixteenth and Seventeenth Centuries* (Notre Dame, IN: University of Notre Dame Press, 2009), 56.

144 ARJBM División 1, leg. 17 fol. 198 Libro de examen de los simples medicinales Antonio de Robles Cornejo 1617.

145 Prieto, *Missionary Scientists*, 41–42. This refers to Jesuit work among the Mapuche but it is no less relevant to Peru.

146 For the extirpation of idolatries in the Andes see Pierre Duviols, *La lutte contre les religions autochtones dans le Pérou colonial: l'extirpation de l'idolâtrie, entre 1532 et 1660* (Lima: Institut Français d'Etudes Andines, 1971); Nicholas Griffiths, *The Cross and the Serpent: Religious Repression and Resurgence in Colonial Peru* (Norman: University of Oklahoma Press, 1995); Kenneth Mills, *Idolatry and Its Enemies: Colonial and Andean Religion and* Extirpation, 1640–1750 (Princeton: Princeton University Press, 1997); and Brosseder, *Power of Huacas*.

practitioners, in theory at least it could have encouraged them to experiment with native plants themselves.

Finally, the failure to adopt native plants may also be viewed in the context of the contemporary debate over the influence of astrology on the natural world and whether local or foreign remedies were the most appropriate to use.[147] The complexion or humoral balance of an individual was thought to be affected by the stars and climate and there was a belief that Spanish bodies should not be treated with exotic or strange plants that were raised under a different constellation. Paracelsians however argued for the universal application of remedies that were appropriate for the treatment of particular diseases rather than for different bodies. The fact that professional medical practitioners, whose business focused, though not exclusively, on Spanish and Creole elites, were continuing to use Old World *materia medica* rather than adopt native medicinal products suggests that at the beginning of the seventeenth century Paracelsian arguments for the universal applicability of remedies were not having a significant impact on medical practice in Lima. However, the procedures involved in testing medicinal products for their efficacy in treating particular ailments, where they did occur, had the effect of encouraging experimentation, a task that fell largely into the hands of apothecaries. Paradoxically, therefore, rather than bolster humoral medical practice that focused on individualised treatments based on a patient's particular constitution, these experimental processes fostered the search for universal remedies that ultimately served to undermine it.[148]

A Medical Marketplace?

These findings raise the question of the applicability of the concept of a "medical marketplace" to medical provision in early colonial Lima. Developed in the context of early modern England, the concept envisaged a unified market where a diversity of practitioners and products competed with each other for custom.[149] The concept emerged at a time when medical historians focussed on the professional and institutional sector, so by including a spectrum of

147 Andrew Wear, "Early Modern Debate," 149–51.

148 Harold J. Cook, "Markets and Cultures: Medical Specifics and the Reconfiguration of the Body in Early Modern Europe," *Transactions of the Royal Historical Society* 21 (2011): 123–45.

149 Roy Porter, "Patient's View," 175–98. For a critique of the concept of a medical market place see: Mark S.R. Jenner and Patrick Wallis, "*The Medical Marketplace," in Medicine and the Market in England and its Colonies, c.1450–1850*, eds. Mark S. R Jenner and Patrick Wallis (Basingstoke: Palgrave Macmillan, 2007), 1–23.

popular healers, it had the advantages both of integrating all forms of health provision under one umbrella and of contributing to knowledge from below. However, it has drawn criticism from a number of standpoints. First, and perhaps most pertinent for this discussion, it is argued that in early modern times the market was not such a competitive free-for-all as the concept implies. In the case of Lima, the market was constrained by the regulation of apothecary shops and the training and licensing of practitioners, even though this may not have been completely effective. In addition, the Inquisition and ecclesiastical courts attempted to control popular medical practices that were regarded as heretical.

Other critics of the concept have noted that the term "market" is less appropriate for the early modern period, when charitable provision and family care were prevalent and treatment of the sick was not driven so much by commercial considerations.[150] Neither were all options freely available to all. Elites with more substantial financial resources would have had a broader choice of treatments, while the care provided by charitable institutions was only available to the poor. Individuals' knowledge of the medical treatments available would have been filtered by their beliefs, tradition, experience, and the information they had acquired from family and friends. Residents of Lima were generally preoccupied with their health and in common with populations world-wide would have been risk-averse in their search for medical care.[151] Hence the sick would have been inclined to seek advice largely though not exclusively from the sector with which they were most familiar. In early modern Lima two broad medical sectors can be identified: a professional or corporate sector, which largely served the elite, and a diverse popular sector. While the two sectors appear essentially distinct and complementary in terms of their medical *practices*, their separation was slightly more blurred in the case of *clienteles*. Individuals, though seeking advice predominantly from medical practitioners in one sector, might also look for treatments in the other.

In the Americas, as in Europe, elites regularly consulted popular healers with specialist skills such as midwives, bonesetters, phlebotomists, tooth-pullers, and oculists, some of whom were partially trained and officially regulated.[152]

150 See Andrew Wear, *Knowledge and Practice*, 28–29.

151 Kenneth J. Arrow, "Uncertainty and the Welfare Economics of Medical Care," *The American Economic Review* 53 (5)(1963): 946.

152 Goodman, "Philip II's Patronage," 54–55; Lanning, *Royal Protomedicato*, 282–86, 290–97, 303; Solano Alonso, *Salud, cultura y sociedad*, 103–04; Brockliss and Jones, *Medical World*, 291–92.

As will be shown in Chapter 7, the medical profession, including *boticarios*, was not held in high regard and members of the elite were not therefore averse to consulting popular healers or herbalists when treatment by a licensed practitioner failed.[153] Within the popular sector several healers might be employed to treat a single condition. Hence, in one redhibitory case involving an African slave in 1608, his owner a carpenter, Juan López, consulted an Indian from El Cercado in the district of San Lázaro who knew how to cure dysentery, and an African slave, Beatriz Criolla, whose healing methods involved placing the beak of a bird on the slave, an African healing practice that aimed at transferring the illness from the person to the bird.[154]

Even though in reality the majority of Lima's population probably could not afford the services of professionally trained practitioners, especially physicians,[155] there is some evidence that members of the popular classes, including slaves, sought advice and treatment by licensed *boticarios*. One such person was Quiomar Biafara, whose name indicates she was of African heritage, who consulted the *boticario* Bernardo Gil in search of a cure for scabies.[156] Outside Lima, in the province of Cuzco, the *corregidor* of Chumbivilcas noted that Indians went to pharmacies in the towns, though they generally preferred to use herbs in their medicinal treatments.[157]

Overall, the structure of medical provision in Lima corresponds closely to that outlined for early modern France by Lawrence Brockliss and Colin Jones. They argue that the market in France was not unstructured, competitive, and open to all. Rather it comprised two sectors: a core comprising a professional and corporatist medical community of practice that was surrounded by a

---

153 Osorio, "'*Callejón de la Soledad*,'" 199–200, 217.

154 AAL Causas de Negros 1609 leg. 1 exp. 31 Juan López, carpintero, contra el Padre Diego de Ybarreta 13 Oct. 1608. For the use of birds and chickens in African healing rituals see Inés Sosadias, "El negro curandero en la Inquisición de Cartagena de Indias siglo XVII." MA in Anthropology, Universidad de los Andes, 1981, 174, 178; Luz Adriana Maya Restrepo "Botánica y medicina africanas en la Nueva Granada, siglo XVII," *Historia crítica* 19 (2000): 39–42; James H. Sweet *Domingos Álvares, African Healing, and the Intellectual History of the Atlantic World* (Chapel Hill: University of North Carolina Press, 2011), 114, 258 n. 32.

155 Juan Lastres (*Historia de la medicina* 2: 81) estimates that in sixteenth-century Lima a medical examination by a physician might cost six *ducados* or by a surgeon or *boticario* four *ducados*.

156 AAL Causas de Negros leg.4 doc. 7 Expediente de la demanda de redivitoria que sigue Hernando de Valdés 1620.

157 RGI 1: 319 Relación fecha por el corregidor de los Chumbibilcas, Don Francisco de Acuña 23 Feb. 1586.

"medical penumbra" of informal and unregulated healers that provided services for the majority of the population.[158]

Using Minerals and Chemicals

Those medical practitioners who advocated experimental techniques in the treatment of illness often employed chemical methods and incorporated minerals in some form. The use of such techniques would have been encouraged in Peru by the region's rich mineral deposits. Indeed, it is clear from Bernabé Cobo's writings that in the early colonial period indigenous people were employing some minerals for medicinal purposes and that some of their treatments dated back to pre-Spanish times.[159] However, Cobo states explicitly that the Indians lacked knowledge of certain minerals, such as copper, tin, magnetite (*piedra imán*) and lead carbonate (*albayalde*),[160] prior to Spanish arrival; in other cases, for example emeralds and pearls, he makes no comment on their indigenous use leaving the question open.

Among the minerals clearly being used by Indians for medicinal purposes was powder made from Armenian bole (*bol arménico*), which the Indians called *tacu*. This was being sold freely in the market and consumed in *chicha* to cure dysentery.[161] According to Robles Cornejo adulterated *bol arménico* was causing many deaths.[162] *Haquimasci*, which Cobo likened to *piedra judaica* (Jews' stone), was also being used to cure dysentery and prevent blood loss, especially from women who had just given birth; it was also employed to heal wounds and treat contagious diseases, in addition to being used as anti-venom and an anti-depressant.[163] Another mineral used by indigenous peoples for medicinal purposes was the copper-based *copaquira*, also known as *piedra lipes* (blue vitriol or copper sulphate), which was employed as an astringent and to treat toothache.[164] A copper-based green stone called *coravari* was also used

158 Brockliss and Jones, *Medical World*, 296. They prefer to use the term "core" and "penumbra" rather than elite and popular, due to the negative connotations of the latter (pp. 8–20, 228–29).

159 Cobo, *Obras*, 1: 108–53.

160 Ibid. 1: 153.

161 Ibid. 1: 116.

162 ARJBM División 1, leg. 17 fols. 619–20 Libro de examen de los simples medicinales Antonio de Robles Cornejo 1617.

163 Cobo, *Obras*, 1: 127.

164 Ibid. 1: 126; Calancha, *Corónic moralizada*, 54.

as an astringent and in the preparation of an eye-wash.[165] Other minerals were used for veterinary purposes. Sulphur was utilised to cure mange in llamas and sheep;[166] initially it was not used to treat humans, though it was later employed as a remedy for skin infections.[167] Some minerals were known to indigenous people but were not used for medicinal purposes. Hence, Cobo claimed that the Indians did not know how to extract *azogue* (mercury) prior to the arrival of the Spanish, but did use vermillion (mercury sulphate) with which it was generally found. However, the vermillion was not being used for medicinal purposes but rather employed as a red pigment in paints, ink, and dyes, while copper sulphate was used with the fruit of *tara* (*Tara spinosa* (Molina) Britton & Rose) to prepare a local ink called *colpa.*[168]

Cobo concluded that God had enriched Peru, not only with innumerable plants and herbs for the benefit of humankind, but also with a great diversity of minerals that could be used to cure illnesses, to manufacture weapons, tools and equipment, and to make ornaments to adorn themselves and their houses.[169] The interaction of native peoples with the mineral world may even have extended to geophagy or the consumption of earth. This is practised in parts of the Peruvian and Bolivian Andes where it is thought that the ingestion of mineral earths provides dietary supplements that counteract the phytotoxins found in local foods.[170]

In Europe, the use of minerals in medicines extended back to classical times. Dioscorides in his *De materia medica* devoted a whole section to the processing of minerals and their use in medicines.[171] Dioscorides was writing before the development of distillation methods, such that the processes he described were based on some form of heating. However, later commentators on Dioscorides sometimes included appendices outlining distillation methods.[172] Robles Cornejo judged that the use of *litargirio* (lead oxide) was so well known

---

165 Cobo, *Obras*, 1: 127.

166 Ibid. 1: 112.

167 Fresquet Febrer, "Uso de productos del reino mineral," 73.

168 Cobo, *Obras*, 1: 116.

169 Ibid. 1: 135–37.

170 David L. Browman, and James N. Gundersen, "Altiplano Comestible Earths: Prehistoric and Historic Geophagy of Highland Peru and Bolivia," *Geoarchaeology* 8 (5) (1993): 413–25.

171 Robert T. Gunther, *The Greek Herbal of Disocorides* (New York: Harner Publishing Co., 1959), 623–60.

172 Robert J Forbes, *A History of the Art of Distillation* (Leiden: E.J. Brill, 1970), 127, 133–34.

that he decided not to discuss it at length in his manual.[173] As noted in Chapter 5, those who developed chemical methods drew on the work of alchemists who were especially interested in mercury, sulphur and antimony, and in the preparation of mineral salts and spirits.[174] Antimony (*stibio* or *antimonio*) in particular became associated with the new experimental forms of medicine and the centre of debates between the Galenists and Paracelsians.[175] The extensive deposits of silver found in Peru and Bolivia were often accompanied by antimony, lead, sulphur, and arsenic; antimony was also found in small quantities on its own.[176] Antimony was one mineral that the Spanish *protomédico general*, Zamudio de Alfaro, indicated that *boticas* should possess,[177] even though it was not commonly used in Spain until the seventeenth century.[178]

A key difference between the Galenists and Paracelsians was that the former only used minerals in medicines that were applied externally, often in ointments and plasters that were used to treat skin infections and wounds, whereas the latter advocated their inclusion in medicines that were taken internally. Antimony was probably used in *unguento de plomo*,[179] but was also a strong purgative.[180] Robles Cornejo writing in Peru at the beginning of the seventeenth century observed that antimony was not only being used externally, but was being taken internally as a purgative, with perhaps 10 or 12, or even 15 grains being used in a single dose; it was also used to treat melancholy.[181] Other hints at the use of antimony by *boticarios* can be seen in Robles Cornejo's

173 ARJBM División 1, leg. 17 fol. 581 Libro de examen de los simples medicinales Antonio de Robles Cornejo 1617.

174 Debus, *Chemical Philosophy*, 1: 20–23; Multhauf, "Significance of Distillation," 330–33; Moran, *Distilling Knowledge*, 12–25. For the relationship between alchemy and chemistry see: Newman, "From Alchemy to 'Chymistry'," 497–517. For the dates at which the processes for separating particular metals and producing mineral acids were discovered see Georgius Agricola, *De re metalica*, trans. Herbert Clark Hoover and Lou Henry Hoover. (New York: Dover Publications, Inc., 1950), 354.

175 Laval, *Botica*, 52–53; Fernández-Carrión and Valverde, *Farmacia y sociedad*, 49.

176 Cobo, *Obras*, 1: 108–53; ARJBM División 1, leg. 17 fol. 588 Libro de examen de los simples medicinales Antonio de Robles Cornejo 1617; Georg G. Peterson, *Mining and Metallurgy in Ancient Perú. The Geological Society of America Special Paper 467* (Boulder, Col.: The Geological Society of America, Inc., 2010), 27–31.

177 Davis and López Terrada, "Protomedicato y farmacia," 593.

178 Fernández-Carrión and Valverde, *Farmacia y Sociedad*, 49, 80.

179 Davis and López Terrada, "Protomedicato y farmacia," 609; Laval, *Botica*, 195.

180 Fresquet Febrer, "Uso de productos del reino mineral," 68.

181 ARJBM División 1, leg. 17 fols. 588–62 Libro de examen de los simples medicinales Antonio de Robles Cornejo 1617.

observation that *boticarios* were not following recipes precisely, but adding ingredients such as *estibio*, scammony, and spurge (*lechetrezna*).[182] According to him, *estibio* was the crude mineral and *antimonio*, also referred to as alcohol, was the name given to the product when it was used in medical treatments.[183] The latter was probably antimony sulphide.[184] Small quantities of antimony were imported by the *boticarios* Juan and Pedro de Bilbao, and when the latter died in 1634 8.5 pounds of antimony and 2.75 pounds of *estibio* were inventoried in his pharmacy.[185] The *boticarios* Francisco Martín Reyna and Gerónimo Pujadas also imported about a dozen pounds of antimony with each fleet. Gerónimo Pujadas regularly imported minerals in larger quantities than other *boticarios*. Two cargoes consigned to him in 1618 and 1619 together contained 37 pounds of antimony, as well as sulphur and arsenic sulphide (*oropimente* and *rejalgar*).[186] Antimony was valued at 20 reals an *arroba* (25 pounds). However, there is no evidence of antimony being imported for hospitals or that they secured it from local suppliers.

Another toxic mineral acid promoted by Paracelsus was *solimán* (mercuric chloride). In Lima this was quite widely employed in the form of unctions to treat syphilis, which in the Hospital of Santa Ana were often applied by African slaves.[187] *Solimán* does not appear among imports for hospitals, but rather the Hospital of Santa Ana acquired it mainly from shops (*tiendas*), though it is not clear whether it was imported or obtained locally. Related to mercury but used externally were *polvos de juanes* or *vigo* containing red precipitate of mercury. These powders had been formulated as an astringent for the treatment of wounds by the Italian surgeon Giovanni da Vigo (ca. 1450–1525).[188] Despite

182 ARJBM División 1, leg. 17 Prohemiales 11 Libro de examen de los simples medicinales Antonio de Robles Cornejo 1617.

183 ARJBM División 1, leg. 17 fol. 588 Libro de examen de los simples medicinales Antonio de Robles Cornejo 1617.

184 Agricola, *De re metallica*, 110, 428.

185 AGNP Protocolos Siglo XVII 1789 Diego Sánchez Vadillo fols. 1372v.–1374v. Inventario de los bienes de Pedro de Bilbao difunto 8 Jul. 1636.

186 AGI Contratación, 1166 N10 425–29 Registro del navío San Pedro 1618; AGI Contratación 1168 N1 191–96 Registro del navío San Salvador 1619.

187 ABPL 9806 fols.104–05 Visita al Hospital de Santa Ana sin fecha [1588]; AAL Causas de Negros leg. 1 doc. 2 Expediente de los autos que sigue el Doctor Vásquez Fajardo contra Gaspar Guerrero 1593; Fresquet Febrer, "Uso de productos del reino mineral," 86.

188 Oviedo, *Methodo*, 441.

their high cost *polvos de juanes*, were acquired in quite large quantities when the *botica* of the Hospital of Santa Ana was established in 1551.[189]

There were more frequent imports of arsenic sulphide (*oropimente*) and red arsenic sulphide (*rejalgar*). These were very toxic minerals and they were generally used in medicines that were applied externally, including in an eyewash called agua de Lanfranc.[190] These mineral products and *solimán* were particularly common among the imports of three private *boticarios* – Francisco Martín Reyna, Gerónimo Pujadas, and Francisco Crespo – where they accounted for about 10 percent of the minerals they imported by value. The proportion is surprisingly high given that these minerals were widely available locally. In fact they were so readily available that in 1551 the *cabildo* of Lima found it necessary to prohibit the sale of "solimán or rejalgar or oropimente or any other product that might be fatal" to any slave and only to Spaniards over 15 years old, because some slaves had died from taking it.[191] Evidence from legal cases resulting from the sale slaves with undeclared illnesses, also reveal that slave owners were regularly using "agua de solimán" to treat their slaves who were suffering from syphilis[192] and employing "piedra lipes" (copper sulphate) to wash their lower parts.[193] In 1634 the *protomedico*, Doctor Juan de Vega, complained that everyone was selling *solimán*, and that the authorities should make it a monopoly and use the proceeds to support the university.[194]

Another mineral product employed in medicines that were taken internally was copper sulphate (*caparrosa*), which Robles Cornejo observed was abundant in the kingdom of Peru especially in Charcas in the valleys of Chaynata, Guantapita and Quilaquila. He suggested that a scruple taken in a drink safeguarded people in an epidemic and a dragma (three scruples) in fennel water

---

189 AGNP Protocolos Siglo XVI 63 Diego Gutiérrez fols. 167–88 Quenta de la botica que va en la nao 20 Oct. 1551. The high price of *polvos de juanes* is evident from the level of *almojarifazgo* charged on their arrival in Lima (AGNP Cajas Reales, Lima H-3 leg. 4 Libro 24-a fols. 1–30 Aranceles para cálculo del almojarifazgo (1817)).

190 Laval, *Botica*, 147–48; Davis and López Terrada, "Protomedicato y farmacia," 601.

191 *Libros de cabildos de Lima*, 3: 416 Ordenanza de solimán 24 Jul. 1551.

192 AAL Causas de Negros leg. 2 doc. 4 Bartolomé Verdugo pone demanda al Bachiller Juan Manuel Carrasco, albacea y tenedor de bienes del Padre Diego de Ybarreta, pues le vendió una negra, Isabel Bañol, con un hijo, 1610.

193 AAL Causas de Negros leg. 2 doc. 29 Diego de Vílchez, marido de Isabel de Landecho, madre de Mariana de Landecho, a su nombre, contra el Licenciado Don Diego Gatica, presbítero, acerca de la venta de Catalina Beafara.

194 AGI Lima 45 N 4 fols. 146–47 Conde de Chinchón 21 Apr. 1634.

helped against poisoning and killed fungus.[195] It is therefore clear that some experimentation with minerals and mineral acids was taking place and that they were being used in wide range of medicines that were taken internally.

Despite these observations on the widespread use of toxic minerals, which probably attracted attention due to their potentially harmful effects, in fact they comprised only a small proportion of the minerals that were either imported or used in recipes in Lima. The minerals that were most commonly utilised were *alumbre* (aluminium potassium sulphate), *cardenillo* (verdigris or basic copper acetate), *albayalde* (lead carbonate or white lead) and *almártaga* (lead oxide – *litargirio*). Hospitals regularly acquired these minerals from *tiendas* and occasionally from apothecaries, who had probably imported them. They were mainly employed in the preparation of ointments and plasters that were used primarily in the treatment of ailments of the skin, such as scabies, but less commonly for venereal disease and muscle strain;[196] those that contained minerals were used more specifically as astringents to dry, clean, and heal wounds and ulcers, or to harden and smooth the skin.[197]

Ointments containing minerals accounted for just over 20 percent of all ointments supplied to Manuel Bautista Pérez for his slaves and household; this was slightly higher than the 15 percent found in prescriptions for other patients, mainly priests.[198] These are very rough estimates that do not take account of the quantity of ointments prepared or of the unknown illnesses that were being treated that would have required different medicines and doses, but they do suggest that ointments containing minerals represented a relatively small proportion of the total. The main ointments containing minerals that were prescribed for slaves incorporated litharge or lead. They included white ointment (*blanco*) that contained lead carbonate. Other common ointments were *egipciaco* prepared from an oximel of copper, honey, sharp vinegar, and *cardenillo*[199] and the more complex Condesa ointment composed of oil and

195 ARJBM División 1, leg. 17 fols. 599–602 Libro de examen de los simples medicinales Antonio de Robles Cornejo 1617.

196 Rojo Vega, *Enfermos y sanadores*, 75; Laval, *Botica*, 189–97.

197 Laval, *Botica*, 45, 49–51, 84; Fresquet Febrer, "Uso de productos del reino mineral," 65 66, 77; Vargas Machuca, *Milicia*, 131; Santiago Díaz Piedrahita and Luis Carlos Mantilla, *La terapéutica en el Nuevo Reino de Granada: un recetario franciscano del siglo XVIII* (Bogotá: Academia Colombiana de Ciencias Exactas, Físicas y Naturales, 2002), 71, 116,131, 135,137, 148.

198 For the bills incurred by Manuel Bautista Pérez with Pedro de Bilbao and Alonso de Carrión see: AGNP SO CO Ca. 57 doc 431 1629, 1635–1640. For the sources of those dispensed to elites associated with the Church see note 96. The precise proportion was 22 percent.

199 Oviedo, *Methodo*, 409; Laval, *Botica*, 192.

berries of myrtle, yellow wax, galls, cypress nuts, pomegranate rind, seeds of senna and plantain, mastic and *alumbre*. The latter was used to treat slackness in the belly, thus for treating hernias and to prevent miscarriage.[200]

Plasters accounted for about five percent of all medicines contained in the prescriptions examined here and of those less than 10 percent contained a mineral. Among the latter the most common were *diaquilón* which contained litharge and was used as an emollient and for tumors, *emplasto confortativo* (containing litharge and *bol arménico*) employed to heal fractures and wounds, and *emplasto geminis* which contained *albayalde* and rose oil, which was also used to treat wounds.[201] These particular types of plaster were applied more commonly to treat Manuel Bautista Pérez's slaves.

Although there is evidence for the employment of minerals in a wide variety of medicines, in fact such treatments remained a minority. An analysis of the set of sixteen lists of prescriptions referred to above, which relate to elite persons mainly associated with the Church, indicates that medicines containing minerals numbered only about three percent of the total number of entries and two percent by value.[202] Those prescribed for internal consumption were generally small quantities of ground precious and semi-precious stones, which had not been produced by distillation but formed part of complex powders or electuaries, such as *confección jacint* and *diamargaritón*.[203] Minerals appear to have been employed more readily to treat Manuel Bautista Pérez's slaves and household. Of medicines supplied to him in 1629 and between 1635 and 1640, about 15 percent (of 2,328 individual medicines) constituted or contained a mineral or chemical.[204] Nearly half of the minerals were to be found in ointments and a further 10 percent in plasters.

Even though the majority of medicines containing minerals were therefore applied externally, they appear to have been employed more extensively in Lima than in Mexico where chemical medicines did not appear until the late seventeenth century at the earliest and the minerals used consisted primarily of precious and semi-precious stones.[205] Minerals also figured more prominently in pharmacies in Peru than in Seville at this time, where mercury was

200 Laval, *Botica*, 193.

201 Ibid. 107–08; Davis and López Terrada, "Protomedicato y farmacia," 610; Oviedo, *Methodo*, 508–10.

202 For the archival sources for the sixteen cases analysed see note 96.

203 Oviedo, *Methodo*, 163, 171.

204 For the bills incurred by Manuel Bautista Pérez with Pedro de Bilbao and Alonso de Carrión see: AGNP SO CO Ca. 57 doc 431 1629, 1635–1640.

205 De Vos, "From Herbs to Alchemy," 141, 144, 154.

not common.[206] In Spain the high cost or shortage of certain minerals may have been factors affecting the extent to which they were employed.[207]

Conclusion

An analysis of the medicines imported and used in Lima prior to the mid-seventeenth century suggests that they were prepared and applied within a humoral framework. Where possible apothecaries used imported *materia medica*; even when they employed locally-produced products, they were often of Old World origin. Their reluctance to adopt native plants was based on a combination of ideological, practical and professional considerations. It reflected the extent to which humoral medicine was entrenched in popular thought and the practical difficulties of working outside the Galenic framework, as well as the social status advantages that professional practitioners might derive from distancing themselves from indigenous healers whose knowledge of native plants was probably superior and whose practices were regarded with suspicion as being harmful and heretical. This is not to say that no experimentation or innovation occurred.

The books possessed by *boticarios* indicate that in preparing medicines they relied on practical manuals rather than scholarly medical texts. This reflected the growing professionalisation and specialisation of pharmacy within the medical profession. Even though apothecaries drew on traditional texts, such as Galen or Dioscorides, later authors who interpreted their works increasingly added their own commentaries based on personal observations and their experiences of the therapeutic value of remedies. They also began writing in the vernacular and simplifying remedies such that they could be applied by the population at large without the intervention of a physician.[208] While there is some evidence for experimentation with *materia medica* in Lima, generally the aim was to establish some consistency or standard of practice rather than

206 Fernández-Carrión and Valverde, *Farmacia y sociedad*, 85.

207 Some costs appear to have been higher in Spain. For example, alum cost 204 maravedís or 6 reals in Seville (Fernández-Carrión and Valverde, *Farmacia y sociedad*, 105) and 2 tomines or 2 reals in Lima (AGNP Cajas Reales, Lima H-3 leg. 4 Libro 24-a fols. 1–30 Aranceles para cálculo del almojarifazgo (1617). Although these lists were compiled to assess the tax to be paid on goods arriving from Spain, they reflected local values. Accounts for the Hospital of Santa Ana in the late sixteenth century suggest that it was paying 2.5 reals a pound for *alumbre* (ABPL 9080 Libro de cuentas del hospital de Santa Ana 1575 a 1585 fols. 254–57).

208 Solomon, *Fictions of Well-Being*, 6–10, 16–39.

prove or disprove propositions or hypotheses. While minerals appear to have been widely available, they were not used extensively in medicines and then generally in treatments that were applied externally. Paula De Vos has argued that the chemical methods that were employed in late seventeenth and eighteenth century Mexico drew on medieval alchemy and did not require the adoption of the new Paracelsian natural philosophy.[209] In fact they were being used alongside traditional methods of preparation. This study echoes her finding but suggests that experimentation with chemical medicines may have been more precocious in Peru than in Mexico reflecting the rich mineral deposits available in the Andes.

209 De Vos, "From Herbs to Alchemy." See also Palmer, "Pharmacy in the Republic of Venice," 117.

CHAPTER 7

The Social World of Apothecaries

> ...the good apothecary should be God-fearing, compassionate, pious, humane, affable, diligent, gentle, and generous to the poor, upright, and prompt to the needs and dangers of the sick; not a player [of cards], nor covetous, or a drinker, or distracted [by entertainment], because from these vices can only follow delays, mistakes, blunders and oversights; things which usually result in a decline in the reputation of doctors, to whom their malice and mistakes are attributed.[1]

∴

The social standing of apothecaries in Lima reflected both the general structure of society in Spain and Peru and the status of the medical profession as a whole within it. Lima's social structure differed in some respects from other colonial cities. As capital of the Viceroyalty of Peru, the city symbolised and promoted the authority of the Spanish state throughout South America and as such its social hierarchy reflected the traditional values that underpinned society in Spain.[2] It was not a mere replication of that in the Peninsula, however. Lima possessed an ethnically diverse population that needed to be incorporated within its social hierarchy, while the opportunities for social advancement were considerable, a process that was facilitated by the weaker exercise of royal authority resulting from Peru's distance from Spain.[3] As such the social hierarchy in Lima was not precisely delineated and individuals jostled to establish their positions in society.[4] The aim here is not to examine the social hierarchy as a means of state control, but rather provide a backdrop to understanding how the medical profession and apothecaries in particular were regarded by

1 Suárez de Figueroa, *Plaza universal*, 302.
2 For the way in which the authority of the king was promoted through ceremonies see Osorio, *Inventing Lima*.
3 Herzog, *Upholding Justice*, 5–8.
4 For studies of the development of social hierarchies and their limitations in Spanish America see Chapter 1 note 59.

 | DOI 10.1163/9789004351271_008

society as a whole and how they attempted to enhance their status, which had implications for the nature of pharmacy practice.

Social stratification in Spain was based on a system of estates, which defined the rights and obligations of different social groups and therefore their role and status.[5] There were three primary estates – the nobility, Church and commoners – and, with the exception of the clergy, the status of individuals was largely determined by birth. However, within each group the status, function, and wealth of individuals varied considerably and it was possible for individuals to ascend the social ladder through entering the Church or military or by providing other services for the Crown. Commoners aspired to become nobles or *hidalgos* and use the title of Don or Doña.[6] It was this hierarchical, estate-based corporative system that was introduced to the New World, but there the social structure was complicated by the presence of other ethnic groups – Native Americans, Africans and *castas*.

This estate system has been contrasted with a class-based form of social stratification, where the status of individuals is based on wealth and where there are no legal restrictions on social mobility. It has been argued that over time the basis of social stratification in the New World shifted from an estate-based system towards one constructed on class.[7] In colonial Lima several factors may have promoted an early shift towards such a class-based hierarchy. The city offered exceptional opportunities for individuals to improve their economic position due to the wealth that could be generated from mining and trade, opportunities that were not available in many other regions of Spanish America. Merchants and miners could become wealthier than many nobles, who became impoverished as their tribute income and access to native labour fell with the decline in the indigenous population.[8] Its distance from Spain and the lack of effective control in many spheres of government meant that social mobility was more easily effected in Peru. In 1637 Viceroy Chinchón advised his successor that because of the vastness of Peru (though possibly referring to the viceroyalty rather than the province), coupled with the relatively small number of Spanish settlers and the lack of an effective judicial system, social

5 See Lyle N. McAlister, "Social Structure and Social Change in New Spain," *Hispanic American Historical Review* 43 (3) (1963): 350–53.

6 Fred Bronner, "Elite Formation in Seventeenth-Century Peru," *Boletín de Estudios Latinoamericanos y del Caribe* 24 (1978): 10–12, 20-; Lockhart, *Spanish Peru*, 34–48.

7 McAlister, "Social Structure," 363; Mörner, *Race Mixture*, 7–8; John K. Chance and William B. Taylor, "Estate and Class in a Colonial City: Oaxaca in 1792," *Comparative Studies in Society and History* 19 (4) (1977): 454–55.

8 Bronner, "Elite Formation," 9–10, 17–19.

control was difficult and people moved freely up and down the social hierarchy.[9] It was this fluidity, which might also be interpreted as instability in the social structure, that it is argued encouraged the Crown to dispense titles to Lima's elites in order to maintain the social order.[10]

From the perspective of an individual raised in an environment where status was based on claims to nobility, the acquisition of wealth in itself was not regarded as sufficient to ensure high social standing. However, wealth could be transmuted into status through the payment of large dowries to secure strategic marriages or could be demonstrated through charitable donations, notably for the support for hospital or convents, or through the sumptuary accumulation and display of precious metals and jewellery. Charitable giving might not only enhance one's social standing, but be seen as a way of obtaining release from purgatory and securing a favourable position in the afterlife.[11] It will be demonstrated below how apothecaries used these mechanisms to boost their public profile and improve their social status.

The Status of the Medical Profession

The medical profession as a whole was not highly regarded. The roots of this lack of esteem lay in the domination of the profession in Spain by Jews and Muslims, even though in theory they were prevented from entering universities due to their inability to demonstrate purity of blood or *limpieza de sangre*.[12] With the expulsion of the Jews from Spain in 1492, some adopted Christianity and became New Christians or *Conversos*, as did some Muslims who converted from Islam to become *Moriscos*, only later to be expelled from Spain in 1609. While persons of Jewish or Muslim ancestry were not permitted to settle in the New World, many did so. They came under the increasing scrutiny of the Inquisition, such that Spaniards, not only those who were New

9 Ibid. 9–10.

10 Ibid. 10–11, 16; Paul Rizo-Patrón, "La nobleza de Lima en tiempos de los Borbones," *Bulletin de l'Institut Français d'Études Andines* 19(1)(1990): 135–36; Osorio, *Inventing Lima,* 24.

11 Magnus Mörner, "Economic Factors and Stratification in Colonial Spanish America with Special Regard to Elites," *Hispanic American Historical Review* 63 (2) (1978): 355–56; Bronner, "Elite Formation," 24–26; Suárez, *Desafíos transatlánticos*, 187–93.

12 Harry Friedenwald, *The Jews and Medicine*, vol. 2 (Baltimore: The John Hopkins Press, 1944), 620, 701–71; Goodman, *Power and Penury*, 219–21; Luis García Ballester, "The Inquisition and Minority Medical Practitioners in Counter Reformation Spain: Judaizing and Morisco Practitioners, 1560–1610," in *Medicine and the Reformation*, eds. Ole Peter Grell and Andrew Cunningham (London: Routledge, 1993), 156–66.

Christians, repeatedly stressed that they were of Old Christian heritage and claimed purity of blood for fear they might be discriminated against or worse brought before the Inquisition. The social value of such claims was enhanced by denying ethnic groups with indigenous, African or mixed blood access to official positions, guilds, religious orders, or entry to universities.[13]

As in Spain, elites in Lima encouraged their sons to enter the Church or the law rather than medicine on account of its low status as a profession that derived from its historic association with Jews and Muslims.[14] In theory the professions of physician, apothecary and surgeon were limited to those who could demonstrate legitimacy and *limpieza de sangre*,[15] but this stipulation was not adhered to consistently in Lima. While those *boticarios* in Lima who aspired to be *familiar* to the Inquisition, such as Francisco de Alva, Jerónimo Rodríguez, Juan de Bilbao, Pedro de Bilbao, and Mateo Pastor,[16] probably needed to demonstrate their *limpieza de sangre*, as the presence of African slaves practising as *boticarios* in Lima's hospitals and working as salaried employees indicates, this was often overlooked. In the early colonial period the shortage of medical

---

13 Lanning, *Royal Protomedicato*, 175–82; Cope, *Limits of Racial Domination*, 24–25; Elliott, *Empires of the Atlantic World*, 171.

14 Ramirez, *Provinical Patriarchs*, 176–77, 226; Zarate, *Inicios de la escuela de medicina*, 27–28, 30. See Chapter 1 for a discussion of the status of the medical profession and of professions involved in science in general in Spain. See also López Piñero, *Ciencia y técnica*, 47–88.

15 *Recopilación de las leyes, pragmáticas* (Muñoz) cap. 6 ordinance 1: 71; Poole, "Politics of *Limpieza de Sangre*," 363, 388; Lanning, "Legitimacy and *Limpieza de Sangre*," 43.

16 For Francisco de Alva and Juan de Bilbao see: *Libros de cabildos de Lima*, 7: 549–50 Título de familiar al bachiller Alba 21 Jan. 1574, *Libros de cabildos de Lima*, 8: 201–02 Familiar del santo oficio al Juan de Bilbao 15 and 24 Feb. 1576. For Pedro de Bilbao's services to the Santo Oficio see: AGNP SO CO 27–277 Pedro de Bilbao, ministro boticario del Santo Oficio contra Don Juan Arévalo de Espinosa, Caballero de Alcántara, Alguacil Mayor del Santo Oficio, (1629). Little is known of Jerónimo Rodríguez, but he made a donation of 30 pesos to the Crown in 1590 (AGI Lima 272 Servicio hecho al rey nuestro señor en la ciudad de los reyes 1590), following a request by Philip II the previous year for a *donativo de servicio* due to Spain's difficult financial position on account of wars with England, France, and Flanders (AGI IG 427, lib. 30, fols. 401r.–403v. real cédula 6 Mar 1589).

Mateo Pastor was *familiar* to the Inquisition in the mid-1630s when he purchased an African slave who was part of the estate of Tomé Cuaresma. The latter was a *Converso* surgeon who was tried by the Inquisition and put to death in 1635 (AGNP SO CO Ca 44 doc. 394 fols. 191–210 no date; Medina, *Historia del tribunal de Santo Oficio*, 2: 137). See also AGNP SO CO 126–1113 1658 El alférez Francisco Fajardo, defensor de los bienes de Mateo Pastor, familiar y boticario del Santo Oficio 14 Sep. 1654.

practitioners meant that the authorities in Lima were forced to be pragmatic and therefore did not press those seeking licenses to present their credentials. Even the respected *boticario*, Bernardo Gil, was not required to produce a certificate of *limpieza de sangre* when he was licensed to practise in 1609.[17]

The Middling Professional Status of the Apothecary

How then did *boticarios* fit into the prevailing social order, including within the medical profession? James Lockhart organises his social history of sixteenth-century Peru around the social categories used at the time, describing the characteristics, functions and status of different social groups.[18] In this study he regards physicians as professionals who fell between noblemen and artisans, whereas he classifies *boticarios* as artisans, though he notes that since they were literate and required specialist training and equipment, they were "near to the professional class."[19] Physicians were accorded higher status on account of their university education and their knowledge of natural philosophy which was deemed to be a higher form of learning than the practical knowledge and skills possessed by apothecaries and surgeons.[20] Although there was no requirement for *boticarios* to attend university, for licensed *boticarios* some knowledge of Latin was essential in order that they could understand physicians' prescriptions and read manuals on how to prepare medicines. Given the requirements for theoretical knowledge as well as technical skills, *boticarios* were regarded as superior to those who practised the more exclusively manual tasks of surgery or phlebotomy and as such they were regarded as having a "middling" status within the medical profession.[21]

Reflecting the availability of archival sources, more is known about those *boticarios* who owned their own pharmacies who came from bourgeois if not elite families. They often attended university and entered the profession to continue the family business. However, probably the majority of *boticarios* were

---

17 AHML Libro 4 de cédulas y provisiones. Título de Bernardo Gil, boticario 7 Nov. 1609. See Chapter 2 for the process of acquiring a title to practise.

18 Lockhart, *Spanish Peru*, 8–9.

19 Ibid. 103.

20 Lanning, *Royal Protomedicato*, 261–62; López Piñero, *Ciencia y técnica*, 50–51; Findlen, *Possessing Nature*, 261–72; Harold J. Cook, "Medicine," in *The Cambridge History of Science*, vol. 3, eds. Katherine Park and Loraine Daston (Cambridge: Cambridge University Press, 2006), 408–16.

21 De Vos, "Art of Pharmacy," 59, 62. See Chapter 2.

what Maher Memarzadeh has called wage pharmacists.[22] These apothecaries possessed the skills to prepare medicines and may even have been examined and possessed title, but lacked the financial resources to establish their own pharmacy. As Chapter 3 has shown the economic standing of *boticarios* would have varied considerably.

Some *boticarios* possessed substantial resources.[23] Francisco de Alva was said to be worth 50,000 *pesos ensayados*, and Mateo Pastor was able to provide goods valued at 2,000 *pesos ensayados* as security for the establishment of the private bank of Juan de la Cueva in 1636.[24] It is important to note that like many individuals at the time, *boticarios* did not earn their income exclusively from their pharmacy business or related trading activities. Juan de Bilbao derived a substantial income from renting out houses and shops. In 1592 he was renting a shop to two tailors for 800 pesos a year and made a contract with the merchant, Pablo de Collaguos, to rent a house for 300 pesos a year.[25] These were only two of the large number of properties he owned. Even though *boticarios* were discouraged from playing cards along with other games and drinking,[26] another *boticario*, Diego de Tineo joint-owned the monopoly for the sale of playing cards (*estanco de naipes*) with the merchant, Juan Ximénez de los Rios.[27] Prominent *boticarios* were often wealthy enough to employ several African slaves in their households. In early colonial Lima household slaves

---

22 Maher Memarzadeh, "Medical practitioners in Early Colonial Mexico," PhD diss., UCLA, 2005, 340–42, 453–54.

23 *Libros de cabildos de Lima*, 7: 549 Título de familiar al bachiller Alba 21 Jan. 1574, *Libros de cabildos de Lima*, 8: 201 Familiar del santo oficio a Juan de Bilbao 24 Feb. 1576 AGNP Real Audiencia. Causas Civiles leg. 16 cuad. 81 fol. 7v., 687 Pleito…contra las bienes y herederos del bachiller Francisco de Alva, boticario morador en la Ciudad de los Reyes. 1576.

24 AGNP Real Audiencia. Causas Civiles leg. 16 cuad. 81 fols. 119–26, 687–715 Pleito…contra las bienes y herederos del bachiller Francisco de Alva, boticario morador en la Ciudad de los Reyes. 1576; *Libros de cabildos de Lima*, 23: 398 Fianzas del banco 22 Dec. 1636. For the bank of Juan de la Cueva see: Suárez, *Comercio y fraude* and *Desafíos transatlánticos*.

25 For example, AGNP Protocolos Siglo XVI 52 Rodrigo Gómez Baeza fols. 2–2v. Arrienda de Juan de Bilbao 4 Jan. 1592, AGNP Protocolos Siglo XVI 52 Rodrigo Gómez Baeza fols. 17–17v. Arrienda de Juan de Bilbao 8 Jan. 1592. See also AGNP Protocolos Siglo XVI 47 Rodrigo Gómez Baeza fols. 731–731v. Arrienda de Juan de Bilbao 4 May 1588 where he rented a house to a shoemaker for 190 pesos a year. Similarly within ten years of arriving in Lima by 1552 the licenced physician, Álvaro de Torres, had acquired nine houses in central Lima which he sold to the city for 15,400 pesos (Lockhart, *Spanish Peru*, 66).

26 ARJBM División 1, leg. 17 Prohemiales 4 Libro de examen de los simples medicinales Antonio de Robles Cornejo 1617.

27 AGNP Protocolos Siglo XVI 51 Rodrigo Gómez Baeza fol. 285–285v. Compañía entre Diego de Tineo boticario y Juan Ximénez del Rio, mercador, sobre el estanco de naipes 8 Mar. 1591.

cost about 500 to 600 pesos or more, about half a year's salary of a minor royal official such as a *corregidor*.[28] When he died in 1576 Francisco de Alva had six female slaves and two male youths living in his household.[29] Clearly those who owned their own *boticas* made a comfortable living, but *oficiales* eked out a more modest existence on an income of several hundred pesos a year or slightly more in the case those who worked in hospitals.[30]

The social status and networks of these different types of *boticarios* were often distinct, but the standing of all was generally enhanced by their association with the medical profession; it also offered opportunities for social advancement for those of less privileged backgrounds, including migrants from Spain.[31] Those with greater financial resources were better placed to improve their social standing, but there were other mechanisms by which this could be achieved, which included the purchase of offices or titles or the payment of dowries to secure favourable marriages.

It was not uncommon for members of Lima's elite to become knights of military orders through government service or purchase, though they remained a minority of the city's *vecinos*.[32] Nevertheless, writing on early sixteenth century Peru, James Lockhart concluded that physicians generally had few pretentions to nobility and seldom sought public office. He suggests that they often came from families in which medicine was a tradition and they were content to dedicate themselves to their profession.[33]

Lockhart's observation would seem to apply equally to *boticarios*; certainly very few used the title Don. The title of Don or Doña was originally the prerogative of the high nobility and those who held high office in government or the Church. In 1560 there were only about 150 nobles in Peru,[34] but over time the title came to be used by a large number of other people, often relatives of true Dons, while some merely assumed the title feeling they had sufficient power

28 Newson and Minchin, *From Capture to Sale*, 225–31.

29 AGNP Real Audiencia. Causas Civiles leg. 16 cuad. 81 fols. 7v–8 Inventario de los bienes del bachiller Alva después de fallecido. 1576. The *boticarios* Juan Matías de Vera and Bernardo Gil both owned four slaves (AAL Testamentos 25-1 fol. 6v. Testamento de Juan Matías de Vera 18 Jun. 1640 (boticario); AAL Testamentos 52-21 fol. 12 Testamento de Bernardo Gil, boticario 1662).

30 See Chapter 3.

31 Memarzadeh, "Medical Practitioners," 347, 349.

32 Lockhart, *Spanish Peru*, 46–47; Bronner, "Elite Formation," 17, provides the figure of 149 *caballeros* (nobles and knights) out of 9–10,000 *vecinos* in mid-seventeenth century Lima.

33 Lockhart, *Spanish Peru*, 65–68.

34 Ibid. 39.

and prestige. In England apothecaries often sought public office to enhance their reputations, but this does not appear to have been the case in Lima.[35]

Even though *boticarios* may not have sought noble status or titles for themselves, they were sufficiently conscious of their social position to pay significant dowries for their daughters to secure husbands of high standing. The amount of dowry paid on marriage reflected the honour of the bride and the economic and social standing of the two families. Dowries could be extremely large leading women in Lima to complain that it was an obstacle to securing a suitable husband. In the seventeenth century dowries among elites were generally between about 10,000 and 40,000 pesos.[36] The *boticario* Pedro de Bilbao provided his daughter with a dowry of 32,000 pesos for her marriage to a lawyer and *relator* of the *Audiencia* Dr Andrés Téllez de Cabrera. Two years later Téllez de Cabrera became *corregidor* of the mining district of Conchucos before dying suddenly in 1634.[37] The post of *corregidor* of Conchucos was worth only 1,000 pesos a year, but it brought status and provided considerable opportunities for enhancing one's income.[38] Daughters of medical practitioners in general, like those of merchants, were commonly married to lawyers or lesser government officials. The dowry paid by Pedro de Bilbao is suggestive of his high economic status, particularly when it is compared to that of 6,000 *pesos de a nueve* paid by the physician Pedro Ramón for the marriage of his daughter Isabel Guzmán to one Antonio del Valle in 1604.[39] However, the dowries paid by even the

---

35 Penelope J. Corfield, "From Poison Peddlers to Civic Worthies: The Reputation of the Apothecaries in Georgian England," *Social History of Medicine* 22(1)(2009): 7–9.

36 Van Deusen, *Between the Scared and Worldly*, 105. For dowries in Peru see: Martín, *Daughters*, 117–27; María Emma Mannarelli, *Private Passions and Public Sins: Men and Women in Seventeenth Century Lima*, trans. Sidney Evans and Meredith D Dodge (Albuquerque: University of New Mexico Press, 2007), 103–05; Jane E. Mangan, *Transatlantic Obligations: Creating the Bonds of Family in Conquest-Era Peru and Spain* (New York, Oxford University Press, 2015), 122–33.

37 *Libros de cabildos de Lima*, 22: 343 Cabildo de Lima receives cédula of appointment of Andrés Téllez de Cabrera as *corregidor* (20 Aug. 1633) on 13 Sep. 1633; Suardo, *Diario de Lima*, 1: 198, 199, 284; 2: 41. He died in 1634 leaving two children as his heirs.

38 Antonio Vázquez de Espinosa, *Compendio y descripción de las Indias occidentales*. Biblioteca de autores españolés 231 (Madrid: Ediciones Atlas, 1969), 507. Salaries for minor officials ranged from 800 to 2,000 pesos (pp. 506–08).

39 AAL Testamentos leg. 7 exp. 18 Testamento de Pedro Ramón, médico 1 Apr.1618. A *peso de a nueve* was worth 306 maravedís compared to the *peso de a ocho* which was 272 maravedís (Bowser, *African Slave*, xiii). It was therefore equivalent to 6,750 pesos. For the marriage see "Perú, matrimonios, 1600–1940," database, *FamilySearch* (https://familysearch.org/ark:/61903/1:1:FNR6-H1M: accessed 21 December 2015), Antonio Del Valle and Ysabel De Gusman Y Sotomayor, 17 Nov 1604; Lima, Peru; FHL microfilm 1,110,202. One Antonio del

wealthiest apothecaries were less than those paid by members of other professional groups, particularly merchants whose daughters might receive a dowry of 60,000 or 80,000 pesos.[40] In the 1630s the largest dowry provided in Peru was by Diego de la Cueva who provided a dowry of 120,000 on the marriage of his daughter to a merchant and hat mill owner, don Antonio Mioño, a Spaniard and knight of the military Order of Santiago.[41]

Criticisms of the Medical Profession

Licensed medical practitioners as a group had a higher status than many other professionals due to their university education, formal training and because their activities were officially regulated. Nevertheless, they were still not held in high esteem. This is exemplified by a letter from Jorge López de Paz, a resident of Arequipa, to a business associate in Lima in which he complained that the medical practitioners attending to him, who had administered syrups, purgatives and other remedies, were "matasanos" (killers of the healthy) who knew no more medicine than an ass.[42] Such feelings towards medical practitioners were widespread and were encapsulated in the late seventeenth century satirical poetry of Juan del Valle y Caviedes. In some fifty poems he condemned professional doctors referring to them as "verdugo en latín" (executioner in Latin), "doctor de la sepultura" (doctor of the grave) and more generally "médicos matantes" (killer doctors).[43] He also levelled charges of corruption against the university for awarding degrees on payment of a fee, suggesting that one doctor Don Melchor Vázquez had paid 3,000 pesos for the title

Valle was given the title of silkworker (*sedero*) in 1608, though it is not certain that this was the same person (*Libros de cabildos de Lima*, 15: 708 Cartas de examen de gorreros y sederos 28 Nov. 1608).

40 For dowries provided by merchants see: Suardo, *Diario de Lima*, 1: 45, 162, 164, 2: 43, 99.

41 Ibid. 1: 164; Manuel de Mendiburu, *Diccionario histórico-biográfico del Perú* (Lima: Imprenta de J. Francisco Solís, 1876) 2: 426.

42 AGNP Tribunal de la Inquisición. Contencioso – Siglo XVII leg. 21 Jorge López de Paz a Manuel Bautista Pérez, Arequipa, 11 May 1635.

43 Daniel R. Reedy, *The Poetic Art of Juan Valle Caviedes* (Chapel Hill: University of North Carolina, 1964), 60–79; Uriel García Cáceres, *Juan del Valle y Caviedes: Cronista de la medicina* (Lima: Banco Central de Reserva del Perú and Universidad Peruana Cayetano Heredia, 1999), 55–119 *passim*. Carlos F. Cabanillas Cárdenas, ed., *Juan del Valle y Caviedes: guerras físicas, proezas medicales, hazañas de la ignorancia* (Madrid: Iberoamericana Editorial Vervuert, 2013), 72–84, identifies the physicians and surgeons in the poems with those practising in Lima at the time.

of *médico*.[44] Although fewer criticisms were directed specifically at *boticarios*, they are generally depicted as accomplices of physicians since they prepared the medicines that physicians prescribed. As such Valle y Caviedes refers to the apothecary as an artilleryman – *boticario artillero*.[45] Such public criticism of medical practice was not exceptional for the time, indeed it was commonplace in Europe, where it was similarly satirised by writers such as Rabelais, Molière and Shakespeare.[46]

These universal complaints probably had as much to do with the limitations of humoral medicine as the shortcomings of physicians or apothecaries, though clearly there were many cases where *boticarios* prepared harmful medicines. In fact Antonio de Robles Cornejo considered this to derive from *boticarios*' ignorance of Latin which led them to rely on their own experience rather than published texts, and thereby produce harmful or ineffective remedies that resulted in further treatments and rising costs. This he argued contributed to the poor reputation of the medical profession as a whole.[47] Even when administered according to traditional manuals, medical treatments had unpredictable outcomes. Medical care was therefore approached from a position of suspicion rather than confidence.

It was not easy for a patient to select a medical practitioner or supplier given their differing abilities and the wide range of *materia medica* available of varying cost and quality.[48] The reputation of particular *boticarios* did not rely wholly on their own skills, for they were supposed to follow the prescriptions issued by physicians. However, they also dispensed medicines on their own account to people who sought their advice and treatment without having previously consulted a physician. In both cases, the actual preparation of medicines required knowledge of the particular qualities and quantities of *materia medica* that were to be employed and combined, and necessitated skill and care in composing them.[49]

The "laws" (*leyes y debidas ordenanzas*) specified by Antonio de Robles Cornejo as being essential for a good *boticario* were that he should purchase

---

44 Cabanillas Cárdenas, *Juan del Valle y Caviedes*, 344–45, 412.

45 Ibid. 227.

46 García Cáceres, *Juan del Valle y Caviedes* 34–35; Tanya Pollard, *Drugs and Theater in Early Modern England* (Oxford University Press: Oxford, 2005), 23–54.

47 ARJBM División 1, leg. 17 Prologo. Libro de examen de los simples medicinales Antonio de Robles Cornejo 1617.

48 Arrow, "Uncertainty," 951 notes that uncertainty about the quality of medicines is more intense than for any other commodity.

49 Michael R. McVaugh, *Medicine before the Plague: Practitioners and their Patients in the Crown of Aragon 1285–1345*. (Cambridge, Cambridge University Press, 1993), 117–18.

good quality simples, prepare compound medicines faithfully according to recipes, and store them correctly so that they did not lose their potency. Other "laws" stressed that they should not overcharge for medicines, noting that sometimes they demanded ten times their value.[50] As the confessional for physicians and surgeons written by Martín de Azpilcueta acknowledged, their sins did not stop at overcharging for medicines but extended to prolonging an illness in order to increase their income or, in collusion with *boticarios*, purchasing more medicines than were needed.[51] Medicine as a practice was a Christian calling and it was expected that medical practitioners' prime interest was in healing patients rather than making profits.[52] In England advice to apothecaries was that they should charge sufficiently high prices for treatments so as to be able them to provide medicines free for the poor.[53] Whether or not this was a consideration for *boticarios* in Lima is not clear, but the popular view was certainly that the prices they charged were excessive.

In an environment where there was a general lack of confidence in the medical profession and where the knowledge and skills of particular physicians or apothecaries was imperfect, the choice of who to turn to for medical care was a hazardous task. Those with reputations for killing or harming patients, overcharging, or whose *boticas* contained old, adulterated products might be avoided.[54] Those aside, the *boticario* to whom an individual might resort would depend on influences other than demonstrated medical expertise or cost; these might include family tradition, knowledge or recommendations from relatives or friends, or merely social standing.[55] Patients might believe that they would receive quality treatment if practitioners possessed official qualifications or were treating people of high status. Bartolomé Díaz Cabeza de Vaca supplied medicines to Diego Núñez de Figueroa, a rich Limeño with an

50 ARJBM División 1, leg. 17 Prohemiales 5, 8, 9, 11,12, 13 Libro de examen de los simples medicinales Antonio de Robles Cornejo 1617. Valle y Caviedes in twelve of his poems made a similar charge against physicians, in one referring to "sentencia de muerte injusta por culpas de mí dinero"(Cabanillas Cárdenas, *Juan del Valle y Caviedes*, 217).

51 Martín de Azpilcueta, *Compendio y summario de confessores y penitentes* (Alcalá: Casa de Iuan Iníguez de Lequerica, 1580).

52 Arrow, "Uncertainty," 949–51.

53 Robert Ralley, "Medical Economies," 29–31.

54 Patrick Wallis, "Consumption, Retailing, and Medicine in Early-Modern London," *Economic History Review* 61(1) (2008): 26, 42–43. For Mexico see De Vos, "Art of Pharmacy," 159–60.

55 See Chapter 6. For England see: Jenner and Wallis, "Medical Marketplace," 12; Ralley, "Medical Economies," 36, 41. For Italy see David Gentilcore's, *Healers and Healing*, 2.

estate worth 200,000 pesos who was appointed governor of Huaylas,[56] as well as a number of royal officials and members of the *cabildo*.[57] Similarly, on his death Pedro de Bilbao was owed some 8,211 pesos by more than 150 individuals, of which a large number held official positions and another 30 possessed the title of Don or Doña.[58] Elites probably continued to seek the advice of professional practitioners despite the debatable efficacy of their humoral treatments and that herbal remedies prepared by popular healers probably inflicted less harm.[59] Indeed, as has been noted in Chapter 3, elite families often made annual contracts with particular physicians and surgeons to treat members of their households.

The Christian Calling of an Apothecary

The status of the medical profession as a whole was enhanced by the fact that it was regarded as a calling by God, within which *boticarios* were seen to have particular responsibilities. According to Ecclesiasticus 38: 4–8, God had created medicinal herbs and given certain people knowledge of how to use them for healing and the relief of pain, which would ensure human health throughout the world and serve to praise God.[60] As such the first of the fourteen "laws" listed by Antonio de Robles Cornejo as being essential for a good *boticario* was that he was to fear and love God with all his heart and comply not only with human laws but also divine ones.[61] The Christian calling of the apothecary was also emphasised in other "laws" which exhorted them to be humane, willing to please, happy, affable, and charitable.[62] According to Robles Cornejo they should not be a player of cards or dice or someone who ate or drank

56 Cook, *Demographic Collapse*, 182–83.

57 AAL Testamentos leg 5 exp. 1 fols. 28–35v. Testamento de Bartolomé Díaz Cabeza de Vaca boticario y autos sobre su cumplimiento con el albacea Juan Manuel Carasco 1608–1626.

58 AGNP Protocolos Siglo XVII 1789 Sánchez Vadillo fols. 2068–2072 Inventario de bienes de Pedro de Bilbao 25 Aug. 1636.

59 Michael Stolberg, *Experiencing Illness and the Sick Body in Early Modern Europe* (Basingstoke: Palgrave Macmillan, 2011), 62–63.

60 Suárez de Figueroa, *Plaza universal*, 300. Different versions of the bible give different translations, but the essence of the verse is the same.

61 ARJBM División 1, leg. 17 Prohemiales 1 Libro de examen de los simples medicinales Antonio de Robles Cornejo 1617.

62 ARJBM División 1, leg. 17 Prohemiales 3 Libro de examen de los simples medicinales Antonio de Robles Cornejo 1617. See also Suárez de Figueroa, *Plaza universal*, 302; Aguilera, *Exposición*, fols. 17v., 21.

excessively.[63] Such behaviour it was argued would lead to "delays, mistakes, blunders, and oversights."[64] *Boticarios* were also exhorted to marry a woman of good blood (*limpia de buena sangre*) or at least an Old Christian of good conduct and reputation.[65]

Given these publically recognised qualities of a good *boticario*, an apothecary might enhance his status by outward expressions of piety and charity, which were seen as a fundamental Christian responsibility.[66] Religion permeated the lives of people in the early modern period, especially in Lima which was capital of the Viceroyalty and the seat of one of the only three archdioceses in Spanish America. Apart from the secular Church, the city housed a tribunal of the Inquisition and possessed monasteries and convents of many religious orders; more than ten percent of the population was associated with the Church.[67] *Cofradías* abounded, religious buildings dominated public space, and religious ceremonies were central to public life in the city. Meanwhile, private houses possessed religious objects, paintings and books.[68]

Piety was publically displayed through membership of *cofradías*, participation in religious ceremonies, and in charitable works. The concept of purgatory featured strongly in religious thought at the time encouraging people to prepare for a "good death." This included provisions in their testaments for the saying of masses for the soul of the deceased and for those in purgatory, or burial in the habit of a particular religious order and the provision of bread, wine and candles.[69] They might also specify donations that were to be made to the church, hospitals, *cofradías*, and other charitable institutions. The desire to demonstrate religiosity and piety was not unique to *boticarios* or the medical profession, but it prevailed among the population at large. However, the particular responsibility of *boticarios* before God for the healing of the sick probably

63 ARJBM División 1, leg. 17 Prohemiales 4 Libro de examen de los simples medicinales Antonio de Robles Cornejo 1617. See also, Aguilera, *Exposición*, fols. 23v–24.

64 Suárez de Figueroa, *Plaza universal*, 302.

65 ARJBM División 1, leg. 17 Prohemiales 6 Libro de examen de los simples medicinales Antonio de Robles Cornejo 1617.

66 Siraisi, *Medieval and Early Renaissance Medicine*, 7–9; Lindemann, *Medicine and Society*, 123–29; Risse, *Mending Bodies*, 73–109; Sowell, *Tale of Healer*, 14–15.

67 Nancy E. Van Deusen, *The Souls of Purgatory: The Spiritual Diary of a Seventeenth-Century Afro-Peruvian Mystic, Ursula de Jesús* (Albuquerque: University of New Mexico Press, 2004), 7.

68 Ibid. 1–49 for insight into the religious life of Lima and its inhabitants.

69 Van Deusen, *Souls of Purgatory*, 36–37; Gabriela Ramos, *Death and Conversion in the Andes: Lima and Cuzco, 1532–1670* (Notre Dame, Indiana: University of Indiana Press, 2010),148–49: Cussen, *Black Saint*, 86–91.

raised public expectations of their actions. It was said that Limeños expended more money on white wax for convents, *cofradías*, masses in one month than the largest cities in Europe did in eight. Antonio de la Calancha described it as the most charitable city in all Christendom.[70]

Boticarios demonstrated their religiosity and social standing through the membership of *cofradías* and participation in public processions. A large number of *cofradías* were founded in Lima, often for separate ethnic and professional groups. In 1619 the city possessed forty-six *cofradías* and there were few people who were not associated in some way with one of them.[71] Certain *cofradías* were considered to be more prestigious than others. Their status depended on their wealth, the Christian devotion of their members publically demonstrated in processions, and on their acts of charity. Individual members might enhance their piety, honour, and status through occupying posts in the *cofradía*, for example as *mayordomo* or *hermanos venticuatro*.[72] At the outset the *hermanos veinticuatro* were the original founders of a *cofradía*. They were responsible for organising its activities, including processions, and they enjoyed certain privileges. Following the death of the original founders they were replaced by new *hermanos venticuatro*, but the privileges they enjoyed were more limited.[73] These posts were always filled by members of the elite.

In the 1570s the *boticario* Francisco de Alva was a *hermano venticuatro* of an unnamed *cofradía*.[74] This was before the foundation in 1603 of the *cofradía* of Nuestra Señora de la Soledad which was particularly associated with medical

70 Calancha, *Crónica moralizada*, lib. 1 cap. 38: 245.

71 Olinda Celestino and Albert Meyers, *Las cofradías en el Perú: región central* (Frankfurt: Editorial Klaus d. Vervuert, 1981), 119–22 and cuadro 6; Walter Vega Jácome, "Cofradías limeñas," in *Lima en el siglo XIV*, ed. Laura Gutiérrez Arbulú (Lima: Pontificia Universidad Católica del Perú, Instituto Riva-Agüero, 2005), 706–07, 731–33. For Indian *cofradías* see: Paul Charney, "A Sense of Belonging: Colonial Indian Cofradías and Ethnicity in the Valley of Lima, Peru," *The Americas* 54(3) (1998): 379–407.

72 Judith Mansilla Justo, "Poder y prestigio social en las cofradías españolas, siglo XVII y XVIII," in *Corporaciones religiosas y evangelización en Iberoamérica, siglos XVI–XVII*, eds. Diego Lévano Medina and Kelly Montoya Estrada (Lima: Universidad Nacional Mayor San Marcos, 2010), 229–32. See Beatriz Garland Ponce, "Las cofradías en Lima durante la colonia: una primera aproximación," in *La venida del reino. Religión, evangelización y cultura en América, Siglos XVI–XX*, ed. Gabriela Ramos (Cuzco: Centro de Estudios Regionales Andinos "Bartolomé de las Casas," 1994), 212–26 for the organisational structure of *cofradías* in Lima.

73 Garland Ponce, "Las cofradías," 217–18.

74 AGNP Real Audiencia leg.16 cuad. 81 fol. 8v. Inventario de los bienes del bachiller Alva después de fallecido 9 Feb. 1576. Among his clothes were a cape and tunic of a *venticuatro* signifying that he was a member of a *cofradía*.

practitioners. The *cofradías's* patron saints were Cosmas and Damián, who were the saints of physicians, pharmacists and surgeons. The *cofradía* de Nuestra Señora de la Soledad was attached to the convent of San Francisco (See Figure 13); its chapel had five altars and was embellished with expensive sculptures. It became one of the most prestigious *cofradías* in the city, playing a leading role in religious celebrations especially during Holy Week, when its members displayed their religious fervour by re-enacting the crucifixion of Christ and flagellating themselves throughout the *cofradía's* procession (See Figure 15).[75] Members of the *cofradía* had to be honourable and of good reputation, while

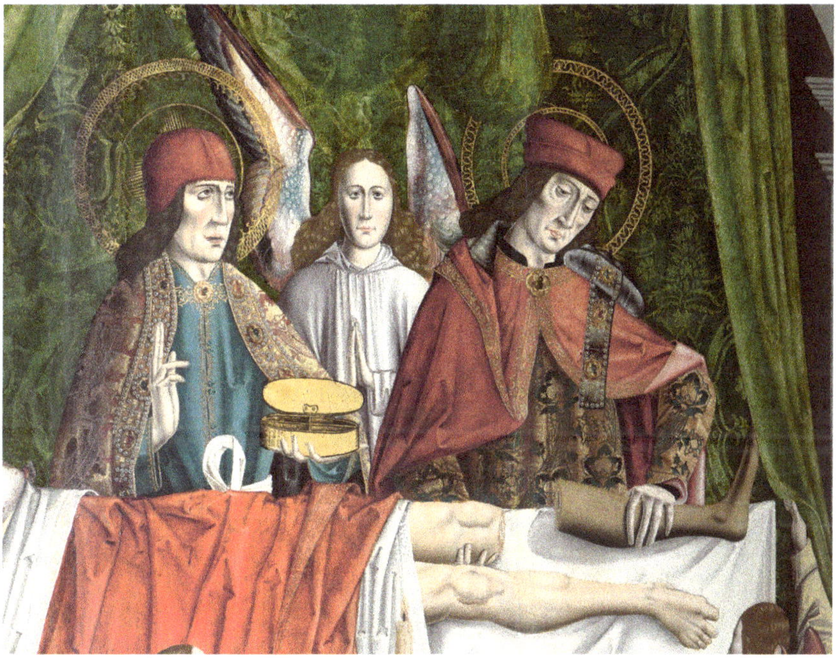

FIGURE 13 *A verger's dream: Saints Cosmas and Damian performing a miraculous cure by transplantation of a leg. Oil painting attributed to the Master of Los Balbases, ca. 1495.*
COURTESY WELLCOME LIBRARY, LONDON.

75 Diego de Córdoba y Salinas, *Crónica franciscana de las provincias del Perú*, ed. Lino Gómez Canedo (Washington DC: American Academy of Franciscan History, 1957), 536–57; Suardo, *Diario de Lima*, 2: 166; Rubén Vargas Ugarte, *Historia de la iglesia en el Perú*. Tomo II (1570–1640) (Burgos: Imprenta de Aldecoa, 1959), 496–97; Kelly Montoya Estrada, "Una procesión de Viernes Santo en Lima XVII," in *Corporaciones religiosas y evangelización en Iberoamérica, siglos XVI–XVII*, eds. Diego Lévano Medina and Kelly Montoya Estrada (Lima: Universidad Nacional Mayor San Marcos, 2010), 145–46.

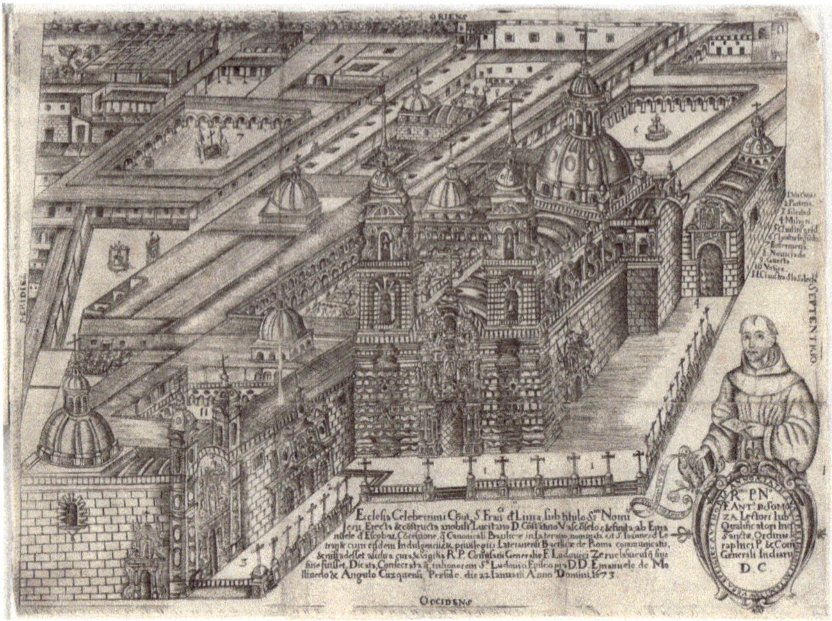

FIGURE 14 *Chapel of the* Cofradía *of Nuestra Señora de la Soledad* (bottom left) *in 1675. Miguel Suárez de Figueroa,* Templo de N. grande patriarca San Francisco de la provincia de los doze apostoles de le Peru en la Ciudad de los Reyes. *Lima, Juan de Benavides, 1675.*
COURTESY OF THE JOHN CARTER BROWN LIBRARY AT BROWN UNIVERSITY.

Blacks, Mulattoes, Mestizos, and Moriscos were, at least in theory, excluded.[76] The obligations of its members were contained in their "carta de esclavitud," which specified the payment of alms, contributions to the *cofradía*, as well as attendance at church services and processions. It also indicated the form in which their religiosity and commitment to the *cofradía* were to be expressed.[77]

Among the founding members of the *cofradía* de Nuestra Señora de la Soledad were a number of known physicians and *boticarios*. They included Francisco Martín Reyna who in 1604 was one of its two *mayordomos*; he was probably

76 Montoya Estrada, "Procesión de Viernes Santo," 147. Montoya Estrada suggests that for the eighteenth century at least, persons from other ethnic groups were buried in the *cofradía's* church.

77 See for example: AAL Cofradías 16 no. 15 Autos seguidos por Juan de Gutiérrez de la Sal contra Pedro Fernandez Valdés 1684. This includes the *carta de esclavitud* of the wife of Gutiérrez de la Sal, Doña Juana Picón.

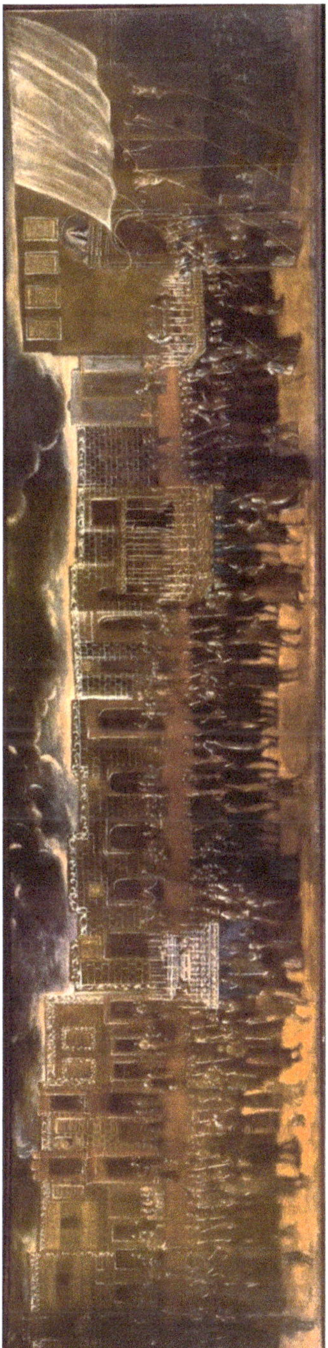

FIGURE 15 *Holy week procession of the* Cofradía *of Nuestra Señora de la Soledad in the late seventeenth century.* The process on leaving the chapel of the Cofradía with the re-enactment of the crucifixion on the right.
PHOTO: KELLY MONTOYA. COURTESY COFRADÍA DE NUESTRA SEÑORA DE LA SOLEDAD, LIMA.

one of its original founders.[78] By 1637 some of the original *hermanos venticuatro* had died, including Francisco Martín Reyna, but among those who remained were known *boticarios* including Bernardo Gil, Francisco de Sandoval, Alonso de Carrión, and Juan Matías de Vera; one of its two *mayordomos* was no less than the *protomedico*, Doctor Juan de la Vega.[79] At that time the *mayordomos* and *hermanos venticuatro* were complaining that the *cofradía* was suffering from an influx of "surgeons, barbers and apothecaries," many of whom were not paying the specified contributions. Not only that, but these new members, who outnumbered the original founders, were electing *mayordomos* from among the guild of surgeons and barbers to detriment of the original founders, who it claimed had committed significant funds to the establishment of the *cofradia*.[80] Apothecaries did not belong to this guild and the documentation suggests that the complaint was essentially against surgeons who were advocating that one of the posts of *mayordomo* should be reserved for them. The association of *cofradías* with particular professions or trades was commonplace in Lima; it served to guarantee support at a time when the number of *cofradías* was expanding rapidly and competition between them was increasing.[81]

Apothecaries might also enhance their social standing through charitable activities. Christian charity given free of charge would signify that an apothecary was a caring person concerned with the relief of suffering and not driven by monetary considerations. Apart from regular alms giving, *boticarios* might make substantial donations to the church or charitable institutions, particularly on their deathbeds. The *boticario* Bernardo Gil expressed his desire to be buried in the chapel of the *cofradía* of Nuestra Señora de la Soledad to which he paid alms.[82] Whether or not they belonged to the *cofradía* of Nuestra

78 AGNP Protocolos Siglo XVII 230 Ramiro Bote fols. 1473–1473v. Escritura de Francisco Martín de Reyna 23 Mar. 1604; *Libros de cabildos de Lima*, 14: 713–14 Piden los mayordomos de la cofradía de la Soledad ...vayan los regidores a la regir 12 Apr. 1604. He is mentioned as a *mayordomo* in AAL Testamentos leg 5 exp. 1 fols. 137–45 Testamento de Bartolomé Díaz Cabeza de Vaca 28 Apr. 1608. In 1604 the other *mayordomo* was Hernán Sánchez.

79 He participated in the *cofradía's* Holy Week procession in 1637 (Suardo, *Diario de Lima*, 2: 166). He died in 1640 (AAL Testamentos 25 no.1 Testamento de Juan Matías de Vera, 1641–1642).

80 AAL Cofradías 16 no. 3 Autos seguidos por los hermanos de venticuatro de la cofradía de Nuestra Señora de la Soledad 1637; AAL Cofradías 16 no. 5 fols. 5–6v., 13–13v. Autos de elección de nuevos mayordomos de la cofradía de Nuestra Señora de la Soledad 1643.

81 Diego Lévano Medina, "La administración de los bienes temporales en las cofradías limeñas del siglo XVII," in *Corporaciones religiosas y evangelización en Iberoamérica, siglos XVI–XVII*, eds. Diego Lévano Medina and Kelly Montoya Estrada (Lima: Universidad Nacional Mayor San Marcos, 2010), 120–22.

82 AAL Testamentos 52–21 fol. 6 Testamento de Bernardo Gil, boticario 1662.

Señora de la Soledad, members of the medical profession often affiliated with the church of San Francisco. The *boticario* Bartolomé Díaz de Cabeza de Vaca, indicated his desire to be buried in a Franciscan habit in the convent de San Francisco where a requiem mass was to be said; he also requested one hundred masses to be said for his soul and another fifty for his ancestors and those who had helped him during his life. Any residual estate was to be used to found a *capellanía* for the saying of masses in the convent of San Francisco.[83]

Capellanías or chaplaincies were capital endowments to a church, generally entrusted to a particular priest, for the saying of masses for the donor's soul or to carry out charitable works. Those founded by elites in Lima reached several thousand pesos.[84] The *boticario* Juan de Urrutia, founded two *capellanías* of unknown value, one to support "the chapel for souls in purgatory" in the Cathedral and the other for the chapel of the Hospital de Nuestra Señora de Atocha for orphan children.[85] More often death-bed donations were much smaller and were pledged for the saying or masses or given to charitable institutions without the establishment of a *capellanía*. In 1618 the physician, Pedro Ramón, who was *familiar* to the Inquisition left 20 pesos to the *cofradía* del Santísimo Sacramento attached to the Cathedral, 100 pesos to the Hospital of San Andrés, 50 pesos to the Hospital of Santa Ana, 50 pesos to the Hospital of La Caridad for the poor, 100 pesos to the female Convent of Las Descalças (San José), and 8 pesos for orphan children.[86] Such donations were not confined to elites and could be quite small. Examples include an Indian tailor from Chachapoyas who in 1578 donated two pesos to the Hospital of Santa Ana and another two pesos to the *cofradía* de Nuestra Señora del Rosario for Indians, while in 1597 a free Black carpenter left 4 pesos to each of the city's four hospitals.[87]

83 AAL Testamentos leg. 5 exp. 1 fols. 12–12v., 20 Testamento de Bartolomé Díaz Cabeza de Vaca 15 Apr. 1608. The surgeon Martín Sánchez, similarly specified that he wished to be buried in a Franciscan habit in the convent of San Francisco and that masses be said in the cathedral for his soul and those of his deceased ancestors (AGNP Protocolos Siglo XVI 154 Pedro de Salinas fols. 258–258v., 721v–722 no date [1547/1548]).

84 Josephe and Francisco Mugaburu, *Chronicle of Colonial Lima: The Diary of Josephe and Francisco Mugaburu, 1640–1697*, trans. and ed. Robert R Miller (Norman: University of Oklahoma Press, 1975), 8, 91, 235.

85 AAL Monasterio de la Concepción leg. 4 exp. 8 Causa seguida por Alonso de Castro en nombre de doña Maria Magdalena, viuda de Gerónimo Pujadas, contra el monasterio de la Concepción 1628.

86 AAL Testamentos leg. 7 exp. 18 Testamento de Pedro Ramón médico 1 Apr. 1618.

87 Quiroz, *Artesanos y manfactureros*, 116–17. For small donations by Indians see: Paul Charney, "'For My Necessities': The Wills of Andean Commoners and Nobles in the Valley of Lima, 1597–1607," *Ethnohistory* 59 (2)(2012): 344.

Despite the large number of people making donations, the financial contribution they made collectively to the running of hospitals was small; most income came from *censos* and properties. Those who lacked the ready cash to make a donation might impose a *censo* on a property. This pledged to the institution an annual income usually set at 5 percent of its capital value. When hospitals were first founded they often received tribute income from *encomiendas*, but as the native population declined they relied increasingly on *censos* and on the rental income from properties that had been donated or acquired; donations made a relatively small contribution.[88] Whereas in 1619 donations to the Hospitals of Santa Ana and San Andrés were 500 pesos and 2,500 pesos respectively, their corresponding income from rents and *censos* were 12,179 pesos and 8,500 pesos.[89] The *boticario* Juan de Bilbao and his wife had a *censo* on four pairs of houses (*pares de casas*) worth 1,558 *pesos ensayados* which generated an annual income of 111 pesos 3 reals for the Hospital of Santa Ana.[90] Over time, *censos* and rents from properties, some of which were donated, came to constitute the main source of income not only for hospitals but also *cofradías*.[91]

Apart from death-bed donations, there were other ways in which charity might be dispensed. As Chapter 3 has demonstrated, *boticarios* often allowed debts to build up, especially those incurred by hospitals and other charitable institutions. In the case of Mexico City, the hesitance of apothecaries to

88 David Cahill, "Financing Health Care in the Viceroyalty of Peru: the Hospitals of Lima in the Late Colonial Period." *The Americas* 52 (2) (1995): 136–54. In fact the growth in the native population towards the end of the eighteenth century meant that tribute income was increasing, but it still represented a minor source of hospital income. Even in the sixteenth century *censos* contributed about a quarter of the income of the hospital of San Andrés (AGI Lima 126 El hospital real de los españoles de la advocación de San Andrés, fols. 9–11 Posesiones, censos y situaciones que tiene el dicho hospital 4 Apr.1582). This may not have included all income, since by 1630 the income of the hospital was recorded as 18,000 ducados. This compared with 24,000 pesos for the hospital of Santa Ana and 6,000 for La Caridad. The most substantial income was of 28,000 for the convents of La Concepción and 16,000 for La Encarnación (Salinas y Córdova, *Memorial*, 196–97). Details of all the income from censos, renting properties and alms from 1575 to the mid seventeenth century can be found in the account books of the Hospital of Santa Ana in the ABPL legajos 9080, 9083–87, 9095–96, 9099–9100.

89 AGI Lima 301 Relación de las ciudades, villas y lugares…20 Apr. 1619. For the sources of income of each hospital in Lima see Guerra, *El hospital*, 429–75 *passim*. The *mayordomo* of the hospital was responsible for setting the value of rents of properties belonging to the hospital and collecting the income (Domingo Angulo, "Las ordenanzas del hospital de Santa Ana." *Revista del Archivo Nacional del Perú* 11 (1938): 144).

90 ABPL 9080 Libro de cuentas del hospital de Santa Ana 1575 a 1585 fols. 45, 123 1583.

91 Lévano Medina, "Administración de los bienes temporales," 128–33.

call in debts has been interpreted as a strategy for enhancing their charitable reputations.[92] The evidence for Lima is more equivocal. While some *boticarios* may have acted in a similar way, there is more evidence for their pursuit of debtors through the courts and for specifying in their wills that monies that they were owed should be collected by their executors.

Apothecaries might also demonstrate their religiosity through objects contained in their pharmacies and homes. Calvaries were commonly displayed in *boticas*,[93] though such displays were not restricted to apothecaries. Francisco de Alva possessed eight paintings, six depicting the history of Samson, one Descent from the Cross and one of Mary Magdalene, as well as eight old canvases depicting the history of Abraham.[94] Even surgeons and barbers of more modest means possessed one or two paintings, almost always depicting the saints or religious scenes.[95] One surgeon, Bartolomé Ortega, had ten canvases, which included paintings of Christ, San Juan Evangelista, Santa Lugarda, and a large painting of San Pedro which was auctioned for 41 pesos.[96] Such religious items may have been displayed more prominently by apothecaries of Portuguese descent and *Converso* status who were at greater risk of being investigated by the Inquisition and charged with Judaizing. It may be significant that when goods belonging to Andres Gonzales, a prominent Portuguese trader in medicines turned *boticario* based in Cartagena, were seized by the Inquisition in 1620, he had four paintings of saints in his possession.[97] However, religious paintings were not exclusive to medical practitioners, but were prominent in elite households in general and were highly valued.[98]

---

92 De Vos, "Art of Pharmacy," 171–81.

93 Bartolomé Díaz Cabeza de Vaca's accounts indicate that he commissioned a calvary for the pharmacy (AAL Testamentos leg. 5 exp. 1 fol. 14 Testamento de Bartolomé Díaz Cabeza de Vaca boticario y autos sobre su cumplimiento con el albacea Juan Manuel Carasco 1608–1626).

94 AGNP Real Audiencia leg. 16 cuad. 81 Inventario de los bienes del bachiller Alva después de fallecido 9 Feb. 1576. The presence of images of Old Testament figures suggests that he might have been a *Converso*, but there is no other evidence that this was the case.

95 AAL Testamentos leg. 15 exp. 13 Testamento de Domingo Pérez Pereira cirujano 16 May 1630; María Dolores Crespo Rodríguez, *Arquitectura doméstica de la Ciudad de los Reyes (1535–1750)* (Seville: Consejo Superior de Investigaciones Científicas, 2006), 353 Testament of Juan Ramírez, barber-surgeon 14 Aug. 1629; AAL Testamentos 46-5 fols. 36–37, 101v.–102 Testamento de Bartolomé de Ortega 1658.

96 AAL Testamentos 46-5 fols. 36–37, 101v.–102 Testamento de Bartolomé de Ortega 1658.

97 AGI Escribanía de Cámara 589B Causa contra Andrés Gonzales, boticario, portugués 1620.

98 Crespo Rodríguez, *Arquitectura doméstica*, 329–37.

Projecting Professionalism

A *boticario* could project his professionalism and social standing to the public through his personal attire. The Spanish Crown and residents of Lima alike were aware that clothing made important statements about status and identity.[99] From the fifteenth century, the Spanish Crown introduced sumptuary laws that restricted the wearing of luxury clothing, bearing of arms, and riding of horses to particular groups. Such laws reflected not only the desire to distinguish social groups, especially the elite from the popular classes, but at the same time embodied a distaste for luxury expressed by moralists and theologians.[100] In Spain, Philip II issued sumptuary laws eight times between 1563 and 1594, and Philip III and Philip IV issued them four times each.[101]

In the Americas, sumptuary laws acquired new dimensions. These laws were guided by concerns to maintain the superior status of Spaniards as conquerors and "civilised" persons while incorporating into the social hierarchy new ethnic groups who were at the same time subjects of the Crown, but were associated with illegitimacy and slavery.[102] In 1571 a law was passed for the Indies, that on pain of confiscation, no Black, whether slave or free, or Mulatto could wear gold, pearls or silk, except if they were married to a Spaniard in which case they could wear some gold earrings with pearls and a necklace, and a dress with velvet trimmings, but not a mantle of crêpe or another cloth, only a small mantilla.[103] Neither were Blacks, Mulattoes or *Zambos* allowed to carry arms, though Mestizos could do so with a licence.[104] As with much colonial legislation, laws followed practice. By then the municipality in Lima had already banned African slaves from wearing a cape and sword twice in 1539

---

99 Karen B. Graubert, *With Our Labor and Our Sweat: Indigenous Women and the Formation of Colonial Society in Peru, 1550–1700* (Stanford: Stanford University Press, 2007), 121–57.

100 Saúl Martínez Bermejo, "Beyond Luxury: Sumptuary Legislation in 17th-Century Castile," in *Making, Using and Resisting the Law in European History*, eds. Günther Lottes, Eero Medijainen, and Jón Vidar Sigurdsson (Pisa: Plus-Pisa University Press, 2008), 93–108.

101 Martínez Bermejo, "Beyond Luxury," 97. For Spanish legislation relating to clothing issued by Philip II see: *Recopilación de las leyes destos reynos, hecha por mandado de la Magestad Catholica del Rey don Philippe Segundo nuestro Señor* (Alcalá de Henares: Casa de Iuan Iñiguez de Lequerica, 1598), lib. 7 tit.12 ley 1: 117–24. For details of dress in Spain in the early sixteenth century see Ruth Matilda Anderson, *Hispanic Costume 1480–1530* (New York: Hispanic Society of America, 1979).

102 McAlister, "Social Structure," 350–55; Mörner, *Race Mixture*, 41–45, 51–68; Cope, *Limits of Racial Domination*, 16.

103 *Recopilación de las leyes de las indias*, lib. 7 tit. 5 ley 28: 290v. 12 Feb. 1571.

104 Ibid. lib. 7 tit. 5 leyes 14–18: 287–88 12 Feb. 1571.

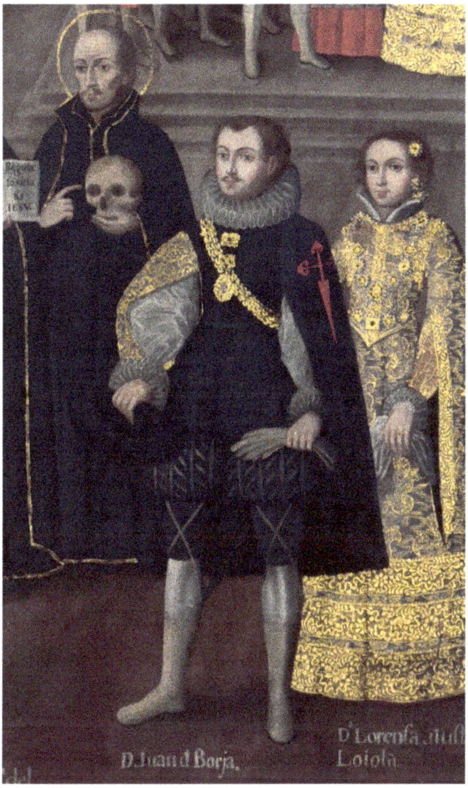

FIGURE 16
Elite formal dress in Lima in the seventeenth century. Extract from painting of the marriage of captain Martín de Loyola to Beatriz Ñusta, ca. 1675–1690. Elite male formal dress was similar to that of Don Juan Henríquez de Borja, who is dressed in black with a ruff and wearing trousers typical of the sixteenth century. He also wears a cape with the emblem of the order of Santiago.
COURTESY MUSEO PEDRO DE OSMA, LIMA.

and 1549.[105] Control over the wearing of particular clothes in Lima was also exercised indirectly through the guilds. Tailors were required to use and sell only silk and woollen cloth, while Blacks, whether slave or free, could be employed in workshops, but could not be masters.[106] The city's markets for imported and locally produced cloth and clothing remained geographically separate. The former operated on the Calle de Mercaderes, where there were some twenty stores (*almacenes*) and two hundred shops, while locally-produced cloth was sold on the Calle de Mantas.[107]

Influences over clothing in Lima were diverse. Legislation emanating from the Counter-Reformation and the Council in Lima in the late sixteenth and early seventeenth centuries generally discouraged the wearing of luxury clothing.[108] (Figure 16).

105 *Libros de cabildos de Lima*, 1: 287 8 Jan. 1539 and Libros de cabildos de Lima, 3: 56 21 Jan 1549.

106 *Libros de cabildos de Lima*, 4: 587–94 Ordenanzas de sastres confirmadas 5 Mar. 1557; Ricardo Cantuarias Acosta, "Las modas limeñas," in *Lima en el siglo XIV*, ed. Laura Gutiérrez Arbulú (Lima: Pontificia Universidad Católica del Perú, Instituto Riva-Agüero, 2005), 296–307 *passim*.

107 Salinas y Córdova, *Memorial*, 255–56.

108 Vargas Ugarte, *Concilios limenses*, 1: 131, 332, 243, 251.

This along with luxury furnishings and the use of silverware was viewed by Licenciado Martel Santoyo, lawyer to the *cabildo* in Lima, as provoking covetousness and discouraging Christianisation.[109] This objection to luxury clothing was reinforced by the personal preference of the Spanish monarchs for sobriety and the desire to protect Spain's textile industry from competition from exotic foreign imports.[110] In Lima an additional deterrent was the high cost of luxury clothing. This arose in part from high transport costs and *almojarifazgo* taxes on imports. The best quality brocade (*brocados de tres altos*) was taxed at 20 pesos a yard, velvet breeches at 40 pesos, and an outer skirt of taffeta at 15 pesos.[111] The scarcity of imports also served to maintain the high demand and both the monetary and non-monetary value of luxury clothing from Europe.[112]

Since imported cloth and clothing were expensive in Lima, from an early date a brisk trade in secondhand clothes emerged.[113] When the *boticario* Bartolomé Díaz Cabeza de Vaca died, his clothing, to be detailed below, most of which was worn, was auctioned and netted some 200 pesos.[114] The items of clothing which commanded the highest prices were those fashioned from luxury cloths imported from Spain, such as a cape of black cloth from Segovia which sold for 21 pesos and two pairs of black velvet collars from Castile, one worn and the other new, together valued at 25 pesos. It is significant that many of these items of used clothing were purchased by his business partner, the *boticario*, Francisco Martín Reyna, suggesting that the second-hand clothes market, particularly for high-priced European goods, was not limited to the popular classes. In fact the market in secondhand clothing was so brisk that it threatened the local textile industry and persuaded the *cabildo* in 1551 to try

109 AGI Patronato 185 no. 31 Relación que hace a su Magestad el Licenciado Martel Santoyo sobre lo que debe proveer y remedian en los reynos del Perú y en otras partes 1542 transcribed and published by Emilio Lissón Chaves, in *La iglesia de España en el Perú: colección de documentos para la historia de la iglesia en el Perú* (Sevilla: Editorial Católica Española, 1943), vol. 1, Part 3, 99–120.

110 Aileen Ribeiro, "Dress in the Early Modern Period, c.1500–1780," in *The Cambridge History of Western Textiles*, ed. David Jenkins (Cambridge: Cambridge University Press, 2003), 665, 672–73; Scarlett O'Phelan, "El vestido como identidad étnica e indicador social de una cultura material," in *El barroco peruano* II, ed. Ramón Mujica Pinilla (Lima: Banco de Crédito del Perú, 2003), 103.

111 AGNP Caja reales: Lima H-3 leg. 4 lib. 24-a fols. 1–30 Aranceles para cálculo del almojarifazgo (1617).

112 Velvet and taffeta were particularly esteemed (Enrique Otte, *Cartas privadas de emigrantes a Indias, 1540–1616* (Mexico: Fondo de Cultura Económica, 1993), 388, 413).

113 *Libros de cabildos de Lima*, 4: 354 Ropa vieja, corredor de tabla 29 Nov. 1555.

114 AAL Testamentos leg. 5 exp. 1 fols. 38–41 Testamento de Bartolomé Díaz Cabeza de Vaca 28 Apr. 1608.

and ban it completely. However, this proved ineffective and two years later it permitted two licensed secondhand dealers to operate.[115]

After 1570 when the Spanish established a permanent presence in the Philippines, cheap silk, satin and damask from China via the Philippines and Mexico made luxury clothing more widely available in Peru. Attempts to restrict this trade proved fruitless.[116] Hence, in 1602 the Mexican Viceroy, the Conde de Monterrey, with an interest in promoting trade between Mexico and Peru reported to the Crown that there [in Peru],

> All these people live very luxuriously. All wear silk, and of the most fine and costly quality. The gala dresses and clothes of the women are so many and so excessive, that in no other kingdom of the world are found such; so that if four merchant-vessels went to Peru annually, all the cloth goods would be sold…[117]

In the early seventeenth century the trade in cloth and clothing with Mexico and China was valued at more than one million pesos, while that from Castile was estimated to be only 5,000 to 6,000 pesos.[118] It was suggested that a *regidor* be commissioned to destroy any Chinese cloth, but this was strongly opposed by Lima's citizens, who added that much of it was used to adorn churches and convents. Chinese fabrics were cheaper than those imported from Europe and were therefore worn mainly by the popular classes, while Spaniards wishing to demonstrate their superior economic and social position preferred clothing from Europe.[119] An anonymous observer of Creole women on the coast of Peru at the beginning of the seventeenth century wrote:

> They are elegantly and expensively dressed; they all generally wear silk and very exquisite cloth and velvet with fine gold and silver. They have thick gold necklaces, strings of pearls, rings, necklaces and headbands of diamonds, rubies, emeralds and amethyst and other valuable and esteemed stones.

115 *Libros de cabildos de Lima*, 3: 460 [Ropavejeros] 16 Oct. 1551, *Libros de cabildos de Lima*, 4: 25 Ropavejeros que haya dos no más 19 May 1553; Cantuarias Acosta, "Modas limeñas," 292.

116 *Libros de cabildos de Lima*, 13: 267–68 Ropa de China 25 May 1599; William Lyle Schurz, "Mexico, Peru and the Manila Galleon," *Hispanic American Historical Review* 1 (1918): 394–402; Borah, *Early Colonial Trade*, 116–27.

117 Emma H. Blair and James A. Robertson, *The Philippine Islands, 1493–1803* (Cleveland, OH: A.H. Clark, 1911), 12: 63 Conde de Monterrey 15 May 1602; Schurz, "Mexico, Peru and the Manila Galleon," 396–97.

118 Salinas y Córdova *Memorial*, 256.

119 Lewin, *Descripción*, 115; *Libros de cabildos de Lima*, 13: 267–71 Ropa de China 25 May 1599.

> While the women are beautiful and graceful, the men are elegant and gallant. They generally all wear good quality clothes of silk and fine cloths from Segovia and collars with costly lace from Flanders. They all wear stockings of silk, are discrete, affable and well bred…they all go through the city on horseback.[120]

The wardrobes belonging to two *boticarios*, Francisco de Alva and Bartolomé Díaz Cabeza de Vaca, exemplify many of these observations, in particular their preference for sober European clothing.[121] While their capes, tunics, doublets, and breeches were generally black, they were often made of satin or taffeta and lined with damask, trimmed with velvet or embroidered with silver thread. The latter also wore black velvet collars. It is also noteworthy that their wardrobes contained little Chinese cloth or clothing and when their Spanish clothes were auctioned following their deaths these commanded high prices. Francisco de Alva also possessed two harquebuses, as well as a sword with a velvet sheath and a dagger with a golden handle. Alva was *familiar* to the Inquisition which gave him licence to wear both offensive and defensive weapons in public and private both day and night and throughout its jurisdiction.[122] His higher status was also evident in his possession of a cape and tunic that signified his position as a *hermano veinticuatro* of a *cofradia*. Not all *boticarios* would have possessed such fine clothing. Wage pharmacists and those who worked in hospitals, who were probably the majority, were of more modest means and in most cases did not write wills.[123] What can be said is that the clothing of surgeons was significantly poorer than that owners of *boticas*. The wardrobe of the surgeon, Domingo Pérez de Pereyra, included a ruff which had become fashionable at the time of his testament in 1637, but few of his clothes were made of luxury fabrics; in fact one set consisted of a suit (*vestido*), waistcoat and long trousers made of "Indian cloth."[124]

---

120 Lewin, *Descripción*, 39. For similar contemporary observations see Fray Diego de Ocaña, *Memoria viva de una tierra de olvido: Relación del viaje al Nuevo Mundo de 1599 a 1607* (Barcelona: CECAL, 2013), 290–91.

121 AGNP Real Audiencia. Causas Civiles leg. 16 cuad. 81 fols. 8v–10 Pleito de ejecución…contra las bienes y herederos del bachiller Francisco de Alva, boticario morador en la Ciudad de los Reyes, 13 Feb. 1576; AAL Testamentos leg. 5 exp. 1 fols. 25–26 Testamento de Bartolomé Díaz Cabeza de Vaca 17 Apr.1608.

122 *Libros de cabildos de Lima*, 8: 202 Familiar del santo oficio a Juan de Bilbao 15 Feb. 1576. This refers to the appointment of Juan de Bilbao to replace Francisco de Alva as familiar to the Inquisition.

123 De Vos, "Art of Pharmacy," 72.

124 AAL Testamentos leg. 15 exp. 13 Inventario de Domingo Pérez de Pereyra 16 May 1637; Ribeiro, "Dress in the Early Modern Period," 662.

Social distances between different ethnic groups in Lima may not have been that discernible from their dress for there were constant complaints that Blacks and those of mixed ethnic origins were wearing luxury clothing and carrying swords and daggers, which resulted in proclamations forbidding these practices to be issued with increasing frequency in the seventeenth century.[125] In 1629 Black and Mulatto women were said to be wearing fine linen blouses with lace, each worth 70 pesos, expensive petticoats, underskirts (*manteo*) worth 200 pesos, and mantles (*manto*) of silk with excessive lace which might reach 100 pesos.[126] At that time the Fiscal reported that ordinances prohibiting Black and Mulatto women from wearing luxury clothing were never observed.[127] This was somewhat exaggerated for in the same year two *Mulatas* were fined for wearing blue silk that was highly decorated with gold trimmings, which was confiscated.[128] Even if there were some prosecutions, the fact that the ordinances were reiterated so frequently suggests they did not act as a deterrent to what was clearly common practice. In 1631 *Mulatas* in Lima, whether slave or free, were not allowed to wear clothes of any kind made of silk or Castilian cloth nor wear slippers with silver decoration.[129] Again in 1667 orders were given that no *Mulata*, *Negra*, or *Zamba*, free or slave, should without exception wear a dress of silk, nor trimming of gold or silver, nor black trim of silk or linen. The penalty for first offence was confiscation of the clothes, for the second a fine of fifty pesos, and for the third two hundred lashes and eight years exile.[130] Even so, slave owners often attempted to display their elevated status by dressing their slaves in fine clothing.[131] In fact although slaves were forbidden from wearing capes or arms, they could do so when accompanying their owners.[132]

In the early seventeenth century, there were some 30,000 Blacks and Mulattoes in Lima and its hinterland,[133] and legislation against Blacks or Mulattoes bearing arms derived essentially from the fear they would revolt.[134] Exceptions

---

125 Mugaburu, *Chronicle of Colonial Lima*, p. 32 (1653), p. 59 (1661), pp. 82–83 (1663), pp. 91–92 (1665), p. 124 (1667).

126 AGI Lima 160 Fiscal Licenciado Varahona Encinillas 30 May 1629.

127 Ibid.

128 Suardo, *Diario de Lima* 1: 17.

129 Ibid. 1: 155.

130 Mugaburu, *Chronicle of Colonial Lima*, 124.

131 Tamara J. Walker, "'He Outfitted his Family in Notable Decency': Slavery, Honour and Dress in Eighteenth-Century Lima," *Slavery and Abolition* 30 (3) (2009): 390–91; O'Phelan, "El vestido," 107–08.

132 *Libros de cabildos de Lima*, 1: 287 Ordenanza sobre los negros 8 Jan. 1539; *Libros de cabildos de Lima*, 2: 56 Negros de cofradía 21 Jan. 1549.

133 AGI Lima 160 Fiscal Licenciado Varahona Encinillas 30 May 1629.

134 Lewin, *Descripción*, 39.

were made for Blacks who were servants of officials who were permitted to wear swords and for Blacks who needed them for their occupation, such as wood cutters and muleteers, who were allowed to carry knives.[135] In terms of style the population at large tried to emulate the upper classes, which in turn followed the fashion in Spain, though the particular fabric and trimmings might be different.[136] Rebecca Earle argues that in the early colonial period, despite sumptuary legislation, there was very little difference in the dress of elites and the popular classes who dressed extravagantly, but that distinctions grew in the Enlightenment period.[137]

Other possessions indicative of a person's social status were jewellery, furniture and furnishings. Perhaps surprisingly, cloth and furnishings figured more commonly than jewellery among Limeños' possessions and they commanded higher prices.[138] Most elite households possessed some pieces of silverware, such as plates, tankards and cutlery, no doubt reflecting the general availability of silver. Gold items were generally rarer and consisted of only small pieces of jewellery, trinkets, or religious items.[139] The apothecary Díaz Cabeza de Vaca possessed over 100 pesos worth of silver, mainly in the form of plates, but only an amethyst ring, gold toothpick, and a purple stain bag embroidered with pearls containing a small gold cross and ornamental chain of steel, which together sold at auction for only 15 pesos 4 reals. Linen sheets on the other hand were each worth 2 to 4 pesos and bedspreads could command over 20 pesos.[140]

The fluidity of early colonial society in Lima meant that individuals employed forms of public display to indicate and enhance their status. This was evident for all social groups, such that Antonio de la Calancha observed that on feast days the artisan would appear as a *regidor*, wearing a cape and velvet, while labourers from Spain pretended to be nobles, and commoners studied

135 Ibid. 40.

136 O'Phelan, "El vestido," 99–100.

137 Rebecca Earle, "Two Pairs of Pink Satin Shoes!!' Race, Clothing and Identity in the Americas (17th–19th centuries)," *History Workshop Journal* 52 (2001): 175–95.

138 For an excellent introduction to the furniture, furnishings and decorations to be found in colonial houses in Lima see Crespo Rodríguez, *Arquitectura doméstica*, 297–340.

139 Ibid. 307–11.

140 AAL Testamentos leg. 5 exp. 1 fols. 38–41 Testamento de Bartolomé Díaz Cabeza de Vaca 28 April 1608. For the belongings of other medical practitioners see: AAL Testamentos 25–1 fols. 4–5v. Testamento de Juan Matías de Vera 18 Jun. 1640 (boticario); AAL Testamentos leg. 15 exp. 13 Testamento de Domingo Perez Pereira cirujano 16 May 1630 (surgeon); AAL Testamentos 28A-1 fols. 79v–81v. Testamento de Juan Gerónimo Navarro 1648 (physician); Crespo Rodríguez, *Arquitectura doméstica,* 353 Testament of Juan Ramírez, barber surgeon 14 Aug. 1629.

how to look like *hidalgos*.[141] This meant that in public places it was difficult to distinguish, the gentleman from the artisan or commoner. This Calancha explained was not policy, but was encouraged by the opportunities of the land.[142] In effect elite ostentation competed with plebeian mimicry.[143] Dress as a symbol of status was generally more important in the New World than the Old,[144] and especially in Lima. The preference of *boticarios* for black and sober clothing thus reflected a desire to emulate the Spanish monarchs and adhere to Church teachings that disdained the wearing of luxury clothing, while their preference for expensive European textiles over cheaper imported Asian cloths both reflected and reinforced their superior social standing.

Conclusion

In many respects, the social standing, religious beliefs and moral compass of *boticarios* in Lima, including their involvement in the Church, demonstrated significant similarities to the life and status of their counterparts in Spain and indeed to other professional groups. However, the opportunities for wealth creation and display that Lima offered as well as the presence of sizeable African, indigenous and *casta* populations, produced a different and more fluid social environment. Apothecaries in Lima sought to reinforce their position among the elite through seldom wearing luxury clothing and maintaining an air of sobriety. They also actively participated in *cofradías*, displayed their piety, and made charitable donations according to public expectations of their profession. While apothecaries in Mexico City were involved in similar religious and charitable activities, those in Lima seem to have been more conscious of the economic gains their businesses could generate.[145] As noted in Chapter 6, apothecaries in Lima also sought to enhance their status by distancing themselves from popular healers by adhering to humoral practices and *materia medica* of Old World origin. Despite such efforts, apothecaries in Lima were not always held in high regard and as in Spain continued to command only a middling status within the medical profession beneath that of university-educated physicians.

141 Calancha, *Crónica moralizada*, lib. 1 cap. 10: 67.

142 Ibid. lib. 1 cap. 38: 245.

143 Osorio, *Inventing Lima*, 149.

144 Solange Alberro, *De gachupín al criollo: o de cómo los españoles de México dejaron* de *serlo* (México: El Colegio de México, 1992), 177–84.

145 De Vos, "Art of Pharmacy," 156–90.

CHAPTER 8

Persistent Practices

> Medical practitioners in New Spain, New France and New England may have borrowed at times from indigenous healers and incorporated some native remedies into their pharmacopoeias, but their theoretical framework and their actual practices remained virtually unchanged. Even when they prescribed novel medicines, they did so for the same reasons that had governed Western medical practice for centuries.[1]

∴

Apothecaries in early colonial Lima embodied both tradition and innovation. Inadequacies in the mechanisms used to control and regulate medical practice in Peru and the opportunities afforded by a whole new world of *materia medica*, should have encouraged scientific enquiry and experimentation. Yet, this study suggests that in the early colonial period humoral medicine predominated. Professional *boticarios* in Lima worked within a humoral framework employing purgatives, laxatives, and other treatments aimed at restoring a balance in the humours. In addition, whether they were treating private clients, slaves or patients in hospitals, they relied largely on Old World plants that were either imported from Europe or were grown locally. They adopted a few native plants as substitutes for Old World imports, such as canafistula and sarsaparilla, and relied on American resins and gums imported from Spanish American regions further north to meet the shortages of these essential products on the Peruvian coast. However, contrary to what might be expected, *boticarios* made relatively little use of local botanical *materia medica*. On the other hand, some *boticarios* began to experiment with minerals to the extent that their use may have been more prevalent in Lima than in Spain at this time. Distillation methods were widely employed and minerals and chemicals were used in medical preparations. However, very few medicines of this kind were employed and they were rarely applied internally.

A complex range of material, social and cultural factors contributed to the absence of native *materia medica* in medicines prepared by apothecaries in

1 Numbers, "Conclusion," 155–56.

 | DOI 10.1163/9789004351271_009

Lima. Of considerable significance was the delay and controversy involved in fitting American plants into the prevailing Galenic framework; extensive testing was required both to identify their appropriate therapeutic use and to allay fears that they might be dangerous or harmful. At the same time, professional medical practitioners, even though they often respected the herbal knowledge of indigenous healers, saw social status advantages in distancing themselves from them and from other popular healers by adhering to Spanish humoral practices and employing *materia medica* of Old World origin. Social status considerations may have been particularly significant in Lima where the social hierarchy was still in the process of consolidation, where royal authority was limited, and where mining and trade provided exceptional opportunities for social advancement. In addition to distancing themselves from popular healers though their professional activities, they also adopted publically visible modes of dress and expressions of piety that emulated the aristocracy.[2]

Despite the predominance of humoral medical practice, this study suggests that some apothecaries were employing empirical and experimental methods, even if this did not signal the adoption of a new natural philosophy. There was a curiosity about Peru's natural world even if it did not involve the extensive adoption of New World *materia medica*. Questions emerged around the efficacy of botanical imports and of Old World plants grown under a different constellation that required reconsideration of the most appropriate products and dosages for the treatment of particular diseases, whose prevalence in Lima also differed from that in Europe, even if they were not unfamiliar. There were some pioneers such as Antonio de Robles Cornejo who was intent on bringing pharmaceutical methods to non-university educated practitioners and whose manuscript, organised by product rather than ailment signified growing specialisation of pharmacy within the medical profession as it diverged from medicine as a practical science. The format of his work also reflected the shift from the diagnosis of illness and personalised treatment following humoral principles to the study of the effectiveness of particular *materia medica*. This process was encouraged by a lack of knowledge and agreement between physicians on the efficacy of humoral treatments and by patients lacking classical training who could grasp the reality of illness and healing and who might treat themselves without the intervention of a physician. Despite the experimental tendencies evident in Robles Cornejo's work, it was written in the Galenic tradition.

2 Lockhart, *Spanish Peru*, 226–27; Bronner, "Elite Formation," 25–26. For Spain see Pike, *Aristocrats and Traders*, 81–93.

From this discussion it will be evident that in the period prior to 1650 apothecaries in Peru saw no contradiction in the employment of experimental methods and humoral beliefs. At this time, their experimental methods focussed on the composition and efficacy of medicines based on Old World plants and their substitutes; they were not, for the most part, directed at testing native products, which with a few exceptions, for example, cinchona, remained largely the preserve of indigenous and popular healers. The focus of apothecaries on Old World *materia medica* was reinforced by their professional training, by the dominance of medical manuals based on Old World products, and by pharmacy inspections. This emphasis effectively separated professional medical practice from other forms of healing, although the distinction was never sharp or absolute.

This finding has two conceptual implications. First, it suggests that medical practitioners did not compete for clients in no single "marketplace," but rather in terms of provision the market was segmented, with a regulated professional sector being largely distinct from the popular sector. Second, recent research on medical practice in early colonial Spanish America has stressed its hybrid nature and even the fusion of healing traditions of European, African and indigenous groups, through a process of medical *mestizaje*.[3] Such studies of the exchange and the interweaving of medical ideas, practices and products, which have generally been grounded in specific social, historical and geographical contexts, have added greatly to knowledge of colonial medicine. However, there is sometimes a tendency to assume that such exchanges were free and simple, when as this study suggests, the process was commonly slowed and constrained by cultural or institutional obstacles. Furthermore, it underlines the necessity not to lose sight of the unequal distribution of power that characterised the social context in which the exchange of ideas and practices took place.

Accounting for the Prevalence of Humoral Medicine

What can account for the prevalence of humoral medicine in Lima? Many interrelated factors were involved. These included attempts by the state working with the Church and Inquisition to bolster humoral beliefs through regulation

3 Martha Few, "Medical *Mestizaje* and the Politics *of Pregnancy in Colonial Guatemala," 1660–1730,* in *Science in the Spanish and Portuguese Empires, 1500–1800*, eds. Daniela Bleichmar, Paula De Vos, Kristine Hufine and Kevin Sheehan (Stanford CA: Stanford University Press, 2009), 133.

and censorship. Perhaps more significant, however, was the fact that humoralism was already embedded in popular Spanish culture.

The state and Church were reluctant to promote new medical practices that implied the adoption of a new natural philosophy, especially one that might challenge the basis of the Catholic faith.[4] It therefore sought to uphold humoral medical practice by establishing a medical infrastructure that was similar to that being developed in Castile. However, as this study has shown, even in Lima, which was capital of the Viceroyalty of Peru, this was only partially achieved. Instead the state relied on the clergy and particularly the religious orders to deliver healthcare.[5] Nevertheless, the fact that the Crown actively promoted the foundation of hospitals served to foster a paternalistic view of Spanish rule and provide legitimisation for its colonial mission.[6]

In the task of maintaining medical orthodoxy, the state was aided by the Inquisition and, in the case of the indigenous population, the ecclesiastical courts. These aimed at suppressing healing practices deemed to be heretical and at controlling the publication and dissemination of literature contrary to the interests of the state and Church. The Inquisition was most active in Lima in the early seventeenth century, but its impact on medical practices in Lima is difficult to evaluate. Only two physicians and two surgeons were brought before the Inquisition and this was for Judaizing or promoting heretical beliefs rather than unorthodox medical practices. Some *curanderos* were also tried by the Inquisition, but due to their healing skills and the general shortage of doctors, they appear to have been allowed to practise as long as they did not employ superstitious or idolatrous methods.[7]

The role of the Inquisition in the realm of censorship is equally difficult to gauge. The medical texts and manuals most widely used by apothecaries were written in the Galenic tradition and there is little evidence for the ownership of medical texts that promoted experimental methods and the use of chemical medicines. It cannot be concluded, however, that the absence of Paracelsian or "modern" texts was due to the effectiveness of the Inquisition's scrutiny.

---

4 Shapin, *Scientific Revolution*, 136.

5 See Cahill, "Financing Health Care" for the role of state finance in medical care in eighteenth-century Lima. For the role of the religious orders in the dissemination of humoral medicine see: Foster, "Origin of Humoral Medicine," 363–64 and *Hippocrates' Latin American Legacy*, 153–55.

6 Risse, "Medicine in New Spain," 42; Warren, *Medicine and Politics*, 20; Ramos, "Indian Hospitals," 204–05.

7 Griffiths, "Andean *Curanderos*," 185–97. For cases against *hechiceras* see, AAL Hechicerías leg. 1 exp. 7 fol. 2 Causa seguida contra Pedro Sayo, acusado de curar enfermos con hierbas 1621; Mannarelli, *Hechicheras*, 38; Sánchez, *Amancebados*, xxxv.

Indeed in Europe as well such texts were not widely available. More likely, as Richard Palmer has noted for Venice, the slow progress of Paracelsianism reflected the extent to which humoralism was entrenched both among medical practitioners and the public at large.

Palmer claims that in Italy Paracelsianism only began to emerge in the late sixteenth century with chemical drugs only becoming widely available in the early seventeenth century. Even then, he argues, they added to rather than replaced traditional remedies.[8] Adding to the delay in the adoption of a new natural philosophy in Spain was existence of a strong alchemic tradition which enabled the development of chemical methods without engagement with Paracelsian philosophy. The existence of copies of the works of the physician and alchemist Arnau de Vilanova in pharmacies in Lima suggests that there too apothecaries were using chemical methods that had been developed by alchemists and were applying chemical medicines within a Galenic framework. In fact the philosophical distinction between Paracelsianism and Galenism may not have been that obvious or seemed so novel at this time.[9] Indeed, Paracelsus himself declared that he had been influenced by the alchemic texts of Vilanova, Llull and Rupescissa. In any case, apothecaries in Lima appear to have been less concerned with challenging the philosophy underlying their methods and more focused on the practical task of preparing medicines that were appropriate for the treatment of particular illnesses.

The significant role played by the clergy in providing medical care had a number of implications not only for its delivery, but also the type of medicine practised. Even though papal decrees in the early thirteenth century discouraged priests from formally studying medicine because it distracted them from their spiritual goals,[10] their Christian responsibility for the relief suffering meant they were actively involved caring for the sick. The knowledge and skills they used would have been acquired through the private study of classical texts such as those of Galen and Hippocrates.[11] In addition to healing the sick themselves,[12] they instructed Indians how to let blood and prepare

8 Palmer, "Pharmacy in the Republic of Venice," 110–17.

9 López Pérez, "Spanish Paracelsus Revisited," 353–57.

10 Siraisi, *Medieval and Early Renaissance Medicine*, 26, 43–44.

11 John Lloyd Mecham, *Church and State in Latin America: A History of Politico-Ecclesiastical Relations* (Chapel Hill: University of North Carolina Press, 1934), 36.

12 Real Academia de Historia, Madrid, Jesuitas 129 fol. 383v. Letras anuas de la provincia del Perú de 1618 años.

medicines,[13] and compiled *recetarios* for use by the population at large.[14] As such, several authors have argued that priests played a more significant role in transmitting humoral medicine to the New World than trained medical practitioners.[15]

Despite the Church's general support for humoral medicine and for the suppression of healing practices deemed heretical, it is clear that some priests, particularly the Jesuits, were using empirical and experimental methods. In fact they saw no contradiction between the methods of scientific enquiry and their religious beliefs, which promised to reveal God's work in nature and support efforts to heal the sick, especially in remote regions where professional medical practitioners were lacking. Their observational and experimental approaches were therefore largely practical in intent and, since they were not seeking to find the *causes* of phenomena, did not challenge the Catholic belief in God's creation.[16]

Professional medical practitioners, the clergy, Inquisition, *protomedicato*, and municipal authorities, were not the only agents promoting humoral medicine. In Europe, medicine was just developing as a specialist occupation, prior to which everyone took responsibility for their own health and acquired a basic knowledge of treatments. Within a community certain individuals, such as a barber or grocer, might develop special skills or knowledge, or might become renowned for the production of simple medicines, such as waters or syrups with effective healing properties. Literate citizens might also collect well-tried recipes in hand-written *recetarios* for domestic use.[17] Unfortunately only a few such *recetarios* exist for Peru and then only from the eighteenth century.[18] Meanwhile some secular elites holding positions of authority, for example, as administrators of hospitals or members of *cofradías*, would have been able to influence the nature medical practice beyond the home. In remote regions they might even teach rudimentary healing skills themselves. In 1586 the *corregidor*

13 AAL Hechicerías 4 27 fol. 3v Cabeza de proceso de oficio por hechicero contra Pablo Ato 3 Dec.1660; Ramos, "Indian Hospitals," 198.

14 See Chapter 6.

15 Guerra, "Role of Religion," 180–81; Foster, *Hippocrates' Latin American Legacy*, 150–51.

16 William B. Ashworth, "Catholicism and Early Modern Science," in *God and Nature: Historical Essays on the Encounter between Christianity and Religion*, eds. David C. Lindberg and Ronald L. Numbers (Berkeley: University of California Press, 1986), 153–58.

17 Elaine Leong, "Making Medicines in the Early Modern Household," *Bulletin of the History of Medicine* 82 (2008): 157–63.

18 See Valdizán and Maldonado, *Medicina popular*, 3: 108–316, 421–87 for various examples of *recetarios* from the late eighteenth or nineteenth century.

of Yauyos, Diego Dávila Briceño, reported that he had been teaching the local residents in his jurisdiction how to let blood.[19] Humoral beliefs were not, therefore, the preserve of a particular occupational group, but came to be widely diffused and understood by the population at large.[20] This extended to the indigenous population, where the failure of native remedies to deal with the major epidemics in the Andes in the late sixteenth and early seventeenth centuries, probably undermined the authority of native healers within their communities, even though the humoral treatments the Spanish introduced were no more effective.[21] This was especially so since the epidemics that afflicted native peoples left Europeans largely unscathed. A final factor that might have facilitated the spread of humoral medicine was that Spanish and indigenous healing traditions were based on similar principles of bodily balance and the humours, even if the qualities attributed to particular substances used in treatments were not always the same. Among Andean peoples the body is viewed as a hydraulic system in which the fluids of air, blood and fat need to be kept in circulation and are affected by whether they are hot or cold.[22]

Accounting for the Slow Adoption of Experimental Methods

State regulation, the Inquisition and entrenched cultural traditions may partially explain why humoral medicine predominated into the early seventeenth century and why experimental approaches appear to have developed less

19 *Relaciones geográficas de Indias* 1: 159 Descripción y relación de la provincia de los Yauyos, Diego Dávila Briceño 15 Jan. 1586.

20 Henry, "Doctors and Healers," 199–202. For a study of the enthusiasm for medical knowledge in Spanish Valencia prior to the professionalization of medicine see McVaugh, *Medicine before the Plague*.

21 Linda A. Newson, "A Historical-Ecological Perspective on Epidemic Disease," in *Advances in Historical Ecology*, ed. William Balée (New York: Columbia University Press, 1998), 56; Daniel T. Reff, *Disease, Depopulation, and Culture Change in Northwestern New Spain, 1518–1764* (Salt Lake City: University of Utah Press, 1991), 280–84; Luz María Hernández Sáenz and George Foster, "Curers and Their Cures in Colonial New Spain and Guatemala: The Spanish Component," in *Mesoamerican Healers* eds. Brad R. Huber and Alan R. Sandstrom. (Austin: University of Texas Press, 2001), 42; Cueto, *Medicine and Public Health*, 16–18. For Andean epidemics see: Cook, *Demographic Collapse* and *Born to Die;* Suzanne A. Alchon, *Native Society and Disease in Colonial Ecuador* (Cambridge: Cambridge University Press, 1991); and Linda A. Newson, *Life and Death in Early Colonial Ecuador* (Norman: University of Oklahoma Press, 1995).

22 Joseph W. Bastien, *Healers of the Andes: Kallawaya herbalists and their medicinal plants* (Salt Lake City: University of Utah Press: 1987), 45–52.

rapidly than might be expected. Studies in the history of medicine have suggested that in order for a significant change in scientific practice to occur it is necessary for a community of scientists to emerge, who can exchange and discuss ideas and methods. Hence George Basalla's model for the spread of western science argues that for colonial science to develop beyond the stage of exploration there needs to be an expansion in the number of scientists and for their ideas to be accepted and validated by a dominant external culture.[23] The number of professional medical practitioners in Lima at this time was small. They would almost certainly have known each other professionally, for example, through trading *materia medica*, lending each other medical texts, inspecting each other's premises, or valuing their medicines for legal cases; they would also have known each other socially even to the extent of sometimes intermarrying. There is also evidence for interactions between medical practitioners and Jesuits at the College of San Pablo. Medical practitioners could borrow books from the College's extensive library which contained both traditional and modern medical texts, many brought to Peru by Jesuits arriving from Europe.[24] On the other hand, the Jesuits might approach apothecaries for the testing of new medicinal products, as was the case with cinchona.

While there appears to have been a growing number of scientists, both secular and ecclesiastical, in Lima in the early colonial period and evidence for at least some exchange in ideas and practices between them, the opportunities for wider dissemination would have been limited by inadequacies in local printing and by scrutiny by the Inquisition. As the seventeenth century progressed, the Inquisition became less active, knowledge of the natural history of Peru accumulated, and the numbers involved in scientific activity, many of whom were Creoles, expanded. This period is outside that studied here, but there are indications from later pharmacy inventories and from the libraries of physicians that experimental methods, including the use of minerals and mineral salts, were becoming more widespread in Lima from the mid-seventeenth.[25] As time progressed local scientists accumulated greater knowledge of the region's geography, flora and mineral resources, and were therefore better placed

23 Basalla, "Spread of Western Science," 611–17.

24 Luis Martín, "La biblioteca del Colegio de San Pablo," 24–29; Guibovich, "Bibliotecas de médicos," 302. See also Chapter 5.

25 See Biblioteca Nacional Perú 1560 Cuenta que da el Cap. Nicólas Navarro mayordomo del hospital de San Andrés 1674–1676; Biblioteca Nacional Peru 1562 Cuenta del mayordomo de San Andrés, Cap. Don José Bernardo de León 1676. See also the inventory of the pharmacy of the Colegio San Pablo when the Jesuits were expelled: AGNP Santo Oficio. Temporalidades. Inventarios leg. 2 cuad. 28 fols. 1–68 1768. See also Chapter 5.

to challenge scientific discourses emanating from the metropolis, making science more relevant to local needs and with scientists spurred on by patriotic sentiments.[26] Such knowledge was founded on empirical methods developed locally rather than in Europe, though the seeds had been sown by the Columbian encounter which forced a revaluation of many ideas and practices and the adaptation of Old World policies, frameworks and institutions to colonial circumstances.[27] This chapter in the history of pharmacy in colonial Lima has yet to be written.

The late seventeenth century is probably the least researched period in colonial Latin American history, yet this study suggests that it may be critical in understanding the development of science, medicine and pharmacy in Peru, and indeed Latin America more generally. It would enable further exploration of the role of different institutions, groups and individuals in scientific practice countering the European narrative that dominates current historiography. The putative role of apothecaries as pioneers in the history of medicine needs further study. An examination of the late seventeenth century when Habsburg power was at its nadir would also throw light on the role of Atlantic connections in understanding colonial medical practice, since in theory weakened state control and reduced intellectual exchange should have encouraged greater local innovation. As such it would throw light on the relationship between empire and medicine more generally.

26 Cañizares-Esguerra, "New World, New Stars"; Lafuente, "Enlightenment Connections."

27 Saldaña, "Science and Public Happiness," 56–59. The Bourbon reforms of the eighteenth century saw the activities of scientists finding validation through alliances with non-medical elites and in the emergence of learned societies and institutions dedicated to it.

Appendices

APPENDIX A

Books Shipped from Spain by the Apothecary Juan Sánchez in 1591

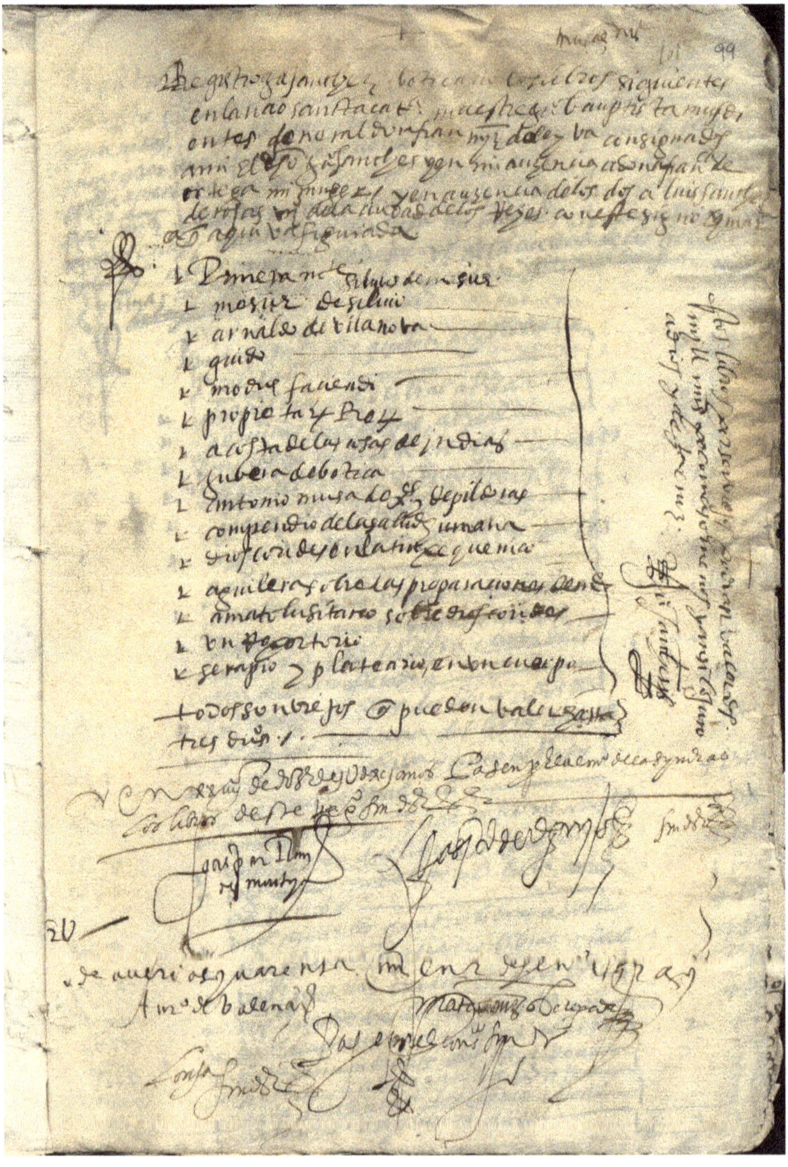

Courtesy Spain. Ministerio de Cultura. Archivo General de Indias, Seville.
SOURCE: AGI CONTRATACI

 | DOI 10.1163/9789004351271_010

Juan Sánchez, apothecary, registers the following books in the ship Santa Catalina, shipmaster Juan Bautista Musdientes and general [of the fleet] Don Francisco Martínez de Leyva consigned to me, the said Juan Sánchez and in my absence to my wife Francisca de Ortega and in the absence of both to Luis Sánchez de Rojas, citizen of the city of kings with this sign and mark entered here.

Primeramente Silvio de Mesue [*Joannis Mesuae Damaceni* … Jacobo Sylvio [Jacques Dubois]], (Paris, 1544)
Mesue de Silvio [ibid.]
Arnaldo de Vilanova [*Antidotarium* (Valencia, 1495)]
Guido [Guy de Chauliac (Guido de Cauliaco) possibly *Chirugía* (Venice, 1480)].
Modus faciendi [Bernardino de Laredo (Seville, 1527)]
Propietarum rerum [Bartolomaeus Anglicus (Bartolomé Anglicus), *De propietatibus rerum* (Cologne, 1472)]
Acosta de las cosas de las indias [José de Acosta, *Historia natural y moral de las indias* (Seville, 1590)]
Jubera de botica [Alfonso Jubera, *Dechado y reformación de todas las medicinas compuestas usuales* (Valladolid, 1578)]
Antonio Musa de jarabes y piladoras [Antonio Musa Brasavola, *Examen omnium syruporum* (Lyon, 1540)]
Compendio de la salud humana [Johann von Ketham (Zaragoza, 1494)]
Dioscórides en latín pequeña. Unspecified small version of Dioscorides in Latin.
Aguilera sobre las preparaciones de Mesue [Antonio de Aguilera, *Exposición sobre las preparaciones de Mesue* (Alcalá de Henares, 1569)]
Amato Lusitano sobre Dioscórides [Amatus Lusitanus, *Index Dioscoridis* (Antwerp, 1536)]
Un reportorio [Jerónimo de Chaves, *Chronographia, o, reportorio de los tiempos* (Seville, 1548)]
Serapio y plateario en un cuerpo [possibly *Practica Io. Serapionis dicta breviarium. Liber Serapionis de simplii medicina. Liber de simplii medicina, dictus circa instans. Practica platearii* (Venice, 1503)]

They are all old and are worth about three ducats [about four pesos]

Source: AGI Contratación 1097 N 5 Image 197 24 Dec. 1591.

APPENDIX B

List of *Materia Medica* Found in Pharmacies in Spain and Lima

	Andrés Zamudio de Alfaro[a] 1590s	Hospital of Santa Ana[b] 1551	Diego de Tineo *botica*[c] 1555	Francisco de Alva *botica*[d] 1576	Bartolomé Díaz Cabeza de Vaca *botica*[e] 1608
Organic Simples					
Abarraz [Albarraz]					X
Abrótano		X	X		
Acacia		X			X
Aceitunas gordas		X			
Acíbar de levante					
Acíbar [de India]	X	X	X	X	X
Acíbar [h]epático			X		
Acíbar secotrino		X	X		
Agallas			X		
Agárico	X	X	X	X	X
Ajalidis					
Alarges [Alarguez?]			X	X	
Alcarabea		X	X		X
Alchechengi					X
Alheña			X	X	
Alholvas		X			X
Alhucema			X		X
Almendras			X		
Almendras amargas			X		X
Almoradux			X		
Ámbar	X		X		

 DOI 10.1163/9789004351271_011

Pedro de Bilbao *botica*[f] 1636	Hospital of Santa Ana[g] 1606	Fernando de Cartagena Cuzco[h] 1618	Common name	Latin name
	X		Stavesacre, larkspur	Delphinium staphisagria L.
			Southern wood	Artemisia abrotanum L.
			Acacia	Acacia sp.
			Large olives	Olea europaea L.
		X	Aloe from the Levant	Aloe vera (L.) Burm.f.
		X	Aloe	Aloe vera (L.) Burm.f.
			Aloe for the liver	Aloe vera (L.) Burm.f.
			Aloe	Aloe from the island of Socotora
X			Galls	
X	X	X	Agaric, mushroom	Polyporus sp.
		X	Unidentified	
		X	Dog-rose	Rosa canina L.
X			Caraway	Carum carvi L.
			Bladder cherry, winter cherry, Chinese lantern	Physalis alkekengi L.
X			Privet	Ligustrum vulgare L.
		X	Fenugreek	Trigonella foenum graecum L.
			Lavender	Lavandula spica L.
			Almonds	Amygdalus spp.
			Bitter almonds	Amygdalus amara Hayne
			Marjoram	Origanum majorana L.
			Amber	

	Andrés Zamudio de Alfaro[a] 1590s	Hospital of Santa Ana[b] 1551	Diego de Tineo *botica*[c] 1555	Francisco de Alva *botica*[d] 1576	Bartolomé Díaz Cabeza de Vaca *botica*[e] 1608
Ameos		X	X		
Anacardos		X			
Anoscastos [Agnus-castus]					
Apio				X	
Arcollo			X		
Aristoloquias [luengo and redondo]		X	X		X
Arrayán		X			X
Aspálato			X		
Avellanas		X	X		
Azafrán		X	X		X
Azafrán romi					X
Azahar					X
Azufeifas [Jujubas]		X	X		
Beleño		X			X
Ben blanco		X	X		
Ben rubio		X	X		X
Bryonia			X		
Cabezuelas de rosas			X		
Cálamo aromático		X	X		
Camepitios					X
Canafistula	X				X
Canela		X	X	X	
Carlina			X		
Cassia [avellanos de cassia]					X

Pedro de Bilbao *botica*[f] 1636	Hospital of Santa Ana[g] 1606	Fernando de Cartagena Cuzco[h] 1618	Common name	Latin name
			Bishop's weed	Ammi majus L
			Cashew	Anacardium sp.
X		X	Chaste tree, Chaste berry, Monk's pepper	Vitex agnus-castus L.
		X	Celery	Apium graveolens L.
			Unidentified	
X		X	Birthwort, Aristolochia	Aristolochia sp.
			Myrtle	Myrtus communis L.
			Rosewood	Dalbergia latifolia Roxb. Simple
			Hazelnut	Corylus avellana L.
			Saffron	Crocus sativus L.
			Bastard saffron, rumin	Carthamus tinctorius L.
			Orange blossom,	Citrus sinensis L.
			Jujube, Chinese or Red Date	Ziziphus zizyphus (L.) H. Karst.
X			Henbane	Hyoscyamus niger L.
			White ben, behen	Moringa arabica Pers.
			Red ben, behen	Moringa arabica Pers.
			Bryony	Bryonia sp.
			Rose buds	Rosa sp.
		X	Calamus, Sweet flag	Acorus calamus L.
			Chamaepitys, cam-epitys, ground pine	Teucrium chamaepitys L
	X	X	Cassia, golden shower tree, drum-stick tree	Cassia fisula L.
		X	Cinnamon	Cinnamomum verum J. Presl
			Carline thistle	Carline sp.
			Cassia	Cinnamomum or Senna sp.

	Andrés Zamudio de Alfaro[a] 1590s	Hospital of Santa Ana[b] 1551	Diego de Tineo *botica*[c] 1555	Francisco de Alva *botica*[d] 1576	Bartolomé Díaz Cabeza de Vaca *botica*[e] 1608
Cebollas albarranas			X		
Cedoaria			X		
Cíperos			X		X
Ciruelas pasas		X	X		
Clavos and madres de clavos		X	X		
Coca de levante		X			
Coloquíntidas	X	X	X	X	X
Cominos rústicos			X	X	
Contra yerba					X
Coriandro			X		
Coronilla del rey		X			
Costo amargo		X	X		
Costos					X
Cubebas		X	X	X	X
Culantro preparado					X
Dauco					X
Dialtea				X	X
Díctamo crético	X		X	X	X
Díctamo real		X	X		X
Doronicus			X	X	
Eléboro blanco		X	X		X
Eléboro negro		X	X		X
Escamonea	X	X	X	X	X
Esclarimente		X			
Espica céltica	X	X	X		
Espicanardo	X	X	X	X	X

Pedro de Bilbao *botica*[f] 1636	Hospital of Santa Ana[g] 1606	Fernando de Cartagena Cuzco[h] 1618	Common name	Latin name
			Maritime squill	Urginea maritima (L.) Baker
			Zedoary	Curcuma zedoaria (Christm.) Roscoe
		X	Cipero sedge	Cyperus spp.
			Prunes	Prunus domestica L.
			Clove	Syzygium aromaticum L.
			Indian berry, levant nut	Anamirta cocculus (L.) Wight & Arn
X		X	Colocynth, bitter apple	Citrullus colocynthis (L.) Schrad
		X	Cumin	Cuminium cyminum L.
			Contrahierba, snakewort	Dorstenia contrajerva L.
			Coriander	Coriandrum sativum L.
			Crown vetch?	Coronilla minima L.
			Bitter costus	Saussurea lappa Decne
			Costus	Costus arabicus L.
		X	Cubeb, Javanese tailed pepper	Piper cubeba L.
	X		Cilantro, coriander	Coriandrum sativum L.
			Carrot	Daucus carota L.
	X		Dialthea, marshmallow	Althaea officinalis L.
		X	Dittany from Crete	Origanum dictamnus L.
			White dittany	Dictamnus albus L.
			Leopard's bane	Doronicum L.
X			White hellebore	Helleborus album L
X			Black hellebore	Helleborus niger L
X	X	X	Scammony	Convulvulus scammonia L.
X			Yellow amber	
X		X	Yellow or Roman Valerian	Valeriana celtica L.
	X	X	Spikenard	Nardostachys grandiflora DC, Nardostachys jatamansi DC

	Andrés Zamudio de Alfaro[a] 1590s	Hospital of Santa Ana[b] 1551	Diego de Tineo *botica*[c] 1555	Francisco de Alva *botica*[d] 1576	Bartolomé Díaz Cabeza de Vaca *botica*[e] 1608
Esquenanto [paja de meca]	X		X	X	X
Estafisagra					X
Ésula			X	X	X
Filipéndula			X		X
Fumaria					
Garbanzos negros			X		X
Guayacán					
Gengibre		X	X	X	X
Habas de mar			X		
Lengua avil [lenguavis]					
Lináloe	X	X	X	X	X
Linaza		X			X
Lingua cervina			X		
Lupinus		X	X		
Macis	X	X		X	X
Malagueta				X	
Maná	X		X	X	X
Maná (Magna) de calabria		X			
Matías			X		
Milium solis		X		X	
Mirabolanos-negros				X	
Mirobolanos-chébulos	X	X	X	X	
Mirobolanos					
Mirobolanos-beléricos	X	X	X	X	
Mirobolanos-citrinos	X	X	X	X	X
Mirobolanos-émblicos	X	X	X	X	X
Mirobolanos-indios	X	X	X	X	

Pedro de Bilbao *botica*[f] 1636	Hospital of Santa Ana[g] 1606	Fernando de Cartagena Cuzco[h] 1618	Common name	Latin name
X	X		Camel grass	Cymbopogon schoenanthus (L.) Spreng.
X			Stavesacre, larkspur	Dephinium staphisagria L.
X			Leafy spurge	Euphorbia esula L.
			Dropwort	Spiraea filipendula L.
X			Fumitory	Fumaria officinalis L.
X			Black chickpeas	Cicer arietinum L.
		X	Lignum vitae	Guaiacum officinale L
		X	Ginger	Zingiber officinale L.
			Sea beans, samphire	Salicornia sp.
X			Unidentified	Bird's tongue?
X	X	X	Linaloe	Bursera aloexylon (Shiede ex Shlecht)
		X	Linseed	Linum usitatissimum L.
			Hart's tongue	Asplenium scolopendrium L.
			Lupin	Lupinus sp
		X	Mace	Holarrhena antidysenterica (Roxb. ex Fleming) Wall. ex A. DC
			Malagueta pepper	Capsicum frutescens L.
X		X	Manna	Fraxinus ornus L.
			Manna from Calabria	Fraxinus ornus L.
			Unidentified	
	X		Gromwell	Lithospermum officinale L.
			Black myrobalan	Terminalia chebula L.
X		X	Chebulic myrobalan	Terminalia chebula L.
	X		Myrobalan unspecified	Terminalia sp.
X		X	Beleric myrobalan	Terminalia bellirica (Gaertn.) Roxb.
X		X	Yellow myrobalan	Terminalia chebula L.
X		X	Emblic myrobalan	Emblica officinalis Gaertn.
X		X	Indian myrobalan	Terminalia chebula L.

	Andrés Zamudio de Alfaro[a] 1590s	Hospital of Santa Ana[b] 1551	Diego de Tineo *botica*[c] 1555	Francisco de Alva *botica*[d] 1576	Bartolomé Díaz Cabeza de Vaca *botica*[e] 1608
Neguillas				X	
Nenúfar			X		
Nísperos			X		
Nuez moscada	X	X	X	X	
Orosus [Regaliz]		X	X	X	
Oruga		X			
Panis pores			X		
Pasas de almunécar			X		
Pelitre					X
Pentafilon			X		X
Peonía		X	X		
Pimienta			X		X
Pimienta blanca	X	X	X	X	
Pimienta larga	X	X	X	X	X
Pimienta negra	X				
Pinas secas			X		
Piñones			X		
Polipodio		X	X	X	X
Rapontico [reupontico]			X		
Ruibarbo	X	X	X	X	X
Sándalos blancos	X	X	X	X	
Sándalos cetrinos		X	X		
Sándalos colorados	X	X	X	X	X
Santónica					
Sasifragia					X
Scordeon			X		
Scrophularia [scrofularia]			X		
Sebesteno			X		

Pedro de Bilbao *botica*[f] 1636	Hospital of Santa Ana[g] 1606	Fernando de Cartagena Cuzco[h] 1618	Common name	Latin name
		X	Nigella, fennel flower	Nigella sativa L.
			Water lily	Nymphaea spp.
			Medlar	Eriobotrya japonica (Thunb.) Lindl.
		X	Nutmeg	Myristica fragrans Houtt.
X		X	Liquorice	Glycyrrhiza glabra L
			Rocket	Eruca sativa (L.) Mill.
			Common stinkhorn?	Phallus impudicus L.
			Raisins from Almuñécar	
	X		Pellitory	Anacyclus officinarum Hayne
			Cinquefoil	Potentilla reptans L.
X			Peony	Paeonia sp.
			Pepper	Unspecified
		X	White pepper	Piper nigrum L.
X		X	Long pepper	Piper longum L.
			Black pepper	Piper nigrum L.
			Dired pine cones	Pinus sp.
			Pinenuts	Pinus sp.
			Polypody	Polypodium vulgare L.
			Rhapontic	Rheum rhaponticum L.
	X	X	Rhubarb	Reum rhabarbarum L.
	X	X	White sandalwood	Santalum album L.
		X	Yellow sandalwood	Santalum citrimum J.B.
X	X	X	Red sandalwood	Santalum rubrum L.
		X	Santonica, wormseed	Artemisia cina Berg & C.F. Schmidt ex Poljakov
			Saxifrage	Saxifraga sp.
			Water germander	Teucrium scordium L.
			Figwort	Scrophularia sp.
			Sebesten plum	Cordia myxa L.

		Andrés Zamudio de Alfaro[a] 1590s	Hospital of Santa Ana[b] 1551	Diego de Tineo *botica*[c] 1555	Francisco de Alva *botica*[d] 1576	Bartolomé Díaz Cabeza de Vaca *botica*[e] 1608
	Selamente				X	
	Sen – oja	X				X
	Sen de luna			X		
	Sen- folículos	X	X		X	
	Sentalis				X	
	Seselios		X			X
	Sínfito			X		
	Stecados					X
	Suelda			X	X	X
	Tamarindo	X	X			
	Taragontía		X			
	Tormentila			X		X
	Turbi[t]		X	X	X	
	Turbit de la tierra					
	Turbit de levante			X		
	Vistorta			X		
	Yeros					
	Yervata			X		
Total	144	28	62	92	42	58
Seeds						
	Acederas			X	X	X
	Adormideras					
	Adormideras blancas	X	X			
	Adormideras montesinas		X			
	Adormideras negras	X	X		X	X
	Agnocasto [anus castus]	X		X		X

Pedro de Bilbao *botica*[f] 1636	Hospital of Santa Ana[g] 1606	Fernando de Cartagena Cuzco[h] 1618	Common name	Latin name
			Unidentified	
	X	X	Senna – leaves	Cassia senna L., Cassia acutifolia Delile
			Senna picked under the moon?	
			Senna – folicules	Senna sp.
			Unidentified	
			Hartwort	Tordylium offcinale L.
			Comfrey	Symphytum sp.
			French lavender	Lavandula stoechas L.
		X	Suelda con suelda, comfrey	Symphytum officinale L.
			Tamarind	Tamrindus indica L.
			Wild arum, lords and ladies	Arum maculatum L
			Tormentil	Potentilla erecta Uspenski ex. Ledeb.
		X	Turpeth	Operculina turpethum L.
	X		Local turpeth	Operculina turpethum (L.) Silva Manso
	X		Turpeth from the Levant	Operculina turpethum (L.) Silva Manso
			Bistort	Persicaria bistorta (L.) Samp.
	X		Bitter vetch	Vicia ervilia L. Willd.
			Unidentified	
30	19	44		
	X	X	Sorrel	Rumex acetosa L.
	X		Poppy unspecified	Papaver sp.
			White poppy	Papaver somniferum L.
			Mountain poppy	Papaver sp.
		X	Black poppy	Papaver somniferum L.
		X	Chaste tree, Chaste berry, Monk's pepper	Vitex agnus castus L.

	Andrés Zamudio de Alfaro[a] 1590s	Hospital of Santa Ana[b] 1551	Diego de Tineo *botica*[c] 1555	Francisco de Alva *botica*[d] 1576	Bartolomé Díaz Cabeza de Vaca *botica*[e] 1608
Albahaca	X	X			X
Alcaparras					
Alegría [sesame]	X		X		
Alexandria			X		X
Alholva	X				
Alquequenje	X				
Anís	X		X	X	
Apio		X			
Arrayán	X		X		X
Bayas del laurel	X		X		X
Beleño	X				
Berbero	X		X		
Brusco	X		X		X
Calabaza	X			X	X
Canamones			X		X
Cardamomo [mayor]	X	X	X	X	X
Cártamo	X		X		
Cebollino				X	X
Cidra	X				X
Cípres [nuez de]	X		X		
Cohombro	X				
Coles		X			
Cominos rústicos					
Cubeba	X				
Culantro	X				
Cuscuta	X		X	X	X
Dauco	X		X		
Endivia	X				
Eneldo	X	X			
Epítimo					

Pedro de Bilbao *botica*[f] 1636	Hospital of Santa Ana[g] 1606	Fernando de Cartagena Cuzco[h] 1618	Common name	Latin name
		X	Sweet basil	Ocimum basilicum L.
X			Caper	Capparis spinosa L.
			Sesame	Sesamum indicum L.
X		X	Alexandrian senna	Senna alexandrina Mill.
			Fenugreek	Trigonella foenum graecum L.
X			Bladder cherry, winter cherry, Chinese lantern	Physalis alkekengi L.
			Aniseed	Pimpinella anisum L.
		X	Celery	Apium graveolens L.
			Myrtle	Myrtus communis L.
	X	X	Bay laurel	Laurus nobilis L.
	X		Henbane	Hyoscyamus niger L.
	X	X	Barberry	Berberis vulgaris L.
		X	Butcher's broom,	Ruscus asculeatus L.
			Calabash	Cucurbita or Lagenaria sp.
			Hemp seed	Cannabis sativa L.
X	X	X	Cardamom	Elettaria cardomomum (L.) Maton
X		X	Safflower	Carthamus tinctorius L.
			Chives	Allium schoenoprasum L.
		X	Citron	Citrus medica L.
		X	Cypress tree	Cupressus sempervirens L.
			Squirting cucumber	Ecballium elaterium (L.) A. Rich.
			Cabbage	Brassica oleracea L.
		X	Cumin	Cuminium cyminum L.
		X	Cubeb	Cubeba officinalis Miquel
			Cilantro, coriander	Coriandrum sativum L.
X		X	Dodder	Cuscuta L.
X			Carrot	Daucus carota L.
			Endive, chicory	Cichorium endivia L.
			Dill	Enethum graveolens L.
		X	Clover dodder	Cuscuta epithymum Murray

	Andrés Zamudio de Alfaro[a] 1590s	Hospital of Santa Ana[b] 1551	Diego de Tineo *botica*[c] 1555	Francisco de Alva *botica*[d] 1576	Bartolomé Díaz Cabez de Vaca *botica*[e] 1608
Escarola	X				
Escarola [fría menor]	X				
Espárrago	X		X		X
Fresno	X				
Fumaria					
Granada	X				
Harmel			X		
Hinojo	X	X		X	X
Jujuba	X				
Junípero [[e]nebro]	X		X		X
Juzquyamo		X	X		
Lechuga	X				X
Lentium			X		
Linaza [lino]	X		X		X
Llantén			X		X
Malvas	X			X	X
Mastuerzo		X			
Melón	X				
Membrillo [cithoniore]	X		X		X
Milium solis [mijo del sol]	X		X	X	X
Nabos		X			
Nasturci[o]			X		
Neguilla [Nigele]			X		X
Orobo			X		
Ortiga	X	X	X		
Peonía	X	X	X		X
Pepino	X		X		X
Perejil	X	X		X	
Petrosilini macedonice			X		

Pedro de Bilbao *botica*[f] 1636	Hospital of Santa Ana[g] 1606	Fernando de Cartagena Cuzco[h] 1618	Common name	Latin name
			Curly endive	Cichorium endivia L.
			Curly endive	Cichorium endivia L.
X		X	Asparagus	Asparagus acutifolius L.
			Ash tree	Fraxinus spp.
X		X	Fumitory	Fumaria officinalis L.
			Pomegranate	Prunus granatum L.
			Harmel	Peganum harmala L.
		X	Sweet fennel	Foeniculum vulgare Mill.
			Jujube	Ziziphus jujuba Mill.
			Juniper	Juniperus communis L.
			Jusquiame, henbane?	Hyoscyamus niger L.
			Lettuce	Lactuca sativa L.
			Mastic?	Pistacia lentiscus L.
		X	Linseed	Linum usitatissimum L.
			Plantain	Plantago major L.
			Mallow	Malva spp.
		X	Garden cress	Lepidium sativum L.
			Melon	Cucumis melo L.
			Quince	Cydonia maliformis Mill.
		X	Gromwell	Lithospermum officinale L.
			Field mustard	Brassica rapa L.
			Watercress	Nasturtium officinale W.T. Aiton
			Nigella, black cumin, fennel flower	Nigella sativa L.
			Spring vetch	Orobus vernus L.
			Nettle	Urtica spp.
		X	Peony	Paeonia sp.
			Cucumber [cocumeris]	Cucumis sativa L.
X		X	Parsley	Petroselinum hortense Hoff.
			Macedonian parsley seed	Petroselinum crispum (Mill.) Nyman

		Andrés Zamudio de Alfaro[a] 1590s	Hospital of Santa Ana[b] 1551	Diego de Tineo *botica*[c] 1555	Francisco de Alva *botica*[d] 1576	Bartolomé Díaz Cabeza de Vaca *botica*[e] 1608
	Psilio [zargatona]	X	X	X	X	
	Puerros					X
	Rábanos		X			X
	Ruda			X		X
	Sauco					
	Verdolaga	X	X	X		
	Verdolaga fría	X				
	Zanahorias					X
Total	73	46	18	34	12	30
Roots						
	Alcaparras	X		X		X
	Aristoloquia larga	X				X
	Aristoloquia redonda	X				X
	Ásaro	X	X	X	X	X
	Beleños secas		X			
	Biznaga [viznaga]	X				
	Cálamo aromatico	X			X	
	Cautibo [cautivo] de mangle					X
	Cipero	X				
	Cohombrillo amargo secas		X			
	Cortezas de cidras	X				
	Díctamo blanco [real]	X			X	
	Ébolo	X				
	Eléboro blanco	X			X	
	Eléboro negro	X			X	

Pedro de Bilbao *botica*[f] 1636	Hospital of Santa Ana[g] 1606	Fernando de Cartagena Cuzco[h] 1618	Common name	Latin name
		X	Psyllium	Plantago pysllium L.
			Leek	Alium porrum L.
			Radish	Raphanus L.
			Rue	Ruta graveleons L.
		X	Elderberry	Sambucus negra L.
X		X	Purslane	Portulaca oleracea L.
			Purslane	Portulaca oleracea L.
			Carrot	Daucus carota L.
11	6	28		
			Caper bush root	Capparis spinosa L.
		X	Long birthwort, aristolochia root	Aristolochia longa L.
		X	Round birthwort, aristolochia root	Aristolochia rotunda L.
	X	X	Asarabacca, European wild ginger, hazelwort root	Asarum europaeum L.
			Dried root of henbane	Hyoscyamus niger L.
			Viznaga, khella root	Ammi visnaga Lam.
X		X	Calamus, sweet flag root	Acorus calamus L.
			Mangrove tree root	Prioria copaifera Griesb.
		X	Cyperus sedge root	Cyperus spp.
			Dried root of bitter cucumber	Ecballium elaterium (L.) A. Rich.
	X		Rind of citron	Citrus medica L.
		X	Dittany root	Dictamnus albus L.
			Red elderberry root	Sambucus racemosa L.
		X	Whitw hellebore root	Helleborus album L
		X	Black hellebore root	Helleborus niger L

		Andrés Zamudio de Alfaro[a] 1590s	Hospital of Santa Ana[b] 1551	Diego de Tineo *botica*[c] 1555	Francisco de Alva *botica*[d] 1576	Bartolomé Díaz Cabeza de Vaca *botica*[e] 1608
	Elemí [helenio, enula]	X				
	Esparraguera		X			
	Espicanardo				X	
	Esquila	X				
	Filipéndula					
	Galanga	X	X	X		X
	Genciana	X		X	X	
	Hermodactil	X	X	X		
	Lignum crucis	X				
	Lirio	X	X	X		X
	Malvavisco			X		
	Mechoacan	X				
	Palo [santo]	X				
	Pelitre	X		X		X
	Peonía	X				X
	Pes columbinus	X				
	Peucédano [perisidano]					
	Pie de palomylla		X			
	Polipodio	X				
	Racimillos de zumaque		X	X		
	Radix mandragore			X	X	
	Rubia [emtores]		X			X
	Rubia tinctorum			X		
	Saxifragia	X		X		
	Sello de santa maría	X				
	Texa blascas [rasuras de]		X			
	Turbit	X			X	X
	Valeriana	X		X	X	
	Zarza	X				
Total	44	30	11	13	10	11

Pedro de Bilbao *botica*[f] 1636	Hospital of Santa Ana[g] 1606	Fernando de Cartagena Cuzco[h] 1618	Common name	Latin name
		X	Elecampane root	Inula helenium L.
			Asparagus root	Asparagus acutifolius L.
X	X		Spikenard root	Nardostachys grandiflora DC, Nardostachys jatamansi DC
			Squill root	Scilla maritima L.
		X	Dropwort	Spiraea filipendula L.
X	X	X	Galangal root	Alpinia galanga (L.) Willd.
		X	Gentian root	Genciana spp.
	X		Hermodactyl, autumn crocus root	Colchicum autumnale L.
		X	Mistletoe root	Viscum album L.
			Lily root	Lilium candidum L.
			Marshmallow	Althaea officinalis L.
			Mechoacan root	Ipomoea purga (Wender.) Hayne
			Lignum vitae root	Guaiacum officinale L
		X	Pellitory root	Anacyclus officinarum Hayne
			Peony root	Paeonia sp.
			Crane's bill root	Geranium columbinum L
		X	Hog's fennel	Peucedanum officinale L.
			Fumitory root	Fumaria officinalis L.
	X		Polypody root	Polypodium vulgare L.
		X	Sumac root	Rhus spp.
			Mandrake root	Mandragora officinarum L.
X		X	Madder root	Rubia spp.
X		X	Madder root	Rubia tinctorum L.
			Saxifrage root	Saxifraga sp.
			Solomon's seal root	Polygonatum odoratum (Mill). Druce
			Yew shavings?	Taxus baccata L.
			Turpeth root	Operculina turpethum L.
			Valerian root	Valeriana offcinalis L.
			Sarsaparilla root	Smilax spp.
5	6	18		

	Andrés Zamudio de Alfaro[a] 1590s	Hospital of Santa Ana[b] 1551	Diego de Tineo *botica*[c] 1555	Francisco de Alva *botica*[d] 1576	Bartolomé Díaz Cabeza de Vaca *botica*[e] 1608
Herbs					
Agrimonia	X		X		
Ajenjo	X				X
Artemisa	X				
Betónica	X				
Calamento	X		X		
Camedrio	X				
Cardo bendito	X				
Centaurea					
Centaurea menor	X				X
Doradilla	X		X		
Escordia	X				
Espliego	X				
Eufrasia	X				
Hierba artética	X		X		
Hipérico	X				
Hisopo	X		X		X
Hoja de laurel	X	X			
Lengua de ciervo	X				
Mastrantes		X			
Mejorana [amoradux]	X	X	X		
Meliloto			X		
Menta	X				
Orégano de la tierra			X		X
Orminio [ormino]					
Poleo	X	X	X		
Romero		X	X		
Ruda	X	X	X		

Pedro de Bilbao *botica*[f] 1636	Hospital of Santa Ana[g] 1606	Fernando de Cartagena Cuzco[h] 1618	Common name	Latin name
			Agrimony	Agrimonia eupatoria L.
X		X	Absinthe wormwood	Artemisia absinthium L.
			Wormwood	Artemisia vulgare L.
			Hedge nettle, betony	Stachyis officinalis Trev.
		X	Calamint	Calamintha officinalis Moench.
			Wall germander	Teucrium chamaedrys L.
			Blessed thistle	Cnicus benedictus L.
	X		Centaury	Centaurea centaurium L.
			Cornflower	Centaurea cyanus L.
			Rustyback fern	Asplenium ceterach L.
			Water germander	Teucrium scordium L.
			Lavender	Lavandula spica L.
			Eyebright	Euphrasia officinalis L.
			Ground pine	Ajuga chamaepitys (L.) Schreber.
			St John's wort	Hypericum perforatum L.
		X	Hyssop	Hyssopus officinalis L.
			Laurel	Laurus nobilis L.
			Hart's-tongue fern	Asplenium scolopendrium Newn.
			Santa Maria, mastrante,	Lantana scabiosiflora Kunth
			Marjoram	Origanum majorana L.
	X		Sweetclover	Melilotus officinalis Medikus.
			Peppermint	Mentha piperita L.
			Oregano	Origanum vulgare L.
X			Clary sage	Salvia sclarea L.
			Pennyroyal	Mentha pulegium L.
			Rosemary	Rosemarinus officinalis L.
			Rue	Ruta graveleons L.

		Andrés Zamudio de Alfaro[a] 1590s	Hospital of Santa Ana[b] 1551	Diego de Tineo *botica*[c] 1555	Francisco de Alva *botica*[d] 1576	Bartolomé Díaz Cabeza de Vaca *botica*[e] 1608
	Sabina	X		X		X
	Salvia	X		X		
	Taray [tamariz]	X		X		
	Tomillo			X		
Total	31	24	6	15	0	5
Flowers						
	Adormidera blanca [papaveris blanci]	X	X	X		X
	Balaustrias	X	X	X		X
	Borrajas	X	X			
	Cantueso [esticados]	X	X	X		
	Epítimo	X	X	X		X
	Lengua de buey	X	X	X		
	Manzanilla	X	X	X	X	
	Nenúfar	X	X			
	Prasio			X		
	Rosas comunes [seca]	X	X		X	
	Rosas cordiales	X				
	Rosas de Toledo			X		
	Violetas	X	X	X	X	X
Total	13	11	10	9	3	4
Gums and resins						
	Alcanfor				X	X
	Almaciga	X	X	X		X
	Alquitira [blanca]	X		X		X
	Ámbar gris		X			
	Amoniaco	X	X	X	X	X
	Asafetida	X	X	X	X	
	Bálsamo		X			
	Bálsamo de romero					

Pedro de Bilbao *botica*[f] 1636	Hospital of Santa Ana[g] 1606	Fernando de Cartagena Cuzco[h] 1618	Common name	Latin name
X		X	Savin juniper, savin	Juniperus sabina L.
			Sage	Salvia officinalis L.
			French tamarisk	Tamarix gallica L.
	X	X	Thyme	Thymus sp.
3	3	5		
			White poppy	Papaver somniferum L.
		X	Flowers of pomegranate	Prunus granatum L.
			Borage	Borago officinalis L.
		X	French lavender	Lavandula stoechas L.
X	X	X	Clover dodder	Cuscuta epithymum Murray
			Bugloss	Anchusa azurea Mill.
			Chamomile	Matricaria chamomilla L.
			Water lily	Nymphaea spp.
		X	Horehound	Marrubium vulgare L.
	X	X	Common rose	Rosa spp.
			Rose for cordial	Rosa spp.
			Roses from Toledo	Rosa spp,
	X	X	Violets	Viola spp.
1	3	6		
X		X	Camphor	Cinnamonum camphora L.
			Mastic	Pistacia lentiscus L.
		X	Gum [white] tragacanth	Astragalus gummifer Labill.
			Ambergris	
X	X	X	Gum ammoniac	Dorema ammoniacum D. Don
	X	X	Asafoetida	Ferula assa-foetida L.
X			Balsam [unspecified]	
X			Rosemary balsam	Rosmarinus officinalis L.

	Andrés Zamudio de Alfaro[a] 1590s	Hospital of Santa Ana[b] 1551	Diego de Tineo *botica*[c] 1555	Francisco de Alva *botica*[d] 1576	Bartolomé Díaz Cabeza de Vaca *botica*[e] 1608
Bodelio [bedelio]		X	X		
Canfora refinada		X	X		
Caraña	X				
Carave [carabe]		X	X		X
Carpo balsamo			X		
Cerrato sandalino					
Copal de méxico					X
Córtamo [cártamo]		X		X	
Estoraque	X	X		X	
Estoraque calamita			X		
Estoraque rubio			X		
Euphorbio	X	X	X	X	X
Gálbano	X	X	X	X	
Gálbano de levante					
Goma aráviga		X	X	X	
Goma de hiedra [yedra]	X	X	X	X	X
Goma de hinojo			X		
Goma elemí			X		
Goma molle				X	
Gomalaca [laca]		X	X		X
Incenso	X	X	X		X
Junípero	X				
Láudano [and purificado]	X	X	X		X
Liquidámbar					X
Menjuy		X	X		
Miera				X	
Mirra	X	X	X	X	X
Opio [fino]	X	X		X	X

Pedro de Bilbao *botica*[f] 1636	Hospital of Santa Ana[g] 1606	Fernando de Cartagena Cuzco[h] 1618	Common name	Latin name
		X	Bdellium	Commiphora sp.
			Refined camphor	Cinnamonum camphora L.
			Gumbo limbo	Bursera simaruba (L.) Sarg.
	X	X	Amber – fossilised resin	
			Torchwood	Amyris balsamifera L.
		X	Sandalwood	Santalum spp.
		X	Copal	Bursera spp.
			Safflower	Carthamus tinctorius L.
X			Storax, Liquidambar	Styrax officnalis L
		X	Calamite storax	Styrax sp.
			Red storax	Styrax sp.
X	X	X	Spurge resin	Euphorbia esula L.
		X	Galbanum	Ferula gummosa Bioss. (F. galbaniflua Bioss & Buhse.)
		X	Galbanum from the Levant	Ferula gummosa Bioss. (F. galbaniflua Bioss & Buhse.)
		X	Gum arabic	Acacia spp.
X	X	X	Gum ivy	Hedera helix L.
			Fennel resin	Foeniculum vulgare Mill.
		X	Gum resin [unspecified]	
			Peruvian peppertree	Schinus molle L.
X	X	X	Goma laca, shellac	Laccifer lacca (Lac beetle)
		X	Frankincense	Boswellia spp.
X			Juniper gum	Ziziphus jujuba Mill.
X		X	Laudanum, tincture of opium	Papaver somniferum L.
			Liquidambar	Liquidambar styraciflua L.
			Benzoin, benjui	Lindera benzoin (L.) Blume
			Juniper oil	Juniperus oxycedrus L.
X	X	X	Myrrh	Commiphora myrrha (Nees) Engl.
X		X	Opium	Papaver somniferum L.

		Andrés Zamudio de Alfaro[a] 1590s	Hospital of Santa Ana[b] 1551	Diego de Tineo *botica*[c] 1555	Francisco de Alva *botica*[d] 1576	Bartolomé Díaz Cabeza de Vaca *botica*[e] 1608
	Opoponaco	X	X	X	X	X
	Resina blanca				X	
	Sangre de drago	X	X	X	X	
	Sangre de drago de gota			X		
	Sarcocola [sarcacola]	X	X	X	X	X
	Serapino	X	X	X	X	
	Tacamaca [tacamahaca]	X				X
	Trementina		X		X	
	Unción					X
	X [j]ilo bálsamo			X		
Total	46	19	25	27	19	18
Animal parts						
	Almizcle	X	X	X		
	Antales		X			
	Blata visansis			X		X
	Canas de vaca	X				X
	Cantárida	X				
	Castóreo	X		X	X	X
	Cebo de mano				X	
	Cuerno de ciervo	X		X		X
	Dentales		X			X
	Enjundia de caballo				X	X
	Enjundia de gallina	X				
	Estiércol de lagarto [hienda]	X				
	Estinco	X				
	Grana chermes [kermes]			X		

Pedro de Bilbao *botica*[f] 1636	Hospital of Santa Ana[g] 1606	Fernando de Cartagena Cuzco[h] 1618	Common name	Latin name
		X	Sweet myrrh, opoponax	Commiphora erythraea (Ehrenb.) Engl.
			White resin	Unspecified
X		X	Dragon's blood	Dracaena spp.
			Drops of dragon's blood	Dracaena spp.
		X	Sarcocolla	Astragalus fasciculifolius Boiss
		X	Gum of giant fennel	Ferula communis L.
		X	Balsam poplar, tacamahaca	Populus balsamifera L.
		X	Turpentine	Pistacia terebinthus L.
		X	Unction [unspecified]	
			Balsam of Gilead	Amyris opobalsamum Forsk.
13	7	27		
			Musk	
			Antlers?	
			Eye powder	Listed as an animal product
			Marrow of beef	
X			Spanish fly, blister bee	
	X	X	Castoreum	
			Animal fat or grease	
			Deer horn	
			Teeth unspecified	
			Horse fat	
			Chicken fat	
X		X	Lizard dung	
			Skink	
			Kermes insect	Coccus ilicis L.

		Andrés Zamudio de Alfaro[a] 1590s	Hospital of Santa Ana[b] 1551	Diego de Tineo *botica*[c] 1555	Francisco de Alva *botica*[d] 1576	Bartolomé Díaz Cabeza de Vaca *botica*[e] 1608
	Grasa		X		X	
	Huesos de corazón de ciervo		X	X		
	Piedra bezar	X				
	Rasuras de marfil [eboris]	X		X	X	
	Sebo de cabrón	X				
Total	19	11	5	7	5	6
Non-organic simples						
Metals and minerals						
	Acero quemado				X	
	Albayalde	X	X	X	X	X
	Alhadida		X			
	Almártaga				X	
	Alquitrán					X
	Alumbre		X	X	X	
	Alumbre de pluma			X	X	
	Antimonio			X		
	Arsénico		X			
	Atutía preparada	X	X		X	X
	Atutía [alejandrina]					
	Azarcón				X	
	Azogue					X
	Azufre			X		X
	Azufre amarillo y verde		X			
	Bol arménico		X	X		
	Bol arménico oriental preparado					X
	Caparrosa de castilla			X		X
	Cardenillo		X	X		

Pedro de Bilbao *botica*[f] 1636	Hospital of Santa Ana[g] 1606	Fernando de Cartagena Cuzco[h] 1618	Common name	Latin name
X	X	X	Grease	
			Deer bones	
			Bezoar stone	
X		X	Ivory shavings	
			Goat's grease	
4	2	4		
			Steel	
		X	White lead, lead carbonate	
			Burnt copper	
		X	Litharge, lead oxide	
		X	Tar, pitch	
		X	Alum, potassium aluminium sulphate	
			Alum in the form of filaments	
X			Antimony	
			Arsenic	
		X	Tutty, zinc oxide, chimney soot from smelting of a mineral	
		X	Tutty, zinc oxide, chimney soot from smelting of a mineral	
		X	Lead oxide	
		X	Mercury	
			Sulphur	
			Yellow and green sulphur	
		X	Armenian bole, aluminium silicate (colored with ferrous oxide to give red earth)	
X		X	Armenian bole from the Levant	
			Copper sulphate, vitriol from Castile	
			Verdigris, acetate of copper	

		Andrés Zamudio de Alfaro[a] 1590s	Hospital of Santa Ana[b] 1551	Diego de Tineo *botica*[c] 1555	Francisco de Alva *botica*[d] 1576	Bartolomé Díaz Cabeza de Vaca *botica*[e] 1608
	Escoria ferri	X			X	
	Espodio	X		X	X	X
	Espodio preparado					
	Estibio de matriolo	X				
	Estibio preparado	X				X
	Lapis hematicus preparado					X
	Lapis judaicus			X		X
	Limadura de cascitis	X				
	Litargirio	X		X		
	Litium			X		
	Minio			X		X
	Mumia			X	X	X
	Oropimente	X	X		X	X
	Panes de oro			X		
	Pez de ávila					
	Piedra lipes					X
	Plomo quemado	X				X
	Rejalgar			X		X
	Sal gema [sar jema]		X	X		
	Solimán crudo		X	X		
	Solimán labrado		X			
	Vermellon			X		X
Total	41	10	12	19	11	18
Stones						
	Albín		X			
	Coral blanco	X		X		X
	Coral blanco preparado					X
	Coral preparado				X	
	Coral rubio [colorado]					X

Pedro de Bilbao *botica*[f] 1636	Hospital of Santa Ana[g] 1606	Fernando de Cartagena Cuzco[h] 1618	Common name	Latin name
			Iron slag	
	X	X	Mineral ash	
		X	Porcessed mineral ash	
X			Antimony	
		X	Processed antimony	
			Bloodstone	
			Jews' stone	
			Filings of copper sulphate or oxide	
			Litharge, almartaga, lead oxide	
			Lithium	
		X	Minium, red lead oxide	
		X	Mummy	
		X	Oropiment, sulphide of arsenic	
			Gold leaf	
		X	Pitch from Avila	
		X	Copper sulphate	
			Burnt lead	
			ReJalgar, arsenic sulphide	
			Halite	
			Crude mercury chloride	
			Processed mercury chloride	
X			Cinnabar	
4	1	18		
			Bloodstone	
		X	White coral	
X			Ground white coral	
			Ground coral	
		X	Coloured coral	

		Andrés Zamudio de Alfaro[a] 1590s	Hospital of Santa Ana[b] 1551	Diego de Tineo *botica*[c] 1555	Francisco de Alva *botica*[d] 1576	Bartolomé Díaz Cabeza de Vaca *botica*[e] 1608
	Coral rubio preparado			X		X
	Cristal	X		X	X	X
	Cristal preparado				X	
	Esmeralda	X	X			X
	Esmeraldas preparados					X
	Granato	X	X	X	X	X
	Hematites	X		X	X	X
	Jacinto [zircón]	X	X	X		
	Jacintos preparados				X	
	Lapis					
	Lapis antalis			X		
	Lapis dentalis			X		
	Lapis lazuli	X	X	X		X
	Lapis lincis			X		X
	Perlas preparados				X	
	Piedra imán	X	X	X	X	
	Rubí	X				
	Sanguinaria			X		
	Topacio	X				
	Zafiro	X				
Total	25	11	6	12	8	11
Chemicals						
	Alcohol					X
	Atincar fino		X	X		
	Sal armoniaco		X			
	Sali[s]tre		X			
	Vitriol		X			X
Total	5	0	4	1	0	2

Pedro de Bilbao *botica*[f] 1636	Hospital of Santa Ana[g] 1606	Fernando de Cartagena Cuzco[h] 1618	Common name	Latin name
X			Ground light coloured coral	
			Crystal	
			Ground crystal	
X			Emerald	
			Ground emeralds	
			Garnet	
		X	Haematite, bloodstone	
			Zircon	
			Ground zircon	
X			Stone [unspecified]	
			Unidentified	
			Tooth tartar	
X		X	Lapis lazuli	
			Lynx stone	
			Ground pearls	
			Magnetite	
			Ruby	
			Bloodstone	
			Topaz	
			Sapphire	
5	0	4		
		X	Alcohol	
		X	Refined tincal, or borax of commerce	
			Salt of ammonium chloride	
			Saltpetre	
		X	Vitriol, sulphuric acid	
0	0	3		

	Andrés Zamudio de Alfaro[a] 1590s	Hospital of Santa Ana[b] 1551	Diego de Tineo *botica*[c] 1555	Francisco de Alva *botica*[d] 1576	Bartolomé Díaz Cabeza de Vaca *botica*[e] 1608
Oils, syrups, juices and waters					
Oils					
[A]beto					X
Absintios [asensios, ajenjos]	X		X		
Adormideras	X	X	X	X	
Alacranes	X	X	X		X
Alcaparras	X	X	X	X	X
Alegría [ajonjolí]	X		X	X	X
Almastiga [almaciga]	X	X	X	X	X
Almendras amargas	X	X	X	X	
Almendras dulces	X	X	X	X	
Amargo					
Aparicio	X				
Aragón					X
Arrayán		X	X	X	
Azafrán	X				
Azahar		X	X		
Azucenas	X				
Bálsamo	X		X		
Bayas			X		X
C[h]ipre			X		
Castóreo	X	X			
Costo [sic]		X	X		
Dialtea					
Dulce					X
Enebro			X		X
Eneldo	X	X	X	X	X
Estoraque		X	X		
Euphorbio	X	X	X		
Higuerilla					X

Pedro de Bilbao *botica*[f] 1636	Hospital of Santa Ana[g] 1606	Fernando de Cartagena Cuzco[h] 1618	Common name	Latin name
			Spruce?	Picea abies (L.) H. Karst.
		X	Absinthe, wormwood	Artemisa absinthium L.
X			Poppy	Papaver somniferum L.
		X	Scorpion	
X		X	Caper	Capparis spinosa L.
		X	Sesame	Sesamum indicum L.
	X	X	Mastic	Pistacia lentiscus L.
	X	X	Biiter almonds	Amygdalus amara Hayne
	X	X	Sweet almonds	Amygdalus dulcis Mill.
X			Bitter oil [unspecified]	
		X	Aparicio oil [of olives]. Oil prepared by Aparicio de Zubia in fifteenth century	
			Recipe prepared with variety of ingredients	
		X	Myrtle	Myrtus communis L.
			Safrron	Crocus sativus
			Orange blossom	Citrus sinensis L.
			Lily	Lilium candidium L.
			Oil of balsam [unspecified]	
		X	Bay laurel	Laurus nobilis L.
			Cypress tree	Cupressus sempervirens L.
			Castoreum	
			Costus	Costus arabicus L.
		X	Dialthea, marshmallow	Althaea officinalis L.
X			Sweet oil	
			Juniper	Juniperus communis L.
X	X	X	Dill	Enethum graveolens L.
			Storax, Liquidambar	Styrax officnalis L
X			Spurge	Euphorbia esula L.
			Castor oil	Ricinis communis L.

	Andrés Zamudio de Alfaro[a] 1590s	Hospital of Santa Ana[b] 1551	Diego de Tineo *botica*[c] 1555	Francisco de Alva *botica*[d] 1576	Bartolomé Díaz Cabeza de Vaca *botica*[e] 1608
Hipérico	X				
Jazmín			X		
Ladrillo			X		
Laurel	X			X	
Linaza [lino]	X	X			X
Liquidámbar				X	
Lirio	X	X	X		
Lombrices	X		X	X	
Manzanilla	X	X	X	X	
Marciatón					X
María					
Mata		X		X	X
Matiolo	X				
Membrillos	X	X	X	X	
Menjuy		X	X		
Menta	X		X		
Mirto	X				
Mostaza [mosta?]		X	X	X	X
Nardino [despique]	X	X	X	X	
Nenúfar			X		
Nueces			X		
Onphancino			X		
Pepitas de calabaza	X		X	X	
Pirión				X	
Rábano			X	X	
Romero			X		
Rosado	X	X	X	X	X
Rosado onfancino	X			X	X
Ruda	X	X	X		X
Sauco	X		X		
Solato	X				

Pedro de Bilbao *botica*[f] 1636	Hospital of Santa Ana[g] 1606	Fernando de Cartagena Cuzco[h] 1618	Common name	Latin name
			St John's wort	Hypericum perforatum L.
			Jasmine	Jasminum sp.
			Brick pieces	
			Laurel	Laurus nobilis L.
	X	X	Flax/Linseed	Linum usitatissimum L.
		X	Liquidambar	Liquidambar styraciflua L.
	X	X	Lily	Lilium candidum L.
	X	X	Worms [unpecified]	
	X	X	Camomile	Matricaria chamomilla L.
		X	Oil invented by Marcianus	Complex
		X	Oil of Santa Maria	Calophyllum mariae Planch et Triana
		X	Bush [unspecified]	
X			Scorpion oil recipe of Andrea Matiolli	
	X	X	Quince	Cydonia maliformis Mill.
			Benzoin, benjui	Lindera benzoin (L.) Blume
			Peppermint	Mentha piperita L.
			Myrtle	Myrtus communis L.
			White mustard	Sinapis alba L.
	X		Spikenard	Spikenard
			Water lily	Nymphaea spp.
			Nuts unspecified	
			Unripe olive	
			Calabash seeds	Cucurbita sp. or Lagenaria sp.
			Piriona insect?	Piriona fasciculata Aldrich 1928
			Radish	Raphanus L.
			Rosemary	Rosemarinus officinalis L.
	X	X	Rose	Rosa spp.
			Rose in oil of unripe olive	
		X	Rue	Ruta graveleons L.
			Elderberry	Sambucus negra L.
			Unidentified	

		Andrés Zamudio de Alfaro[a] 1590s	Hospital of Santa Ana[b] 1551	Diego de Tineo *botica*[c] 1555	Francisco de Alva *botica*[d] 1576	Bartolomé Díaz Cabeza de Vaca *botica*[e] 1608
	Sopilativo [opilativo?]			X		
	Trementina		X	X		
	Unguento agripa		X	X		
	Víboras	X				
	Violado	X	X	X		
	Vulpino [raposo]	X	X	X		
	Yerba buena					X
	Ynsensias [incensio]				X	
	Yrino [irino]		X			
	Zorra		X			
Total	69	35	29	42	22	19
Syrups (*jarabe, lamedor*)						
	[Al]miba[r] aromática					X
	Absintios [ajenjo, asensios]	X		X		X
	Acederas	X				X
	Acetoso	X			X	X
	Acetoso y diarrodón				X	X
	Achichoria con ruibarbo	X				X
	Ácido de cidras	X				
	Adormideras	X				X
	Agraz	X			X	X
	Agrega					
	Almíbar de membrillos	X		X	X	
	Apestado					
	Arrayán			X	X	X
	Arrope		X			
	Arrope de moras		X		X	X

Pedro de Bilbao *botica*[f] 1636	Hospital of Santa Ana[g] 1606	Fernando de Cartagena Cuzco[h] 1618	Common name	Latin name
X			Unspecified	To remove obstruction
			Turpentine	Pistacia terebinthus L.
			Agrippa ointment	Based on bryonia (Bryonia sp.) and invented by the King of Agrippa
			Snake oil	
	X		Violet	Viola spp.
			Fox oil	
		X	Mint	Mentha spp.
			Frankincense	Hyssopus officinalis L.
			Iris	Iris germanica L.
		X	Fox oil	
8	12	25		
			Aromatic syrup, possibly of quince	
X			Absinthe, wormwood	Artemisa absinthium L.
			Sorrel	Rumex acetosa L.
			Vinegar and sugar	
			Vinegar, sugar and roses	
			Chicory and rhubarb	Cichorium endivia L. and Reum rharbarbarum L.
	X		Citron	Citrus medica L.
	X	X	Poppy	Papaver somniferum L.
		X	Verjuice [unripe grapes]	Vitis vinifera L.
	X		Unidentified	
	X		Quince syrup	Cydonia maliformis Mill.
	X		Unidentified	
X		X	Myrtle	Myrtus communis L.
			Syrup [unspecified]	
		X	Blackberry syrup	Rubus sp or Morus sp.

	Andrés Zamudio de Alfaro[a] 1590s	Hospital of Santa Ana[b] 1551	Diego de Tineo *botica*[c] 1555	Francisco de Alva *botica*[d] 1576	Bartolomé Díaz Cabeza de Vaca *botica*[e] 1608
Arrope de nueces	X	X			
Artemisa	X				
Bisancis	X		X		
Borrajas	X			X	X
Calabaca[s]					X
Camuesas				X	X
Cantueso [Estecados]	X				X
Cinco raíces [con vinagre]	X				X
Cortezas de cidras	X				X
Culantrillo	X			X	
Culantrillo de conserva	X				
Diamorón	X		X		
Dos raíces				X	X
Endivia [Chicoria]	X		X	X	
Epítimo	X		X		
Escoria ferri	X				
Eupatorio	X		X		
Fumaria compuesto	X				
Fumaria simple (Funisterra)	X	X	X		X
Granadas	X				
Guayacán					X
Hisopo	X		X		
Incensios				X	
Infusión de rosas	X		X		
Infusión violar	X				

Pedro de Bilbao *botica*[f] 1636	Hospital of Santa Ana[g] 1606	Fernando de Cartagena Cuzco[h] 1618	Common name	Latin name
			Nut syrup [unspecified]	
			Wormwood	Artemisa vulgare L.
			Endive, borage, celery and hops	Hops are Humerus lupulus L.
	X	X	Borage	Borago officinalis L.
			Calabash	Cucurbita or Lagenaria sp.
			Apples	Pyrus malus L.
	X		French lavender	Lavandula stoechas L.
			Five roots [parsley, celery, asparagus and butcher's broom	
	X	X	Rind of Citron	Citrus medica L.
	X	X	Maidenhair fern	Adiantrum capillus-veneris L.
			Maidenhair fern conserve	Adiantrum capillus-veneris L.
			Blackberry syrup	Rubus sp or Morus sp.
			Two roots [unspecified]	
	X	X	Endive, chicory	Cichorium endivia L.
			Clover dodder	Cuscuta epithymum Murray
			Iron slag	
X			Agrimony	Eupatorium sp.
			Complex fumitory syrup	Fumaria officinalis L.
		X	Simple fumitory syrup with fumaria, canafistula and tamarind	Fumaria officinalis L.
			Pomegranate	Prunus granatum L.
			Lignum vitae	Guaiacum officinale L
			Hyssop	Hyssopus officinalis L.
			Frankincense	Boswellia spp.
			Rose	Rosa spp.
			Violet	Viola spp.

	Andrés Zamudio de Alfaro[a] 1590s	Hospital of Santa Ana[b] 1551	Diego de Tineo *botica*[c] 1555	Francisco de Alva *botica*[d] 1576	Bartolomé Díaz Cabeza de Vaca *botica*[e] 1608
Jujubas [Azofeifas]	X		X		X
Laca	X				
Limones	X				X
Liquiricia [orosus]	X				X
Llantén			X		X
Membrillos	X			X	X
Menta [compuesto]	X		X		X
Miel de abejas					X
Miel de sentaura [centaurea?]					
Miel rosada	X		X	X	
Miel rosada colada			X		
Miel rosado pérsica	X				
Mirto y tusilago	X				
Nueve infusiones				X	
Oxicara			X		
Oximel	X				X
Oximel esquélitico	X				X
Oxizacara			X		
Polipodio					
Prasio			X		
Raíces				X	
Raíces con vinagre	X				
Raíces sin vinagre	X				
Rosado	X		X	X	X
Rosas secas	X			X	X
Sabor regis [rey sabor]					X
Sen					

Pedro de Bilbao *botica*[f] 1636	Hospital of Santa Ana[g] 1606	Fernando de Cartagena Cuzco[h] 1618	Common name	Latin name
			Jujube, Chinese or Red Date	Ziziphus zizyphus
			Goma laca, shellac	Laccifer lacca (Lac beetle)
	X		Lemon	Citrus limon (L.) Burm. f.
			Liquorice	Glycyrrhiza glabra L.
	X		Plantain	Plantago major L.
	X	X	Quince	Cydonia maliformis Mill.
			Peppermint	Mentha piperita L.
		X	Bee honey	
X			Centuary	Centaurea centaurium L.
	X	X	Rose honey	
			Strained rose honey	
			Rosa persica honey	Rosa persica J.F. Gmel.
			Myrtle and coltsfoot	Myrthus communis L. And Tussilago farfara L.
			Nine infusions [based on rose]	Rosa spp.
			Type of insect, unidentified	
		X	Honey in white wine vinegar	
	X		Honey in vinegar of squill	Scilla maritima L.
			Citric acid (agrio) with milk, honey and sugar	
	X		Polypody	Polypodium vulgare L.
			Horehound	Marrubium vulgare L.
	X	X	Roots [unspecified]	
			Roots with vinegar	
			Roots without vinegar	
	X	X	Rose	Rosa spp.
		X	Dried roses	Rosa spp.
			King Sabor syrup	Syrup of apples, borage, bugloss, aniseed, saffron
	X		Senna – leaves	Cassia senna L., Cassia acutifolia Delile

		Andrés Zamudio de Alfaro[a] 1590s	Hospital of Santa Ana[b] 1551	Diego de Tineo *botica*[c] 1555	Francisco de Alva *botica*[d] 1576	Bartolomé Díaz Cabeza de Vaca *botica*[e] 1608
	Tamarindos				X	
	Verdolagas	X				
	Vino					X
	Violado	X		X		X
	Violado de conserva	X				
	Vizenzis				X	
	Yerba buena				X	
	Zarzaparilla				X	
	Zumo de limón	X				
Total	76	47	4	21	22	33
Juices and infusions (*zumo, infusion*)						
	Acat[c]ia			X		
	Acederas					X
	Agraz	X			X	X
	Ajenjos [abcensios, absintios]	X		X	X	X
	Almirones				X	
	Borrajas	X			X	X
	Culantrillo				X	
	Endivia	X				X
	Eupatorio	X		X	X	X
	Fumaria [Funisterra]	X		X		
	Granadas	X	X	X		
	Hipoquistidos	X		X		
	Limones	X				
	Liquiricia	X				
	Lúpulos	X				
	Manzanas					X
	Membrillos	X	X	X	X	X
	Miel de centaurea	X				X
	Miel rosada colada				X	
	Opio	X		X		

Pedro de Bilbao *botica*[f] 1636	Hospital of Santa Ana[g] 1606	Fernando de Cartagena Cuzco[h] 1618	Common name	Latin name
			Tamarind	Tamrindus indica L.
			Purslane	Portulaca oleracea L.
			Wine	
	X	X	Violet	Viola spp.
			Violet conserve	Viola spp.
			Unidentified [bisantis?]	
			Mint	Mentha spp.
	X	X	Sarsaparilla	Smilax spp.
			Lemon	Citrus limon (L.) Burm. f.
4	21	18		
			Acacia	Acacia sp.
			Sorrel	Rumex acetosa L.
			Verjuice [unripe grapes]	Vitis vinifera L.
		X	Absinthe wormwood	Artemisia absinthium L.
			Chicory, endive	Cichorium intybus L.
			Borage	Borago officinalis L.
			Maiden hair fern	Adiantrum capillus-veneris L.
			Endive, chicory	Cichorium endivia L.
		X	Agrimony	Eupatorium sp.
			Fumitory	Fumaria officinalis L.
			Pomegranate	Prunus granatum L.
		X	Daisy	Bellis sp.
			Lemon	Citrus limon (L.) Burm.f.
			Liquorice	Glycyrrhiza glabra L
			Hops	Humerus lupulus L.
			Apple	Pyrus malus L.
		X	Quince	Cydonia maliformis Mill.
			Honey of centaury	Centaurea centaurium L.
			Strained rose honey	
			Opium	Papaver somniferum L.

		Andrés Zamudio de Alfaro[a] 1590s	Hospital of Santa Ana[b] 1551	Diego de Tineo *botica*[c] 1555	Francisco de Alva *botica*[d] 1576	Bartolomé Díaz Cabeza de Vaca *botica*[e] 1608
	Orosus		X			
	Planpina				X	
	Regaliz			X		
	Rosa seca					X
	Rosas		X	X	X	X
Total	25	14	4	10	10	11
Waters						
	[En]senape		X			
	Agua ardiente de cabeza		X		X	
	Alidonia [alidona]		X			
	Almirones		X			
	Apio		X			
	Arrayán	X				
	Asensios			X		
	Azaderas [acederas]				X	X
	Azahar		X		X	X
	Borrajas		X			
	Cabezas de rosas	X			X	X
	Celidonia	X		X		
	Cerrajes					
	Colirio					X
	Culantrillo				X	
	Endivia		X		X	X
	Eufrasia	X	X	X		
	Fumisterra			X		
	Galia[sic] moscata			X		
	Guindas	X				
	Hinojo	X	X		X	X
	Incensio		X			
	Lanfranco	X				

Pedro de Bilbao *botica*[f] 1636	Hospital of Santa Ana[g] 1606	Fernando de Cartagena Cuzco[h] 1618	Common name	Latin name
		X	Liquorice	Glycyrrhiza glabra L
			Duckweed, chickweed, pimpernel	
			Licorice extract	Glycyrrhiza glabra L.
			Dried rose	Rosa spp.
		X	Rose	Rosa spp,
0	0	6		
			White mustard seed	Sinapis alba L.
			Water for head fever	
			Stone in the intestines of a swalllow	
			Chicory, endive	Cichorium intybus L.
			Celery	Apium graveolens L.
			Myrtle	Myrtus communis L.
			Absinthe, wormwood	Artemisa absinthium L.
			Sorrel	Rumex acetosa L.
	X		Orange blossom	Citrus sinensis L.
	X	X	Borage	Borago officinalis L.
			Rose buds	Rosa spp.
			Celandine	Chelidonium majus L.
	X		Sow thistle	Sonchus oleraceus L.
			Eye wash	
			Maiden hair fern	Adiantrum capillus-veneris L.
			Endive	Cichorium endivia L.
			Eyebright	Euphrasia officinalis L.
			Fumitory	Fumaria officinalis L.
			Muscat wine	
			Sour cherry	Prunus cerasus L.
	X	X	Sweet fennel	Foeniculum vulgare Mill.
			Frankincense	Boswellia spp.
			Eye wash composed of wine, rose water, plantain water, oropiment and cardenillo	

		Andrés Zamudio de Alfaro[a] 1590s	Hospital of Santa Ana[b] 1551	Diego de Tineo *botica*[c] 1555	Francisco de Alva *botica*[d] 1576	Bartolomé Díaz Cabeza de Vaca *botica*[e] 1608
	Lengua de buey		X			
	Llantén	X	X		X	
	Luminosa	X				
	Malvas					X
	Manzanilla			X	X	
	Membrillos			X	X	X
	Panplina		X			
	Rosada	X		X	X	X
	Trébol				X	
	Vinagre esquilítico	X				X
	Vinagre rosado	X		X	X	X
	Yerba buena [hierba buena]		X			
Total	35	12	15	9	13	11
Complex medicines						
Electuaries						
	Atriaca de valencia		X	X		
	Benedicta	X		X	X	
	Confección [h]amech simple y compuesto	X	X	X	X	X
	Confección de genys			X		
	Diacatolicón	X		X	X	X
	Diafinicón	X		X		X
	Diaprunus laxativo	X		X	X	
	Diaprunus simple	X		X		X
	Diasén	X		X		
	Diaseterón			X		
	Hiera logodion	X	X	X		
	Hiera picra simple (gerapliega)	X		X		X
	Indio menor (mayor)	X		X	X	X

Pedro de Bilbao *botica*[f] 1636	Hospital of Santa Ana[g] 1606	Fernando de Cartagena Cuzco[h] 1618	Common name	Latin name
			Bugloss	Anchusa azurea Mill.
	X		Plantain	Plantago major L.
			Syrup of plantain and purslane mixed with alum and beaten egg white.	
			Mallow	Malva spp.
			Chamomile	Matricaria chamomilla L.
			Quince	Cydonia maliformis Mill.
			Chickweed	Stellaria media (L.) Vill.
	X	X	Rose	Rosa spp.
			Trefoil, clover	Trefolium L.
			Vinegar with squill	Scilla maritima L.
			Rose vinegar	
			Mint	Mentha spp.
0	6	3		
			Complex	
		X	Complex	
	X	X	Complex	
			Unidentified	
	X	X	Complex	
	X	X	Date and vinegar	
		X	Plum and white wine	
	X	X	Complex	
			Burnt silk, pearls, coral and lapis lazuli	
			Complex of satiron (ragwort)	Senecio jacobaea L.
			Complex	
	X	X	Complex	
		X	Complex	

		Andrés Zamudio de Alfaro[a] 1590s	Hospital of Santa Ana[b] 1551	Diego de Tineo *botica*[c] 1555	Francisco de Alva *botica*[d] 1576	Bartolomé Díaz Cabeza de Vaca *botica*[e] 1608
	Magistral de tor[r]es				X	
	Psilio			X		
	Rosado mesue	X		X	X	
	Tamaros yndos [tamarindos?]					X
	Triaca de diaseteron			X		
	Zumo de rosas [de nicolao]	X		X		
Total	19	12	3	17	7	7
Opiates and others						
	Antídoto emagogo	X				
	Confección de galanga					X
	Diacurcuma magna	X		X		
	Dialaca magna	X		X		
	Filonio pérsico	X	X		X	
	Filonio romano	X	X		X	X
	Llitontripon	X		X		X
	Micleta	X		X	X	X
	Mitridato	X	X			
	Requies magna	X				
	Triaca de toledo					X
	Triaca magna (con y sin opio)	X	X	X		
	Trifera magna	X				
Total	13	11	4	5	3	5
Cordials and others						
	Confección alquermes	X		X		
	Confección de jacintos	X				X
	Diambra	X				

Pedro de Bilbao *botica*[f] 1636	Hospital of Santa Ana[g] 1606	Fernando de Cartagena Cuzco[h] 1618	Common name	Latin name
	X		Complex	
			Psyllium	Plantago pysllium L.
	X	X	Complex	
		X	Based on tamarind	
			Complex based on satiron (ragwort)	Senecio jacobaea L.
	X		Complex	
0	8	10		
			Emmenagogue of Nicolau	
			Based on galangal	
			Based on saffron	
			Based on laca	
		X	Complex of Mesue	
		X	Complex	
			Complex	
			Based on myrobolans	
			Complex	
			Based on opium and mandrake	
		X	Complex	
X			Complex	
			Complex	
1	0	3		
	X	X	Dried bodies of the insect Kermes ilicis	
	X	X	Complex	
			Based on ambar	

		Andrés Zamudio de Alfaro[a] 1590s	Hospital of Santa Ana[b] 1551	Diego de Tineo *botica*[c] 1555	Francisco de Alva *botica*[d] 1576	Bartolomé Díaz Cabeza de Vaca *botica*[e] 1608
	Diamusco dulce	X				
	Diarrodón abatis	X			X	X
	Aromático rosado	X			X	X
	Polvos cetrinos			X		
	Polvos de bizma	X		X		X
	Polvos de diacimino	X			X	X
	Polvos de diadraganto	X				X
	Polvos de diairis	X				
	Polvos de diamargariton frío	X			X	X
	Polvos de diamusco	X				X
	Polvos de diatrion piperon	X				
	Polvos de gera				X	
	Polvos de vigo [de juanes]	X	X	X		X
	Polvos restrictivos				X	
	Triaca de esmeraldas	X				X
	Triasándalos	X				
Total	19	16	1	4	6	10
Pills						
	Agárico	X				X
	Agregativos	X			X	
	Alefanginas	X		X		
	Artéticas	X				
	Asaharayet [asegered]	X				X
	Aúreas	X				X
	Coquias (Cochias)	X				X
	Fétidas	X				
	Fumaria [fumisterra]	X		X		X

Pedro de Bilbao *botica*[f] 1636	Hospital of Santa Ana[g] 1606	Fernando de Cartagena Cuzco[h] 1618	Common name	Latin name
		X	Based on musk	
		X	Based on rose	
		X	Based on rose	
X			Citrinous powder	
			Complex	
		X	Based on cumin	
		X	Based on gum tragacanth	
			Based on iris or lily	
	X	X	Complex	
		X	Complex	
			Based on pepper	
		X	Complex	
X		X	Red precipitate of mercury	
		X	Restrigent	
	X		Anti-venom of emeralds	
		X	Three types of sandalwood	
2	4	13		
	X	X	Agaric, mushroom	Polyporus sp.
	X	X	Complex	
			Complex	
			Complex	
			Complex	
	X	X	Complex	
	X	X	Colocynth, scammony and hiera picra	
	X		Leek	Alium porrum L.
	X	X	Fumitory	Fumaria officinalis L.

		Andrés Zamudio de Alfaro[a] 1590s	Hospital of Santa Ana[b] 1551	Diego de Tineo *botica*[c] 1555	Francisco de Alva *botica*[d] 1576	Bartolomé Díaz Cabeza de Vaca *botica*[e] 1608
	Hermodactiles	X				X
	Hiera simple	X				
	Indias	X				
	Lapis lazuli	X				
	Lucis	X				
	Mastique	X				X
	Nitro					
	Ruibarbo	X				X
	Sine quibus	X				
	Stomaticas					X
Total	19	17	0	2	1	9
Powders						
	Hiera simple de Galeno					
	Empello de bacas lauri (Baccis lauri]					X
	Alexandria					X
	Almaciga					X
	Almártaga					X
	Arrayán					X
	Coloquíntida					X
	Lirios					X
	Margaritas					
	Minio					X
	Mirra					X
	Oropimento					X
	Rosa					X
	Sándalos citrinos					X
	Sándalos colorados					X

Pedro de Bilbao *botica*[f] 1636	Hospital of Santa Ana[g] 1606	Fernando de Cartagena Cuzco[h] 1618	Common name	Latin name
			Hermodactyl, autumn crocus	Colchicum autumnale L.
			Complex	
			Prepared with salt from India	
		X	Lapis lazuli	
		X	Complex	
			Mastic	Pistacia lentiscus L.
	X		Potassium nitrate	
		X	Rhubarb	Rheum rhabarbarum L.
		X	Aloe	Aloe vera
			Stomach pills	
0	7	9		
	X		Complex Galenic mixture	
			Complex	
			Alexandrian senna	Senna alexandrina Mill.
			Mastic	Pistacia lentiscus L.
			Litharge, lead oxide	
			Myrtle	Myrtus communis L.
	X		Colocynth, bitter apple	Citrullus colocynthis (L.) Schrad.
			Lily	Lilium candidum L.
		X	Pearls	
		X	Minium, red lead oxide	Commiphora myrrha (Nees) Engl.
			Myrrh	
			Oropiment, sulphide of arsenic	
			Rose	Rosa spp.
			Yellow sandalwood	Santalum rubrum L.
			Red sandalwood	Symphytum officinale L.

		Andrés Zamudio de Alfaro[a] 1590s	Hospital of Santa Ana[b] 1551	Diego de Tineo *botica*[c] 1555	Francisco de Alva *botica*[d] 1576	Bartolomé Díaz Cabeza de Vaca *botica*[e] 1608
	Suelda					X
	Unguento citrino			X		
Total	17	0	0	1	0	14
Plasters						
	Apostilcón cirújico					X
	Cartagines					X
	Centaurea	X		X		X
	Ceroto de hisopo	X		X		X
	Ceroto confortativo de vigo	X	X	X		X
	Contrarotura	X	X	X		
	De pele arietine					X
	Diafinicón	X	X	X		
	Dialthea					
	Diapalma	X	X	X	X	
	Diaquilón armóniaco			X		
	Diaquilón mayor y menor	X	X	X	X	X
	Empello ceroneo			X		X
	Empello relato					X
	Estomaticón	X				
	Filhi zacahariae [empello zacharias?]	X				X
	Geminis	X		X		X
	Gracia dei		X	X		X
	Griego			X		
	Guillen serven	X	X	X		
	Gumado	X				

Pedro de Bilbao *botica*[f] 1636	Hospital of Santa Ana[g] 1606	Fernando de Cartagena Cuzco[h] 1618	Common name	Latin name
			Suelda con suelda, comfrey	Santalum citrimum J.B.
			Ointment of citron peel	
0	2	2		
			Surgical ointment	
	X	X	Complex	
		X	Centaury	Centaurea centaurium L.
			Hyssop	Hyssopus officinalis L.
		X	Complex	
		X	Complex	
			Sheep's skin	
		X	Based on dates	
		X	Dialthea, marshmallow	Althaea officinalis L.
	X	X	Based on litharge and palm oil	
			With ammonium chloride	
	X	X	Complex	
			Complex	
			Unidentified	
	X	X	Complex	
		X	Complex	
			Based on albayalde	
		X	Based on turpentine and incense	
	X		Based on verdgris and litharge	
		X	Complex	
	X		Based on resins of bdellio, fennel and gum amoniaco	

		Andrés Zamudio de Alfaro[a] 1590s	Hospital of Santa Ana[b] 1551	Diego de Tineo *botica*[c] 1555	Francisco de Alva *botica*[d] 1576	Bartolomé Díaz Cabeza de Vaca *botica*[e] 1608
	Isi aedigonis (Isis epigoni)	X				
	Madre					
	Meliloto	X	X	X		X
	Mundificativo de nido de golondrina	X				
	Negro					
	Nicolao massa					X
	Oxicrocio	X		X		X
	Pro matrice [Admatorcini]	X		X		
	Raíz					
	Ranas	X				X
	Sándalos colorados					X
	Triafármaco	X				X
Total	33	19	8	16	2	18
Ointments						
	Agripa	X	X	X	X	
	Almártaga					X
	Apostolorum	X	X		X	X
	Aragón	X		X	X	
	Armoniaco				X	
	Atutía			X	X	X
	Aúreo	X			X	
	Azahar					X
	Basilicón	X				X
	Blanco	X			X	X
	Castaña	X				
	Ceroto litargirio	X				

Pedro de Bilbao *botica*[f] 1636	Hospital of Santa Ana[g] 1606	Fernando de Cartagena Cuzco[h] 1618	Common name	Latin name
			Complex	
		X	No fixed ingredients, chosen by particular apothecaries	
		X	Sweetclover	Melilotus officinalis Medikus.
			Based on swallow's nests	
		X	Based on albayalde	
	X	X	Recipe of Nicolao Massa	
	X	X	Complex	
			Complex	
		X	Unspecified	
	X	X	Frogs and other ingredients	
			Red sandalwood	Santalum rubrum L.
	X		Based on litharge	
0	10	19		
	X	X	Complex	
	X	X	Litharge, lead oxide	
	X	X	Complex	
		X	Complex	
		X	Ammonium chloride	
	X		Tutty, zinc oxide, chimney soot from smelting of a mineral	
	X		Slag from gold smelting	
	X	X	Orange blossom	Citrus sinensis L.
			Complex	
	X	X	Based on white lead	
			Chestnut	Castanea sativa L.
			Litharge, almartaga	

	Andrés Zamudio de Alfaro[a] 1590s	Hospital of Santa Ana[b] 1551	Diego de Tineo *botica*[c] 1555	Francisco de Alva *botica*[d] 1576	Bartolomé Díaz Cabeza de Vaca *botica*[e] 1608
Cetrino		X			
Comitisse			X		
Condesa				X	
Confortativo [de vigo?]		X			
Cordial	X				
Deopilativo del bazo	X			X	
Deopilativo del higado	X				X
Dialthea	X	X	X		
Dolor de costado					
Egipciaco	X				
Estoraque			X		
Goma elemí	X				
Hiera logadion					X
Hisopo húmedo	X		X		
León					X
Litargirio	X				
Marciatón	X	X	X	X	
Media confección	X				X
Minio	X				X
Plomo	X				
Pompholigos [de tutía]	X		X		
Populeón	X	X	X	X	X
Pro morbo					
Resuntivo		X			
Rosado	X	X	X	X	X
Rubio de vigo	X				
Sandalino	X		X	X	X

Pedro de Bilbao *botica*[f] 1636	Hospital of Santa Ana[g] 1606	Fernando de Cartagena Cuzco[h] 1618	Common name	Latin name
			Yellow ointment unspecified	
			Complex	
	X	X	Complex	
		X	Red precipitate of mercury	
			Complex	
			Ointment to remove obstructions to spleen	
			Ointment to remove obstructions to liver	
			Dialthea, marshmallow	Althaea officinalis L.
		X	Ointment for pain in the side	
	X	X	Alum, verdigris	
			Storax, Liquidambar	Styrax officnalis L
			Diverse resins	
			Complex	
			Complex	
			Unidentified	Recipe of Doctor Leon?
			Litharge, almartaga	
	X	X	Complex ointment invented by Marcianus	
			Mastic, frankincense	
	X	X	Minium, red lead oxide	
		X	Lead	
			Tutty, lead, frankincense	
X			Complex	
	X		Ointment to treat syphilis	
			Restorative	
	X	X	Rose	Rosa spp.
		X	Red precipitate of mercury	
	X		Sandalwood	Santalum spp.

		Andrés Zamudio de Alfaro[a] 1590s	Hospital of Santa Ana[b] 1551	Diego de Tineo *botica*[c] 1555	Francisco de Alva *botica*[d] 1576	Bartolomé Díaz Cabeza de Vaca *botica*[e] 1608
	Sopilativo [desopilativo]		X	X		
	Terbenta			X		
	Trementina de abeto	X		X		
	Unción					X
	Verde			X	X	
Total	44	26	10	16	14	15
Other						
Conserves						
	Borrajas	X	X	X		
	Cantueso	X	X	X		
	Carne de ciruela	X	X		X	
	Carne de ciruelas silvestres	X				
	Carne de dátiles			X		X
	Culantrillo de pozo	X				
	Hierbabuena	X				
	Higos negros			X		
	Lengua de buey	X		X		
	Mirabolanos			X		
	Nueces de nogal			X		
	Rosada	X		X		
	Rosada de pérsica de miel y azúcar	X		X		
	Servas			X		
	Violada	X	X	X		
Total	15	10	4	11	1	1

Pedro de Bilbao *botica*[f] 1636	Hospital of Santa Ana[g] 1606	Fernando de Cartagena Cuzco[h] 1618	Common name	Latin name
	X	X	Unspecified	To remove obstruction
			Turpentine, terebinth?	Pistacia terebinthus L
			Turpentine from spruce	Picea abies (L.) H. Karst.
			Unction unspecified	
			Green	
1	15	17		
			Borage	Borago officinalis L.
			French lavendar, spike	Lavandula stoechas L.
			Plum	Prunus spp.
			Wild plums	Prunus spp.
X		X	Date palm	Phoenix dactylifera L.
			Fern from the well	Adiantum capillus-veneris L.
			Mint	Mentha spp.
			Black fig	Ficus carica L.
			Bugloss	Anchusa azurea Mill.
			Myrobalan	Terminalia chebula L.
			Walnut	Junglans regia L.
			Rose	Rosa spp.
			Rosa persica	Rosa persica J.F. Gmel.
			Fruits of serbal (rowan)	Scorbus sp.
		X	Violet	Viola spp.
1	0	2		

		Andrés Zamudio de Alfaro[a] 1590s	Hospital of Santa Ana[b] 1551	Diego de Tineo *botica*[c] 1555	Francisco de Alva *botica*[d] 1576	Bartolomé Díaz Cabeza de Vaca *botica*[e] 1608
Medicinal pieces and ingredients (trociscos)						
	Absintios	X				X
	Alcaparras	X				
	Alquequenje	X				
	Bérbero	X	X			
	Blancos de rasis	X				
	Carabe	X				X
	Diarrodon	X	X			X
	Espodio con simientes	X	X			X
	Eupatorio	X				
	Galia alefangina	X				X
	Galia moscata de mesue	X	X			
	Galia moscata de nicolao	X				
	Mirica [mirra]	X	X			
	Ramich	X				
	Rasis con/sin opio					X
	Ruibarbo	X				X
	Terra sigillata	X		X		
Total	17	16	5	1	0	7
Flour						
	Abenate [avenate]			X		
	Almidón		X			
	Almortas	X				

Pedro de Bilbao *botica*[f] 1636	Hospital of Santa Ana[g] 1606	Fernando de Cartagena Cuzco[h] 1618	Common name	Latin name
			Absinthe, wormwood	Artemisa absinthium L.
			Caper	Capparis spinosa L.
	X		Bladder cherry, winter cherry, Chinese lantern	Physalis alkekengi L.
		X	Barberry	Berberis vulgaris L.
			Lead carbonate prepared after Rasis	
			Amber – fossilised resin	
			Rose	Rosa spp.
			Mineral ash with seeds	
			Agrimony	Eupatorium sp.
			Complex based on myrobolanos	
			Complex based on nutmeg after Mesue	
			Complex based on nutmeg after Nicolao	
			Myrrh	Commiphora myrrha (Nees) Engl.
			Sorrel and others	Rumex acetosa L.
	X	X	Resin with/out opium	
			Rhubarb	Rheum rhabarbarum L.
	X		A clay mineral	
0	3	2		
			Oatmeal	
			Flour unspecified	
			White pea	Lathyrus sativus L.

		Andrés Zamudio de Alfaro[a] 1590s	Hospital of Santa Ana[b] 1551	Diego de Tineo *botica*[c] 1555	Francisco de Alva *botica*[d] 1576	Bartolomé Díaz Cabeza de Vaca *botica*[e] 1608
	Bizcocho blanco [del coro]		X			
	Cebada	X				
	Habas	X				
	Lenteja	X				
	Tortas de rosas			X		
	8	4	2	2	0	0
Miscellaneous						
	Aguardiente		X			
	Amento dulce			X		
	Aureo pigmento			X		
	Azúcar cande		X		X	
	Azúcar quebrados				X	
	Azúcar rosado		X			X
	Capullos de seda					X
	Cera amarilla					
	Rasuras blancas [de vino]			X		
	Rasuras tintas			X		
	Seda cruda			X		
	Sumu terra				X	
	Taco almagra					
Total	13	0	3	5	3	2
Total	863	429	251	391	214	325

Sources:

a Recommendations of the Spanish *protomédico* Andrés Zamudio de Alfaro in the 1590s: *Catálogo de las cosas que los boticarios han de tener en sus boticas* in Davis and López Terrada, "Protomedicato y farmacia," 591–612.

b First pharmacy of the hospital of Santa Ana: AGNP Protocolos Siglo XVI 63 Diego Gutiérrez fols. 177v.-178 Quenta de la botica 20 Oct. 1551. See also: Miguel Rabí Chara, "La primera botica de los hospitales de la ciudad de Lima en el siglo XVI," *Asclepio* 52 (2000): 276–77.

Pedro de Bilbao *botica*[f] 1636	Hospital of Santa Ana[g] 1606	Fernando de Cartagena Cuzco[h] 1618	Common name	Latin name
			White biscuit	
			Barley flour	Hordeum vulgare L.
			Bean flour	Vicia faba L.
			Lentils	Lens culinaris Medikus
			Rose cakes	
0	0	0		
			Aguardiente	
			Nut wine	
			Gold pigment	
			Sugar candy	
			Brown sugar	
	X	X	Rose sugar	
X			Silkworm cacoon	
		X	Yellow wax	
		X	White wine residue dye	
			Red wine residue dye	
			Raw silk	
			Unidentified	
		X	Unidentified	
1	1	4		
94	136	290		

c *Botica* imported by Diego de Tineo: JCB Mss codex Sp 136 fols. 861–868 Francisco Martínez y compañía obligación – Diego de Tineo y consortes 1555.

d Inventory of the *botica* of Francisco de Alva: AGNP Real Audiencia. Causas Civiles legajo 16 cuad. 81 fols. 10v-15 Inventario de los bienes del bachiller Alba [sic], después de fallecido. 1576.

e Inventory of the *botica* of Bartolomé Diaz Cabeza de Vaca: AAL Testamentos 5 exp. 1 fols. 44–49v. Memoria de drogas y medicinas … 6 Sep. 1608.

f Inventory of the *botica* of Pedro de Bilbao: AGNP Protocolos Siglo XVII 1789 Sánchez Vadillo fols. 1372v.-1378v. Inventario de bienes de Pedro de Bilbao 25 Aug. 1636.

g Inspection of the pharmacy of the hospital of Santa Ana in 1606. ABPL 9086 fols. 118–123 Visita of the *botica* of the hospital of Santa Ana by Doctor Melchor Romero 9 and 10. Oct. 1606.

h Inventory of the *botica* of Fernando de Cartagena, Cuzco 1618: "Una botica colonial," *Revista del archivo histórico del Cuzco* 4 (1953): 263–82.

The total number of plant species found in pharmacy inventories is slightly smaller than is indicated in the above table. Pharmacies often listed different parts of the same plant separately, for example, as simples, seeds and roots, so that some are counted more than once. Since duplicate species entries accounted for less than ten per cent of the total number of botanical products listed above and since pharmacists distinguished the different forms in which they were stored, they are retained here as separate entries.

While every attempt has been made to identify the *materia medica* and provide English names, it is recognised that this is not always an easy task. This applies also to the Latin names for plants, some of which have changed over time. The names of products in different pharmacies varied slightly. A large number of texts and databases were used, among the most useful were:

The Plant List. http://www.theplantlist.org/ [Accessed 1 Nov. 2015]; USDA United States Department of Agriculture, Plants Database. http://plants.usda.gov/java/ [Accessed 1 Nov. 2015]; International Plant Names Index. http://www.ipni.org/[Accessed 1 Nov. 2015]; Lily Y. Beck (trans.) *Pedanius Dioscorides of Anazarbus: De Materia Medica* (Hildesheim, Zurich, New York: Olms-Weidmann); Hermilio Valdizán and Angel Maldonado, *La medicina popular peruana* (Lima: Torres Aguirre, 1922); Enrique Laval, *Botica de los Jesuitas de Santiago* (Santiago: Asociación Chilena de Asistencia Social, 1953); Paula De Vos, "European Materia Medica in Historical Texts: Longevity of a Tradition and Implications for Future Use," *Journal of Ethnopharmacology*, 132 (2010): 31–39; Charles Davis, and María Luz López Terrada, "Protomedicato y farmacia en Castilla a finales del siglo XVI: edición crítica del *Catálogo de las cosas que los boticarios han de tener en sus boticas*, de Zamudio de Alfaro, protomédico general (1592–1599)," *Asclepio* 62 (2) (2010): 579–626.

For the composition of complex medicines the following were used: Enrique Laval, *Botica de los Jesuitas de Santiago* (Santiago: Asociación Chilena de Asistencia Social, 1953) and Luis de Oviedo, *Methodo de la colección, y reposición de las medicinas simples, de su corrección, y preparación* (Madrid: Luis Sánchez, 1622). Although first published in 1581, the 1622 edition of Oviedo is used since it is more comprehensive. The second edition in 1595 added electuaries, syrups, pills, oils and medicinal ingredients, and the third edition in 1609 included ointments and plasters.

APPENDIX C

Books Shipped from Spain to Doctor Melchor de Amusco in Nombre de Dios, 1584

Title in manuscript	Author	First date and place of publication	Suggested title of book
un gualtero bruelo practico	Gualtherus Bruele	Antwerp, 1579	Praxis medicinae theorica et empirica familiarissima
controversias de valles dos pares	Francisco Valles	Alcalá, 1556	Controversiarum medicarum et philosophicarum libri decem.
los galenos en quatro cuerpos	Galen		Four unspecified volumes of Galen
un avicena	Avicenna		Unspecified
tabula consilios joanes mater y de gracia			Unidentified
donato antonio	Donato Antonio Altomare	Venice, 1562	De medendis febribus ars medica
las obras de vega	Cristóbal de Vega	Lyon, 1564	Opera, nempe, Liber de arte medendi
paulo	Paulus Aegineta	Basel, 1556	Medicinæ totius enchiridion
gordonio	Bernardo de Gordonio	Sevilla, 1495	Lilio de medicina
savanorola y herculano			Unidentified
arnaldo	Arnau de Vilanova		Unspecified
consiliador	Petrus de Abano	Venice, 1565	Conciliator differentiarum quae inter philosophos et medicos versantur
practica de savanarola	Joannes Michael (Savonarola)	Venice, 1497	Practica maior
una biblia			A bible

 | DOI 10.1163/9789004351271_012

Title in manuscript	Author	First date and place of publication	Suggested title of book
laguna	Andrés Laguna		Unspecified
galeno de sanitate tuenda y otros cuerpos chicos todos de galeno	Galen	Paris, 1517	De sanitate tuenda: libri sex
sensuras de mesue	Bartolomaeus Angelo Paglia	Venice, 1543	In Antidotarium Joannis filii Mesue censura cum declaratione simplicium medicinarum
bernaldo de senio	Bernardino de Siena		Sermons, unspecified
tagavejo	Vittore Trincavelli	Basel, 1571	De compositione et usu medicinalium
articela	Franciscus Argilagnes	Venice, 1483	Articella, seu, Opus artis medicinae.
nicolao proposito	Nicole Prévost	Lyon, 1491	Dispensarium magistri Nicolai prepositi ad aromatarios
estilo descrevir cartas	Juan de Icíar	Zaragoza, 1552	Nuevo estilo descreuir cartas mensageras sobre diversas materias
mercado de tavardillo	Luis Mercado	Valladolid, 1574	De essentia causis signis et curatione febris malignae in qua maculae rubentes similes morsibus pulicum per cutem erumpunt.
valerio	Valerio Cordo	Venice, 1546	Dispensatorium, hoc est Pharmacorum conficiendorum ratio
guerra de portugal	Francisco Díaz de Vargas	Zaragoza, 1581	Discurso y summario de la guerra de Portugal y successos della

Title in manuscript	Author	First date and place of publication	Suggested title of book
coloquio sobre la dentadura	Francisco Martínez de Castrillo	Valladolid, 1557	Coloquio breve y compendioso sobre la materia de la dentadura y maravillosa obra de la boca
aviso de sanidad	Francisco Núñez de Oria	Madrid, 1572	Auiso de sanidad que trata de todos los géneros de alimentos y del regimiento de la sanidad co[m]prouado por los más insignes y graues doctore
libro de cozina	Ruberto de Nola	Toledo, 1525	Libro de cozina [sic]
el parto de la virgen	Jacopo Sannazaro	Salamanca, 1569	El parto de la virgen
metafora de medicina	Bernardino de Laredo	Sevilla, 1522	Metaphora medicine
modus facendi	Bernardino de Laredo	Sevilla, 1527	Modus faciendi cum ordine medicandi
batalla de roncesvalles	Francisco Garrido de Villena	Valencia, 1555	El verdadero sucesso de la famosa batalla de Roncesualles
problemas de aristoteles	Aristotle	Unspecified	Problemata Aristotelis ac philosophorum medicorumque complurium
franco de peste	Francisco Franco	Sevilla, 1569	Libro de enfermedades contagiosas y de la preservación dellas
Manuscript torn			
Manuscript torn			
marco aurelio	Antonio de Guevara	Sevilla, 1528	Libro aureo de Marco Aurelio
lucio apuleyo	Lucio Apuleyo	Sevilla, 1520	Libro del Lucio Apuleyo del asno de oro
galateo espanol	Lucas Gracián Dantisco	Madrid, ca 1582	Galateo español
luzman	Jerónimo de Contreras	Barcelona, 1565	Selva de aventuras

Title in manuscript	Author	First date and place of publication	Suggested title of book
viaje y nufragio del macedonico	Juan Bautista de Loyola	Salamanca, 1578	Viaje y naufragio del macedonio de Loyola
filonio de taranta	Valesco de Tarenta	Barcelona, 1484	Practica, quae alias Philonium dicitur
collado de indicatione	Luis Collado	Valencia, 1572	De indicationibus librum unum
joanes de vigo	Giovanni de Vigo	Rome, 1514	Practica in arte chirurgica continens novem libros infra scriptos
virgilio en romance			Virgil in Spanish
pedraza de conciencia	Iuan de Pedraza	Barcelona, 1566	Summa de casos de conciencia
valles de revictus in acutis	Francisco Valles	Alcalá, 1569	Commentaria in libros Hippocratis de Ratione victus in morbis acutis
antonio musa de morbo galico	Antonio Musa Brasavola	Venice, 1553	De morbo gallico
farmacopaea de silvio	Jacobo Sylvio	Lyons, 1548	Pharmacopoeae Iacobi Sylvii
rondoleto	Guillaume Rondelet	Paris, ca 1545	Methodus curandorum omnium morborum corporis humani in tres libros distincta
dino florentino sobre avicena	Dino del Garbo	Ferrara, 1489	Expositio super tertia, quarta, et parte quintae fen IV: Canonis Avicennae.
anatomia de montanana [sic]	Bernardino Montana de Monserrate	Valladolid, 1551	Libro de la anothomía del hombre
lemos sobre el metodo	Luis de Lemos	Salamanca, 1581	Methodus medendi
araucana primera y segunda parte	Alonso de Ercilla y Çuñiga	Madrid, 1569	La Araucana, primera y segunda partes
silvio sobre me [mesue]	Jacobo Sylvio	Paris, 1542	Joannis Mesuae Damaceni ... Jacobo Sylvio

Title in manuscript	Author	First date and place of publication	Suggested title of book
fragoso de botica	Juan Fragoso	Alcalá, 1566	Catalogus simplicium medicamentorum
actuario de urinis	Joannes Actuarius	Venice, 1519	De urinis
antonio musa de simples	Antonio Musa Brasavola	Lyon, 1537	Examen omnium simplicium medicamentorum
valdes de la utilidad de la sangria	Fernando de Valdés	Sevilla, 1582	Tratado de la utilidad de la sangría en las viruelas y otras enfermedades de los muchachos
reportorio de chaves	Jerónimo de Chaves	Sevilla, 1548	Chronographía o repertorio de los tiempos
gaynero	Antonio Guainerio	Pavia, 1481	Opera medica
petro bacitano			Unidentified
joanes bacanelus	Giovanni Battista Baccanelli	Venice, 1553	De consensu medicorum in curandis morbis libri quatuor
epidemias	Hippocrates	Paris, 1546	Libri epidemiorum Hippocratis primus, tertius, et sextus, cum Galeni in eos commentariis
daca de urinis	Alfonso Díez Daza	Sevilla, 1577	Artium et medicinae doctoris
aphorisimos de hipocrates 2 pares	Hippocrates	Unspecified	Aphorismi
cornelio celso	Aulus Cornelius Celso	Florence, 1478	De medicina
inquiridion	Alfonso López Corella	Zaragoza, 1549	Enchiridion medicinae
antonio musa de simples	Antonio Musa Brasavola	Rome, 1536	Examen omnium simplicium medicamentorum
pronosticos			Unspecified almanac
la conquista del penon	Baltasar de Collazos	Valencia, 1566	Commentarios de la fundación y conquistas y toma del Peñon

Title in manuscript	Author	First date and place of publication	Suggested title of book
pronosticos de valles	Francisco Valles	Alcalá, 1567	Commentaria in prognosticum Hippocratis
carta pacio para confesar			Copy book for confession
merino practico	Diego Merino	Burgos, 1574	De morbis internis libri sex

SOURCE: AGI CONTRATACIÓN 1081 N2 R1 FOLS. 67–68 REGISTRO DEL NAVÍO NUESTRA SEÑORA DE CANDELARIA 1584.

Note: The titles are the author's interpretation and are not definitive. The dates and place of publication are those of known first editions and not necessarily the editions contained in the shipment.

Glossary

For the names of all plants and minerals see Appendix B

Alambique	Glass still used for distillation
Alcalde	Magistrate
Almojarifazgo	Ad valorem tax
Alquitara	Metal still used for distillation
Aposento	Room or store
Arancel	Schedule or list, here of prices
Armada	Armed fleet
Avería	Tax levied to support the *armadas*
Bachiller	Holder of bachelor's degree
Barbero	Barber
Barrio	Neighbourhood or suburb
Beata	Nun who lived outside a convent
Beaterio	Residence for *beatas*
Benemérito	Worthy citizen
Botica	Pharmacy
Boticario	Apothecary
Cabildo	Town council
Capellanía	Chaplaincy
Casa de Contratación	Board of Trade
Casta	Person of mixed ethnic background
Cédula	Decree
Censo	Agreement for the payment of an annuity
Cerero	Wax worker or trader
Chácara	Small holding or farm
Cirujano	Surgeon
Cofradía	Brotherhood
Colegio	College, school
Collación	District of a parish
Compañía	Company or co-partnership
Compuesto	Compound medicine
Confitero	Confectioner
Converso	New Christian or Crypto-Jew
Corregidor	Provincial magistrate
Droguero	Druggist
Ducado	Ducat, 375 maravedís

Educanda	Secular student at convent school
Encomienda	An allocation of Indians to an individual who was entitled to exact tribute and labour from them in return for Christian instruction.
Escribano	Notary, scribe
Especiero	Spicer, grocer
Espumadera	Skimmer
Estanco	Monopoly
Estanco de naipes	Monopoly for the sale of playing cards
Familiar	Officer of the Inquisition
Fiel ejecutor	Public inspector, often of weights and measures
Gremio	Guild
Hábito	Dress of a person belonging to a military order
Hechicera/o	Witch, sorcerer
Hermano venticuatro	Original founder of a cofradía
Hidalgo	Noble
Jarabe	Syrup
Lamedor	Thick medicinal syrup
Licenciado	Title given to a person with a bachelor's degree or licenciate.
Licenciatura	Degree, licence
Limpieza de sangre	Purity of blood
Maestro	Master tradesman/artisan
Maravedí	Small Spanish coin
Mayordomo	Steward, administrator
Médico	Physician
Mercader	Merchant
Mita de plaza	Forced labour system
Morisco	Person of Moorish heritage
Obraje	Textile workshop
Oficial	Skilled journeyman
Perulero	Peruvian born trader with Spain
Peso corriente	272 maravedís
Peso de oro	450 maravedís
Peso de plata de a nueve	450 maravedís, used in business accounts
Peso de plata ensayada	307 maravedís, used in business accounts
Protomedicato	Medical board, entrusted with examining and licensing medical practitioners.
Protomédico	Chief medical officer and examiner
Pulpero	Owner of a general store

Rebotica	Back room of a pharmacy used for preparing medicines
Quarterón	A quarter, in this case of indigenous of African ancestry
Receta	Recipe, prescription
Recetario	Book of récipes or prescriptions
Regidor	Councillor, member of the town council
Sarna	Scabies
Seglar	Secular student at convent school
Tienda	Shop
Trastienda	Back room of a shop
Unguento	Ointment
Vale	Promissary note
Vecino	Citizen
Velero	Tallow chandler
Vestido	Suit
Visita	Inspection
Yanacona	Indigenous person who had left his/her community and worked for a Spaniard
Zambo/a (also Zambahigo)	Person of mixed African and Indian descent

Bibliography

Primary Sources

Acosta, José de. *Historia natural y moral de las Indias in Obras del Padre José de Acosta*. Biblioteca de autores españoles 73, 1–247. Madrid: Ediciones Atlas, 1954 [1590].

Agricola, Georgius. *De re metallica*. Translated by Herbert Clark Hoover and Lou Henry Hoover. New York: Dover Publications, Inc., 1950 [1556].

Aguilera, Antonio de. *Exposición sobre las preparaciones de Mesue*. Alcalá: Juan de Villanueva, 1569.

Angulo, Domingo. "Las ordenanzas del hospital de Santa Ana." *Revista del Archivo Nacional del Perú* 11 (1938): 131–56.

Antúnez y Acevedo, Rafael. *Memorias históricas sobre la legislación y gobierno del comercio de los españoles con sus colonias en las Indias occidentales*. Madrid: Imprenta de Sancha, 1797.

Arriaga, Pablo Joseph de. *La extirpación de idolatrías del Perú*. Lima: Geronymo de Contreras, 1621.

Azpilcueta, Martín de. *Compendio y summario de confessores y penitentes*. Alcalá: Casa de Iuan Iñíguez de Lequerica, 1580.

Blair, Emma H. and James A. Robertson. *The Philippine Islands, 1493–1803*. 55 vols. Cleveland, OH: A.H. Clark, 1903–1909.

Calancha, Antonio de la. *Corónica moralizada del orden de San Agustín en el Perú*. Barcelona: Pedro Lacavallería, 1639.

Cardano, Girolamo. *Book of My Life*. Translated by Jean Stoner. New York: New York Review Books, 2002 [1575].

Castillo, Juan de. *Pharmacopoea, universa medicamenta in officinis pharmaceuticis usitata complectens, et explicans*. Cádiz Gadibus: Apud Joannem de Borja, 1622.

Cieza de León, Pedro. *Obras completas*. 2 vols. Madrid: Consejo Superior de Investigaciones Científicas, 1984.

Cobo, Bernabé. *Obras*, 2 vols. Biblioteca de autores españoles 91–92. Madrid: Ediciones Atlas, 1956 [1653].

Colmenero, José. *Reprobación de pernicioso abuso de los polvos de la corteza de quarango o China china*. Salamanca, Eugenio Antonio Garcia, 1697.

Constituciones y ordenanças de la Vniuersidad, y Studio General de la Ciudad de los Reyes del Piru, 1602. https://archive.org/details/constitucionesy001univ [Accessed 28 Oct. 2015].

Constituciones y ordenanzas del hospital real de Santa Ana, Lima, 28 Feb. 1609. https://archive.org/details/constitucionesy000hosp [Accessed 2 Jul. 2016].

Córdoba y Salinas, Diego de. *Crónica franciscana de las provincias del Perú*. Edited by Lino Gómez Canedo. Washington, DC: American Academy of Franciscan History, 1957.

Figueroa, Juan de. *Opusculo de astrología en medicina*. Lima. No publisher. 1660.

Fragoso, Juan. *Discursos de las cosas aromáticas, árboles y frutales, y de otras muchas medicinas simples, que se traen de la India oriental y sirven al uso de medicina*. Madrid: Francisco Sánchez, 1572.

Garzoni, Tomaso. *La piazza universale di tutte le professioni del mondo*, 2 vols. Edited by Paolo Cherchi and Beatrice Collina. Turin: Giulio Einaldi, 1996 [1587].

Hernández, Francisco. *Quatro libros: De la natvraleza, y virtvdes de las plantas, y animales que estan receuidos en el vso de medicina en la Nueua España, y la methodo, y correcion, y preparacion, que para administrallas se requiere con lo que el Doctor Francisco Hernandez escriuio en lengua Latina*. Mexico: Casa de la viuda de Diego Lopez Daualos, 1615.

Hidalgo Agüero, Bartolomé de. *Thesoro de la verdadera cirugía*. Seville: En Casa de Francisco Pérez, 1604.

Index et catalogus librorum prohibitorum. Madrid: Apud Alphonsum Gomezium, 1583.

Laredo, Bernardino de. *Modus faciendi: cum ordine medicandi: a médicos y boticarios muy común y necesario*. Seville: Jacobo Cromberger, 1527.

León, Andrés de. *Tratados de medicina, cirugía, y anatomía*. Valladolid: Luis Sánchez, 1605.

Lewin, Boleslao, ed. *Descripción del Virreinato del Perú; crónica inédita de comienzos del siglo XVII* [Pedro de León Portocarrero]. Rosario: Universidad Nacional del Litoral, Facultad de Filosofía, Letras y Ciencias de la Educación, 1958.

Libros de cabildos de Lima. Edited by Bertram T. Lee, Juan Bromley, Sophy E. Schofield, and Emilio Harth-Terré. 23 vols. Lima: Torres Aguirre, 1935–1963.

Lizárraga, Reginaldo de. *Descripción breve de toda la tierra del Perú, Tucumán, Río de la Plata y Chile*. Biblioteca de autores españoles 216. Madrid: Ediciones Atlas, 1968.

López de León, Pedro. *Prática [sic] y teórica de las apostemas en general y particular: questiones y prácticas de cirugía, de heridas, llagas, y otras cosas nuevas, y particulares*. Seville: Oficina de Luys Estupiñan, 1628.

Méndez Nieto, Juan. *Discursos medicinales*. Edited by Luis S. Granjel. Salamanca: Universidad de Salamanca, 1989.

Mendiburu, Manuel de. *Diccionario histórico-biográfico del Perú*. 2 vols. Lima: Imprenta de J. Francisco Solís, 1876.

Monardes, Nicólas. *Primera y segunda y tercera parte de la historia medicinal de las cosas que se traen de nuestras Indias Occidentales, que sirven en medicina*. Seville: Alonso Escriuano, 1574.

Monardes, Nicolas. *Joyfull Newes Out of the Newfound World*. Edited by John Frampton. London: William Norton, 1580.

Mugaburu, Josephe and Francisco. *Chronicle of Colonial Lima: The Diary of Josephe and Francisco Mugaburu, 1640–1697*. Translated and edited by Robert R. Miller. Norman: University of Oklahoma Press, 1975.

Muñoz, Miguel Eugenio. *Recopilación de las leyes, pragmáticas, reales decretos, y acuerdos del Proto-medicato*. Valencia: Imprenta de la Viuda de Antonio Bordazar, 1751.

Murillo, Jerónimo. *Therapeutica, método de Galeno en lo que toca a cirugía*. Zaragoza, 1561.

Murúa, Martín de. *Historia general del Perú*. 2 vols. Madrid: Instituto Gonzalo Fernández de Oviedo, 1962–1964 [1616].

Novísima recopilación de las leyes de España. Madrid, 1805.

Ocaña, Fray Diego de. Memoria viva de una tierra de olvido: Relación del viaje al Nuevo Mundo de 1599 a 1607. Barcelona: CECAL, 2013.

Ortega, Francisco de. *Directorio de boticarios, en que se ponen ocho advertencias*. Seville: Matías Clavijo, 1625.

Oviedo, Luis de. *Methodo de la colección, y reposición de las medicinas simples, de su corrección, y preparación*. Madrid: Luis Sánchez, 1622 [1581].

Padrón de los Indios de Lima en 1613. Comp. Miguel de Contreras. Edited by Noble David Cook. transcribed by Mauro Escobar Gamboa. Lima: Universidad Nacional de San Marcos, 1968.

Palacios, Felix. *Palestra pharmaceutica chymico-galenica*. Madrid: Juan Garcia Infançon, 1706.

Porres, Matías de. *Breve advertencias para beber frío con nieve*. Lima, 1621.

Recopilación de las leyes de los reynos de las indias. 3 vols. Madrid: Gráficas Ultra, 1943 [1681].

Recopilación de las leyes destos reynos, hecha por mandado de la Magestad Catholica del Rey don Philippe Segundo nuestro Señor. Alcalá de Henares: Casa de Iuan Iñiguez de Lequerica, 1598.

Recopilación de las leyes, pragmáticas reales, decretos, y acuerdos del Real Proto-Medicato: hecha por encargo y dirección del mismo Real Tribunal por Don Miguel Eugenio Muñoz. Valencia: Imprenta de la Viuda de Antonio Bordazar, 1751.

Recopilación de los ordenamientos de Sevilla. Seville: Juan Varela de Salamanca, 1527. http://bvpb.mcu.es/es/consulta/registro.cmd?id=451883 [Accessed 17 Mar. 2016].

Relaciones geográficas de Indias: Peru. Biblioteca de autores españoles 183–185. Edited by Marcos Jiménez de Espada. Madrid: Ediciones Atlas, 1965.

Saladino de Ascoli. *Compendio de los boticarios*. Translated by Alonso Rodríguez Tudela. Valladolid: Arnao Guillén de Brocar, 1515.

Salinas y Córdova, Fray Buenaventura de. *Memorial de las historias del Nuevo Mundo Pirú* [sic]. Vol. 1. Lima: Universidad Nacional Mayor de San Marcos, 1957 [1630].

Suardo, José Antonio. *Diario de Lima (1629–1639)*. Edited by Rubén Vargas Ugarte. 2 vols. Lima: "Lumen", 1936.

Suárez de Figueroa, Christóval. *Plaza universal de todas ciencias y artes*. Madrid: Luis Sánchez, 1615.

Susio, Giovanni Battista. *Libro del conoscere la pestilenza*. Mantova: Giacomo Ruffinello, 1576.

"Una botica colonial." *Revista del archivo histórico del Cuzco* 4 (1953): 263–82.

Valles, Francisco de. *Tratado de las aguas destiladas, pesos y medidas de que los boticarios deuen vsar por nueva ordenança y mandato de su Magestad y su Real Consejo*. Madrid: Luis Sánchez, 1592.

Vargas Machuca, Captain Bernardo de. *Milicia y descripción de las Indias*. Madrid: Librería de Victoriano Suárez, 1892.

Vargas Machuca, Captain Bernardo de. *The Indian Militia and Description of the Indies*. Edited by Kris Lane, translated by Timothy F. Johnson. Durham, NC: Duke University Press, 2008.

Vargas Ugarte, Rubén. *Concilios limenses (1551–1772)*. 3 vols. Lima: Imp. Juan Cardenal Guevara, 1951–1954.

Vázquez de Espinosa, Antonio. *Compendio y descripción de las Indias occidentales*. Biblioteca de autores españoles 231. Madrid: Ediciones Atlas, 1969.

Veitia Linage, Joseph de. *Norte de la contratación de las Indias Occidentales*. Seville: Imprenta de Francisco de Blas, 1672.

Secondary Sources

Aguirre Beltrán, Gonzalo. *Medicina y magia: el proceso de aculturación en la estructura colonial.* México: Universidad Veracruzana, Instituto Nacional Indigenista, 1992 [1963].

Alberro, Solange. *De gachupín al criollo:* o *de cómo los españoles* de *México dejaron de serlo*. México: El Colegio *de* México, 1992.

Alchon, Suzanne A. *Native Society and Disease in Colonial Ecuador*. Cambridge: Cambridge University Press, 1991.

Alperrine-Bouyer, Monica. *La educación de las élites indígenas en el Perú colonial*. Lima: Instituto de Estudios Peruanos, 2007.

Altman, Ida. *Emigrants and Society: Extremadura and Spanish America in the Sixteenth Century*. Berkeley: University of California, 1989.

Anagnostou, Sabine. "Jesuits in Spanish America: Contributions to the Exploration of the American Materia Medica." *Pharmacy in History* 47 (1) (2005): 5–10.

Anderson, Ruth Matilda. *Hispanic Costume 1480–1530*. New York: Hispanic Society of America, 1979.

Aragón Noriega, Ilana. "El pan, el vino, y otros negocios: aspectos laborales de la mujer." In *Lima en el siglo XIV*, edited by Laura Gutiérrez Arbulú, 257–85. Lima: Pontificia Universidad Católica del Perú, Instituto Riva-Agüero, 2005.

Armus, Diego, ed. *Disease in the History of Modern Latin America: From Malaria to Aids*. Duke University Press: Durham, 2003.

Armus, Diego. "Legados y tendencias en la historiografía sobre la enfermedad en América Latina moderna." In *Higienizar, medicar, gobernar: historia, medicina y sociedad en Colombia*, edited by Jorge Márquez, Álvaro Casa, and Victoria Estrada, 13–39. Medellín: Universidad Nacional de Colombia, 2004.

Arnold, David, ed. *Imperial Medicine and Indigenous Societies*. Manchester: Manchester University Press, 1988.

Arrebola Nacle, Pilar and Guillermina López Andújar. "Suministro de medicamentos a la gente de mar y guerra de la Real Armada (1636)." *Boletin de la sociedad española de historia de la farmacia* 27 (1986): 43–52.

Arrow, Kenneth J. "Uncertainty and the Welfare Economics of Medical Care." *The American Economic Review* 53 (5) (1963): 941–73.

Ashworth, William B. "Catholicism and Early Modern Science." In *God and Nature: Historical Essays on the Encounter between Christianity and Religion*, edited by David C. Lindberg and Ronald L. Numbers, 136–66. Berkeley: University of California Press, 1986.

Attfield, Robin. "Christian Attitudes to Nature." *Journal of the History of Ideas* 44 (3) (1983): 369–86.

Aulet Sastre, Guillermo. "Precios autorizados de libros españoles en Indias." *Revista de Indias* 24 (1946): 311–12.

Azzolini, Monica. "Reading Health in the Stars: Politics and Medical Astrology in Renaissance Milan." In *Horoscopes and Public Spheres: Essays in the History of Astrology*, edited by Günter Oestmann, H. Dareel Rytkin, and Kocku von Stukrad, 183–205. Berlin: Walter de Gruyter, 2005.

Barrera-Osorio, Antonio. *Experiencing Nature: The Spanish American Empire and the Early Scientific Revolution*. Austin: University of Texas Press, 2006.

Barrera-Osorio, Antonio. "Knowledge and Empiricism in the Sixteenth-century Spanish Atlantic World." In *Science in the Spanish and Portuguese Empires: 1560–1800*, edited by Daniela Bleichmar, Paula De Vos, Kristin Huffine, and Kevin Sheehan, 219–32. Stanford: Stanford University Press, 2009.

Basalla, George. "The Spread of Western Science." *Science* 156 (1967): 611–22.

Bastien, Joseph W. *Healers of the Andes: Kallawaya Herbalists and Their Medicinal Plants*. University of Utah Press: Salt Lake City, 1987.

Bauer, Arnold J. "The Church in the Economy of Spanish America: Censos and Depósitos in the Eighteenth and Nineteenth Centuries." *Hispanic American Historical Review* 63 (4) (1983): 707–33.

Binde, Per. "Nature in Roman Catholic Tradition." *Anthropological Quarterly* 74 (1) (2001): 15–27.

Bleichmar, Daniela. "Books, Bodies, and Fields: Sixteenth-Century Transatlantic Encounters with New World *Materia Medica*." In *Colonial Botany: Science, Commerce, and Politics in the Early Modern World*, edited by Londa Schiebinger and Claudia Swan, 83–99. Philadelphia, PA: University of Pennsylvania Press, 2004.

Bleichmar, Daniela, Paula De Vos, Kristine Hufine and Kevin Sheehan, eds. *Science in the Spanish and Portuguese Empires, 1500–1800*. Stanford: Stanford University Press, 2009.

Borah, Woodrow. Early *Trade and Navigation between Mexico and Peru, Ibero-Americana* 38. Berkeley and Los Angeles: University of California, 1954.

Boumediene, Samir. *La colonisation du savoir: une histoire des plantes medicinales de "Nuevo Mundo"* (1492–1750). Vaulx-en-Velin: Éditions des mondes à faire, 2016.

Bowers, Kristy Wilson "Tradition and Innovation in Spanish Medicine: Bartolomé Hidalgo de Agüero and the Vía Particular." *The Sixteenth Century Journal* 41(1) (2010): 29–47.

Bowers, Kristy Wilson. *Plague and Public Health in Early Modern Seville*. Rochester: University of Rochester Press, 2013.

Bowser, Frederick P. *The African Slave in Colonial Peru, 1524–1650*. Stanford CA: Stanford University Press, 1974.

Boyd-Bowman, Peter. "Spanish Patterns of Emigration to the Indies to 1600." *Hispanic American Historical Review* 56 (4) (1976): 580–604.

Brockliss, Lawrence and Colin Jones. *The Medical World of Early Modern France*. Oxford: Clarendon Press, 1997.

Bromley, Juan. "La ciudad de Lima en el año 1630." *Revista histórica* 24 (1959): 268–317.

Bromley, Juan. *Las Viejas Calles de Lima*. Lima: Municipalidad Metropolitana de Lima, 2005. At: http://www.limateca.org/uploads/tinymce/2005_Las_viejas_calles_de_Lima_-_Juan_Bromley.pdf [Accessed 28 Feb. 2017].

Bronner, Fred. "Elite Formation in Seventeenth-Century Peru." *Boletín de estudios latinoamericanos y del caribe* 24 (1978): 3–26.

Brosseder, Claudia. "Astrology in Seventeenth-century Peru." *Studies in History and Philosophy of Biological and Biomedical Sciences* 41 (2) (2010): 146–57.

Brosseder, Claudia. *The Power of Huacas: Change and Resistance in the Andean World of Colonial Peru*. Austin: University of Texas Press, 2014.

Browman, David L. and James N. Gundersen. "Altiplano Comestible Earths: Prehistoric and Historic Geophagy of Highland Peru and Bolivia." *Geoarchaeology* 8 (5) (1993): 413–25.

Burns, Kathryn. *Colonial Habits: Convents and the Spiritual Economy of Cuzco, Peru*. Durham: Duke University Press, 1999.

Burns, Kathryn. "Andean Women in Religion: *Beatas*, 'Decency', and the Defence of Honour in Colonial Cuzco." In *Gender, Race and Religion in the Colonization of the Americas*, edited by Nora E. Jaffary, 81–91. Aldershot: Ashgate, 2007.

Cabanillas Cárdenas, Carlos F., ed. *Juan del Valle y Caviedes: guerras físicas, proezas medicales, hazañas de la ignorancia*. Madrid: Iberoamericana Editorial Vervuert, 2013.

Cagle, Hugh. "Cultures of Inquiry, Myths of Empire: Natural History in Colonial Goa." In *Medicine, Trade and Empire: Garcia de Orta's Colloquies on the Simples and*

Drugs of India (1563), edited by Palmira Fontes da Costa, 107–28. Farnham: Ashgate, 2015.

Cahill, David. "Financing Health Care in the Viceroyalty of Peru: The Hospitals of Lima in the Late Colonial Period." *The Americas* 52 (2) (1995): 123–54.

Cañizares-Esguerra, Jorge. "New World, New Stars: Patriotic Astrology and the Invention of Indian and Creole Bodies in Colonial Spanish America, 1600–1650." *The American Historical Review* 104 (1) (1999): 33–68.

Cañizares-Esguerra, Jorge. "Spanish America: From Baroque to Modern Colonial Science." In *The Cambridge History of Science*, vol. 4, edited by Roy Porter, 718–38. Cambridge: Cambridge University Press, 2003.

Cañizares-Esguerra, Jorge. "Iberian Science in the Renaissance: Ignored How Much Longer?." *Perspectives on Science* 12 (1) (2004): 86–124. Also, modified in *Nature, Empire, and Nation: Explorations of the History of Science in the Iberian World* as "The Colonial Iberian Roots of the Scientific Revolution," 14–45. Stanford: University of Stanford Press, 2006.

Cañizares-Esguerra, Jorge. "Iberian Colonial Science." *Isis* 96 (2005): 64–70.

Cantuarias Acosta, Ricardo. "Las modas limeñas." In *Lima en el siglo XIV*, edited by Laura Gutiérrez Arbulú, 287–307. Lima: Pontificia Universidad Católica del Perú, Instituto Riva-Agüero, 2005.

Celestino, Olinda and Albert Meyers. *Las cofradías en el Perú: región central*. Frankfurt: Editorial Klaus d. Vervuert, 1981.

Chakrabarti, Pratik. *Medicine and Empire 1600–1960*. Basingstoke: Palgrave Macmillan, 2014.

Chance, John K. and William B. Taylor. "Estate and Class in a Colonial City: Oaxaca in 1792." *Comparative Studies in Society and History* 19 (4) (1977): 454–87.

Charles, John. "Trained by Jesuits: Indigenous *Letrados* in Sixteenth-Century Peru." In *Indigenous Intellectuals: Knowledge, Power and Colonial Culture in Mexico and the Andes*, edited by Gabriela Ramos and Yanna Yannakakis, 60–78. Durham: Duke University Press, 2014.

Charney, Paul. "A Sense of Belonging: Colonial Indian Cofradías and Ethnicity in the Valley of Lima, Peru." *The Americas* 54 (3) (1998): 379–407.

Charney, Paul. *Indian Society in the Valley of Lima, Peru, 1532–1765*. Lanham, MD: University Press of America, 2001.

Charney, Paul. "'For My Necessities': The Wills of Andean Commoners and Nobles in the Valley of Lima, 1597–1607." *Ethnohistory* 59 (2) (2012): 323–51.

Chaunu, Huguette and Pierre Chaunu. *Séville et l'Atlantique, 1450–1650*. 8 vols. Paris: A. Colin, 1955–1959.

Chirlone, Quintín and Carlos Mallaína. "Biografía Antonio Robles Cornejo." *El restaurador farmacéutico*, año 11 no. 8 20 Mar. 1855. On line at: http://bibliotecavirtual.ranf.com/es/catalogo_imagenes/grupo.cmd?path=2010122 [Accessed 11 May 2016].

Chirlone, Quintín and Carlos Mallaína. *Historia de la farmacia*. 2nd ed. Madrid: Imp. José M. Ducazcal, 1865.

Clayton, Lawrence A. "Trade and Navigation in the Seventeenth-Century Viceroyalty of Peru." *Journal of Latin American Studies* 7 (1) (1975): 1–21.

Clouse, Michele. *Medicine, Government and Public Health in Philip II's Spain: Shared Interests, Competing Authorities*. Farnham: Ashgate, 2011.

Colmeiro, Miguel. "Noticias acerca de un manuscrito perteneciente al licenciado Antonio Robles Cornejo." *Revista de los progresos de las ciencias exactas, físicas y naturales* (Madrid) 9 (7) (1859): 440–44.

Cook, Harold J. "Medicine." In *The Cambridge History of Science*, vol. 3, edited by Katherine Park and Loraine Daston, 407–34. Cambridge: Cambridge University Press, 2006.

Cook, Harold J. *Matters of Exchange: Commerce, Medicine, and Science in the Dutch Golden Age*. New Haven: Yale University Press, 2007.

Cook, Harold J. "Physicians and Natural History." In *Cultures of Natural History*, edited by Nicholas Jardine, James A. Secord and Emma C. Spary, 91–105. Cambridge: Cambridge University Press, 2008.

Cook, Harold J. "Markets and Cultures: Medical Specifics and the Reconfiguration of the Body in Early Modern Europe." *Transactions of the Royal Historical Society* 21 (2011): 123–45.

Cook, Harold J. and Timothy D. Walker. "Circulation of Medicine in the Early Modern Atlantic World." *Social History of Medicine* 26 (3) (2013): 337–51.

Cook, Noble David. *Demographic Collapse: Indian Peru 1520–1620*. Cambridge: Cambridge University Press, 1981.

Cook, Noble David. *Born to Die: Disease and New World Conquests, 1492–1650*. Cambridge University Press: Cambridge, 1998.

Cooper, Alix. *Inventing the Indigenous: Local Knowledge and Natural History in Early Modern Europe*. Cambridge: Cambridge University Press, 2007.

Cope R. Douglas. *The Limits of Racial Domination: Plebeian Society in Colonial Mexico City, 1660–1720*. Madison: The University of Wisconsin Press, 1994.

Cordero del Campillo, Miguel. *Crónicas de Indias: ganadería, medicina y veterinaria*. Salamanca: Junta de Castilla y León, 2001.

Corfield, Penelope J. "From Poison Peddlers to Civic Worthies: The Reputation of the Apothecaries in Georgian England." *Social History of Medicine* 22 (1) (2009): 1–21.

Crawford, Matthew J. *The Andean Wonder Drug: Cinchona Bark and Imperial Science in the Spanish Atlantic, 1630–1800*. Pittsburgh, PA: University of Pittsburgh Press, 2016.

Crespo Rodríguez, María Dolores. *Arquitectura doméstica de la Ciudad de los Reyes (1535–1750)*. Seville: Consejo Superior de Investigaciones Científicas, 2006.

Crosby, Alfred W. "Virgin Soil Epidemics as a Factor in the Aboriginal Depopulation in America." *The William and Mary Quarterly* 33 (2) (1976): 289–99.

Cueto, Marcus and Stephen Palmer. *Medicine and Public Health in Latin America: A History*. New York: Cambridge University Press, 2015.

Cunningham, Andrew. "The Culture of Gardens." In *Cultures of Natural History*, edited by Nicholas Jardine, James A. Secord and Emma C. Spary, 38–56. Cambridge: Cambridge University Press, 2008.

Cunningham, Andrew and Bridie Andrews, eds. *Western Medicine as Contested Knowledge*. Manchester University Press: Manchester, 1997.

Curtin, Philip D. *Death by Migration: Europe's Encounter with the Tropical World in the Nineteenth Century*. Cambridge University Press: Cambridge, 1989.

Cushner, Nicholas P. *Lords of the Land: Sugar, Wine, and Jesuit Estates of Coastal Peru, 1600–1767*. New York: SUNY Press, 1980.

Cussen, Celia. *Black Saint of the Americas: The Life and Afterlife of Martín de Porres*. Cambridge: Cambridge University Press, 2014.

Daston, Lorraine and Katharine Park. *Wonders and the Order of Nature 1150–1750*. New York: Zone Books, 1998.

Davis, Charles and María Luz López Terrada. "Protomedicato y farmacia en Castilla a finales del siglo XVI: edición crítica del *Catálogo de las cosas que los boticarios han de tener en sus boticas*, de Zamudio de Alfaro, protomédico general (1592–1599)." *Asclepio* 62 (2) (2010): 579–626.

De Vos, Paula S. "The Art of Pharmacy in Seventeenth- and Eighteenth-Century Mexico." PhD diss., University of California, Berkeley, 2001.

De Vos, Paula S. "The Apothecary in Seventeenth- and Eighteenth-Century Mexico: Historiography and Case Studies in Medical Regulation, Charity, and Science." *Colonial Latin American Historical Review* 13 (3) (2004): 249–83.

De Vos, Paula S. "The Science of Spices: Empiricism and Economic Botany in the Early Spanish Empire." *Journal of World History* 17 (4) (2006): 399–427.

De Vos, Paula S. "From Herbs to Alchemy: the Introduction of Chemical Medicine to Mexican Pharmacies in the Seventeenth and Eighteenth Centuries." *Journal of Spanish Cultural Studies* 8 (2) (2007): 135–68.

De Vos, Paula S. "European Materia Medica in Historical Texts: Longevity of a Tradition and Implications for Future Use." *Journal of Ethnopharmacology*, 132 (1) (2010): 28–47.

De Vos, Paula S. "The 'Prince of Medicine', Yūhannā ibn Māsawayh and the Foundations of the Western Pharmaceutical Tradition." *Isis* 104 (4) (2013): 667–712.

De Vos, Paula S. "Apothecaries, Artists and Artisans: Early Industrial Material Culture in the Biological Old Regime." *Journal of Interdisciplinary History*, 45 (3) (2015): 277–336.

Debus, Allen G. *The English Paracelsians*. New York: Franklin Watts, Inc., 1968.

Debus, Allen G. *The Chemical Philosophy: Paracelsian Science and Medicine in the Sixteenth and Seventeenth Centuries* vol. 1. New York: Science History Publication, 1977.

Debus, Allen G. "Chemists, Physicians and the Changing Perspectives on the Scientific Revolution." *Isis* 89 (1) (1998): 66–81.

Debus, Allen G. "Paracelsus and the Delayed Scientific Revolution in Spain: A Legacy of Philip II." In *Reading the Book of Nature: the Other Side of the Scientific Revolution*, edited by Allen G. Debus and Michael T. Walton, 147–61. Kirksville-Missouri: Sixteenth Century Journal Publishers, Inc., 1998.

Delgado Matallana, Gustavo. *Historia de la enseñanza médica en el Perú*. Lima: Universidad Nacional Mayor de San Marcos, Fondo Editorial, 2008.

Deza Bringas, Luis. *Testimonios del linaje médico peruano en los libros del cabildo de Lima, siglo XVI*. Lima: Universidad de San Martín de Porres, Facultad de Medicina Humana, 2004.

Díaz Piedrahita, Santiago and Luis Carlos Mantilla. *La terapéutica en el Nuevo Reino de Granada: un recetario franciscano del siglo XVIII*. Bogotá: Academia Colombiana de Ciencias Exactas, Físicas y Naturales, 2002.

Drayton, Richard. *Nature's Government: Science, Imperial Britain and the "Improvement" of the World*. New Haven: Yale University Press, 2000.

Dueñas, Alcira. *Indians and Mestizos in the "Lettered City"*. Boulder: University Press of Colorado, 2010.

Durán Montero, María Antonia. *Lima en el siglo XVII: arquitectura, urbanismo y vida cotidiana*. Seville: Diputación Provincial, 1994.

Duviols, Pierre. *La lutte contre les religions autochtones dans le Pérou colonial: l'extirpation de l'idolâtrie, entre 1532 et 1660*. Lima: Institut Français d'Études Andines, 1971.

Eamon, William. *Science and the Secrets of Nature: Books of Secrets in Medieval and Early Modern Culture*. Princeton: Princeton University Press, 1994.

Earle, Rebecca. "'Two Pairs of Pink Satin Shoes!!' Race, Clothing and Identity in the Americas (17th–19th centuries)." *History Workshop Journal* 52 (2001): 175–95.

Earle, Rebecca. "'If You Eat Their Food': Diets and Bodies in Early Colonial Spanish America." *American Historical Review* 115 (3) (2010): 688–713.

Earle, Rebecca. *The Body of the Conquistador: Food, Race and the Colonial Experience in Spanish America, 1492–1700*. Cambridge: Cambridge University Press, 2012.

Eguiguren, Luis Antonio. *Alma mater: origines de la Universidad de San Marcos (1551–1579)*. Lima 1939. No publisher.

Eguiguren, Luis Antonio. *Diccionario histórico cronológico de la universidad real y pontificia de San Marcos y sus colegios*, Tomo I. Lima 1940. Printer: Torres Aguirre.

Elliott, John H. *Empires of the Atlantic World: Britain and Spain in America 1492–1830*. New Haven: Yale University Press, 2006.

Estes, J. Worth. "The European Reception of the First Drugs from the New World." *Pharmacy in History* 37 (1) (1995): 3–23.

Fernández-Carrión, Mercedes and David Martín-Castilla. "Francisco de Ortega y la profesión farmacéutica sevillana en el primer tercio del siglo XVII." *Boletín de la sociedad española de historia de la farmacia* 37 (148) (1986): 289–301.

Fernández-Carrión, Mercedes and José Antonio Pérez Romero. "Visitas de inspección sanitaria en especierías, confiterías, cererías y aguardenterías de Antequera durante el siglo XVII." *Baética* 8 (1985): 435–46.

Fernández-Carrión, Mercedes and José Luis Valverde. *Farmacia y sociedad en Sevilla en el siglo XVI*. Seville: Servicio de Publicaciones del Ayuntamiento de Sevilla. 1985.

Fernández-Carrión, Mercedes and José Luis Valverde. "Research Notes on Spanish American Drug Trade." *Pharmacy in History* 30–31 (1988–1989): 27–32.

Few, Martha. *Women Who Live Evil Lives: Gender, Religion and the Politics of Power in Colonial Guatemala*. Austin: University of Texas Press, 2002.

Few, Martha. "Medical *Mestizaje* and the Politics *of Pregnancy in Colonial Guatemala, 1660–1730*" In *Science in the Spanish and Portuguese Empires, 1500–1800*, edited by Daniela Bleichmar, Paula De Vos, Kristine Hufine and Kevin Sheehan, 132–46. Stanford: Stanford University Press, 2009.

Findlen, Paula. *Possessing Nature: Museums, Collecting, and Scientific Culture in Early Modern Italy*. Berkeley and Los Angeles: University of California Press, 1994.

Findlen, Paula. "Courting Nature." In *Cultures of Natural History*, edited by Nicholas Jardine, James A. Secord and Emma C. Spary, 57–74. Cambridge: Cambridge University Press, 2008.

Fisher, Andrew B. and Matthew D. O'Hara, "Introduction: Racial Identities and Their Interpreters in Colonial Latin America." In *Imperial Subjects: Race and Identity in Colonial Latin America*, edited by Andrew B. Fisher and Matthew D. O'Hara, 15–23. Durham: Duke University Press, 2009.

Flores Hernández, Benjamín. "Medicina de los conquistadores, en la *Milicia Indiana* de Bernardo de Vargas Machuca." *Boletín mexicano de historia y filosofía de la médicina* 6 (1) (2003): 5–10.

Forbes, Robert J. *A History of the Art of Distillation*. Leiden: E.J. Brill, 1970.

Ford, Thayne R. "Stranger in a Foreign Land: José de Acosta's Scientific Realisations in Sixteenth-century Peru." *Sixteenth Century Journal* 29 (1) (1998): 19–33.

Foster, George M. "Relationship between Spanish and Spanish-American Folk Medicine." *Journal of American Folklore* 66 (1953): 201–17.

Foster, George M. "On the Origin of Humoral Medicine in Latin America." *Medical Anthropology Quarterly* NS 1 (4) (1987): 355–93.

Foster, George M. *Hippocrates' Latin American Legacy: Humoral Medicine in the New World*. Langhorne, PA: Gordon and Breach, 1994.

Foust, Clifford M. *Rhubarb: The Wondrous Drug*. Princeton: Princeton University Press, 1992.

Freedman, Paul. *Out of the East: Spices and the Medieval Imagination*. New Haven: Yale University Press, 2008.

Fresquet Febrer, José Luis. "Uso de productos del reino mineral en la terapéutica del siglo XVI: el libro de los *Medicamentos Simples* de Juan Fragoso (1581) and el *Antidotario* de Juan Calvo (1580)." *Asclepio* 51 (1999): 55–92.

Fresquet Febrer, José Luis. "*Juan Fragoso y los 'Discursos de las cosas aromáticas, árboles y frutales…'(1572)*." Valencia: CISC – Universitat de Valencia, 2001.

Friedenwald, Harry. *The Jews and Medicine*, vol. 2. Baltimore: The John Hopkins Press, 1944.

Garcia Ballester, Luis. "The Inquisition and Minority Medical Practitioners in Counter Reformation Spain: Judaizing and Morisco Practitioners, 1560–1610." In *Medicine and the Reformation*, edited by Ole Peter Grell and Andrew Cunningham, 156–91. London: Routledge, 1993.

García Ballester, Luis. *La búsqueda de la salud: sanadores y enfermos en la España medieval.* Barcelona: Ediciones Peninsula, 2001.

García Cáceres, Uriel. *Juan del Valle y Caviedes: Cronista de la medicina*. Lima: Banco Central de Reserva del Perú and Universidad Peruana Cayetano Heredia, 1999.

García Fuentes, Lutgardo. *Los peruleros y el comercio de Sevilla con las Indias, 1580–1630*. Seville: Universidad de Sevilla, 1997.

Garland Ponce, Beatriz. "Las cofradías en Lima durante la colonia: una primera aproximación." In *La venida del reino. Religión, evangelización y cultura en América, Siglos XVI–XX*, edited by Gabriela Ramos, 199–228. Cuzco: Centro de Estudios Regionales Andinos "Bartolomé de las Casas", 1994.

Garofalo, Leo. "Conjuring with Coca and the Inca: the Andeanisation of Lima's Afro-Peruvian Ritual Specialists, 1580–1690." *The Americas* 63 (1) (2006): 53–80.

Gentilcore, David. *Healers and Healing in Early Modern Italy*. Manchester: Manchester University Press, 1998.

Giglioni, Guido. "Girolamo Cardano: University Student and Professor." *Renaissance Studies* 27 (4) (2013): 517–32.

Gómez, Pablo F. "The Circulation of Bodily Knowledge in the Seventeenth-century Black Spanish Caribbean," *Social History of Medicine* 26 (3) (2013): 383–402.

González Arce, José Damián. "Los proyectos de ordenanzas generales de médicos, cirujanos y boticarios de Castilla (ca.1491–1513)." *Dynamis* 31 (1) (2011): 207–26.

González Sánchez, Carlos A. "El libro y la carrera de Indias: registro de ida de navíos." *Archivo hispalense* 72 (1989): 93–103.

González Sánchez, Carlos A. "Los libros de los españoles el virreinato del Perú. Siglos XVI y XVI." *Revista de Indias*, 56 (no. 206) (1996): 7–47.

González Sánchez, Carlos A. "Consideraciones sobre el comercio de libros en Lima a principios del siglo XVII." *Anuario de Estudios Americanos* 54 (2) (1997): 665–92.

González Sánchez, Carlos A. *New World Literacy: Written Culture across the Atlantic, 1500–1700*. Translated by Tristan Platt, 46–54. Lewisburg: Bucknell University Press, 2011.

Goodman, David C. "Philip II's Patronage of Science and Engineering." *The British Journal for the History of Science* 16 (1) (1983): 49–66.

Goodman, David C. *Power and Penury: Government, Technology and Science in Philip II's Spain*. Cambridge: Cambridge University Press, 1988.

Grafton, Anthony and Nancy Siraisi. "Between the Election and My Hopes: Girolamo Cardano and Medical Astrology." In *Secrets of Nature: Astrology and Alchemy in Early Modern Europe,* edited by William R. Newman and Anthony Grafton, 69–132. Cambridge, MA: MIT Press, 2001.

Granjel, Luis S. *La medicina española renacentista*. Salamanca: Ediciones Universidad de Salamanca, 1980.

Granjel, Luis S. *Discursos medicinales: vida y obra de Juan Méndez Nieto*. Salamanca: Universidad de Salamanca y Junta de Castilla y León, 1989.

Grant, Edward. "When Did Modern Science Begin?" *The American Scholar* 66 (1997): 105–13.

Graubert, Karen B. *With Our Labor and Our Sweat: Indigenous Women and the Formation of Colonial Society in Peru, 1550–1700*. Stanford: Stanford University Press. 2007.

Green, Monica. "Bodies, Gender, Health, Disease: Recent Work on Medieval Women's Medicine." *Studies in Medieval and Renaissance History*, 3rd ser. 5 (2005): 1–46.

Griffiths, Nicholas. *The Cross and the Serpent: Religious Repression and Resurgence in Colonial Peru*. Norman: University of Oklahoma Press, 1995.

Griffiths, Nicholas. "Andean *Curanderos* and their Repressors: The Persecution of Native Healing in Late Seventeenth- and Early Eighteenth-Century Peru." In *Spiritual Encounters: Interactions between Christianity and Native Religions in Colonial America*, edited by Nicholas Griffiths and Fernando Cervantes, 185–97. Birmingham: University of Birmingham Press, 1999.

Guerra, Francisco. *Nicolás Bautista Monardes: su vida y su obra (ca. 1493–1588)*. Mexico City: Compañía Fundidora de Cierro y Acero de Monterrey, 1961.

Guerra, Francisco. "Drugs from the Indies and the Political Economy of the Sixteenth Century." In *Analecta medico-historica: materia medica in the XVIth century*, edited by M. Florkin, 29–55. Oxford: Pergamon, 1966.

Guerra, Francisco. "The Role of Religion in Spanish American Medicine." In *Medicine and Culture*, edited by F.N.L. Poynter, 179–88. Wellcome Institute: London, 1969.

Guerra, Francisco. *El Tesoro de Medicinas de Gregorio López* 1542–1596. Madrid: Ediciones Cultura Hispánica del Instituto de Cooperación Iberoamericana, 1982.

Guerra, Francisco. *El hospital en hispanoamérica y filipinas 1492–1898*. Madrid: Ministerio de Sandiad y Consumo, 1994.

Guibovich, Pedro. Autores, censores y producción de libros en el virreinato peruano (2015). Unpublished manuscript at: https://escriturasvirreinales.files.wordpress.com/2015/05/guibovich-autores_y_censores-u-c.pdf [Accessed 2 Jul. 2016].

Guibovich Pérez, Pedro M. "Printing Press in Colonial Peru: Production Process and Literary Categories in Lima." *Colonial Latin American Review* 10 (2) (2001): 167–88.

Guibovich Pérez, Pedro M. "Bibliotecas de médicos en Lima colonial." In *Del autor al lector*, edited by Carmen Castañeda, 293–304. Mexico City: CIESAS, 2002.

Guibovich Pérez, Pedro M. *Censura, libros e inquisición en el Perú colonial, 1570–1754*. Seville: Universidad de Sevilla, Secretariado de publicaciones, 2004.

Gunther, Robert T. *The Greek Herbal of Disocorides*. New York: Harner Publishing Co., 1959.

Gutiérrez de Pineda, Virginia. *Medicina tradicional de Colombia: el triple llegado*. 2 vols. Bogotá: Universidad Nacional de Colombia, 1985.

Halikowski-Smith, Stefan. "'Profits Sprout Like Tropical Plants': A Fresh Look at What Went Wrong with the Eurasian Spice Trade c. 1550–1800." *Journal of Global History* 3 (2008): 389–418.

Hamnett, Brian R. "Church Wealth in Peru: Estates and Loans in the Archdiocese of Lima in the Seventeenth Century." *Jahrbuch für Geschichte Lateinamerikas* 10 (1973): 113–32.

Hampe-Martínez, Teodoro. "The Diffusion of Books and Ideas in Colonial Peru: A Study of Private Libraries in the Sixteenth and Seventeenth Centuries." *Hispanic American Historical Review* 273 (2) (1993): 211–33.

Haring, Clarence H. *Trade and Navigation between Spain and the Indies*. Cambridge, Mass.: Harvard University Press, 1918.

Harris, Steven J. "Jesuit Scientific Activity in the Overseas Missions, 1540–1773." *Isis* 96 (1) (2005): 71–79.

Hellmer, Marie. "Le Callao (1617–1815)" *Jahrbuch für Geschicte von Staat, Wirtschaft und Gesellschaft Lateinamerikas* 2 (1965): 145–95.

Henry, John. "Doctors and Healers: Popular Culture and the Medical Profession." In *Science, Culture and Popular Belief in Renaissance Europe*, edited by Stephen Pumfrey, Paolo L. Rossi and Maurice Slawinski, 191–221. Manchester: Manchester University Press, 1991.

Hernández Sáenz, Luz María. *Learning to Heal: The Medical Profession in Colonial Mexico, 1767–1831*. New York: Peter Lang, 1997.

Hernández Sáenz, Luz María and Foster, George M. "Curers and Their Cures in Colonial New Spain and Guatemala: The Spanish Component." In *Mesoamerican Healers*, edited by Brad R. Huber and Alan R. Sandstrom, 19–46. Austin: University of Texas Press, 2001.

Herrera Dávila, Joaquín. "Las boticas sevillanas de 1631." *Boletín de la sociedad española de historia de la farmacia* 39 (nos. 154–155) (1988): 63–81.

Herrera Hinojo, Pilar. "Contratos de aprendizaje en farmacia en el siglo XVI. Notas para la historia de la farmacia española." *Boletín de la sociedad española de historia de farmacia* 19 (no. 73) (1968): 73–79.

Herzog, Tamar. *Upholding Justice: Society, State, and the Penal System in Quito (1650–1750)*. Ann Arbor: University of Michigan Press, 2004.

Horkheimer, Max and Theodor Adorno. *Dialectic of Enlightenment.* New York: Herder and Herder, 1972.

Israel, Jonathan I. "Counter Reformation, Economic Decline, and the Delayed Impact of the Medical Revolution in Catholic Europe." In *Health Care and Relief in Counter-Reformation Europe*, edited by Ole Peter Grell, Andrew Cunningham, with Jon Arrizabalaga, 40–55. London: Routledge, 1999.

Jarcho, Saul. "Medicine in Sixteenth Century New Spain as Illustrated by the Writings of Bravo, Farfán and Vargas Machuca." *Bulletin of the History of Medicine* 31 (1957): 425–41.

Jarcho, Saul. "Origin of the American Indian as Suggested by Fray Joseph de Acosta (1589)." *Isis* 50 (4) (1959): 430–38.

Jenner, S.R. Mark and Patrick Wallis. *The Medical Marketplace.* In *Medicine and the Market in England and its Colonies, c.1450–1850*, 1–23. Basingstoke: Palgrave Macmillan, 2007.

Jouve Martín, José R. *The Black Doctors of Colonial Lima: Science, Race, and Writing in Colonial and Early Republican Peru.* Montreal: McGill-Queen's University Press, 2014.

Kamen, Henry. *The Spanish Inquisition: An Historical Revision.* London: Weidenfeld and Nicolson, 1997.

Katzew, Ilona. *Casta Painting: Images of Race in Eighteenth-Century Mexico.* New Haven: Yale University Press, 2004.

Kremers and Urdang's History of Pharmacy. Revised by Glenn Sonnedecker. 4th ed. Madison, WI: American Institute for the History of Pharmacy, 1986.

Lafuente, Antonio. "Enlightenment Science in an Imperial Context: Local Science in the Late-Eighteenth-Century Hispanic World." *Osiris* 15 (2001): 155–73.

Lanning, John Tate. *Academic Culture in the Spanish Colonies.* Oxford: Oxford University Press, 1940.

Lanning, John Tate. "Legitimacy and *Limpieza de Sangre* in the Practice of Medicine in the Spanish Empire." *Jahrbuch für Geschichte von Staat, Wirtschaft und Gesellschaft Lateinamerikas* 4 (1967): 37–60.

Lanning, John Tate. *The Royal Protomedicato: The Regulation of the Medical Professions in the Spanish Empire*, edited by John Jay TePaske. Durham: Duke University Press, 1985.

Lastres, Juan B. *Historia de la medicina peruana*. 3 vols. Lima: Impr. Santa María, 1951.

Laval, Enrique. *Botica de los Jesuitas de Santiago*. Santiago: Asociación Chilena de Asistencia Social, 1953.

Lavrin, Asunción. "Female Religious." In *Cities and Society in Colonial Latin America*, edited by Louisa Schell Hoberman and Susan Migden Socolow, 165–95. Albuquerque: University of New Mexico Press, 1986.

Leonard, Irving A. "Best Sellers of the Lima Book Trade." *Hispanic American Historical Review* 22 (1) (1942): 5–33.

Leonard, Irving A. "On the Lima Book Trade, 1591." *Hispanic American Historical Review* 33 (4) (1953): 511–25.

Leonard, Irving A. *Books of the Brave: Being an Account of Books and of Men in the Spanish Conquest and Settlement of the Sixteenth-century New World*. Berkeley and Los Angeles: University of California, 1992 [1949].

Leonard, Irving A. *Los libros del conquistador*. Mexico: Fondo de Cultura Económica, 1996 [1949].

Leong, Elaine. "Making Medicines in the Early Modern Household." *Bulletin of the History of Medicine* 82 (2008): 145–68.

Lévano Medina, Diego. "La administración de los bienes temporales en las cofradías limeñas del siglo XVII." In *Corporaciones religiosas y evangelización en Iberoamérica, siglos XVI–XVII*, edited by Diego Lévano Medina and Kelly Montoya Estrada, 111–42. Lima: Universidad Nacional Mayor San Marcos, 2010.

Lewis, Laura A. *Hall of Mirrors: Power, Witchcraft, and Caste in Colonial Mexico*. Durham, NC: Duke University Press, 2003.

Lindemann, Mary. *Medicine and Society in Early Modern Europe*. Cambridge: Cambridge University Press, 1999.

Lissón Chaves, Emilio, ed. *La iglesia de España en el Perú: colección de documentos para la historia de la iglesia en el Perú, que se encuentran en varios archivos*. 5 vols. Seville: Editorial Católica Española, 1943–1947.

Livingstone, David N. *Putting Science in its Place: Geographies of Scientific Knowledge*. Chicago: The University of Chicago Press, 2003.

Livingstone, David N. and Charles W.J. Withers, eds. *Geography and Enlightenment*. Chicago: The University of Chicago Press, 1999.

Lockhart, James. *Spanish Peru 1532–1560: A Colonial Society*. Madison: The University of Wisconsin Press, 1968.

Lohmann Villena, Guillermo. *Plata del Perú, riqueza de Europa: los mercaderes peruanos y el comercio con la metropolí en el siglo XVII*. Lima: Fondo Editorial del Congreso del Perú, 2004.

Lohmann Villena, Guillermo and María Justina Sarabia Viejo. *Francisco de Toledo: disposiciones gubernativas para el virreinato del Perú 1575–1580*. Seville: Escuela de Estudios Hispano-Americanos, 1989.

López Pérez, Miguel. "La influencia de la alquimia medieval hispana en la Europa moderna." *Asclepio* 54 (2002): 211–29.

López Pérez, Miguel. "Spanish Paracelsus Revisited and Decontaminated." *Azogue* 7 (2013) URL: http://www.revistaazogue.com. [Accessed 23 May 2016].

López Pérez, Miguel and Mar Rey Bueno. "Simón de Tovar (1528–1596): redes familiares, naturaleza Americana y comercio de maravillas en la Sevilla del XVI." *Dynamis* 26 (2006): 69–91.

López Piñero, José María. "Paracelsus and His Work in Sixteenth and Seventeenth Century Spain." *Clio Medica* 8 (2) (1973): 113–41.

López Piñero, José María. *Ciencia y técnica en la sociedad española de los siglos XVI y XVII*. Barcelona: Labor Universitaria 1979.

López Piñero, José María. "Las 'nuevas medicinas' americanos en la obra (1565–1574) de Nicolás Monardes." *Asclepio* 42 (1) (1990): 3–67.

López Piñero, José María and Francesc Bujosa Homar. "Tradición y renovación en la medicina española del siglo XVI." *Asclepio* 30–31 (1978–1979): 285–306.

López Piñero, José María and Francisco Calero, eds. *De pulvere febrifugo Occidentalis Indiae (1663) de Gaspar Caldera de Heredia y la introducción de la quina en Europa*. Valencia: Instituto de Estudios Documentales e Históricos sobre la Ciencia, Universidad de Valencia-CSIC, 1992.

López Terrada, María Luz. "Medical Pluralism in the Iberian Kingdoms: The Control of Extra-academic Practitioners in Valencia." *Medical History Supplement* 29 (2009): 7–25.

Lowry, Lyn Brandon. "Forging an Indian Nation: Urban Indians under Spanish Colonial Control, Peru 1535–1765." PhD diss. University of California, Berkeley, 1991.

Lozoya, Xavier. "Natural History and Herbal Medicine in Sixteenth-century America." In *Science in Latin America: A History*, edited by Juan José Saldaña, 29–50. Austin: University of Texas Press, 2006.

Lynch, John. *Spain under the Habsburgs*. 2 vols. Oxford: Blackwell, 1965.

MacCormack, Sabine. *On the Wings of Time: Rome, the Incas, Spain and Peru*. Princeton: Princeton University Press, 2009.

MacLeod, Roy. "Introduction." In *Disease, Medicine and Empire: Perspectives on Western Medicine and the Experience of European Expansion*, edited by Roy MacLeod and Milton Lewis, 1–18. London: Routledge, 1988.

MacLeod, Roy. "Nature and Empire: Science and the Colonial Enterprise." *Osiris* 15 (2000): 1–13.

Mangan, Jane E. *Trading Roles: Gender, Ethnicity and the Urban Economy in Colonial Potosí*. Durham, NC: Duke University Press, 2005.

Mangan, Jane E. *Transatlantic Obligations: Creating the Bonds of Family in Conquest-Era Peru and Spain*. New York: Oxford University Press, 2015.

Mannarelli, María Emma. "Inquisición y mujeres: las hechiceras en el Perú durante el siglo XVII." *Revista Andina* 3 (1) 1985: 141–56.

Mannarelli, María Emma. *Hechiceras, beatas y expósitas: mujeres y poder inquisitorial en Lima*. Lima: Fondo Editorial del Congreso del Perú, 1998.

Mannarelli, María Emma. *Private Passions and Public Sins: Men and Women in Seventeenth Century Lima*. Translated by Sidney Evans and Meredith D. Dodge. Albuquerque: University of New Mexico Press, 2007.

Mansilla Justo, Judith. "Poder y prestigio social en las cofradías españolas, siglo XVII y XVIII." In *Corporaciones religiosas y evangelización en Iberoamérica, siglos XVI–XVII*, edited by Diego Lévano Medina and Kelly Montoya Estrada, 229–72. Lima: Universidad Nacional Mayor San Marcos, 2010.

Marañón, Pedro Manuel Alonso. "Constituciones del colegio real de San Felipe y San Marcos de Lima." *Estudios de historia social y económica de América* 15 (1997): 419–34.

Martín, Luis. *The Intellectual Conquest of Peru: The Jesuit College of San Pablo, 1568–1767*. New York: Fordham University Press, 1968.

Martín, Luis. *Daughters of the Conquistadores: Women of the Viceroyalty of Peru*. Albuquerque: University of New Mexico Press, 1983.

Martín, Luís. "La biblioteca del Colegio de San Pablo (1568–1767), antecedente de la Biblioteca Nacional." In *La Biblioteca Nacional: aportes para su historia*, 25–37. http://www.comunidadandina.org/bda/docs/PE-CA-0015.pdf [Accessed 2 Jul. 2016].

Martín, Luis and Jo Ann Geurin Pettas. *Scholars and Schools in Colonial Peru*. Dallas, TX: Southern Methodist University, 1973.

Martínez, María Elena. *Genealogical Fictions: Limpieza de Sangre, Religion, and Gender in Colonial Mexico*. Stanford: Stanford University Press, 2008.

Martínez Bermejo, Saúl. "Beyond Luxury: Sumptuary Legislation in 17th-Century Castile." In *Making, Using and Resisting the Law in European History*, edited by Günther Lottes, Eero Medijainen, and Jon Vidar Sigurdsson, 94–108. Pisa: Plus-Pisa University Press, 2008.

Matallana, Gustavo Delgado. *Historia de la enseñanza médica en el Perú*. Lima: Universidad Nacional Mayor de San Marcos, 2008.

Maya Restrepo, Luz Adriana. "Botánica y medicina africanas en la Nueva Granada, siglo XVII." *Historia crítica* 19 (2000): 27–47.

McAlister, Lyle N. "Social Structure and Social Change in New Spain." *Hispanic American Historical Review* 43 (3) (1963): 349–70.

McClellan, James E. III. *Colonialism and Science: Saint Domingue in the Old Regime*. Baltimore: Johns Hopkins University Press, 1992.

McNeill, J.R. *Mosquito Empires: Ecology and War in the Greater Caribbean, 1620–1914*. Cambridge: Cambridge University Press, 2010.

McVaugh, Michael R. *Medicine before the Plague: Practitioners and their Patients in the Crown of Aragon 1285–1345*. Cambridge, Cambridge University Press, 1993.

McVaugh, Michael R. "Chemical Medicine in the Medical Writings of Arnau de Vilanova." II *Trobada Internacional d'Estudis sobre Arnau de Vilanova. Arxiu de Textos Catalans Antics* 23–24: (2004–2005): 239–64.

McVaugh, Michael R. "The 'Experience-Based Medicine' of the Thirteenth Century." *Early Science and Medicine* 14 (2009): 105–30.

Mecham, John Lloyd. *Church and State in Latin America: A History of Politico-Ecclesiastical Relations*. Chapel Hill: University of North Carolina Press, 1934.

Medina, José Toribio de. *La imprenta en Lima,* 1584–1824. 4 vols. Santiago: Impreso y grabado en casa del autor, 1904–1907.

Medina, José Toribio de. *Historia del tribunal de Santo Oficio de la Inquisición de Lima (1569–1820)*. Vol. 1. Santiago, Chile: Fondo Histórico y Bibliográfico J.T. Medina, 1956.

Meléndez, Mariselle and Karen Stolley. "Introduction: Enlightenments in Ibero-America." *Colonial Latin American Review* 24 (1) (2015): 1–16.

Memarzadeh, Maher. "Medical Practitioners in Early Colonial Mexico." PhD diss., UCLA, 2005.

Millones-Figueroa, Luis. "La historia natural del padre Bernabé Cobo: algunas claves para su lectura." *Colonial Latin American Review* 12 (1) (2003): 85–97.

Mills, Kenneth. *Idolatry and Its Enemies: Colonial and Andean Religion and* Extirpation, 1640–1750. Princeton: Princeton University Press, 1997.

Montes, Javier Alejo and María Carmen Rodríguez García. "Los estudios de la facultad de medicina en la Universidad de Salamanca de finales del siglo XVI." In *Espacio, tiempo y forma, Serie IV, Historia moderna* 7 (1994): 37–50.

Montoya Estrada, Kelly. "Una procesión de Viernes Santo en Lima XVII." In *Corporaciones religiosas y evangelización en Iberoamérica, siglos XVI–XVII*, edited by Diego Lévano Medina and Kelly Montoya Estrada, 143–60. Lima: Universidad Nacional Mayor San Marcos, 2010.

Moran, Bruce T. "The *Herbarius* of Paracelsus." *Pharmacy in History*, 35 (3) (1993): 99–127.

Moran, Bruce T. *Distilling Knowledge. Alchemy, Chemistry, and the Scientific Revolution*. Cambridge, Mass.: Harvard University Press, 2005.

Moreau, Emmanuelle. "Le Père Bernabé Cobo et la nomenclature botanique." *Caravelle* 82 (2004): 195–204.

Mörner, Magnus. *Race Mixture in the History of Latin America*. Boston: Little, Brown & Company, 1967.

Mörner, Magnus. "Economic Factors and Stratification in Colonial Spanish America with Special Regard to Elites." *Hispanic American Historical Review* 63 (2) (1978): 335–69.

Muldrew, Craig. *The Economy of Obligation: The Culture of Credit and Social Relations in Early Modern England*. Basingstoke: Macmillan, 1998.

Multhauf, Robert P. "John of Rupescissa and the Origin of Medical Chemistry." *Isis* 45 (2) (1954): 359–67.

Multhauf, Robert P. "Medical Chemistry and 'the Paracelsians'." *Bulletin of the History of Medicine* 28 (1954): 101–26.

Multhauf, Robert P. "The Significance of Distillation in Renaissance Medical Chemistry." *Bulletin of the History of Medicine* 30 (1956): 329–46.

Navarro Brotóns, Victor and William Eamon. "Spain and the Scientific Revolution: Questions and Conjectures." In *Más allá de la Leyenda Negra: España y la revolución científica*, edited by Victor Navarro Brotons and William Eamon, 27–38. Valencia: Instituto de Historia de la Ciencia y Documentación López Piñero, 2007.

Newman, William R. "From Alchemy to 'Chymistry'." *The Cambridge History of Science*. Vol. 3, edited by Katharine Park and Lorraine Daston, 497–517. Cambridge: Cambridge University Press, 2006.

Newson, Linda A. "A Historical-Ecological Perspective on Epidemic Disease." In *Advances in Historical Ecology*, edited by William Balée, 42–63. New York: Columbia University Press, 1998.

Newson, Linda A. *Life and Death in Early Colonial Ecuador*. Norman: University of Oklahoma Press, 1995.

Newson, Linda A. and Minchin, Susie. *From Capture to Sale: The Portuguese Slave Trade to Spanish South America in the Early Seventeenth Century*. Leiden: Brill, 2007.

Nieto Olarte, Mauricio. "Scientific Practices in the Sixteenth-Century Iberian Atlantic." In *Theorising the Ibero-American Atlantic*, edited by Harald E. Braun and Lisa Vollendorf, 141–58. Leiden: Brill, 2013.

Numbers, Ronald L. "Conclusion." In *Medicine in the New World: New Spain, New France, and New England*, edited by Ronald L. Numbers, 154–58. Knoxville: University of Tennessee Press, 1987.

O'Phelan, Scarlett. "El vestido como identidad étnica e indicador social de una cultura material." In *El barroco peruano* II, edited by Ramón Mujica Pinilla, 99–133. Lima: Banco de Crédito del Perú, 2003.

O'Toole, Rachel S. *Bound Lives: Africans, Indians, and the Making of Race in Colonial Peru*. Pittsburgh: University of Pittsburgh Press, 2012.

Osorio, Alejandra B. "'El callejón de la soledad': Vectors of Cultural Hybridity in Seventeenth-century Lima." In *Spiritual Encounters: Interactions between Christianity and Native Religions in Colonial America*, edited by Nicholas Griffiths and Fernando Cervantes, 198–229. Birmingham: University of Birmingham Press, 1999.

Osorio, Alejandra B. "Hechicerías y curanderías en la Lima del siglo XVII: Formas femeninas de control y acción social." In *Mujeres y género en la historia del Perú*, edited by Margarita Zegarra, 59–75. Lima: CENDOC-Mujer, 1999.

Osorio, Alejandra B. *Inventing Lima: Baroque Modernity in Peru's South Sea Metropolis*. New York: Palgrave Macmillan, 2008.

Otte, Enrique. *Cartas privadas de emigrantes a Indias, 1540–1616*. Mexico: Fondo de Cultura Económica, 1993.

Palmer, Richard. "Pharmacy in the Republic of Venice in the Sixteenth Century." In *The Medical Renaissance of the Sixteenth Century*, edited by A. Wear, R.K. French and I.M. Lonie, 100–17. Cambridge: Cambridge University Press, 1985.

Pardo-Tomás, José. "Autores médicos en los índices inquisitoriales españoles del siglo XVI." *Dynamis* 5–6 (1985–1986): 201–14.

Pardo-Tomás, José. *Ciencia y censura: la inquisición española y los libros científicos en los siglos* XVI *y* XVII. Madrid: CSIC, 1991.

Pardo-Tomás, José. "Two Glimpses of America from a Distance: Carolus Clusius and Nicolás Monardes." In *Carolus Clusius: Towards a Cultural History of a Renaissance Naturalist*, edited by Florike Egmond, Paul Hoftijzer and Robert Visser, 173–93. Amsterdam: Edita, 2007.

Pardo-Tomás, José. "'Antiguamente vivían más sanos que ahora': Explanations of Native Mortality in the *Relaciones Geográficas de Indias*." In *Medical Cultures of the Early Modern Spanish Empire*, edited by John Slater, Mariluz López Terrada and José Pardo-Tomás, 41–65. Farnham: Ashgate, 2014.

Pastor Frechoso, Feliz Francisco. *Boticas, boticarios y materia médica en Valladolid: siglos XVI y XVI*. Salamanca: Junta de Castilla y León. Salamanca: Consejería de Cultura y Turismo, 1993.

Perdiguero, Enrique. "Protomedicato y curanderismo." *Dynamis* 16 (1996): 91–108.

Peterson, Georg G. *Mining and Metallurgy in Ancient Perú. The Geological Society of America Special Paper 467*. Translation of *Minería y metalurgia en el antiguo Perú*, by William E. Brooks. Boulder, Col.: The Geological Society of America, Inc., 2010.

Pike, Ruth. *Aristocrats and Traders: Sevillian Society in the Sixteenth Century*. Ithaca, NY: Cornell University Press, 1972.

Pomata, Gianna. "Practising between Heaven and Earth: Women Healers in Seventeenth-century Bologna." *Dynamis* 19 (1999): 119–43.

Poole, Stafford. "The Politics of *Limpieza de Sangre*: Juan de Ovando and His Circle in the Reign of Philip ll." *The Americas* 55 (1999): 359–89.

Porter, Roy. "The Patient's View." *Theory and Society* 14 (2) (1985): 175–98.

Porter, Roy. *The Greatest Benefit to Mankind: The Medical History of Humanity from Antiquity to the Present*. London: HarperCollins, 1997.

Portuondo, María M. *Secret Science: Spanish Cosmography and the New World*. Chicago: University of Chicago Press, 2009.

Premo, Bianca. *Children of the Father King: Youth, Authority and Legal Minority in Colonial Lima*. Chapel Hill: University of North Carolina, 2005.

Prieto, Andrés I. *Missionary Scientists: Jesuit Science in Spanish South America, 1570–1810*. Nashville, TN: Vanderbilt University Press, 2011.

Puerto Sarmiento, Francisco Javier. "La farmacia renacentista española y la botica de El Escorial." In *La ciencia en el Monasterio del Escorial*, edited by Francisco Javier Campos and Fernández de Sevilla, 73–132. Madrid: Real Universitario Escorial-María Cristina, 1993.

Puerto Sarmiento, Francisco Javier. "Alquimia áurea: alquimia y destilación en la corte de Felipe II (1527–1598)." *Dynamis* 17 (1997): 107–40.

Quezada, Noemí. *Enfermedad y maleficio: el curandero en el México colonia*, 2nd ed. México: Universidad Nacional Autónoma de México, Instituto de Investigaciones Antropológicas, 2000.

Quiroz Chueca, Francisco. *Gremios coloniales peruanos*. Lima: Universidad Nacional Mayor de San Marcos, Seminario de Historia Rural Andina, 1991.

Quiroz Chueca, Francisco. "Compañías y gremios artesanales, Lima siglo XVI." *Sequilao* 1 (1992): 1–14.

Quiroz Chueca, Francisco. *Gremios, razas y libertad de industria: Lima colonial*. Lima: Universidad Nacional Mayor de San Marcos, 1995.

Quiroz Chueca, Francisco. "Gremios en Lima." In *Lima en el siglo XVI*, edited by Laura Gutiérrez Arbulú, 493–525. Lima: Instituto Riva-Agüero, 2005.

Quiroz Chueca, Francisco. *Artesanos y manufactureros*. Lima: Instituto de Estudios Peruanas, 2008.

Quiroz Chueca, Francisco. Artisans and Journeymen in Colonial Lima. Unpublished manuscript, 2014.

Rabí Chara, Miguel. *Del hospital de Santa Ana (1549 a 1924) al hospital nacional Arzobispo Loayza (1925 a 1999): 450 años de protección de la salud de las personas*. Lima: INDECOPI, 1999.

Rabí Chara, Miguel. "La primera botica de los hospitales de la ciudad de Lima en el siglo XVI." *Asclepio* 52 (2000): 269–80.

Rabí Chara, Miguel. *El hospital de San Bartolomé de Lima : la protección y asistencia de la gente de color de 1646 a 1821 y evolución posterior. Examen de un proceso histórico, social y sanitaria*. Lima: Grahuer, 2001.

Raina, Dhruv. "From West to Non-West Basalla's Three-stage Model Revisited." *Science as Culture* 8 (4) (1999): 497–516.

Ralley, Robert. "Medical Economies in Fifteenth Century England." In *Medicine and the Market in England and its Colonies, c.1450–1850*, edited by Mark Jenner and Patrick Wallis, 24–46. New York: Palgrave Macmillan, 2007.

Ramírez, Susan E. *Provincial Patriarchs: Land Tenure and the Economics of Power in Colonial Peru*. Albuquerque: University of New Mexico Press, 1985.

Ramos, Gabriela. *Death and Conversion in the Andes: Lima and Cuzco, 1532–1670*. Notre Dame, Indiana: University of Indiana Press, 2010.

Ramos, Gabriela. "Indian Hospitals and Government in the Colonial Andes." *Medical History* 57 (2) (2013): 186–205.

Reedy, Daniel R. *The Poetic Art of Juan Valle Caviedes*. Chapel Hill: University of North Carolina, 1964.

Reff, Daniel T. *Disease, Depopulation, and Culture Change in Northwestern New Spain, 1518–1764*. Salt Lake City: University of Utah Press, 1991.

Rey Bueno, Mar. "El informe Valles: los desdibujados límites del arte de boticarios a finales del siglo XVI (1589–1594)." *Asclepio* 56 (2) (2004): 243–68.

Rey Bueno, Mar. "Concordias medicinales de entrambos mundos." *Revista de Indias* 66 (no. 237) (2006): 347–62.

Rey Bueno, Mar. "Los proyectos sobre materia medica peruana de Antonio de Robles Cornejo y Matías de Porres (1617–1621)." In *Rotas da Natureza: cientistas, vaigens, expedições, instituições*, edited by Ana Leonor Pereira and João Pita, 27–31. Coimbra: Universidade de Coimbra, 2006.

Rey Bueno, Mar. "Los paracelsistas españoles: medicina química en la España moderna." In *Más allá de la Leyenda Negra: España y la revolución científica*, edited by Victor Navarro Brotons and William Eamon, 41–55. Valencia: Instituto de Historia de la Ciencia y Documentación López Piñero, 2007.

Rey Bueno, Mar and María Esther Alegre Pérez. "Los distiladores de Su Magestad: distilación, espagiria y paracelsismo en la corte de Felipe II." *Dynamis* 21 (2001): 323–50.

Rey Bueno, Mar and María Esther Alegre Pérez. "Renovación en la terapéutica real: los destiladores de su magestad, maestros simplicistas y médicos herbolarios de Felipe II." *Asclepio* 53 (1) (2001): 27–55.

Ribeiro, Aileen. "Dress in the Early Modern Period, c.1500–1780." In *The Cambridge History of Western Textiles*, edited by David Jenkins, 659–90. Cambridge: Cambridge University Press, 2003.

Ricardo, Antonio. "Testamento de don Antonio Ricardo." *Revista del Archivo Nacional del Perú* 19 (1955): 293–305.

Risse, Guenter B. "Transcending Cultural Barriers: the European Reception of Medicinal Plants from the Americas." In *Botanical Drugs of the Americas in the Old and New Worlds: Invitational Symposium at the Washington-Congress, 1983*, edited by Wolfgang-Hagen Hein, 31–42. (Amerikanische pflanzliche Arzneien in der Alten und Neuen Welt : Einladungs-Symposium anlässlich des Kongresses in Washington, 1983). Stuttgart: Wissenschaftliche Verlagsgesellschaft, 1984.

Risse, Guenter B. "Medicine in New Spain." In *Medicine in the New World: New Spain, New France, and New England*, edited by Ronald L. Numbers, 12–63. Knoxville: University of Tennessee Press, 1987.

Risse, Guenter B. *Mending Bodies, Saving Souls: A History of Hospitals*. New York: Oxford University Press, 1999.

Rizo-Patrón, Paul. "La nobleza de Lima en tiempos de los Borbones." *Bulletin de l'Institut Français d'Études Andines* 19 (1) (1990): 129–63.

Rocco, Fiammetta. *Miraculous Fever-Tree: Malaria, Medicine and the Cure That Changed the World*. New York: HarperCollins, 2003.

Rodríguez Guerrero, José. "Censura y Paracelsismo durante el reinado de Felipe II."*Azogue* 4 (2001) URL: http://www.revistaazogue.com [Accessed 2 Jul. 2016].

Rodríguez-Buckingham, Antonio. "Change and the Printing Press in Sixteenth-Century Spanish America." In *Agent of Change: Print Culture Studies after Elizabeth L. Einstein*, edited by Sabrina Alcorn Baron, Eric N. Lindquist and Eleanor F. Shevlin, 216–37. Amherst and Boston: University of Massachusetts Press, 2007.

Rojo Vega, Anastasio. *Enfermos y sanadores en la Castilla del siglo XVI*. Valladolid: Universidad De Valladolid, 1993.

Romero Romero, Catalina. "Libros, cultura y sociedad en el Perú Virreinal: Las bibliotecas de los colegios jesuitas de Arequipa, Potosí y las misiones de Moxos en el siglo XVIII." 2 vols. PhD diss., Universidad de Complutense de Madrid, 1992.

Ronderos, Paula. "El arte de boticarios durante la primera mitad del siglo XVII en el Nuevo Reino de Granada." *Fronteras de historia* 12 (2007): 175–96.

Ronderos, Paula. *El dilema de los rótulos: Lectura del inventario de una botica santafereña de comienzos del siglo XVII*. Bogotá: Pontificia Universidad Javeriana, 2007.

Sabater, Pilar Gardeta. "El nuevo modelo del Real Tribunal del Protomedicato en la América española: trasformaciones sufridas ante las Leyes de Indias y el cuerpo legislativo posterior." *Dynamis* 16 (1996): 237–59.

Saldaña, Juan José. "Science and Public Happiness during the Latin American Enlightenment." In *Science in Latin America: A History*, edited by Juan José Saldaña, 50–92. Austin: University of Texas Press, 2006.

Sánchez, Ana. *Amancebados, hechicheros y rebeldes (Chancay, siglo XVII)*. Cuzco: Centro de estudios regionales andinos, Bartolomé de las Casas, 1991.

Sánchez-Menchero, Mauricio. "'From Where They Are Now to Whence They Came From': News About Health and Disease in New Spain (1550–1615)." In *Medical Cultures of the Early Modern Spanish Empire*, edited by John Slater, Mariluz López Terrada and José Pardo-Tomás, 91–105. Farnham: Ashgate, 2014.

Sayre, Meredith Beck. "Cultivating Soils and Souls: The Jesuit Garden in the Americas." MA diss., Simon Fraser University, 2005.

Schiebinger, Londa. *Plants and Empire: Colonial Bioprospecting in the Atlantic World*. Cambridge, Mass.: Harvard University Press, 2004.

Schiebinger, Londa and Claudia Swan, eds. *Colonial Botany: Science, Commerce, and Politics in the Early Modern World*. Philadelphia: University of Pennsylvania Press, 2005.

Schurz, William Lyle. "Mexico, Peru and the Manila Galleon." *Hispanic American Historical Review* 1 (1918): 389–402.

Scott, Heidi V. *Contested Territory: Mapping Peru in the Sixteenth and Seventeenth Centuries*. Notre Dame, IN: University of Notre Dame Press, 2009.

Shapin, Steven. *The Scientific Revolution*. Chicago: University of Chicago Press, 1996.

Silverblatt, Irene. *Modern Inquisitions: Peru and the Colonial Origins of the Civilized World*. Durham: Duke University Press, 2004.

Siraisi, Nancy G. *Medieval and Early Renaissance Medicine: An Introduction to Knowledge and Practice*. Chicago: University of Chicago, 1990.

Slater, John. "The Green Gold Fallacies: Myth and Reality in the Transatlantic Trade in Medicinal Plants (1493–1663)." In *Geografías médicas: orillas y fronteras culturales de la medicina hispanomericana (siglos XVI y XVII)*, edited by José Pardo-Tomás and Mauricio Sánchez Menchero, 99–122. Mexico DF: Universidad Autónoma de México, 2014.

Slater, John and Andrés Prieto. "Was Spanish Science Imperial?" *The Colorado Review of Hispanic Studies* 7 (2009): 3–10.

Smith, Pamela H. *The Business of Alchemy: Science and Culture in the Holy Roman Empire*. Princeton: Princeton University Press, 1997.

Smith, Pamela H. "Science on the Move: Recent Trends in the History of Early Modern Science." *Renaissance Quarterly* 62 (2) (2009): 345–75.

Smith, Pamela H., Amy R. Meyers and Harold J. Cook, eds. *Ways of Making and Knowing: The Material Culture of Empirical Knowledge*. Ann Arbor: University of Michigan Press, 2014.

Socolow, Susan Migden. *The Women of Colonial Latin America*. Cambridge: Cambridge University Press, 2000.

Solano Alonso, J. *Salud, cultura y sociedad en Cartagena de Indias siglos XVI y XVII*. Universidad del Atlántico: Barranquilla, 1998.

Solomon, Michael. *Fictions of Well-Being: Sickly Readers and Vernacular Medical Writing in Late Medieval and Early Modern Spain*. Philadelphia: University of Pennsylvania Press, 2010.

Sorní, Javier and José María Suñe. "Barcelona. Baja edad media: especieros o boticarios?" *Boletín de la sociedad española de historia de la farmacia* 34 (no. 136) (1983): 139–50.

Sorní, Javier and José María Suñe. "La farmacia en Barcelona desde *Alfons el Benigne* a *Pere el Ceremoniós* (1327–1387)." *Boletín de la sociedad española de historia de la farmacia* 36 (nos. 141–42) (1985): 67–79.

Sosadias, Inés. "El negro curandero en la Inquisición de Cartagena de Indias siglo XVII." MA diss., Universidad de los Andes, 1981.

Sowell, David. *The Tale of Healer Miguel Perdomo Neira: Medicine, Ideologies, and Power in the Nineteenth-Century Andes*. Wilmington, Delaware: Scholarly Resources Inc., 2001.

Spargo, John Webster. *Virgil the Necromancer: Studies in Virgilian Legends*. Cambridge, Mass.: Harvard University Press, 1934.

Stephenson, Marcia. "From Marvelous Antidote to the Poison of Idolatry: The Transatlantic Role of Andean Bezoar Stones during the Late Sixteenth and Early Seventeenth Centuries." *Hispanic American Historical Review* 90 (1) (2010): 3–39.

Stolberg, Michael. *Experiencing Illness and the Sick Body in Early Modern Europe.* Basingstoke: Palgrave Macmillan, 2011.

Strochhia, Sharon T. "The Nun Apothecaries of Renaissance Florence: Marketing Medicines in the Convent." *Renaissance Studies* 25 (5) (2011): 627–47.

Studnicki-Gizbert, Daviken. A Nation Upon the Ocean Sea*: Portugal's Atlantic Diaspora and the Crisis of the Spanish Empire, 1492–1640*. Oxford: Oxford University Press, 2007.

Suárez, Margarita. *Comercio y fraude el en Perú colonial: las estrategias mercantiles de un banquero*. Lima: Banco Central de Reserva del Perú, Fondo Editorial: Instituto de Estudios Peruanos, 1995.

Suárez, Margarita. *Desafíos transatlánticos: mercaderes, banqueros y el estado en el Perú virreinal, 1600–1700*. Lima: Pontificia Universidad Católica del Perú, Instituto Riva-Agüero: Fondo de Cultura Económica: Instituto Francés de Estudios Andinos, 2001.

Sweet, James H. *Domingos Álvares, African Healing, and the Intellectual History of the Atlantic World.* Chapel Hill: University of North Carolina Press, 2011.

Urdang, George. "The Development of Pharmacopoeias." *Bulletin of the World Health Organisation* 4 (4) (1951): 577–603.

Urdang, George. "How Chemicals Entered the Official Pharmacopoeias." *Archives internationales d'histoire des sciences* 7 (1954): 303–14.

Valcarcel, Carlos Daniel. *Historia de la educación colonial.* Lima: Editorial Universo, 1968.

Valdizán, Hermilio and Angel Maldonado. *La medicina popular peruana*. 3 vols. Lima: Torres Aguirre, 1922.

Valle y Caviedes, Juan del. *Obra completa.* Edited by Daniel R. Reedy. Caracas: Biblioteca Ayacucho, 1984.

Valverde, José Luis. "Regulaciones de farmacia contenidas en las ordenanzas municipales de las ciudades españolas." *Sonderdruck aus Veröffentlichungen der Internationalen Gesellschaft für Geschichte der Pharmazie* [Die Vörträge der Hauptversammlung in Luxemburg] 36: 135–57. Stuttgart, 1970.

Valverde, José Luis and Guillermina López Andújar. "Los disposiciones legales sobre el certificado de 'limpieza de sangre' en relación al ejército profesional farmacéutico." *Boletín de la sociedad española de la historia de la farmacia* 31 (1981): 259–71.

Van Deusen, Nancy E. *Between the Sacred and the Worldly: The Institutional and Cultural Practice of Recogimiento in Colonial Lima.* Stanford: Stanford University Press, 2001.

Van Deusen, Nancy E. *The Souls of Purgatory: The Spiritual Diary of a Seventeenth-Century Afro-Peruvian Mystic, Ursula de Jesús*. Albuquerque: University of New Mexico Press, 2004.

Van Deusen, Nancy E. "Circuits of Knowledge among Women in Early Seventeenth-Century Lima." In *Gender, Race and Religion in the Colonization of the Americas*, edited by Nora E. Jaffary, 137–50. Aldershot: Ashgate, 2007.

Varey, Simon, ed. *The Mexican Treasury: The Writings of Dr. Francisco Hernández*. Translated by Cynthia L. Chamberlain and Simon Varey. Stanford: Stanford University Press, 2002.

Varey, Simon, Rafael Chabrán and Dora B. Weiner, eds. *Searching for the Secrets of Nature: The Life and Works of Dr. Francisco Hernández*. Stanford: Stanford University Press, 2002.

Vargas Ugarte, Rubén. *Impresos peruanos (1584–1650)*. Lima: Universidad Nacional San Marcos, 1953.

Vargas Ugarte, Rubén. *Historia de la iglesia en el Perú*. Tomo II (1570–1640). Burgos: Imprenta de Aldecoa, 1959.

Vega Jácome, Walter. "Cofradías limeñas." In *Lima en el siglo XIV*, edited by Laura Gutiérrez Arbulú, 703–52. Lima: Pontificia Universidad Católica del Perú, Instituto Riva-Agüero, 2005.

Vergara, Teresa C. "Growing Up Indian: Migration, Labor, and Life in Lima (1570–1640)." In *Raising an Empire: Children in Early Modern Iberia and Colonial Latin America*, edited by Ondina E. González and Bianca Premo, 75–106. Albuquerque: University of New Mexico Press, 2007.

Vila Vilar, Enriqueta. *Hispanoamérica y el comercio de esclavos: los asientos Portugueses*. Seville: Escuela de Estudios Hispanoamericanos, 1977.

Vila Vilar, Enriqueta. "Las ferias de Portobelo: apariencia y realidad del comercio con Indias." *Anuario de estudios americanos* 39 (1982): 275–340.

Walker, Tamara J. "'He Outfitted his Family in Notable Decency': Slavery, Honour and Dress in Eighteenth-Century Lima." *Slavery and Abolition* 30 (3) (2009): 383–402.

Walker, Timothy D. *Doctors, Folk Medicine and the Inquisition: the Repression of Magical Healing in Portugal during the Enlightenment*. Leiden: Brill, 2005.

Wallis, Patrick. "Consumption, Retailing, and Medicine in Early-Modern London." *Economic History Review* 61 (1) (2008): 26–53.

Ward, Christopher. *Imperial Panama: Commerce and Conflict in Isthmian America, 1550–1800*. Albuquerque: University of New Mexico Press, 1994.

Warren, Adam. *Medicine and Politics in Colonial Peru: Population Growth and the Bourbon Reforms*. Pittsburgh, PA: University of Pittsburgh Press, 2010.

Wear, Andrew. "The Early Modern Debate about Foreign Drugs: Localism versus Universalism in Medicine." *The Lancet* 354 (1999): 149–51.

Wear, Andrew. *Knowledge and Practice in English Medicine, 1550–1680*. Cambridge University Press, Cambridge, 2000.

Whittet, T.D. "Pepperers, Spicers and Grocers – Forerunners of the Apothecaries." *Proceedings of the Royal Society of Medicine* 61 (1968): 25–30.

Winterbottom, Anne E. "Of the China Root: A Case study of the Early Modern Circulation of Materia Medica." *Social History of Medicine*, 28 (1) (2015): 22–44.

Withers, Charles W.J. *Placing the Enlightenment: Thinking Geographically about the Age of Reason*. Chicago: the University of Chicago Press, 2007.

Withers, Charles W.J. and David N. Livingstone. "Introduction: On Geography and Enlightenment." In *Geography and Enlightenment*, edited by David N. Livingstone and Charles W.J. Withers, 1–28. Chicago: The University of Chicago Press, 1999.

Zarate, Eduardo C. *Inicios de la escuela de medicina de Lima*. Lima: No publisher, 2005.

Index